Neurologic Intervention for Physical Therapist Assistants

Neurologic Intervention for Physical Therapist Assistants

Suzanne "Tink" Martin, MACT, PT
Professor
Department of Physical Therapy
University of Evansville
Evansville, Indiana

Mary Kessler, MHS, PT
Associate Professor
Department of Physical Therapy
University of Evansville
Evansville, Indiana

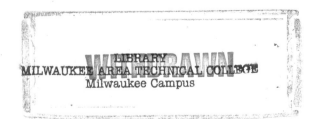
W.B. SAUNDERS COMPANY
A Harcourt Health Sciences Company
Philadelphia • London • New York • St. Louis • Sydney • Toronto

W.B. SAUNDERS COMPANY
A Harcourt Health Sciences Company

The Curtis Center
Independence Square West
Philadelphia, Pennsylvania 19106

Library of Congress Cataloging-in-Publication Data

Martin, Suzanne.
  Neurologic intervention for physical therapist assistants/Suzanne "Tink" Martin, Mary Kessler.—1st ed.

    p.; cm.

  ISBN 0–7216–3176–2

    1. Nervous system—Diseases—Physical therapy. 2. Neuromuscular diseases—Physical therapy. 3. Physical therapy assistants. I. Kessler, Mary. II. Title.

  [DNLM: 1. Nervous System Diseases—rehabilitation. 2. Motor Skills. 3. Physical Therapy—methods. 4. Trauma, Nervous System—rehabilitation. WL 140 M383n 2000]

  RC350.P48 M37 2000

  616.8'0462—dc21   00–028499

Acquisitions Editor: Andrew Allen
Developmental Editor: Scott W. Weaver
Manuscript Editor: Amy Norwitz
Production Manager: Linda R. Garber
Illustration Specialist: Lisa Lambert
Book Designer: Jonel Sofian

NEUROLOGIC INTERVENTION FOR PHYSICAL THERAPIST ASSISTANTS   ISBN 0–7216–3176–2

Printed in the United States of America

Last digit is the print number: 9   8   7   6   5   4   3   2   1

To my husband, Terry, who has shared me all too often with my professional pursuits and the profession that I regard so highly—we will have more time for movies, travel, and gourmet cooking.

To my parents, "Boots" and Sue Delker, whose love and care have nurtured me all my life. Thank you for your guidance and direction.

To Carol, who taught me that with more education comes more responsibility.

Tink

To Craig, my husband, who has always provided me with love, support, and encouragement to pursue this and other professional goals, and to Kyle and Kaitlyn, who have waited patiently to see this project completed and their photographs in print.

A final word of thanks to my parents, John and Judy Oerter, who have through the years encouraged me to work hard and strive for excellence. You have always believed in me and my ability to succeed.

Mary

Acknowledgments

I must acknowledge the dedication and hard work of my colleague, friend, and coauthor, Mary Kessler. She has kept her eye on the quality of the project and has kept working to make it better. I thank all the adults and children and their families who graciously agreed to put up with the photo sessions. A special thank-you to Janet Szczepanski for demonstrating techniques with Marie in the stroke chapter and with Mary in the spinal cord chapter. Thank you to Dr. Catherine McGraw, Donna Cech, Barbara Hahn, and Mary Kay Solon for reading drafts of manuscripts and providing valuable feedback. The physical therapist assistant students at the University of Evansville should be commended for providing the stimulus for the idea and for their tenacity in reading and critiquing earlier versions. Thank you to those physical therapist assistants who have attended our presentations on this and related topics. You all provided us with feedback.

Tink

I must thank my good friend, mentor, colleague, and coauthor, Tink Martin. Without Tink, this project would never have been conceptualized or completed. Tink has taken care of many of the details, always trying to keep us focused on the end result. Her words of encouragement and support have been most appreciated.

A special thanks to our colleague, Janet Szczepanski, who read all of the drafts of the adult chapters and provided valuable insight, suggestions, and editorial changes. She also demonstrated many of the interventions in the CVA and SCI Chapters. Other recognition is needed for Jessica Dugan, a 2000 graduate from our MPT program, who graciously allowed one of her assignments (a TBI SOAP note) to appear in this text. Additional thanks to Sandy Pritchett, a dear friend and colleague, who reviewed the CVA chapter and has always offered a supportive ear and heart.

Mary

Reviewers

Denise Marie Abrams, BS, PT
Broome Community College
Binghamton, New York

S. Renea Akin, MHS, PT
Paducah Community College
Paducah, Kentucky

Candace A. Bahner, MS, PT
Washburn University
Topeka, Kansas

Delores B. Bertoti, MS, PT, PCS
Alvernia College
Reading, Pennsylvania
Beaver College
Glenside, Pennsylvania

Mary Sue Ingman, PT
College of St. Catherine–Minneapolis
Minneapolis, Minnesota

Mary Theresa Moretti, PT
PTA Program Director
PTA Program ACCE
Stanly Community College
Albermarle, North Carolina

Pamela Lehmann Taft, MS, PT
Maria College
Albany, New York

Julie A. Toney, PT, ACCE
Owens Community College
Toledo, Ohio

Preface

Physical therapist assistants are providing more and more of the physical therapy care to individuals with neurologic dysfunction. There was no textbook that we thought specifically covered neurologic interventions for the physical therapist assistant, so we took on the challenge. Because we have taught physical therapist assistants about neurologic treatment interventions for adults and children for many years, it seemed a logical step to put the anatomy, pathology, and treatment together in a textbook.

This textbook provides a link between the pathophysiology of neurologic conditions and possible interventions to improve movement outcomes. What started as a techniques book has, we hope, transcended a cookbook approach, to provide background information regarding interventions that can be used in the rehabilitation of adults and children. We are hopeful that this text will assist student physical therapist assistants in their acquisition of knowledge regarding the treatment of adults and children with neurologic dysfunction.

Writing is not the easiest thing to do, as Tink had previously experienced in authoring an entry-level text. However, we thought a second book would be manageable. Colleagues encouraged us, students critiqued it, reviewers reviewed it, and our spouses tacitly supported all the extra hours given to the writing. Although the task seemed daunting, we thought the project could realistically be completed in three years. Five years later, we feel joy, relief, happiness, and a real sense of accomplishment that the project is finally completed.

One always embarks hoping for clear sailing with a quick passage to the destination. As with most things, life intervenes. We have persevered and hope that the end result will meet its intended purpose—to teach and provide a basis for physical therapist assistants to learn how to implement interventions within their knowledge base and abilities. In addition, it is our hope that academicians involved in the education of physical therapist assistants will find this text to be a useful reference.

The mark of sophistication of any society is how well it treats the young and the old, the most vulnerable segments of the population. We hope in some small measure that our efforts will make it easier to unravel the mystery of directing movement, guiding growth and development, and relearning lost functional skills to improve the quality of life of the people we serve.

Tink Martin
Mary Kessler

Contents

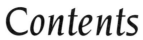

SECTION 2: ADULTS

SECTION 3: CHILDREN

SECTION 1

FOUNDATIONS

CHAPTER 1

The Role of the Physical Therapist Assistant in Neurologic Rehabilitation

OBJECTIVES

After reading this chapter, the student will be able to

1. Understand Nagi's Disablement Model.
2. Describe the role of the physical therapist assistant in the treatment of adults and children with neurologic dysfunction.

INTRODUCTION

The practice of physical therapy in the United States continues to change to meet the demands placed on service provision by managed care and federal regulations. The profession has seen an increased number of physical therapist assistants providing physical therapy intervention for adults and children with neurologic deficits. Physical therapist assistants are now employed in outpatient clinics, inpatient rehabilitation centers, extended care and pediatric facilities, school systems, and home health care agencies. Traditionally, the rehabilitation management of adults and children with neurologic dysfunction consisted of treatment derived from the knowledge of disease and interventions directed at the amelioration of patient signs and symptoms. The current view of health and disease has evolved from a traditional model based solely on pathology and clinical course to a health status model based on the disablement process.

Sociologist Saad Nagi developed a model of health status that is used to describe the relationship between health and function (Nagi, 1991). The four components of this model (disease, impairments, functional limitations, and disability) evolve as the individual loses health. Disease is defined as a pathologic state manifested by the presence of signs and symptoms that disrupt an individual's homeostasis or internal balance. Impairments are alterations in anatomic, physiologic, or psychologic structures or functions. Functional limitations occur as a result of impairments and become evident when an individual is unable to perform everyday activities that are considered part of the person's daily routine. Examples of physical impairments include a loss of strength in the anterior tibialis muscle or a loss of 15 degrees of active shoulder flexion. These physical impairments may or may not limit the individual's ability to perform functional tasks. Inability to dorsiflex the ankle may prohibit the patient from achieving toe clearance and heelstrike during ambulation, whereas a 15-degree limitation in shoulder range will have little impact on the person's ability to perform self-care or dressing tasks.

According to the disablement model, a disability results when functional limitations become so great that the person is unable to meet age-specific expectations within the social or physical environment (Verbrugge and Jette, 1994). Society can erect physical and social barriers to hinder a person with a disability from participating in expected roles. The societal attitudes encountered by a person with a disability can result in society's perceiving that the individual is handicapped. Figure 1–1 depicts Nagi's classification system of health status. The use of the disablement model di-

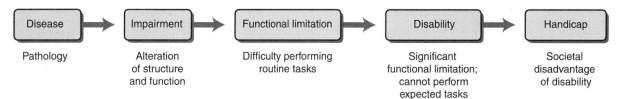

FIGURE 1–1 ■ Nagi classification system of health status.

rects health care practitioners to focus on the relationship between impairment and functional limitation and the patient's ability to perform everyday activities. Improved function in the home or the community thus becomes the preferred outcome of any therapeutic intervention.

Function is defined by the Guide to Physical Therapist Practice (APTA, 1997) as "those activities identified by an individual as essential to support physical, social and psychological well-being and to create a personal sense of meaningful life." Function is related to age-specific roles in a given social context and physical environment. Function is defined differently for a child of 6 months, an adolescent of 15 years, and a 65-year-old adult. Factors that define an individual's functional performance include personal characteristics such as physical ability, emotional status, and cognitive ability; the environment the person functions within such as the home, school, or community; and the social expectations placed on the person's performance by family, community, or society in general (Fig. 1–2).

Various functional skills are needed in domestic, vocational, and community environments. Performing these skills enhances the individual's physical and psychologic well-being. Individuals define themselves by what they are able to do. Performance of functional tasks not only depends on one's physical abilities but also is affected by emotional status, cognitive ability, and social and cultural expectations (Cech and Martin, 1995).

THE PHYSICAL THERAPIST ASSISTANT'S ROLE IN TREATING PATIENTS WITH NEUROLOGIC DEFICITS

Little or no debate exists on whether physical therapist assistants have a role in treating adults with neurologic deficits, as long as the individual needs of the patient are taken into consideration. The primary physical therapist is still ultimately responsible for the patient. It is the responsibility of the supervising physical therapist to determine which patients or proce-

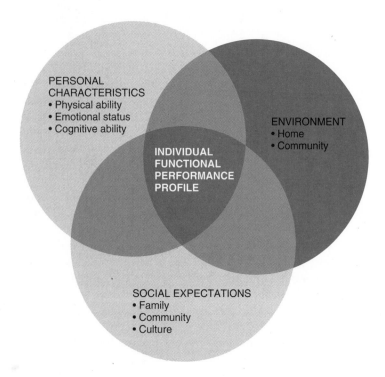

FIGURE 1–2 ■ Factors defining an individual's functional performance. (From Cech D, Martin S [eds]. Functional Movement Development Across the Life Span. Philadelphia, WB Saunders, 1995.)

dures require the expertise and decision-making capacity of the physical therapist and which tasks may be safely delegated to the physical therapist assistant. Prior to delegating any patient or portion of the patient's care, the physical therapist must critically evaluate the patient's condition (stability of the patient) and consider the practice setting, the type of intervention to be provided, and the patient's probable outcome (APTA, 1998a). In addition, the knowledge base of the physical therapist assistant and his or her level of experience must be considered when determining which activities can be appropriately delegated. Consequently, decisions regarding delegation should be based solely on the patient's needs and not on convenience or financial remuneration.

Although physical therapist assistants work with adults who have had cerebrovascular accidents, spinal cord injuries, and traumatic brain injuries, some physical therapists still view pediatrics as a specialty area of practice. This narrow perspective is held even though physical therapist assistants are working with children in hospitals, schools, and the community. Although some areas of pediatric physical therapy are specialized, many areas are well within the scope of practice of the generalist physical therapist and physical therapist assistant (Miller and Ratliffe, 1998). To assist in resolving this controversy, the Pediatric Section of the American Physical Therapy Association (APTA) developed a draft position statement outlining the use of physical therapist assistants in various pediatric settings. The original position paper stated that "physical therapist assistants could be appropriately utilized in pediatric settings with the exception of the medically unstable, such as neonates in the ICU" (Section on Pediatrics, APTA, 1995). This document was revised in 1997 and is available from the Section on Pediatrics. The most recent position paper now states that "the physical therapist assistant is qualified to assist in the provision of pediatric physical therapy services under the direction and supervision of a physical therapist. It is recommended that physical therapy services to children who are physiologically unstable not be delegated to the physical therapist assistant" (Section on Pediatrics, APTA, 1997). In addition, this position paper also states that "delegation of physical therapy procedures to a physical therapist assistant should not occur when a child's condition requires multiple adjustments of sequences and procedures due to rapidly changing physiologic status and/or response to treatment" (Section on Pediatrics, APTA, 1997). The guidelines proposed in this document follow those suggested by Nancy Watts in her 1971 article on task analysis and division of responsibility in physical therapy (Watts, 1971). This article was written to assist physical therapists with guidelines for delegating patient care activities to support personnel. The principles of patient or client delegation as defined by Watts can be applied to the provision of physical therapy services for adults and children with neuromuscular dysfunction. Physical therapists and physical therapist assistants unfamiliar with this article are encouraged to review it because the guidelines set forth are still applicable to today's clinicians.

THE PHYSICAL THERAPIST ASSISTANT AS A MEMBER OF THE HEALTH CARE TEAM

The physical therapist assistant functions as a member of the rehabilitation team in all treatment settings. Members of this team include the primary physical therapist; the physician; speech, occupational, and recreation therapists; nursing personnel; the psychologist; and the social worker. However, the two most important members of this team are the patient and family. In a rehabilitation setting, the physical therapist assistant is expected to provide therapeutic interventions to improve the patient's functional independence. Relearning motor activities such as bed mobility, transfers, ambulation skills, and wheelchair negotiation, if appropriate, is emphasized to enhance the patient's functional mobility. In addition, the physical therapist assistant is required to participate in patient and family teaching and patient care conferences and is expected to provide input into the patient's discharge planning. As is the case for all team activities, open and honest communication among all team members is crucial to achieve an optimal functional outcome for the patient.

The rehabilitation team working with a child with a neurologic deficit usually consists of the child, his or her parents, the various physicians involved in the child's management, and other health care professionals such as an audiologist, physical and occupational therapists, a speech pathologist, and the child's classroom teacher. The physical therapist assistant is expected to bring certain skills to the team and to the child, including knowledge of positioning and handling, use of adaptive equipment, management of abnormal muscle tone, and the knowledge of developmental activities that foster acquisition of functional motor skills and movement transitions. Family teaching and instruction are expected within a family-centered approach to the delivery of various interventions. Because the physical therapist assistant may be providing services to the child in his or her home or school, the assistant may be the first to observe additional problems or be told of a parent's concern. These observations or concerns should be communicated to the supervising physical therapist in a timely manner.

Physical therapists and physical therapist assistants are valuable members of a patient's health care team.

To optimize the relationship between the two and to maximize patient outcomes, each practitioner must understand the educational preparation and experiential background of the other. The preferred relationship between physical therapists and physical therapist assistants is one characterized by "trust, mutual respect, adaptability, cooperation, and an appreciation for individual and cultural differences" (APTA, 1998b). This relationship involves delegation, communication, and supervision and culminates in more clearly defined identities for both practitioners (APTA, 1998b).

CHAPTER SUMMARY

Changes in physical therapy practice have led to a growth in the number of physical therapist assistants and greater variety in the types of patients treated by these clinicians. Physical therapist assistants are actively involved in the treatment of adults and children with neurologic deficits. After a thorough evaluation of the patient's status, the primary physical therapist may determine that the patient's treatment or a portion of the treatment may be safely delegated to the assistant. The physical therapist assistant functions as a member of the patient's rehabilitation team and works with the patient to minimize the effects of physical impairments and functional limitations. Improved function in the home, school, or community remains the primary goal of physical therapy interventions.

REVIEW QUESTIONS

1. Define the term impairment according to the Nagi Disablement Model.
2. List the factors that affect an individual's performance of functional activities.
3. Identify those factors that the physical therapist must consider prior to delegating a patient to the physical therapist assistant.
4. Discuss the roles of the physical therapist assistant when working with adults or children with neurologic dysfunction.

REFERENCES

American Physical Therapy Association. Guide to physical therapist practice. Phys Ther 77:1177–1187, 1625–1636, 1997.

American Physical Therapy Association. Direction, delegation, and supervision in physical therapy services, HOD 06-96-30-42. House of Delegates: Standards, Policies, Positions and Guidelines. Alexandria, VA, American Physical Therapy Association, 1998a, pp 34–36.

American Physical Therapy Association Education Division. A Normative Model of Physical Therapist Assistant Education, 1st rev. Alexandria, VA, American Physical Therapy Association, 1998b.

Cech D, Martin S (eds). Functional Movement Development Across the Life Span. Philadelphia, WB Saunders, 1995, pp 3–17.

Miller ME, Ratliffe KT. The emerging role of the physical therapist assistant in pediatrics. In Ratliffe KT (ed). Clinical Pediatric Physical Therapy. St. Louis, CV Mosby, 1998, pp 15–22.

Nagi SZ. Disability concepts revisited: implications for prevention. In Pope AM, Tarlox AR (eds). Disability in America: Toward a National Agenda for Prevention. Washington, DC, National Academy Press, 1991, pp 309–327.

Section of Pediatrics, American Physical Therapy Association. Draft position statement on utilization of physical therapist assistants in the provision of pediatric physical therapy. Section on Pediatrics Newsletter 5:14–17, 1995.

Section on Pediatrics, American Physical Therapy Association. Utilization of Physical Therapist Assistants in the Provision of Pediatric Physical Therapy. Alexandria, VA, American Physical Therapy Association, 1997.

Verbrugge L, Jette A. The disablement process. Soc Sci Med 38:1–14, 1994.

Watts NT. Task analysis and division of responsibility in physical therapy. Phys Ther 51:23–35, 1971.

CHAPTER 2

Neuroanatomy

OBJECTIVES

After reading this chapter, the student will be able to

1. Differentiate between the central and peripheral nervous systems.
2. Identify significant structures within the nervous system.
3. Understand primary functions of structures within the nervous system.
4. Describe the vascular supply to the brain.
5. Discuss components of the cervical, brachial, and lumbosacral plexuses.

INTRODUCTION

The purpose of this chapter is to provide the student with a review of neuroanatomy. Basic structures within the nervous system are described and their functions discussed. This information is important to physical therapists and physical therapist assistants who treat patients with neurologic dysfunction because it assists clinicians with identifying clinical signs and symptoms. Additionally, it allows the physical therapist assistant to develop an appreciation of the patient's prognosis and potential functional outcome. It is, however, outside the scope of this text to provide a comprehensive discussion of neuroanatomy. The reader is encouraged to review the works of Cohen (1999), Curtis (1990), Farber (1982), FitzGerald (1996), Littell (1990), Lundy-Ekman (1998), and others for a more in-depth review of these concepts.

MAJOR COMPONENTS OF THE NERVOUS SYSTEM

The nervous system is divided into two parts, the central nervous system (CNS) and the peripheral nervous system (PNS). The CNS is composed of the brain, the cerebellum, the brain stem, and the spinal cord, whereas the PNS comprises all the components out-

side the cranium and spinal cord. Physiologically, the PNS is divided into the somatic nervous system and the autonomic nervous system (ANS). Figure 2–1 illustrates the major components of the CNS.

The nervous system is a highly organized communication system that serves the body. Nerve cells within the nervous system receive, transmit, analyze, and communicate information to other areas throughout the body. For example, sensations such as touch, proprioception, pain, and temperature are transmitted from the periphery as electrochemical impulses to the CNS through sensory tracts. Once information is processed within the brain, it is relayed as new electrochemical impulses to peripheral structures through motor tracts. This transmission process is responsible for an individual's ability to interact with the environment. Individuals are able to perceive sensory experiences, to initiate movement, and to perform cognitive tasks as a result of a functioning nervous system.

Types of Nerve Cells

The brain, brain stem, and spinal cord are composed of two basic types of nerve cells called neurons and neuroglia. Three different subtypes of neurons have been identified based on their function: (1) afferent neurons, (2) interneurons, and (3) efferent neurons. Afferent or sensory neurons are responsible for

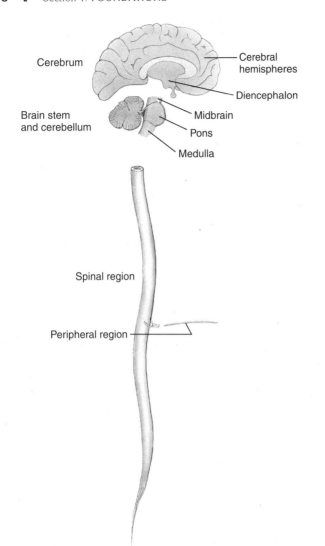

FIGURE 2–1 ■ Regions of the nervous system. Regions are listed on the left, and subdivisions are listed on the right. (From Lundy-Ekman L. Neuroscience: Fundamentals for Rehabilitation. Philadelphia, WB Saunders, 1998.)

receiving sensory input from the periphery of the body and transporting it into the CNS. Interneurons connect neurons to other neurons. Their primary function is to organize information received from many different sources for later interpretation. Efferent or motor neurons transmit information to the extremities to signal muscles to produce movement.

Neuroglia are non-neuronal supporting cells that provide critical services for neurons. Three different types of neuroglia (astrocytes, oligodendroglia, and microglia) have been identified. Astrocytes are responsible for maintaining the capillary endothelium and as such provide a vascular link to neurons. Oligodendroglia wrap myelin sheaths around axons in the white matter and produce satellite cells in the gray matter that participate in ion exchange between neurons. Microglia are known as the phagocytes of the CNS. They engulf and digest pathogens and assist with nervous system repair after injury.

Neuron Structures

As depicted in Figure 2–2, a neuron consists of a cell body, dendrites, and an axon. The dendrite is responsible for receiving information and transferring it to the cell body, where it is processed. Dendrites bring impulses into the cell body from other neurons. The number and arrangement of dendrites present in a neuron vary. The cell body or soma is composed of a nucleus and a number of different cellular organelles. The cell body is responsible for synthesizing proteins and supporting functional activities of the neuron, such as transmitting electrochemical impulses and repairing cells. Cell bodies that are grouped together in the CNS appear gray and thus are called gray matter. Groups of cell bodies with similar functions are assembled together to form nuclei. The axon is the message-sending component of the nerve cell. It extends from the cell body and is responsible for transmitting impulses from the cell body to target cells that can include muscle cells, glands, or other neurons.

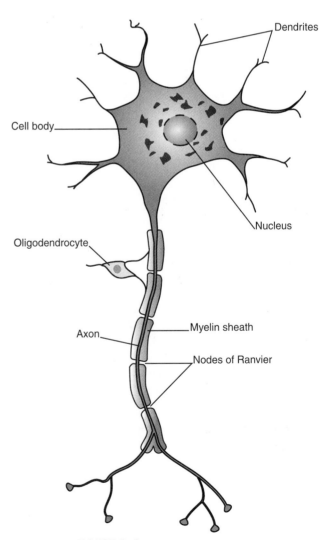

FIGURE 2–2 ■ Diagram of a neuron.

Synapses

The space between the axon of one neuron and the dendrite of the next neuron is called the synapse. Synapses are the connections between neurons that allow different parts of the nervous system to communicate with and influence each other. An axon transports electrical impulses or chemicals called neurotransmitters to and across the synapse. The relaying of information from one neuron to the next takes place at the synapse.

Axons

Once information is processed, it is conducted to other neurons, muscle cells, or glands by the axon. Axons can be myelinated or unmyelinated. Myelin is a lipid/protein that encases and insulates the axon. The presence of a myelin sheath increases the speed of impulse conduction, thus allowing for increased responsiveness of the nervous system. The myelin sheath surrounding the neuron is not continuous; it contains interruptions or spaces within the myelin called the nodes of Ranvier. Saltatory conduction is the process whereby electrical impulses are conducted along an axon by jumping from one node to the next (Fig. 2–3). This process increases the velocity of nervous system impulse conduction. Unmyelinated axons send messages more slowly than myelinated ones.

White Matter

Areas of the nervous system with a high concentration of myelin appear white because of the fat present within the myelin. Consequently, white matter is composed of axons that carry information away from cell bodies. White matter is found in the brain and spinal cord. Myelinated axons are bundled together within the CNS to form fiber tracts.

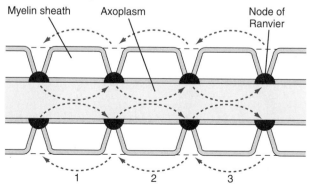

FIGURE 2–3 ■ Saltatory conduction along a myelinated axon. (Redrawn from Guyton AC. Textbook of Medical Physiology, 8th ed. Philadelphia, WB Saunders, 1991.)

Gray Matter

Gray matter refers to areas that contain large numbers of nerve cell bodies and dendrites. Collectively, these cell bodies give the region its grayish coloration. Gray matter covers the entire surface of the cerebrum and is called the cerebral cortex. Gray matter is also present deep within the spinal cord and is discussed in more detail later in this chapter.

Fibers and Pathways

Major sensory or afferent tracts carry information to the brain, and major motor or efferent tracts relay transmissions from the brain to smooth and skeletal muscles. Sensory information enters the CNS through the spinal cord or by the cranial nerves as the senses of smell, sight, hearing, touch, taste, heat, cold, pressure, pain, and movement. Information travels in fiber tracts composed of axons that ascend in a particular path from the sensory receptor to the cortex for interpretation. Motor signals descend from the cortex to the spinal cord through efferent fiber tracts for muscle activation. Fiber tracts are designated by their point of origin and by the area in which they terminate. Thus, the corticospinal tract, the primary motor tract, originates in the cortex and terminates in the spinal cord. The lateral spinothalamic tract, a sensory tract, begins in the lateral white matter of the spinal cord and terminates in the thalamus. A more thorough discussion of motor and sensory tracts is presented later in this chapter.

Brain

The brain consists of the cerebrum, which is divided into two cerebral hemispheres (the right and the left), the cerebellum, and the brain stem. The surface of the cerebrum or cerebral cortex is composed of depressions (sulci) and ridges (gyri). These convolutions increase the surface area of the cerebrum without requiring an increase in the size of the brain. The outer surface of the cerebrum is composed of gray matter, whereas the inner surface is composed of white matter fiber tracts. Therefore, information is conveyed by the white matter and is processed and integrated within the gray matter.

Supportive and Protective Structures

The brain is protected by a number of different structures and substances to minimize the possibility of injury. First, the brain is surrounded by a bony structure called the skull or cranium. The brain is also covered by three layers of membranes called meninges, which provide additional protection. The outermost layer is the dura mater. The dura is a thick, fibrous connective tissue membrane that adheres to the cranium. The area between the dura mater and the skull is known as the epidural space. The next or middle layer is the arachnoid. The space between the dura and the arachnoid is called the subdural space. The third protective layer is the pia mater. This is the innermost layer and adheres to the brain itself. The pia mater also contains the cerebral circulation. The cranial meninges are continuous with the membranes that cover and protect the spinal cord. Cerebrospinal fluid bathes the brain and circulates within the subarachnoid space. Figure 2–4 shows the relationship of the skull with the cerebral meninges.

Lobes of the Cerebrum

The cerebrum is divided into four lobes—frontal, parietal, temporal, and occipital—each having unique functions, as shown in Figure 2–5A. The hemispheres of the brain, although apparent mirror images of one another, have specialized functions as well. This sidedness of brain function is called hemispheric specialization or lateralization.

Frontal Lobe. The frontal lobe is frequently referred to as the primary motor cortex. The frontal lobe is responsible for voluntary control of complex motor activities. In addition to its motor responsibilities, the frontal lobe also exhibits a strong influence over cognitive functions including judgment, attention, awareness, abstract thinking, mood, and aggression. The principal motor region responsible for speech (Broca's area) is located within the frontal lobe. In the left hemisphere, Broca's area plans movements of the mouth to produce speech. In the opposite hemisphere, this same area is responsible for nonverbal communication including gestures and adjustments of the individual's tone of voice.

Parietal Lobe. The parietal lobe is the primary sensory cortex. Incoming sensory information is processed and meaning is provided to stimuli within this lobe. Perception is the process of attaching meaning to sensory information. Much of our perceptual learning requires a functioning parietal lobe. Specific body regions are assigned locations within the parietal lobe for this interpretation. This mapping is known as the sensory homunculus (Fig. 2–5B). The parietal lobe also plays a role in short-term memory functions.

Temporal Lobe. The temporal lobe is the primary auditory cortex. Wernicke's area of the temporal lobe allows an individual to hear and comprehend spoken language. Visual perception, musical discrimination, and long-term memory capabilities are all functions of the temporal lobe.

Occipital Lobe. The occipital lobe is the primary visual cortex providing for the organization, integration, and interpretation of visual information. The eyes take in visual information and then send it to the occipital cortex for interpretation.

Association Cortex

Association areas are areas within the parietal, temporal, and occipital lobes that horizontally link different parts of the cortex. For example, the sensory association cortex integrates and interprets information from all the lobes receiving sensory input and allows individuals to perceive and attach meaning to sensory experiences. Additional functions of the association areas include personality, memory, intelligence (problem solving and comprehension of spatial relationships), and the regulation of mood and affect (Lundy-Ekman, 1998). Figure 2–5C depicts association areas within the cerebral hemispheres.

Motor Areas of the Cerebral Cortex

The primary motor cortex, located in the frontal lobe, is primarily responsible for contralateral voluntary control of upper extremity and facial movements. Thus, a greater proportion of the total surface area of this region is devoted to neurons that control these body parts. Other motor areas include the premotor area, which controls muscles of the trunk and anticipatory postural adjustments, and the supplementary mo-

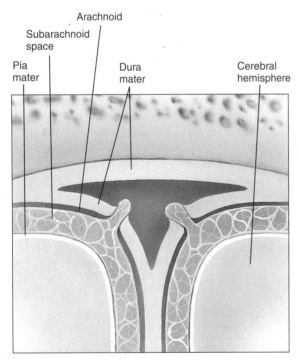

FIGURE 2–4 ■ A coronal section through the skull, meninges, and cerebral hemispheres. The section shows the midline structures near the top of the skull. The three layers of meninges are indicated. (From Lundy-Ekman L. Neuroscience: Fundamentals for Rehabilitation. Philadelphia, WB Saunders, 1998.)

Arachnoid

Subarachnoid space

Pia mater

Dura mater

Cerebral hemisphere

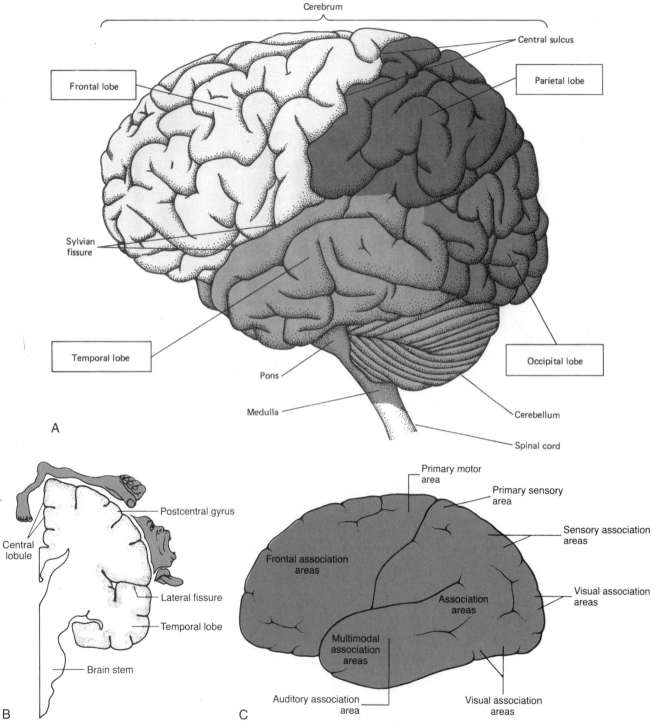

FIGURE 2–5 ∎ The brain. *A,* Left lateral view of the brain, showing the principal divisions of the brain and the four major lobes of the cerebrum. *B,* Sensory homunculus. *C,* Primary and association sensory and motor areas of the brain. (*A,* From Guyton AC. Basic Neuroscience: Anatomy and Physiology, 2nd ed. Philadelphia, WB Saunders, 1991; *B* and *C,* from Cech D, Martin S [eds]. Functional Movement Development Across the Life Span. Philadelphia, WB Saunders, 1995.)

tor area, which controls initiation of movement, orientation of the eyes and head, and bilateral, sequential movements. The supplemental motor area also plays a role in preprogramming movement sequences that are already part of the individual's motor memories (Lundy-Ekman, 1998).

Hemispheric Specialization

The cerebrum can be further divided into the right and left cerebral hemispheres. Gross anatomic differences have been demonstrated within the hemispheres. In 95% of the population, including all right-handed individuals and 50% of those who are left-hand dominant, the left hemisphere is the location of the primary speech center (Geschwind and Levitsky, 1968; Guyton, 1991; Lundy-Ekman, 1998). Table 2–1 lists primary functions of both the left and right cerebral hemispheres.

Left Hemisphere Functions. The left hemisphere has been described as the verbal or analytic side of the brain. The left hemisphere allows for the processing of information in a sequential, organized, logical, and linear manner. The processing of information in a step by step or detailed fashion allows for thorough analysis. For the majority of people, language is produced and processed in the left hemisphere, specifically the frontal and temporal lobes. The left parietal lobe allows an individual to recognize words and to comprehend what has been read. In addition, mathematical calculations are performed in the left parietal lobe. An individual is able to sequence and perform movements and gestures as a result of a functioning left frontal lobe. A final activity of the left cerebral hemisphere is the expression of positive emotions including happiness and love. Common impairments seen in patients with left hemispheric injury include an inability to plan motor tasks (apraxia); difficulty in initiating, sequencing, and processing a task; compulsiveness; difficulty in producing or comprehending speech; perseveration of speech or motor behaviors; and distractibility (O'Sullivan, 1994).

Right Hemisphere Functions. The right cerebral hemisphere is responsible for an individual's nonverbal and artistic abilities. The right side of the brain allows individuals to process information in a complete or holistic fashion without specifically reviewing all the details. The individual is able to grasp or comprehend general concepts. Visual-perceptual functions including eye-hand coordination, spatial relationships, and perception of one's position in space are carried out in the right hemisphere. The ability to communicate

nonverbally and to comprehend what is being expressed is also assigned to the right parietal lobe. Nonverbal skills including understanding facial gestures, recognizing visual-spatial relationships, and being aware of body image are processed in the right side of the brain. Other functions include mathematical reasoning and judgment, sustaining a movement or posture, and perceiving negative emotions including anger and unhappiness (O'Sullivan, 1994). Specific deficits that can be observed in patients with right hemisphere damage include poor judgment, unrealistic expectations, denial of disability, disturbances in body image, irritability, and lethargy.

Hemispheric Connections

Even though the two hemispheres of the brain have discrete functional capabilities, they perform many of the same actions. Communication between the two hemispheres is constant, so individuals can be analytic and yet still grasp broad general concepts. It is possible for the right hand to know what the left hand is doing and vice versa. The corpus callosum is a large group of axons that connect the right and left cerebral hemispheres and allow communication between the two cortices.

Deeper Brain Structures

Subcortical structures lie deep within the brain and include the internal capsule, the diencephalon, and the basal ganglia. These structures are briefly discussed because of their functional significance to motor function.

Internal Capsule. All descending fibers leaving the motor areas of the frontal lobe travel through the internal capsule, a deep structure within the cerebral hemisphere. The internal capsule is made up of axons that project from the cortex to the white matter fibers (subcortical structures) located below and from sub-

Table 2–1 ▌ BEHAVIORS ATTRIBUTED TO THE LEFT AND RIGHT HEMISPHERES

BEHAVIOR	LEFT HEMISPHERE	RIGHT HEMISPHERE
Cognitive style	Processing information in a sequential, linear manner Observing and analyzing details	Processing information in a simultaneous, holistic, or gestalt manner Grasping overall organization or pattern
Perception/cognition	Processing and producing language	Processing nonverbal stimuli (environmental sounds, speech intonation, complex shapes, and designs) Visual-spatial perception Drawing inferences, synthesizing information
Academic skills	Reading: sound-symbol relationships, word recognition, reading comprehension Performing mathematical calculations	Mathematical reasoning and judgment Alignment of numerals in calculations
Motor	Sequencing movements Performing movements and gestures to command	Sustaining a movement or posture
Emotions	Expressing positive emotions	Expressing negative emotions Perceiving emotion

From O'Sullivan SB. Stroke. In O'Sullivan SB, Schmitz TJ (eds). Physical Rehabilitation Assessment and Treatment, 3rd ed. Philadelphia, FA Davis, 1994, p 337.

cortical structures to the cerebral cortex. The capsule is shaped like a less-than sign (⟨), with an anterior and a posterior limb. The corticospinal tract travels in the posterior part of the capsule and allows information to be transmitted from the cortex to the brain stem and spinal cord. A lesion within this area can cause contralateral loss of voluntary movement and conscious somatosensation, which is the ability to perceive tactile and proprioceptive input. The internal capsule is pictured in Figure 2–6.

Diencephalon. The diencephalon is situated deep within the cerebrum and is composed of the thalamus and hypothalamus. The diencephalon is the area where the major sensory tracts (dorsal columns and lateral spinothalamic) and the visual and auditory pathways synapse. The thalamus consists of a large collection of nuclei and synapses. In this way, the thalamus serves as a central relay station for sensory impulses traveling upward from other parts of the body and brain to the cerebrum. It receives all sensory impulses except those associated with the sense of smell and channels them to appropriate regions of the cortex for interpretation. Moreover, the thalamus relays sensory information to the appropriate association areas within the cortex. Motor information received from the basal ganglia and cerebellum is transmitted to the correct motor region through the thalamus. Sensations of pain and peripheral numbness can also be identified at the level of the thalamus.

Hypothalamus. The hypothalamus is a group of nuclei that lie at the base of the brain, underneath the thalamus. The hypothalamus regulates homeostasis, which is the maintenance of a balanced internal environment. This structure is primarily involved in automatic functions including the regulation of hunger, thirst, body temperature, blood pressure, and sleep-wake cycles. Regulation of these bodily functions is often carried out by the ANS or by the endocrine system through the release of hormones. The hypothalamus is responsible for integrating the functions of both the endocrine system and the nervous system through its control over the pituitary gland.

Basal Ganglia. Another group of nuclei located at the base of the cerebrum comprise the basal ganglia. The basal ganglia form a subcortical structure made up of the caudate, putamen, globus pallidus, substantia nigra, and subthalamic nuclei. The basal ganglia are primarily responsible for the regulation of posture and muscle tone and play a role in the control of volitional and automatic movement. This motor circuit is essential for normal movement because of its effects on the motor planning areas of the cerebral cortex. The most common condition that results from dysfunction within the basal ganglia is Parkinson's disease. Patients with Parkinson's disease exhibit bradykinesia (slowness initiating movement), akinesia (difficulty in initiating movement), rigidity, and a flexed posture.

Limbic System. The limbic system is a group of deep brain structures in the diencephalon and cortex that includes parts of the thalamus and hypothalamus and a portion of the frontal and temporal lobes. The hypothalamus controls primitive emotional reactions including rage and fear. The limbic system guides the emotions that regulate behavior and is involved in learning and memory. More specifically, the limbic sys-

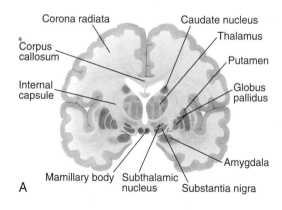

A

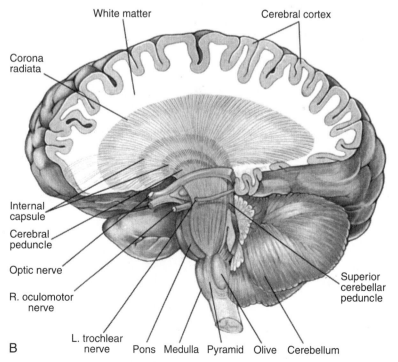

B

FIGURE 2–6 ■ The cerebrum. *A,* Diencephalon and cerebral hemispheres. *B,* A deep dissection of the cerebrum showing the radiating nerve fibers, the corona radiata, that conduct signals in both directions between the cerebral cortex and the lower portions of the central nervous system. (*A,* From Lundy-Ekman L. Neuroscience: Fundamentals for Rehabilitation. Philadelphia, WB Saunders, 1998; *B,* from Guyton AC. Basic Neuroscience: Anatomy and Physiology, 2nd ed. Philadelphia, WB Saunders, 1991.)

tem appears to control memory, pain, pleasure, rage, affection, sexual interest, fear, and sorrow.

Cerebellum

The cerebellum controls balance and complex muscular movements. It is located below the occipital lobe of the cerebrum and is posterior to the brain stem. It fills the posterior fossa of the cranium. Like the cerebrum, it also consists of two symmetric hemispheres. The cerebellum is responsible for the integration, coordination, and execution of multijoint movements. The cerebellum regulates the initiation, timing, sequencing, and force generation of muscle contractions. It sequences the order of muscle firing when a group of muscles work together to perform a movement such as stepping or reaching. The cerebellum also assists with balance and posture maintenance and has been identified as a comparator of actual motor performance to that which is anticipated. The cerebellum monitors and compares the movement requested, for instance, the step, with the movement actually performed (Horak, 1991).

Brain Stem

The brain stem is located between the base of the cerebrum and the spinal cord and is divided into three sections (Fig. 2–7). Moving cephalocaudally, the three areas are the midbrain, pons, and medulla. Each of the different areas is responsible for specific functions. The midbrain connects the diencephalon to the pons and acts as a relay station for tracts passing between the cerebrum and the spinal cord or cerebellum. The midbrain also houses reflex centers for visual, auditory, and tactile responses. The pons contains bundles of axons that travel between the cerebellum and the rest of the CNS and functions with the medulla to regulate the breathing rate. It also contains

reflex centers that assist with orientation of the head in response to visual and auditory stimulation. Cranial nerve nuclei can also be found within the pons, specifically, cranial nerves V through VIII, which carry motor and sensory information to and from the face. The medulla is an extension of the spinal cord and contains the fiber tracts that run through the spinal cord. Motor and sensory nuclei for the neck and mouth region are located within the medulla, as well as the control centers for heart and respiration rates. Reflex centers for vomiting, sneezing, and swallowing are also located within the medulla.

The reticular activating system is also situated within the brain stem and extends vertically throughout its length. The system maintains and adjusts an individual's level of arousal including sleep-wake cycles. In addition, the reticular activating system facilitates the voluntary and autonomic motor responses necessary for certain self-regulating, homeostatic functions and is involved in the modulation of muscle tone throughout the body.

Spinal Cord

The spinal cord has two primary functions: coordination of motor information and movement patterns and communication of sensory information. Subconscious reflexes including withdrawal and stretch reflexes are integrated within the spinal cord. Additionally, the spinal cord provides a means of communication between the brain and the peripheral nerves. The spinal cord is a direct continuation of the brain stem, specifically the medulla. The spinal cord is housed within the vertebral column and extends approximately to the level of the first lumbar vertebra. The spinal cord has two enlargements, one that extends from the third cervical segment to the second

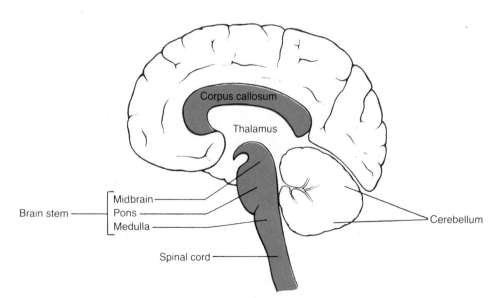

FIGURE 2–7 ■ Midsagittal view of the brain. (Redrawn from Farber SD. Neurorehabilitation: A Multisensory Approach. Philadelphia, WB Saunders, 1982.)

thoracic segment and another that extends from the first lumbar to the third sacral segment. These enlargements accommodate the great number of neurons needed to innervate the upper and lower extremities located in these regions. At approximately the L1 level, the spinal cord becomes a cone-shaped structure called the conus medullaris. The conus medullaris is composed of sacral spinal segments. Below this level, the spinal cord becomes a mass of spinal nerve roots called the cauda equina. The cauda equina consists of the nerve roots for spinal nerves L2 through S5. Figure 2–8 depicts the spinal cord and its relation to the brain. A thin filament, the filum terminale, extends from the caudal end of the spinal cord and attaches to the coccyx. In addition to the bony protection offered by the vertebrae, the spinal cord is also covered by the same protective meningeal coverings as in the brain.

Internal Anatomy

The internal anatomy of the spinal cord can be visualized in cross-sections and is viewed as two distinct areas. Figure 2–9A illustrates the internal anatomy of the spinal cord. Like the brain, the spinal cord is composed of gray and white matter. The center of the spinal cord, the gray matter, is distinguished by its H-shaped or butterfly-shaped pattern. The gray matter contains cell bodies of motor and sensory neurons and synapses. The upper portion is known as the dorsal or posterior horn and is responsible for transmitting sensory stimuli. The lower portion is referred to as the anterior or ventral horn. It contains cell bodies of lower motor neurons, and its primary function is to transmit motor impulses. The lateral horn is present at the T1 to L2 levels and contains cell bodies of preganglionic sympathetic neurons. It is responsible for processing autonomic information. The periphery of the spinal cord is composed of white matter. The white matter is composed of sensory (ascending) and motor (descending) fiber tracts. A tract is a group of nerve fibers that are similar in origin, destination, and function. These fiber tracts carry impulses to and from various areas within the nervous system. In addition, these fiber tracts cross over from one side of the body to the other at various points within the spinal cord and brain. Therefore, an injury to the right side of the spinal cord may produce a loss of motor or sensory function on the contralateral side.

Major Afferent (Sensory) Tracts

Two primary ascending sensory tracts are present in the white matter of the spinal cord. The dorsal or posterior columns carry information about position sense (proprioception), vibration, two-point discrimination, and deep touch. Figure 2–10 shows the location of this tract. The fibers of the dorsal columns cross in the brain stem. Pain and temperature sensations are transmitted in the spinothalamic tract located anterolaterally in the spinal cord (see Fig. 2–10). Fibers from this tract enter the spinal cord, synapse, and cross within three segments. Sensory information must be relayed to the thalamus. Touch information has to be processed by the cerebral cortex for discrimination to occur. Light touch and pressure sensations enter the spinal cord, synapse, and are carried in the dorsal and ventral columns.

Major Efferent (Motor) Tract

The corticospinal tract is the primary motor pathway. This tract originates in the frontal lobe from the primary and premotor cortices and continues through interconnections and various synapses, finally to synapse on anterior horn cells in the spinal cord. This tract also crosses from one side to the other in the brain stem. A common indicator of corticospinal tract damage is the Babinski sign. To test for this sign, the clinician takes a blunt object such as the back of a pen and runs it along the lateral border of the patient's foot (Fig. 2–11). The sign is present when the great toe extends and the other toes splay. The presence of

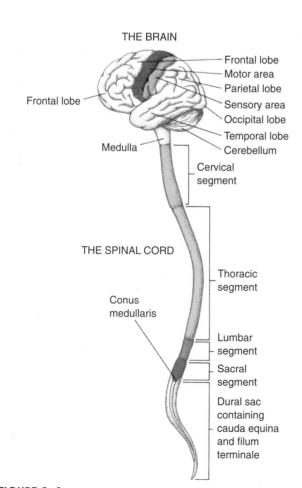

FIGURE 2–8 ■ The principal anatomic parts of the nervous system. (From Guyton AC. Basic Neuroscience: Anatomy and Physiology, 2nd ed. Philadelphia, WB Saunders, 1991.)

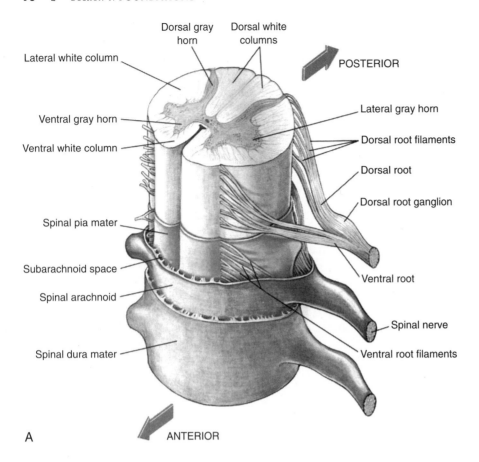

A

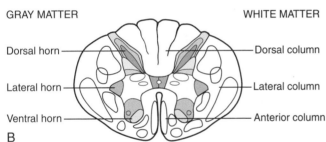

B

GRAY MATTER   WHITE MATTER

Dorsal horn — — Dorsal column

Lateral horn — — Lateral column

Ventral horn — — Anterior column

FIGURE 2-9 ■ The spinal cord. *A*, Structures of the spinal cord and its connections with the spinal nerve by way of the dorsal and ventral spinal roots. Note also the coverings of the spinal cord, the meninges. *B*, Cross-section of the spinal cord. The central gray matter is divided into horns and a commissure. The white matter is divided into columns. (*A*, From Guyton AC. Basic Neuroscience: Anatomy and Physiology, 2nd ed. Philadelphia, WB Saunders, 1991.)

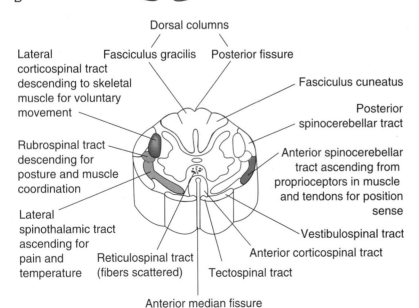

Dorsal columns

Lateral corticospinal tract descending to skeletal muscle for voluntary movement

Fasciculus gracilis

Posterior fissure

Fasciculus cuneatus

Posterior spinocerebellar tract

Rubrospinal tract descending for posture and muscle coordination

Anterior spinocerebellar tract ascending from proprioceptors in muscle and tendons for position sense

Lateral spinothalamic tract ascending for pain and temperature

Vestibulospinal tract

Reticulospinal tract (fibers scattered)

Anterior corticospinal tract

Tectospinal tract

Anterior median fissure

FIGURE 2-10 ■ Cross-section of the spinal cord showing tracts. (From Gould BE. Pathophysiology for the Health-Related Professions. Philadelphia, WB Saunders, 1997.)

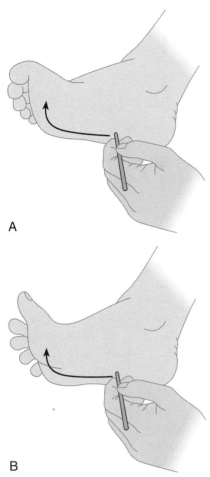

A

B

FIGURE 2-11 ■ *A,* Stroking from the heel to the ball of the foot along the lateral sole, then across the ball of the foot, normally causes the toes to flex. *B,* Babinski sign in response to the same stimulus. In corticospinal tract lesions, or in infants less than 6 months old, the big toe extends, and the other toes fan outward. (From Lundy-Ekman L. Neuroscience: Fundamentals for Rehabilitation. Philadelphia, WB Saunders, 1998.)

a Babinski sign indicates that damage to the corticospinal tract has occurred.

Other Descending Tracts

Other descending motor pathways that affect muscle tone are the rubrospinal, lateral and medial vestibulospinal, tectospinal, and medial and lateral reticulospinal tracts. The rubrospinal tract originates in the red nucleus of the midbrain and terminates in the anterior horn, where it synapses with lower motor neurons that primarily innervate the upper extremities. Fibers from this tract facilitate flexor motor neurons and inhibit extensor motor neurons. Proximal muscles are primarily affected, although the tract does exhibit some influence over more distal muscle groups. The rubrospinal tract has been said to assist in the correction of movement errors. The lateral vestibulospinal

tract assists in postural adjustments through facilitation of proximal extensor muscles. Regulation of muscle tone in the neck and upper back is a function of the medial vestibulospinal tract. The medial reticulospinal tract facilitates limb extensors, whereas the lateral reticulospinal tract facilitates flexors and inhibits extensor muscle activity. The tectospinal tract provides for orientation of the head toward a sound or a moving object.

Anterior Horn Cell

An anterior horn cell is a large neuron located in the gray matter of the spinal cord. An anterior horn cell sends out axons through the ventral or anterior spinal root; these axons eventually become peripheral nerves and innervate muscle fibers. Thus, activation of an anterior horn cell stimulates skeletal muscle contraction. Alpha motor neurons are a type of anterior horn cell that innervates skeletal muscle. Because of axonal branching, several muscle fibers can be innervated by one neuron. A motor unit consists of an alpha motor neuron and the muscle fibers it innervates. Gamma motor neurons are also located within the anterior horn. These motor neurons transmit impulses to the intrafusal fibers of the muscle spindle.

Muscle Spindle

The muscle spindle is the sensory organ in muscle and is composed of motor and sensory endings and muscle fibers. These fibers respond to stretch and therefore provide feedback to the nervous system regarding the muscle's length.

The easiest way to conceptualize how the muscle spindle functions within the nervous system is to review the stretch reflex mechanism. Stretch or deep tendon reflexes can easily be facilitated in the biceps, triceps, quadriceps, and gastrocnemius muscles. If a sensory stimulus such as a tap on the patellar tendon is applied to the muscle and its spindle, the input will enter through the dorsal root of the spinal cord to synapse on the anterior horn cell (alpha motor neurons). Stimulation of the anterior horn cell elicits a motor response, reflex contraction of the quadriceps (extension of the knee), as information is carried through the anterior root to the skeletal muscle. An important note about stretch or deep tendon reflexes is that their activation and subsequent motor response can occur without higher cortical influence. The sensory input coming into the spinal cord does not have to be transmitted to the cortex for interpretation. This has clinical implications because it means that a patient with a cervical spinal cord injury can continue to exhibit lower extremity deep tendon reflexes despite lower extremity paralysis.

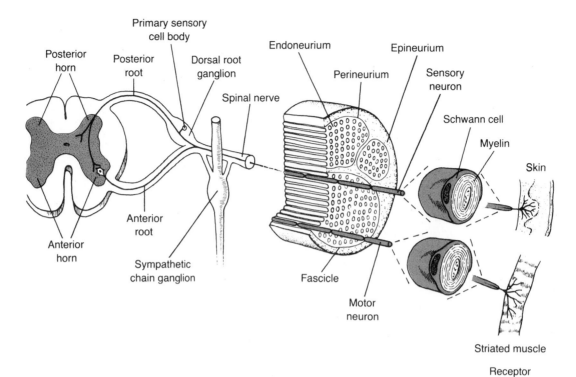

FIGURE 2-12 ∎ Schematic representation of the peripheral nervous system and the transition to the central nervous system. (From Cech D, Martin S [eds]. Functional Movement Development Across the Life Span. Philadelphia, WB Saunders, 1995.)

Peripheral Nervous System

The PNS consists of the nerves leading to and from the CNS, including the cranial nerves exiting the brain stem and the spinal roots exiting the spinal cord, many of which combine to form peripheral nerves. These nerves connect the CNS functionally with the rest of the body through sensory and motor impulses. Figure 2–12 provides a schematic representation of the PNS and its transition to the CNS.

The PNS is divided into two primary components: the somatic (body) nervous system and the ANS. The somatic or voluntary nervous system is concerned with reactions to outside stimulation. This system is under conscious control and is responsible for skeletal muscle contraction by way of the 31 pairs of spinal nerves. By contrast, the ANS is an involuntary system that innervates glands, smooth (visceral) muscle, and the myocardium. The primary function of the ANS is to maintain homeostasis or an optimal internal environment. Specific functions include the regulation of digestion, circulation, and cardiac muscle contraction.

Somatic Nervous System

Within the PNS are 12 pairs of cranial nerves, 31 pairs of spinal nerves, and the ganglia or cell bodies associated with the cranial and spinal nerves. The cranial nerves are located in the brain stem and can be either sensory or motor nerves. Primary functions of the cranial nerves include eye movements, smell, sensations perceived by the face and tongue, and innervation of the sternocleidomastoid and trapezius muscles. See Table 2–2 for a more detailed list of cranial nerves and their major functions.

The spinal nerves consist of 8 cervical, 12 thoracic, 5 lumbar, and 5 sacral nerves and 1 coccygeal nerve. Cervical spinal nerves C1 through C7 exit above the corresponding vertebrae. Because there are only 7 cervical vertebrae, the C8 spinal nerve exits above the T1 vertebra. From that point on, each succeeding spinal nerve exits below its respective vertebra. Figure 2–13 shows the distribution and innervation of the peripheral nerves.

Spinal nerves, consisting of sensory and motor components, exit the intervertebral foramen. Once through the foramen, the nerve divides into two primary rami. This division represents the beginning of the PNS. The dorsal or posterior rami innervate the paravertebral muscles, the posterior aspects of the vertebrae, and the overlying skin. The ventral or anterior primary rami innervate the intercostal muscles, the muscles and skin in the extremities, and the anterior and lateral trunk.

The 12 pairs of thoracic nerves do not join with other nerves and maintain their segmental relationship. However, the anterior primary rami of the other spinal nerves join together to form local networks known as the cervical, brachial, and lumbosacral plex-

Table 2-2 ▌ CRANIAL NERVES

NUMBER	NAME	FUNCTION	CONNECTION TO BRAIN
I	Olfactory	Smell	Inferior frontal lobe
II	Optic	Vision	Diencephalon
III	Oculomotor	Moves eye up, down, medially; raises upper eyelid; constricts pupil	Midbrain (anterior)
IV	Trochlear	Moves eye medially and down	Midbrain (posterior)
V	Trigeminal	Facial sensation, chewing, sensation from temporomandibular joint	Pons (lateral)
VI	Abducens	Abducts eye	Between pons and medulla
VII	Facial	Facial expression, closes eye, tears, salivation, taste	Between pons and medulla
VIII	Vestibulocochlear	Sensation of head position relative to gravity and head movement; hearing	Between pons and medulla
IX	Glossopharyngeal	Swallowing, salivation, taste	Medulla
X	Vagus	Regulates viscera, swallowing, speech, taste	Medulla
XI	Accessory	Elevates shoulders, turns head	Spinal cord and medulla
XII	Hypoglossal	Moves tongue	Medulla

From Lundy-Ekman L. Neuroscience: Fundamentals for Rehabilitation. Philadelphia, WB Saunders, 1998, p 251.

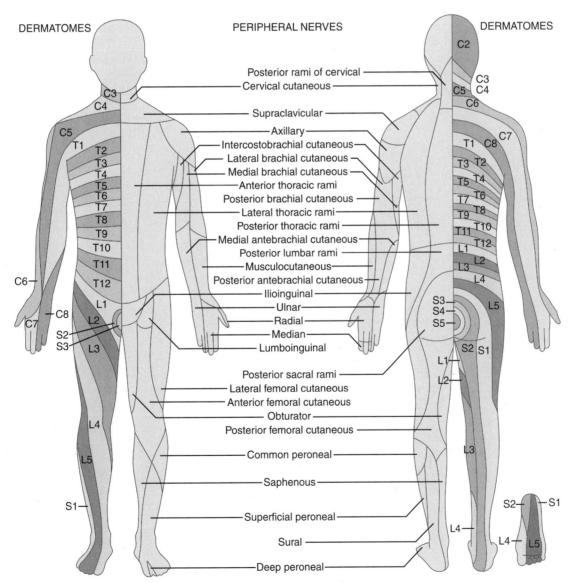

FIGURE 2-13 ▌ Dermatomes and cutaneous distribution of peripheral nerves. (From Lundy-Ekman L. Neuroscience: Fundamentals for Rehabilitation. Philadelphia, WB Saunders, 1998.)

uses (Guyton, 1991). The reader is given only a brief description of these nerve plexuses, because a detailed description of these structures is beyond the scope of this text.

Cervical Plexus. The cervical plexus is composed of the C1 through C5 spinal nerves. These nerves primarily innervate the deep muscles of the neck, the superficial anterior neck muscles, the levator scapulae, and portions of the trapezius and sternocleidomastoid. The phrenic nerve, one of the specific nerves within the cervical plexus, is formed from branches of C3 through C5. This nerve innervates the diaphragm, the primary muscle of respiration, and is the only motor and main sensory nerve for this muscle (Guyton, 1991). Figure 2–14 identifies components of the cervical plexus.

Brachial Plexus. The anterior primary rami of C5 through T1 form the brachial plexus. The plexus divides and comes together several times, providing muscles with motor and sensory innervation from more than one spinal nerve root level. The five primary nerves of the brachial plexus are the musculocutaneous, axillary, radial, median, and ulnar nerves. Figure 2–15 depicts the constituency of the brachial plexus. These five peripheral nerves innervate the majority of the upper extremity musculature, with the exception of the medial pectoral nerve (C8), which innervates the pectoralis muscles; the subscapular nerve (C5 and C6), which innervates the subscapularis; and the thoracodorsal nerve (C7), which supplies the latissimus dorsi muscle (Guyton, 1991).

The musculocutaneous nerve innervates the forearm flexors. The elbow, wrist, and finger extensors are innervated by the radial nerve. The median nerve supplies the forearm pronators and the wrist and finger flexors, and it allows thumb abduction and opposition. The ulnar nerve assists the median nerve with wrist and finger flexion, abducts and adducts the fingers, and allows for opposition of the fifth finger (Guyton, 1991).

Lumbosacral Plexus. Although some authors discuss the lumbar and sacral plexuses separately, they are discussed here as one unit because together they innervate lower extremity musculature. The anterior primary rami of L1 through S3 form the lumbosacral plexus. This plexus innervates the muscles of the thigh, lower leg, and foot. This plexus does not undergo the same separation and reuniting as does the brachial plexus. The lumbosacral plexus has eight roots, which eventually form six primary peripheral

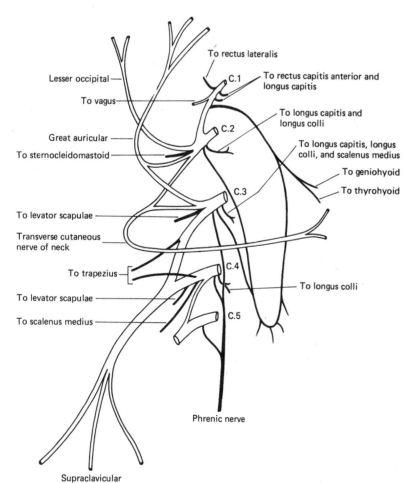

FIGURE 2–14 ▮ The cervical plexus and its branches. (From Guyton AC. Basic Neuroscience: Anatomy and Physiology, 2nd ed. Philadelphia, WB Saunders, 1991.)

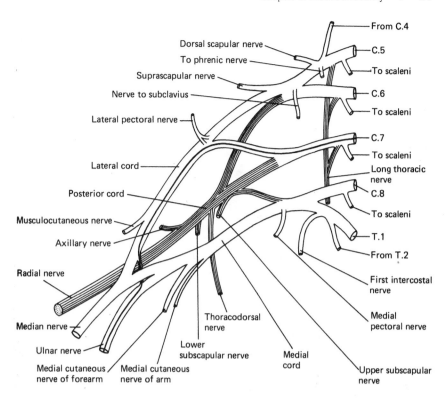

FIGURE 2-15 ■ The brachial plexus and its branches. (From Guyton AC. Basic Neuroscience: Anatomy and Physiology, 2nd ed. Philadelphia, WB Saunders, 1991.)

nerves: obturator, femoral, superior gluteal, inferior gluteal, common peroneal, and tibial. The sciatic nerve, which is frequently discussed in physical therapy practice, is actually composed of the common peroneal and tibial nerves encased in a sheath. This nerve innervates the hamstrings and causes hip extension and knee flexion. The sciatic nerve separates into its components just above the knee (Guyton, 1991). The lumbosacral plexus is also shown in Figures 2–16 and 2–17.

Peripheral Nerves. Two major types of nerve fibers are contained in peripheral nerves: motor (efferent) and sensory (afferent) fibers. Motor fibers have a large cell body with multiple branched dendrites and a long axon. The cell body and the dendrites are located within the anterior horn of the spinal cord. The axon exits the anterior horn through the white matter and is located with other similar axons in the anterior root, which is located outside the spinal cord in the intervertebral foramen. The axon then eventually becomes part of a peripheral nerve and innervates a motor end plate in a muscle. The sensory neuron, on the other hand, has a dendrite that originates in the skin, muscle tendon, or Golgi tendon organ and travels all the way to its cell body, which is located in the dorsal root ganglion within the intervertebral foramen (Fig. 2–18). Golgi tendon organs are encapsulated nerve endings found at the musculotendinous junction. They are sensitive to tension within muscle tendons and transmit this information to the spinal cord. The axon travels through the dorsal (posterior) root of a spinal

nerve and into the spinal cord through the dorsal horn. The axon may terminate at this point, or it may enter the white matter fiber tracts and ascend to a different level in the spinal cord or brain stem. Thus, a sensory neuron sends information from the periphery to the spinal cord.

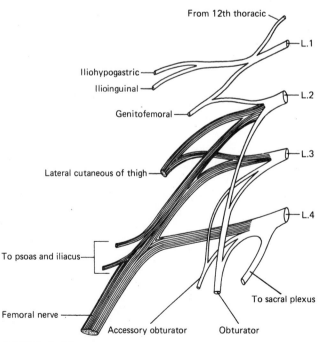

FIGURE 2-16 ■ The lumbar plexus and its branches, especially the femoral nerve. (From Guyton AC. Basic Neuroscience: Anatomy and Physiology, 2nd ed. Philadelphia, WB Saunders, 1991.)

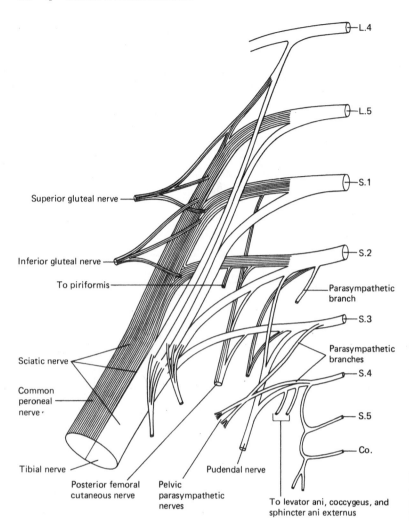

Figure labels:
- L.4
- L.5
- S.1
- S.2
- S.3
- S.4
- S.5
- Co.
- Superior gluteal nerve
- Inferior gluteal nerve
- To piriformis
- Sciatic nerve
- Common peroneal nerve
- Tibial nerve
- Posterior femoral cutaneous nerve
- Pelvic parasympathetic nerves
- Pudendal nerve
- To levator ani, coccygeus, and sphincter ani externus
- Parasympathetic branch
- Parasympathetic branches

FIGURE 2–17 ■ The sacral plexus and its branches, especially the sciatic nerve. (From Guyton AC. Basic Neuroscience: Anatomy and Physiology, 2nd ed. Philadelphia, WB Saunders, 1991.)

Autonomic Nervous System

Functions of the ANS include the regulation of circulation, respiration, digestion, metabolism, secretion, body temperature, and reproduction. Control centers for the ANS are located in the hypothalamus and the brain stem. The ANS is composed of motor neurons located within spinal nerves that innervate smooth muscle, cardiac muscle, and glands, which are also called effectors or target organs. The ANS is divided into the sympathetic and parasympathetic divisions. Both the sympathetic and parasympathetic divisions innervate internal organs, use a two-neuron pathway and one-ganglion impulse conduction, and function automatically. Autoregulation is achieved by integrating information from peripheral afferents with information from receptors within the CNS. The two-neuron pathway (preganglionic and postganglionic neurons) provides the connection from the CNS to the autonomic effector organs. Cell bodies of the preganglionic neurons are located within the brain or spinal cord. The myelinated axons exit the CNS and synapse with collections of postganglionic cell bodies. Unmyelinated axons from the postganglionic neurons ultimately innervate the effector organs (Farber, 1982).

The sympathetic fibers of the ANS arise from the thoracic and lumbar portions of the spinal cord. Axons of preganglionic neurons terminate in either the sympathetic chain or the prevertebral ganglia located in the abdomen. The sympathetic division of the ANS assists the individual in responding to stressful situations and is often referred to as the fight-or-flight response. Sympathetic responses help the individual to prepare to cope with the perceived stimulus by maintaining an optimal blood supply. Activation of the sympathetic system stimulates smooth muscle in the blood vessels to contract, thereby causing vasoconstriction. Norepinephrine, also known as noradrenaline, is the major neurotransmitter responsible for this action. Consequently, heart rate and blood pressure are increased as the body prepares for a fight or to flee a dangerous situation. Blood flow to muscles is increased by being diverted from the gastrointestinal tract.

The parasympathetic division maintains vital bodily functions or homeostasis. The parasympathetic division receives its information from the brain stem, specifically cranial nerves III (oculomotor), VII (facial), IX (glossopharyngeal), and X (vagus), and from lower

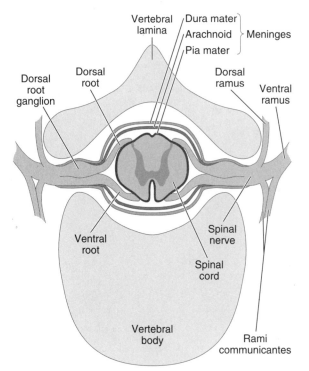

FIGURE 2–18 ■ Spinal region. The spinal nerve is formed of axons from the dorsal and ventral roots. The bifurcation of the spinal nerve into dorsal and ventral rami marks the transition from the spinal to the peripheral region. (From Lundy-Ekman L. Neuroscience: Fundamentals for Rehabilitation. Philadelphia, WB Saunders, 1998.)

sacral segments of the spinal cord. The vagus nerve is a parasympathetic preganglionic nerve. Motor fibers within the vagus nerve innervate the myocardium and the smooth muscles of the lungs and digestive tract. Activation of the vagus nerve can produce the following effects: bradycardia, decreased force of cardiac muscle contraction, bronchoconstriction, increased mucus production, increased peristalsis, and increased glandular secretions. Efferent activation of the sacral components results in emptying of the bowels and bladder and arousal of sexual organs. Acetylcholine is the chemical transmitter responsible for sending nervous system impulses to effector cells in the parasympathetic division. Acetylcholine is used for both divisions at the preganglionic synapse and dilates arterioles. Thus, activation of the parasympathetic division produces vasodilation. When an individual is calm, parasympathetic activity decreases heart rate and blood pressure and signals a return of normal gastrointestinal activity. Figure 2–19 shows the influence of the sympathetic and parasympathetic divisions on effector organs (Farber, 1982; Lundy-Ekman, 1998).

The CNS also exerts influence over the ANS. The regions most closely associated with this control are the hypothalamus, which regulates functions such as digestion, and the medulla, which controls heart and respiration rates.

Cerebral Circulation

A final area that must be reviewed when discussing the nervous system is the circulation to the brain. The cells within the brain completely depend on a continuous supply of blood for glucose and oxygen. The neurons within the brain are unable to carry out glycolysis and to store glycogen. It is therefore absolutely essential that these neurons receive a constant supply of blood. Knowledge of cerebrovascular anatomy is essential to understand the clinical manifestations, diagnosis, and management of patients who have had cerebrovascular accidents and traumatic brain injuries.

Anterior Circulation

All arteries to the brain arise from the aortic arch. The first major arteries ascending anteriorly and laterally within the neck are the common carotid arteries. The carotid arteries are responsible for supplying the

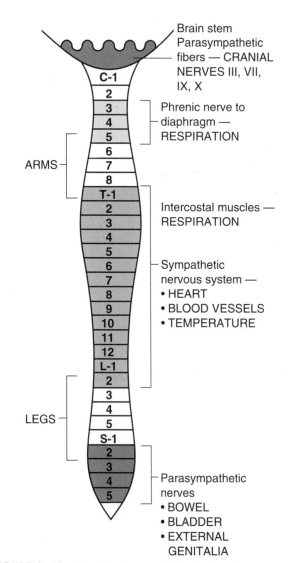

FIGURE 2–19 ■ Functional areas of the spinal cord. (From Gould BE. Pathophysiology for the Health-Related Professions. Philadelphia, WB Saunders, 1997.)

bulk of the cerebrum with circulation. The right and left common carotid arteries bifurcate just behind the posterior angle of the jaw to become the external and internal carotids. The external carotid arteries supply the face, whereas the internal carotids enter the cranium and supply the cerebral hemispheres including the frontal lobe, the parietal lobe, and parts of the temporal lobe. In addition, the internal carotid artery supplies the optic nerves and the retina of the eyes. At the base of the brain, the internal carotid bifurcates into the right and left anterior and middle cerebral arteries. The middle cerebral artery is the largest of the cerebral arteries and is most often occluded. It is responsible for supplying the lateral surface of the brain with blood and also the deep portions of the frontal and parietal lobes. The anterior cerebral artery supplies the superior border of the frontal and parietal lobes. Both the middle cerebral artery and the anterior cerebral artery make up what is called the anterior circulation to the brain. Figures 2–20 and 2–21 depict the cerebral circulation.

Posterior Circulation

The posterior circulation is composed of the two vertebral arteries, which are branches of the subclavian. The vertebral arteries supply blood to the brain stem and cerebellum. The vertebral arteries leave the

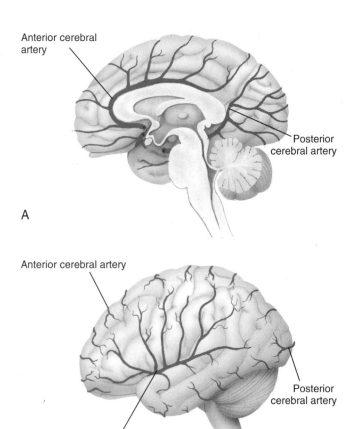

A

B

FIGURE 2–21 ■ The large cerebral arteries: anterior, middle, and posterior. (From Lundy-Ekman L. Neuroscience: Fundamentals for Rehabilitation. Philadelphia, WB Saunders, 1998.)

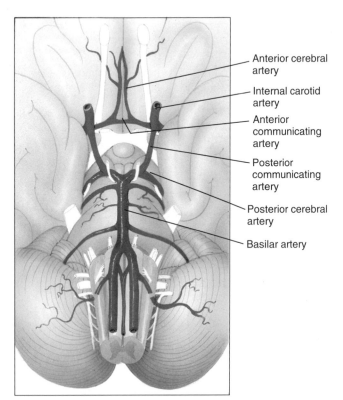

FIGURE 2–20 ■ From anterior to posterior, the arteries that form the circle of Willis are the anterior communicating, two anterior cerebral, two internal carotid, two posterior communicating, and two posterior cerebral arteries. (From Lundy-Ekman L. Neuroscience: Fundamentals for Rehabilitation. Philadelphia, WB Saunders, 1998.)

base of the neck and ascend posteriorly to enter the skull through the foramen magnum. The two vertebral arteries then unite to form the basilar artery. The basilar artery supplies the brain stem and the medial portion of the temporal and occipital lobes with circulation. This artery also bifurcates to form the right and left posterior cerebral arteries. The two posterior cerebral arteries supply blood to the occipital and temporal lobes.

The carotid arteries, through the anterior cerebral artery, and the vertebral arteries, through the posterior cerebral arteries, are interconnected at the base of the brain and form the circle of Willis. This connection of blood vessels provides a protective mechanism to the structures within the brain. Because of the circle of Willis, failure or occlusion of one cerebral artery does not critically decrease blood flow to that region. Consequently, the occlusion can be circumvented or bypassed to meet the nutritional and metabolic needs of cerebral tissue.

REACTION TO INJURY

What happens when the CNS or the PNS is injured? The CNS and the PNS are prone to different types of injury, and each system reacts differently. Within the CNS, artery obstruction of sufficient duration produces tissue death within minutes. However, changes within the neurons themselves are not evident for 12 to 24 hours. By 24 to 36 hours, the damaged area becomes soft and edematous. An inflammatory reaction takes place within the brain tissue and is characterized by an influx of macrophages to clean up the necrotic debris. Liquefaction and cavitation begin, and the area of dead tissue is eventually converted into a cyst. In time, the infarct will eventually retract, and the cystic cavity will by surrounded by a glial scar. The damaged neurons will not be replaced, and the original function of the area will be lost (Branch, 1987).

Nearby undamaged axons demonstrate collateral sprouting in 4 to 5 days after injury. These sprouts replace the damaged synaptic area, thus increasing input to other neurons. Although these collateral sprouts do not replace original circuits, they do develop from systems most closely associated with the injured area.

Conversely, peripheral nerve injuries often result from means other than vascular compromise. Common causes of peripheral nerve injuries include stretching, laceration, compression, traction, disease, chemical toxicity, and nutritional deficiencies. The response of a peripheral nerve to the injury is different from that in the CNS. If the cell body is destroyed, regeneration is not possible. The axon undergoes necrosis distal to the site of injury, the myelin sheath begins to pull away, and the Schwann cells phagocytize the area, producing wallerian degeneration (Fig. 2–22). If the damage to the peripheral nerve is not too significant and occurs only to the axon, regeneration is possible. Axonal sprouting from the proximal end of the damaged axon can occur. The axon regrows at the rate of 1.0 mm per day depending on the size of the nerve fiber (Lundy-Ekman, 1998). To have a return of function, the axon must grow and reinnervate the appropriate muscle. Failure to do so results in degeneration of the axonal sprout. The rate of recovery from a peripheral nerve injury depends on the age of the patient and the distance between the lesion and the destination of the regenerating nerve fibers. A discussion of the physical therapy management of peripheral nerve injuries is beyond the scope of this text.

Injury to a motor neuron can result in variable findings. If an individual experiences damage to the corticospinal tract from its origin in the frontal lobe to its end within the spinal cord, the patient is classified as having an upper motor neuron injury. Clinical signs of an upper motor neuron injury include spasticity (increased resistance to passive stretch), hyperreflexia, the presence of a Babinski sign, and possible clonus. Clonus is a repetitive stretch reflex that is elicited by passive dorsiflexion of the ankle or passive wrist extension. If the injury is to the anterior horn, the anterior

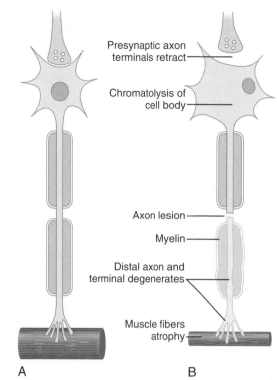

FIGURE 2–22 ■ Wallerian degeneration. *A*, Normal connections before an axon is severed. *B*, Degeneration following severance of an axon. Degeneration following axonal injury involves several changes: (1) the axon terminal degenerates, (2) myelin breaks down and forms debris, and (3) the cell body undergoes metabolic changes. Subsequently, (4) presynaptic terminals retract from the dying cell body, and (5) postsynaptic cells degenerate. (From Lundy-Ekman L. Neuroscience: Fundamentals for Rehabilitation. Philadelphia, WB Saunders, 1998.)

horn cell, the spinal root, or the spinal nerve, the patient is recognized as having a lower motor neuron injury. Clinical findings of this type of injury include flaccidity, marked muscle atrophy, muscle fasciculations, and hyporeflexia.

CHAPTER SUMMARY

An understanding of the structures and functions of the nervous system is necessary for physical therapists and physical therapist assistants. This knowledge assists practitioners in working with patients with neuromuscular dysfunction because it allows one to have a better appreciation of the patient's pathologic condition, deficits, and potential capabilities. In addition, an understanding of neuroanatomy is helpful when educating patients and their families regarding the patient's condition and possible prognosis.

REVIEW QUESTIONS

1. Describe the major components of the nervous system.
2. What is the function of the white matter?
3. What are some of the primary functions of the parietal lobe?
4. What is Broca's aphasia?
5. Discuss the primary function of the thalamus.
6. What is the primary function of the corticospinal tract?
7. What is an anterior horn cell? Where are these cells located?
8. Discuss the components of the PNS.
9. Where is the most common site of cerebral infarction?
10. What are some clinical signs of an upper motor neuron injury?

REFERENCES

Branch EF. The neuropathology of stroke. In Duncan PW, Badke MB (eds). Stroke Rehabilitation: The Recovery of Motor Control. St. Louis, Year Book, 1987, pp 49–77.

Cohen H. Neuroscience for Rehabilitation, 2nd ed. Philadelphia, Lippincott Williams & Wilkins, 1999.

Curtis BA. Neurosciences: The Basics. Philadelphia, Lea & Febiger, 1990.

Farber SD. Neurorehabilitation: A Multisensory Approach. Philadelphia, WB Saunders, 1982, pp 1–59.

FitzGerald MJT. Neuroanatomy Basic and Clinical, 3rd ed. Philadelphia, WB Saunders, 1996.

Geschwind N, Levitsky W. Human brain: left-right asymmetries in temporal speech regions. Science 161:186–187, 1968.

Guyton AC. Basic Neuroscience: Anatomy and Physiology, 2nd ed. Philadelphia, WB Saunders, 1991, pp 1–24, 39–54, 244–245.

Horak FB. Assumptions underlying motor control for neurologic rehabilitation. In Contemporary Management of Motor Control Problems: Proceedings of the II Step Conference. Alexandria, VA, Foundation for Physical Therapy, 1991, pp 11–27.

Littell EH. Basic Neuroscience for the Health Professions. Thorofare, NJ, Slack Incorporated, 1990.

Lundy-Ekman L. Neuroscience: Fundamentals for Rehabilitation. Philadelphia, WB Saunders, 1998, pp 132–143, 227–230, 322–330, 335.

O'Sullivan SB. Stroke. In O'Sullivan SB, Schmitz TJ (eds). Physical Rehabilitation Assessment and Treatment, 3rd ed. Philadelphia, FA Davis, 1994, pp 329–337.

CHAPTER 3

Motor Control and Motor Learning

INTRODUCTION

Motor abilities and skills are acquired during the process of motor development through motor control and motor learning. Once a basic pattern of movement is established, it can be varied to suit the purpose of the task or the environmental situation in which the task is to take place. Early motor development displays a fairly predictable sequence of skill acquisition through childhood. However, the ways in which these motor abilities are used for function are highly variable. Individuals rarely perform the movement exactly the same way every time. This variability must be part of any model used to explain how posture and movement are controlled.

Any movement system must be able to adapt to the changing demands of the individual mover and environment in which the movement takes place. The individual mover must be able to learn from prior movement experiences. Different theories of motor control emphasize different developmental aspects of posture and movement. Development of postural control and balance is embedded in the development of motor control. Understanding the relationship among motor control, motor learning, and motor development pro-

vides a valuable framework for understanding the treatment of individuals with neurologic dysfunction at any age.

Motor development is a product as well as a process. The products of motor development are the milestones of the developmental sequence and the kinesiologic components of movement such as head and trunk control necessary for these motor abilities. These products are discussed in Chapter 4. The process of motor development is the way in which those abilities emerge. The process and the product are affected by many factors such as time (age), maturation (genes), adaptation (physical constraints), and learning. Motor development is the result of the interaction of the innate or built-in species blueprint for posture and movement and the person's experiences with moving afforded by the environment. Sensory input is needed for the mover to learn about moving and the results of moving. Motor development is the combination of the nature of the mover and the nurture of the environment. Part of the genetic blueprint for movement is the means to control posture and movement. Motor development, motor control, and motor learning contribute to an ongoing process of change throughout the life span of every person who moves.

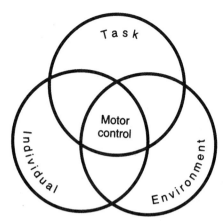

FIGURE 3–1 ▪ Motor control emerges from an interaction between the individual, the task, and the environment. (From Shumway-Cook A, Woollacott MH. Motor Control: Theory and Practical Applications. Baltimore, Williams & Wilkins, 1995.)

MOTOR CONTROL

Motor control, the ability to maintain and change posture and movement, is the result of a complex set of neurologic and mechanical processes. Those processes include motor, cognitive, and perceptual development. "The development of motor control begins with the control of self movements, and proceeds to the control of movements in relationship to changing conditions" (VanSant, 1995). Control of self-movement largely results from the development of the neuromotor systems. As the nervous and muscular systems mature, movement emerges. Motor control allows the nervous system to direct what muscles should be used, in what order, and how quickly, to solve a movement problem. The infant's first movement problem relates to overcoming the effect of gravity. A second but related problem is how to move a larger head as compared with a smaller body to establish head control. Later, movement problems are related to controlling the interaction between stability and mobility of the head, trunk, and limbs. Control of task-specific movements such as stringing beads or riding a tricycle depends on cognitive and perceptual abilities. The task to be carried out by the person within the environment dictates the type of movement solution that is going to be needed.

Because the motor abilities of a person change over time, the motor solutions to a given motor problem may also change. The motivation of the individual to move may also change over time and may affect the intricacy of the movement solution. An infant encountering a set of stairs sees a toy on the top stair. She creeps up the stairs but then has to figure out how to get down. She can cry for help, bump down on her buttocks, creep down backward, or even attempt creeping down forward. A toddler faced with the same dilemma may walk up the same set of stairs one step at a time holding onto a railing, and descend in sitting holding the toy, or she may be able to hold the toy with one hand and the railing with the other and descend the same way she came up the stairs. The child will walk up and down without holding on, and an even older child may run up those same stairs. The relationship among the task, the individual, and the environment is depicted graphically in Figure 3–1. All three components must be considered when thinking about motor control.

Motor Control Time Frame

Motor control happens not in the space of days or weeks, as is seen in motor development, but in fractions of seconds. Figure 3–2 illustrates a comparison of time frames associated with motor control, motor learning, and motor development. Motor control occurs because of physiologic processes that happen at cellular, tissue, and organ levels. Physiologic processes

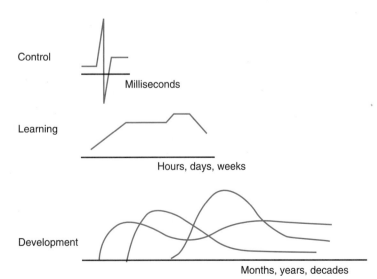

FIGURE 3–2 ▪ Time scales of interest from a motor control, motor learning, and motor development perspective. (From Cech D, Martin S [eds]. Functional Movement Development Across the Life Span. Philadelphia, WB Saunders, 1995.)

have to happen quickly to produce timely and efficient movement. What good does it do if you extend an outstretched arm after having fallen down? Extending your arm in a protective response has to be quick enough to be useful, that is, to break the fall. Persons with nervous system disease may exhibit the correct movement pattern, but they have impaired timing, producing the movement too slowly to be functional, or they have impaired sequencing of muscle activation, producing a muscle contraction at the wrong time. Both of these problems, impaired timing and impaired sequencing, are examples of deficits in motor control.

Role of Sensation in Motor Control

Sensory information plays an important role in motor control. Initially, sensation cues reflexive movements in which few cognitive or perceptual abilities are needed. A sensory stimulus produces a reflexive motor response. Touching the lip of a newborn produces head turning, whereas stroking a newborn's outstretched leg produces withdrawal. Sensation is an ever-present cue for motor behavior in the seemingly reflex-dominated infant. As voluntary movement emerges during motor development, sensation provides feedback accuracy for hand placement during reaching and later for creeping. Sensation from weight bearing reinforces maintenance of developmental postures such as the prone on elbows position and the hands and knees position. Sensory information is crucial to the mover when interacting with objects and maneuvering within an environment. Figure 3–3 depicts how sensation provides the necessary feedback for the body to know whether a task such as reaching or walking was performed and how well it was accomplished.

Theories of Motor Control

Many theories of motor control have been posited, but only those most closely related to early motor development are discussed in this chapter. The first theoretic model of motor control presented is the traditional hierarchic one. Second, a systems model of motor control is outlined.

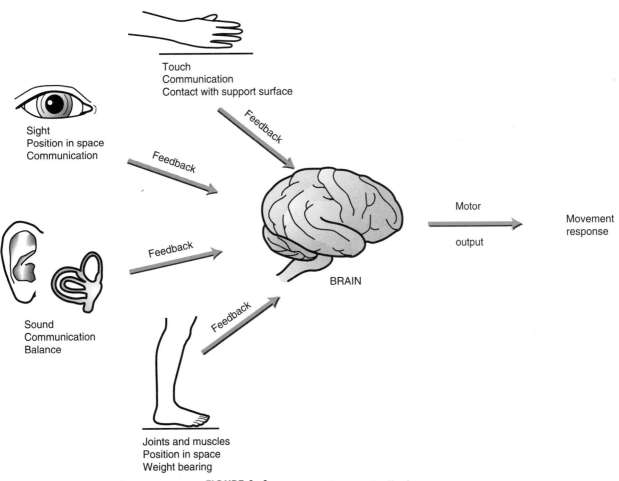

FIGURE 3–3 ■ Sources of sensory feedback.

Hierarchic Theory

Many theories of motor control exist, but the most traditional one is that of a hierarchy. Characteristics of a hierarchic model of motor control include a top-down perspective. The cortex of the brain is seen as the highest level of control, with all subcortical structures taking orders from it. The cortex can and does direct movement. A person can generate an idea about moving in a certain way and the nervous system carries out the command. The ultimate level of motor control, voluntary movement, is achieved by maturation of the cortex.

In the hierarchic model, a relationship exists between the maturation of the developing brain and the emergence of motor behaviors seen in infancy. One of the ways in which nervous system maturation has been routinely gauged is by the assessment of reflexes. The reflex is seen as the basic unit of movement in this motor control model. Movement is acquired from the chaining together of reflexes and reactions. A reflex is the pairing of a sensory stimulus with a motor response, as shown in Figure 3–4. Some reflexes are simple and others are complex. The simplest reflexes occur at the spinal cord level. An example of a spinal cord level reflex is the flexor withdrawal. A touch or noxious stimulus applied to the bottom of the foot produces lower extremity withdrawal. These reflexes are also referred to as primitive reflexes because they occur early in the life span of the infant. Another example is the palmar grasp. Primitive reflexes are listed in Table 3–1.

The next higher level of reflexes comprises the tonic reflexes, which are associated with the brain stem of the central nervous system. These reflexes produce changes in muscle tone and posture. Examples of tonic reflexes exhibited by infants are the tonic labyrinthine reflex and the asymmetric tonic neck reflex. In the latter, when the infant's head is turned to the right, the infant's right arm extends and the left arm flexes. The tonic labyrinthine reflex produces increased extensor tone when the infant is supine and increased flexor tone in the prone position. In this

Table 3–1 ▌ PRIMITIVE REFLEXES

REFLEX	AGE AT ONSET	AGE AT INTEGRATION
Suck-swallow	28 weeks' gestation	2–5 months
Rooting	28 weeks' gestation	3 months
Flexor withdrawal	28 weeks' gestation	1–2 months
Crossed extension	28 weeks' gestation	1–2 months
Moro	28 weeks' gestation	4–6 months
Plantar grasp	28 weeks' gestation	9 months
Positive support	35 weeks' gestation	1–2 months
Asymmetric tonic neck	Birth	4–6 months
Palmar grasp	Birth	9 months
Symmetric tonic neck	4–6 months	8–12 months

From Cech D, Martin S (eds). Functional Movement Development Across the Life Span. Philadelphia, WB Saunders, 1995, p 81.

model, most infantile reflexes (sucking and rooting), primitive spinal cord reflexes, and tonic reflexes are integrated by 4 to 6 months. Exceptions do exist. Integration is the mechanism by which less mature responses are incorporated into voluntary movement.

In the hierarchic model, nervous system maturation is seen as the ultimate determinant of the acquisition of postural control. As the infant develops motor control, brain structures above the spinal cord begin to control posture and movement until the ultimate balance reactions are achieved. The ultimate balance reactions are the righting, protective, and equilibrium reactions.

Righting and equilibrium reactions are complex postural responses that continue to be present even in adulthood. These postural responses involve the head and trunk and provide the body with an automatic way to respond to movement of the center of gravity within and outside the body's base of support. Extremity movements in response to quick displacements of the center of gravity out of the base of support are called protective reactions. These are also considered postural reactions and serve as a back-up system should the righting or equilibrium reaction fail to compensate for a loss of balance. According to the hierarchic model of motor control, automatic postural responses are associated with the midbrain and cortex (Fig. 3–5).

The farther up one goes in the hierarchy, the more inhibition there is of lower structures and the movements they produce, that is, reflexes. Tonic reflexes inhibit spinal cord reflexes, and righting reactions inhibit tonic reflexes. Inhibition allows previously demonstrated stimulus-response patterns of movement to be integrated or modified into more volitional movements. A more complete description of these postural responses is given as part of the development of postural control from a hierarchic perspective.

Development of Motor Control. Development of motor control can be described by the relationship of mobility and stability of body postures (Sullivan et al,

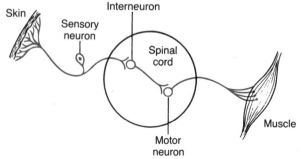

FIGURE 3–4 ▪ Three neuron nervous system. (Redrawn from Romero-Sierra C. Neuroanatomy: A Conceptual Approach. New York, Churchill Livingstone, 1986.)

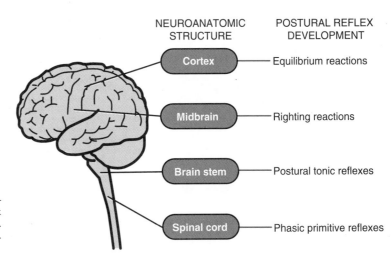

NEUROANATOMIC STRUCTURE — POSTURAL REFLEX DEVELOPMENT

Cortex — Equilibrium reactions

Midbrain — Righting reactions

Brain stem — Postural tonic reflexes

Spinal cord — Phasic primitive reflexes

FIGURE 3–5 ■ The classic reflex hierarchy in which central nervous system maturation is linked to postural reflex development. (Modified from Cech D, Martin S [eds]. Functional Movement Development Across the Life Span. Philadelphia, WB Saunders, 1995.)

1982) and by the acquisition of automatic postural responses (Cech and Martin, 1995). Initial random movements (mobility) are followed by maintenance of a posture (stability), movement within a posture (controlled mobility), and finally, movement from one posture to another posture (skill). The sequence of acquiring motor control is seen in key developmental postures in Figure 3–6. With acquisition of each new posture comes the development of control within that posture. For example, weight shifting in prone precedes rolling prone to supine; weight shifting on hands and knees precedes creeping; and cruising, or sideways weight shifting in standing, precedes walking. The actual motor accomplishments of rolling, reaching, creeping, cruising, and walking are skills in which mobility is combined with stability and the distal parts of the body, that is, the extremities, are free to move. The infant develops motor and postural control in the following order: mobility; stability; controlled mobility; and finally, skill.

Stages of Motor Control

Stage One. Stage one is mobility, when movement is initiated. The infant exhibits random movements within an available range of motion for the first 3 months of development. Movements during this stage are erratic. They lack purpose and are often reflex based. Random limb movements are made when the infant's head and trunk are supported in the supine position. Mobility is present before stability. In adults, mobility refers to the availability of range of motion to assume a posture and the presence of sufficient motor unit activity to initiate a movement.

Stage Two. Stage two is stability, the ability to maintain a steady position in a weight-bearing, antigravity posture. It is also called static postural control. Developmentally, stability is further divided into tonic holding and co-contraction. Tonic holding occurs at the end of the shortened range of movement and usually involves isometric movements of antigravity postural

extensors (Stengel et al, 1984). Tonic holding is most evident when the child maintains the pivot prone position (prone extension), as seen in Figure 3–6. Postural holding of the head begins asymmetrically in prone, is followed by holding the head in midline, and progresses to holding the head up past 90 degrees from the support surface. In the supine position, the head is turned to one side or the other; then it is held in midline; and finally, it is held in midline with a chin tuck while the infant is being pulled to sit at 4 months (Fig. 3–7).

Co-contraction is the simultaneous static contraction of antagonistic muscles around a joint to provide stability in a midline position or in weight bearing. Various groups of muscles, especially those used for postural fixation, allow the developing infant to hold such postures as prone extension, prone on elbows and hands, all fours, and semi-squat. Co-contraction patterns are shown in Figure 3–6. Once the initial relationship between mobility and stability is established in prone and later in all fours and standing, a change occurs to allow mobility to be superimposed on the already established stability.

Stage Three. Controlled mobility is mobility superimposed on previously developed postural stability by weight shifting within a posture. Proximal mobility is combined with distal stability. This controlled mobility is the third stage of motor control and occurs when the limbs are weight bearing and the body moves, such as in weight shifting on all fours or in standing. The trunk performs controlled mobility when it is parallel to the support surface or when the line of gravity is perpendicular to the trunk. In prone and all fours positions, the limbs and the trunk are performing controlled mobility when shifting weight.

The infant's first attempts at weight shifts in prone happen accidentally with little control. As the infant tries to reproduce the movement and practices various movement combinations, the movement becomes more controlled. Another example of controlled mo-

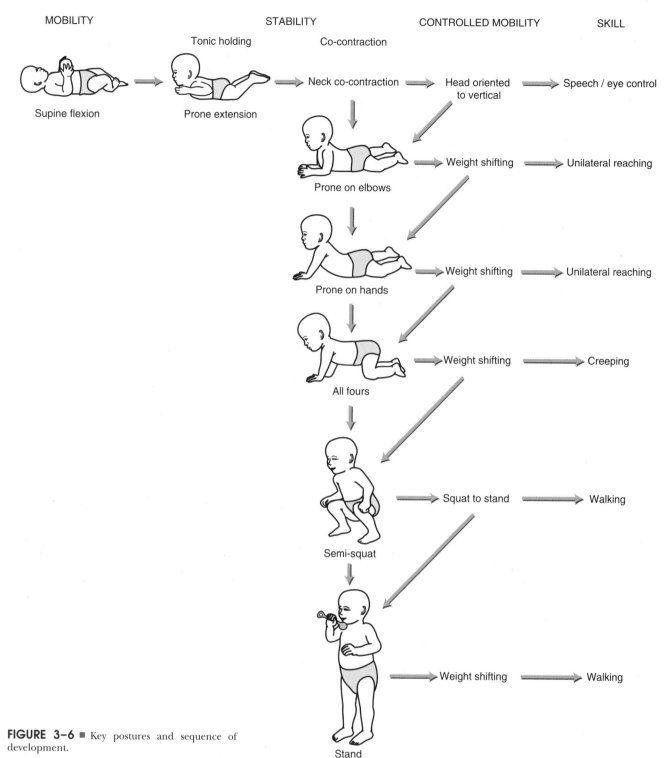

FIGURE 3–6 ▪ Key postures and sequence of development.

bility is demonstrated by an infant in a prone on elbows position who sees a toy. If the infant attempts to reach for the toy with both hands, which she typically does before reaching with one hand, the infant is likely to fall on her face. If she perseveres and learns to shift weight onto one elbow, she has a better chance of obtaining the toy. Weight bearing, weight shifting, and co-contraction of muscles around the

shoulder are crucial to the development of shoulder girdle stability. Proximal shoulder stability supports upper extremity function for skilled distal manipulation. If this stability is not present, distal performance may be impaired. Controlled mobility is also referred to as dynamic postural control.

Stage Four. Skill is the most mature type of movement and is usually mastered after controlled mobility

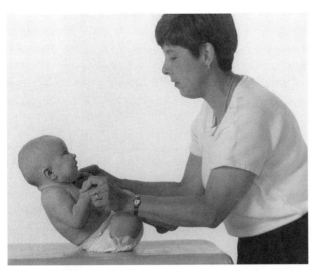

FIGURE 3–7 ■ Chin tuck when pulled to sit.

within a posture. For example, after weight shifting within a posture such as in a hands and knees position, the infant frees the opposite arm and leg to creep reciprocally. Creeping is a skilled movement. Other skill patterns are also depicted in Figure 3–6. Skill patterns of movement occur when mobility is superimposed on stability in non-weight bearing; proximal segments stabilize while distal segments are free for movement. The trunk does skilled work when it is upright or parallel to the force of gravity. In standing, only the lower extremities are using controlled mobility when weight shifting occurs. If the swing leg moves, it performs skilled work while the stance limb performs controlled mobility. When an infant creeps or walks, the limbs that are in motion are using skill, and those in contact with the support surface are using controlled mobility. Creeping and walking are considered skilled movements. Skilled movements involve manipulation and exploration of the environment.

Development of Postural Control. Postural control develops in a cephalocaudal direction in keeping with Gesell's developmental principles, which are discussed in Chapter 4. Postural control is demonstrated by the ability to maintain the alignment of the body—specifically, the alignment of body parts relative to each other and the external environment. "The functions that maintain or preserve alignment have been called 'equilibrium' or 'balance'" (VanSant, 1995). The infant learns to use a group of automatic postural responses to attain and maintain an upright erect posture. These postural responses are continuously used when balance is lost in an effort to regain equilibrium.

The sequence of development of postural reactions entails righting reactions, followed by protective reactions, and last, equilibrium reactions. In the infant, head righting reactions develop first and are followed by the development of trunk righting reactions. Pro-

tective reactions of the extremities emerge next in an effort to safeguard balance in higher postures such as sitting. Finally, equilibrium reactions develop in all postures beginning in prone. One way of looking at these postural reactions is based on a hierarchic view of how the nervous system works, as seen in Figure 3–5. As the nervous system matures, ever higher centers are responsible for coordinating the infant's postural responses to shifts of center of mass within the base of support. Figure 3–8 shows a hierarchic representation of how muscle tone, reflexes, and reactions are related to attainment of selective voluntary movement, postural control, and equilibrium reactions. Traditionally, posture and movement develop together in a cephalocaudal direction, so balance is achieved in different positions relative to gravity. Head control is followed by trunk control; control of the head on the body and in space comes before sitting and standing balance.

Righting Reactions. Righting reactions are responsible for orienting the head in space and keeping the eyes and mouth horizontal. This normal alignment is maintained in upright vertical position and when the body is tilted or rotated. Righting reactions involve head and trunk movements to maintain or regain orientation or alignment. Some righting reactions begin at birth, but most are evident between 4 and 6 months of age, as listed in Table 3–2. Gravity and change of head or body position provide cues for the most frequently used righting reactions. Vision cues an optical righting reaction, gravity cues the labyrinthine righting reaction, and touch of the support surface to the abdomen cues the body-on-the-head reaction. These

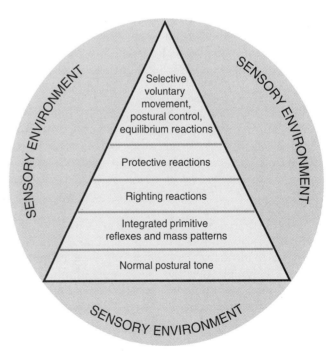

FIGURE 3–8 ■ Normal postural reflex mechanism. (Courtesy of Jan Utley.)

Table 3-2 ∎ RIGHTING AND EQUILIBRIUM REACTIONS

REACTION	AGE AT ONSET	AGE AT INTEGRATION
Head righting		
Neck (immature)	34 weeks' gestation	4–6 months
Labyrinthine	Birth–2 months	Persists
Optical	Birth–2 months	Persists
Neck (mature)	4–6 months	5 years
Trunk righting		
Body (immature)	34 weeks' gestation	4–6 months
Body (mature)	4–6 months	5 years
Landau	3–4 months	1–2 years
Protective		
Downward lower extremity	4 months	Persists
Forward upper extremity	6–7 months	Persists
Sideways upper extremity	7–8 months	Persists
Backward upper extremity	9 months	Persists
Stepping lower extremity	15–17 months	Persists
Equilibrium		
Prone	6 months	Persists
Supine	7–8 months	Persists
Sitting	7–8 months	Persists
Quadruped	9–12 months	Persists
Standing	12–24 months	Persists

From Cech D, Martin S (eds). Functional Movement Development Across the Life Span. Philadelphia, WB Saunders, 1995, p 83.

three head righting reactions assist the infant in developing head control.

Head turning can produce neck-on-body righting, in which the body follows the head movement. If either the upper or lower trunk is turned, a body-on-body righting reaction is elicited. Either neck-on-body righting or body-on-body righting can produce log rolling or segmental rolling. Log rolling is the immature righting response seen in the first 3 months of life; the mature response emerges around 4 months of age. The purpose of righting reactions is to maintain the correct orientation of the head and body in relation to the ground. Head and trunk righting reactions occur when weight is shifted within a base of support; the amount of displacement determines the degree of response. For example, in the prone position, slow weight shifting to the right produces a lateral bend or righting of the head and trunk to the left. If the displacement is too fast, a different type of response may be seen, a protective response. Slower displacements are more likely to elicit head and trunk righting. These can occur in any posture and in response to anterior, posterior, or lateral weight shifts.

Righting reactions have their maximum influence on posture and movement between 10 and 12 months of age, although they are said to continue to be present until the child is 5 years old. Righting reactions are no longer considered to be present if the child can come to standing from a supine position without using trunk rotation. The presence of trunk rotation indicates a righting of the body around the long axis. Another explanation for the change in mo-

tor behavior could be that the child of 5 years has sufficient abdominal strength to perform the sagittal plane movement of rising straight forward and attaining standing without using trunk rotation.

Protective Reactions. Protective reactions are extremity movements that occur in response to rapid displacement of the body by diagonal or horizontal forces. They have a predictable developmental sequence, which can be found in Table 3-2. By extending one or both extremities, the individual prepares for a fall or prepares to catch himself. A 4-month-old infant's lower extremities extend and abduct when the infant is held upright in vertical and quickly lowered toward the supporting surface. At 6 months, the upper extremities show forward protective extension, followed by sideways extension at 7 to 8 months and backward extension at 9 months. Protective staggering of the lower extremities is evident by 15 to 17 months (Barnes et al, 1978). Protective reactions of the extremities should not be confused with the ability of the infant to prop on extended arms, a movement that can be self-initiated by pushing up from prone or by being placed in the position by a caregiver. Because the infant must be able to bear weight on extended arms to exhibit protective extension, propping or pushing up can be useful as a treatment intervention.

Equilibrium Reactions. Equilibrium reactions are the most advanced postural reactions and are the last to develop. These reactions allow the body as a whole to adapt to slow changes in the relationship of the center of gravity with the base of support. By incorporating the already learned head and trunk righting reactions, the equilibrium reactions add extremity responses to flexion, extension, or lateral head and trunk movements to regain equilibrium. In lateral weight shifts, the trunk may rotate in the opposite direction of the weight shift to further attempt to maintain the body's center of gravity within the base of support. The trunk rotation is evident only during lateral displacements. Equilibrium reactions can occur if the body moves relative to the support surface, as in leaning sideways, or if the support surface moves, as when one is on a tilt board. In the latter case, these movements are called tilt reactions. The three expected responses to a lateral displacement of the center of gravity toward the periphery of the base of support in standing are as follows: (1) lateral head and trunk righting occurs away from the weight shift; (2) the arm and leg opposite the direction of the weight shift abduct; and (3) trunk rotation away from the weight shift may occur. If the last response does not happen, the other two responses can provide only a brief postponement of the inevitable fall. At the point at which the center of gravity leaves the base of support, protective extension of the arms may occur, or a protective step or stagger may reestablish a stable base. Thus, the order in which the reactions are acquired developmentally is different from the order in which they are used for balance.

Equilibrium reactions also have a set developmental sequence and timetable (see Table 3–2). Because prone is a position from which to learn to move against gravity, equilibrium reactions are seen first in prone at 6 months, then supine at 7 to 8 months, sitting at 7 to 8 months, on all fours at 9 to 12 months, and standing at 12 to 21 months. The infant is always working on more than one postural level at a time. For example, the 8-month-old infant is perfecting supine equilibrium reactions while learning to control weight shifts in sitting, freeing first one hand and then both hands. Sitting equilibrium reactions mature when the child is creeping. Standing and cruising are possible as equilibrium reactions are perfected on all fours. The toddler is able to increase walking speed as equilibrium reactions mature in standing.

Systems Models of Motor Control

A systems model of motor control is currently used to describe the relationship of various brain and spinal centers working together to control posture and movement. However, because more than one "systems" theory of motor control exists, some of the features that make these approaches different from the traditional top-down hierarchic model are identified. Inherent in any systems theory is the view that motor control is accomplished by the complex interaction of many systems of the body, not just the nervous system. The musculoskeletal system and the cardiopulmonary system as well as the nervous system are involved in motor control. If movement were to be considered a system of the body such as the pulmonary system, posture would be listed as one of the components. Posture should be considered its own system. Depending on the task to be carried out, such as playing the piano or walking, different postures would be required, such as sitting or standing, respectively. Certain activities such as walking can be done only in certain postures. The complex interaction of postural control's component processes is discussed in further detail in the next section.

A second characteristic of systems theories of motor control is that posture and movement are thought to be self-organizing. As the body grows and various body systems mature, the speed of nervous system responses increases, and the changing relationship among the body systems produces different motor responses. The basic functional unit in the systems theories is the movement pattern. Movement emerges from this complex interaction of the changing body's systems. Prior to attaining upright standing, other means of mobility are generated in movement patterns such as rolling or creeping. Erect standing is the body's answer to how to achieve mastery over gravity, and walking is the logical solution to finding an efficient means of mobility.

Feedback is a third fundamental characteristic of systems models of motor control. To control movements, the individual needs to know whether the movement has been successful in the past. In a closed-loop model of motor control, sensory information is used as feedback to the nervous system to provide assistance with the next action. A person engages in closed-loop feedback when playing a video game that requires guiding a figure across the screen. This type of feedback provides self-control of movement. A loop is formed from the sensory information that is generated as part of the movement and is fed back to the brain. This sensory information influences future motor actions. Errors that can be corrected with practice are detected, and performance can be improved. This type of feedback is shown in Figure 3–9.

By contrast, in an open-loop model of motor control, movement is cued either by a central structure, such as a motor program, or by sensory information from the periphery. The movement is performed without feedback. When a baseball pitcher throws a favorite pitch, the movement is too quick to allow feedback. Errors are detected after the fact. An example of action spurred by external sensory information is what happens when a fire alarm sounds. The person hears the alarm and moves before thinking about moving. This type of feedback model is also depicted in Figure 3–9 and is thought to be the way in which fast movements are controlled. Another way to think of the difference between closed-loop and open-loop motor control can be exemplified by someone who learns to play a piano piece. The piece is played slowly while the student is learning and receiving feedback, but once it is learned, the student can sit down and play it through quickly, from beginning to end.

Components of the Postural Control System. In the systems models, both posture and movement are considered systems that represent the interaction of other biologic and mechanical systems and movement components. The relationship between posture and movement is also called postural control. As such, posture implies a readiness to move, an ability not only to react to threats to balance but also to anticipate postural needs to support a motor plan. A motor plan is a plan to move, usually stored in memory. Seven components have been identified as part of a postural control system, as depicted in Figure 3–10. These are limits of stability, environmental adaptation, the musculoskeletal system, predictive central set, motor coordination, eye-head stabilization, and sensory organization. Postural control is a complex process that must be ongoing.

Limits of Stability. Limits of stability are the boundaries of the base of support of any given posture. As long as the center of gravity is within the base of

A CLOSED LOOP

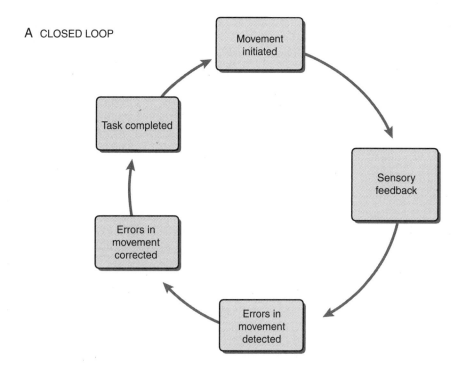

B OPEN LOOP

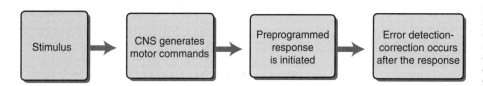

FIGURE 3–9 ▪ *A* and *B,* Models of feedback. (Redrawn from Montgomery, PC, Connolly BH. Motor Control and Physical Therapy: Theoretical Framework and Practical Application. Hixson, TN, Chattanooga Group, Inc, 1991.)

support, the person is stable. An infant's base of support is constantly changing relative to the body's size and amount of contact the body has with the supporting surface. Supine and prone are more stable postures by virtue of having so much of the body in contact with the support surface. However, in sitting or standing, the size of the base of support depends

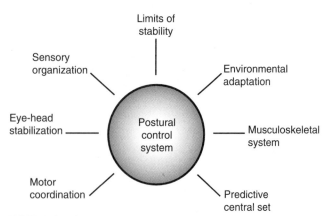

FIGURE 3–10 ▪ Components of normal postural control. (Redrawn from Duncan P [ed]. Balance: Proceedings of the APTA Forum. Alexandria, VA, American Physical Therapy Association, 1990, with permission of the APTA.)

on the position of the lower extremities and on whether the upper extremities are in contact with the supporting surface. In standing, the area in which the person can move within the limits of stability or base of support is called the cone of stability, as shown in Figure 3–11. The central nervous system perceives the body's limits of stability through various sensory cues.

Environmental Adaptation. Our posture adapts to the environment in which the movement takes place in much the same way as we change our stance if riding on a moving bus and have nothing stable to grasp. Infants have to adapt to moving in a gravity-controlled environment after being in utero. The body's sensory systems provide input that allows the generation of a movement pattern that dynamically adapts to current conditions. In the systems model, this movement pattern is not limited to the typical postural reactions.

Musculoskeletal System. The two major systems that contribute most to postural control and therefore to balance are the musculoskeletal and neurologic systems. The musculoskeletal system provides the mechanical structure for any postural response. This response includes postural alignment and musculoskeletal flexibility of all body segments such as the neck,

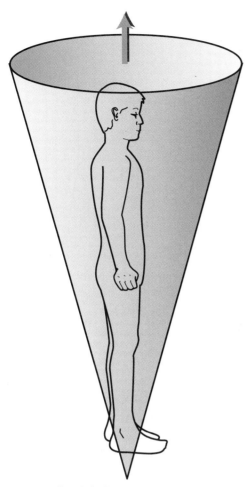

FIGURE 3-11 ■ Cone of stability.

thorax, pelvis, hip, knee, and ankle. The neurologic system processes vital sensory information to choose the correct postural and motor response, to plan for the response, and to execute the response. When both the nervous and muscular systems are functioning optimally, postural responses are appropriate and adequate to maintain balance.

Predictive Central Set. Predictive central set is that component of postural control that can best be described as postural readiness. Sensation and cognition are used as an anticipatory cue prior to movement as a means of establishing a state of postural readiness. This readiness or postural set must be present to support movement. Think of how difficult it is to move in the morning when first waking up; the body is not posturally ready to move. Contrast this state of postural unpreparedness with an Olympic competitor who is so focused on the motor task at hand that every muscle has been put on alert, ready to act at a moment's notice. Predictive central set is critical to postural control. Mature motor control is characterized by the ability of the body, through the postural set, to anticipate what movement is to come, such as when you tense your arm muscles prior to picking up a

heavy weight. Anticipatory preparation is an example of feedforward processing, in which sensory information is sent ahead to prepare for the movement to follow, in contrast to feedback, in which sensation from a movement is sent back to the nervous system for comparison and error detection. Many adult patients with neurologic deficits lack this anticipatory preparation, so postural preparedness is often a beginning point for treatment. Children with neurologic deficits may never have experienced using sensation in this manner.

Motor Coordination. Motor coordination is the ability to sequence muscle responses in a timely fashion to respond to displacements of the center of gravity within the base of support. According to Maki and McIllroy (1996), the process by which the central nervous system generates the patterns of muscle activity required to regulate the relationship between the center of gravity and the base of support is postural control. Postural sway in standing is an example of such motor coordination. Sway strategies have been described by Nashner (1990) in his systems model of postural control.

Eye-Head Stabilization. The visual system must provide accurate information about the surrounding environment during movement and gait. The vestibular system also coordinates with the visual system, so if the head is moving either with or without the body's moving, a stable visual image of the environment continues to be transmitted to the brain. If the head or eyes cannot be stable, movement can be impaired. Clinical examples can be seen in the individual with nystagmus or lack of head control.

Sensory Organization. Sensory organization is the province of the nervous system. Three sensory systems are primarily used for posture and balance and therefore motor control: visual, vestibular, and somatosensory. Vision is critical for the development of balance during the first 3 years of life. Development of head control is impeded in infants with inaccurate visual input. Researchers have also demonstrated how powerful vision is in directing movement by using a visual cliff. A baby will stop creeping across a floor because of the visual illusion that the depth of the surface has changed.

Vestibular input is relayed to the brain by the structures within the middle ear whenever the head moves. The tonic labyrinthine reflex is cued by the labyrinths within the ear that detect the head's relation to gravity. Head lifting behavior in infants is related to maintaining the correct orientation of the head to gravity. Early motor behaviors stimulate vestibular receptors. A close relationship also exists between eye and head movements, to provide a stable visual image even when the body or head is moving. The eyes have to be able to move separately from the head, to dissociate, and to scan the surroundings to assess environmental conditions. In adults, information from the vestibular system can resolve a postural response dilemma when sensory data are conflicting about whether the body is moving.

Somatosensation is the combination of touch and proprioceptive information the body receives from being in contact with the support surface and from joint position. The ability of an individual to use this information for postural responses occurs first in the form of reflexes and then as more sophisticated input from the unconscious movement of weight-bearing joints in contact with the support surface. Not until middle to late childhood is this source of information consistently used for balance.

Nashner's Model of Postural Control

Nashner's (1990) model for the control of standing balance describes three common sway strategies seen in quiet standing: the ankle strategy, the hip strategy, and the stepping strategy. An adult in a standing position sways about the ankles. This strategy depends on having a solid surface in contact with the feet and intact visual, vestibular, and somatosensory systems. If the person sways backward, the anterior tibialis fires to bring the person forward; if the person sways forward, the gastrocnemius fires to bring the person back to midline.

A second sway strategy, called the hip strategy, is usually activated when the base of support is narrower, as when standing crosswise on a balance beam. The ankle strategy is not effective in this situation because the entire foot is not in contact with the support surface. In the hip strategy, muscles are activated in a proximal-to-distal sequence, that is, muscles around the hip are activated to maintain balance before those muscles at the ankles. The last sway strategy is that of stepping. If the speed and strength of the balance disturbance are sufficient, the individual may take a step to prevent loss of balance or a fall. This stepping response is the same as a lower extremity protective reaction. The ankle and the hip strategies are shown in Figure 3–12.

The visual, vestibular, and somatosensory systems previously discussed provide the body with information about movement and cue appropriate postural responses in standing. For the first 3 years of life, the visual system appears to be the dominant sensory system for posture and balance. Vision is used both as feedback as the body moves and as feedforward to anticipate that movement will occur. Children as young as 18 months demonstrate an ankle strategy when quiet standing balance is disturbed (Forssberg and Nashner, 1982). However, the time it takes for them to respond is longer than in adults. Results of studies of 4- to 6-year-old children's responses to disturbances of standing balance were highly variable, al-

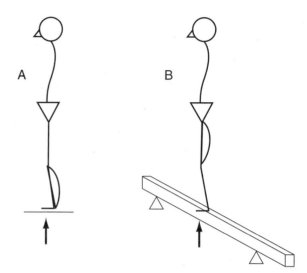

FIGURE 3–12 ■ Sway strategies. *A,* Postural sway about the ankle in quiet standing. *B,* Postural sway about the hip in standing on a balance beam. (Modified from Cech D, Martin S [eds]. Functional Movement Development Across the Life Span. Philadelphia, WB Saunders, 1995.)

most as if balance was worse than in younger children. Sometimes the children demonstrated an ankle strategy, and sometimes they demonstrated a hip strategy (Shumway-Cook and Woollacott, 1985). Not until 7 to 10 years of age were children able to demonstrate consistent ankle strategies as quickly as adults (Shumway-Cook and Woollacott, 1985). This finding is in keeping with the knowledge that the nervous system appears to be mature in its myelination of major tracts by age 10. Adult sway strategies can be expected to be present in 7- to 10-year-old children.

RELATIONSHIP OF MOTOR CONTROL WITH MOTOR DEVELOPMENT

Motor control is the control of posture and movement that supports the initial acquisition of motor abilities and their continual adaptation to the changing physical demands encountered throughout the life span. Without appropriate motor control, motor development would not proceed normally. Children and adults with neuromuscular disorders exhibit abnormal motor control and subsequent abnormal patterns of movement. Whether these abnormal patterns of movement are learned or are the result of factors that hinder (constrain) movement because of existing disease remains to be proven. Constraints can be such things as lack of strength, endurance, and range of motion. Constraints to developmental change are further discussed at the end of the next section on motor learning.

Two views of motor control and their relation to the development of posture and movement have been presented. Although the two views of postural control, the classic hierarchic-maturational view and the action-oriented systems view, may seem to be in conflict, they are not. The infant may initially learn the automatic postural system through maturation and the action system through experience, so both possibilities are available to the mover. We know that the nervous system is organized in many different ways to respond to varying movement demands.

Which model of motor control, hierarchic or systems, best explains changes in posture and movement seen across the life span depends on the age and experience of the mover, the physical demands of the task to be carried out, and the environment in which the task is to be performed. The way in which a 2-year-old child may choose to solve the movement problem of how to reach the cookie jar in the middle of the kitchen table will be different from the solution devised by a 12-year-old child. The younger the child, the more homogenous the movement solutions are. As the infant grows into a child, the movement solutions seem to become more varied, and that, in and of itself, may reflect the self-organizing properties of the systems of the body involved in posture and movement. A comparison of the two models of control is found in Table 3–3.

Posture has a role in movement before, during, and after a movement. Posture should be thought of as preparation for movement. A person would not think of starting to learn to in-line skate from a seated position. The person would first stand with the skates on and try to balance while standing before taking off on the skates. The person's body tries to anticipate the posture that will be needed before the movement. Therefore, with patients who have movement dysfunction, the clinician must prepare them to move before movement is initiated.

When learning to in-line skate, the person continually tries to maintain an upright posture. Postural control maintains alignment while the person moves forward. If the person loses balance and falls, posture is reactive. When falling, an automatic postural response comes from the nervous system, arms are extended in protection. Stunt performers have learned to avoid injury by landing on slightly bent arms, then tucking and rolling. Through the use of prior experience and knowledge of present conditions, the end result is modified and a full-blown protective response is prevented. In many instances, automatic postural responses must be unlearned to learn and perfect fundamental motor skills. Think of a broad jumper who is airborne and moving forward in a crouch position. To prevent falling backward he must keep his arms forward and counteract the natural tendency to reach back.

MOTOR LEARNING

Motor learning is defined as the process that brings about a permanent change in motor performance as a result of practice or experience (Schmidt, 1988). Infants practice many movements during the first year of life to achieve upright locomotion. Part of learning tasks that involve self-movement is to learn the rules of moving. Motor learning occurs when the rules and the tasks are perfected. Early in life, these tasks are the motor milestones, whereas later in life, these tasks involve other motor skills. Task-specific abilities, other than walking, that must be learned in infancy include self-feeding and object play. Fundamental motor patterns such as running, hopping, throwing, and catching are learned in childhood. Many sports-related skills begun in childhood are often carried over into leisure activities. Motor tasks in adolescence and adulthood are primarily related to jobs and leisure. These tasks may require manipulation of a computer keyboard, driving a car, or playing golf.

Motor Learning Time Frame

The process by which a person learns the skills that make up the developmental sequence and learns how to execute and control movement, automatically and voluntarily, is motor learning. Motor learning takes place within a time frame that is somewhere between the two extremes of the milliseconds seen in motor control and the months needed for motor development (see Fig. 3–2). How long it takes to learn a motor task depends on several factors: the difficulty of the task; the amount of practice and feedback received; and the motivation to learn the task. We have all experienced trying to learn something that was un-

Table 3–3 ■ COMPARISON OF HIERARCHIC AND SYSTEMS MODELS OF MOTOR CONTROL

FEATURES	HIERARCHIC MODEL	SYSTEMS MODEL
Basis of control	CNS maturation	Self-organizing systems (MS, CNS, CP)
Type of postural response	Reactive	Steady state and anticipatory
Examples of postural response	Righting, equilibrium, protective reactions	Standing sway strategies, postural readiness

CNS, central nervous system; CP, cardiopulmonary; MS, musculoskeletal.

interesting and not useful as opposed to learning to play a game. Infants are interested in learning to move and work hard to learn to move. They have an innate interest in moving and a need to move that occupies their first year of life.

To understand the time frame for motor learning, one only has to look at how long it takes for the typically developing infant to attain an upright posture and to walk. The entire first year of life is spent learning to move safely against gravity. At no other time in life is so much time devoted to learning one motor skill. Each motor milestone, such as rolling, sitting, and creeping, is practiced and partially perfected as the infant moves from postures in prone and supine, to sitting, and to four point. Once standing and walking are achieved, it seems as though there is no looking back as the child spends the next 5 years learning more complex motor skills such as running, jumping, hopping, and skipping. The child refines upper extremity movements to learn to throw, catch, and strike objects, in addition to mastering cursive writing. These upper extremity skills also require total body control and eye-hand and eye-foot coordination. Motor learning takes place over a span of hours, days, and weeks. The perfection of some skills takes years; ask anyone trying to improve a batting average or a soccer kick. Even though motor development, motor control, and motor learning take place within different time frames, these time frames do not exclude one or the other processes from taking place. In fact, it is possible that because these processes do have different time bases for action, they may be mutually compatible.

Phases of Motor Learning

Three phases of motor learning have been identified by Fitts and Posner (1967). They are the cognitive phase, the associative phase, and the autonomous phase. From the previous discussion of motor control, it may be apparent that these three phases of learning may be linked to different types of motor control. The phases of motor learning are found in Table 3–4.

Cognitive Phase

When a task is completely new to a learner, cognition has to play a major role in learning what the task

entails. The first phase of motor learning can be associated with a closed-loop model of control because sensory input is used by the nervous system to learn about moving and about the desired movement. To learn any new movement, such as driving a car or knitting, the task must be thought about; hence, the phase is called cognitive. Others refer to this as the verbal-cognitive stage because verbal directions are given in the form of instructions to someone old enough to understand them. Remember being taught to ride a bike or swing on a swing; verbal directions were useful regarding the speed to pedal or when to pump the legs. Children with cognitive deficits acquire motor milestones at a slower rate. Patients who have difficulty thinking and processing verbal information, such as after a traumatic brain injury or a cerebrovascular accident, have difficulty in this stage of motor learning. You cannot be thinking about what your name is when trying to learn to transfer. In this stage, a great deal of attention must be devoted to learning a new motor task or relearning a previously known task. The ability to attend may be lacking in a person after a traumatic brain injury or cerebrovascular accident. Consider the look of concentration on an infant's face as she is trying to turn over, reach for an object, or walk for the first time. The slightest distraction can interrupt concentration and may result in an unsuccessful attempt. Consider, too, how much a patient with a neurologic deficit must concentrate to try to relearn a movement that was once performed easily. Mastery of the task is not the goal of this first stage of motor learning. The learner must understand "what to do," so visually guided movements may be helpful during this phase. The goal is to obtain an overall idea or gestalt of what the task is all about, and again, this goal may be difficult in individuals with cognitive deficits.

Associative Phase

The second stage of motor learning is the associative phase. Cognition is still important, but now the person associates aspects of the motor performance of the task with success or failure. Learning takes place with each new trial, and errors are detected and corrected with the next attempt. Sensory feedback is a crucial part of this phase. Schmidt (1991) called this

Table 3–4 ▌ **PHASES OF MOTOR LEARNING**

FEATURES	COGNITIVE	ASSOCIATIVE	AUTONOMOUS
Degree of attention to task	High	Medium	Low
Sensory assistance used for learning	Verbal directions	Proprioception	Very little
	Gestalt of the task	Error detection	
	Visually guided	Error correction	
		Less visual dependence	
Type of feedback	Open loop	Open loop	Closed loop

the motor stage of motor learning. Success comes with practice and the ability of the person to detect errors and to correct them. As small details of the movement task are perfected, speed and efficiency of movement improve. For example, once an infant learns to creep forward on hands and knees, she may appear to be quicker than the adult who is trying to race across the living room before some knickknack can be reached. Further improvement in movement efficiency comes through practice in a variety of settings. This stage of motor learning lasts longer than the first one. Now the learner is concentrating on "how to do" the task. Difficulties may arise in this stage of motor learning when the person has a low frustration tolerance for failure or has problems detecting or correcting errors because of sensory or motor deficits.

Autonomous Phase

The third and last phase of motor learning is the autonomous phase. Once the task is mastered, it can be carried out with little attention to the details. For instance, have you ever driven home and arrived at your destination only to realize that you did not recall what occurred en route because you were thinking of other things? Your driving was autonomous, independent of outside interference. Although this may not be the safest example of an autonomous motor skill, it is relevant because almost everyone has done it. Walking becomes autonomous or automatic; the recital piano piece you endlessly practiced as a child can be played through to completion without your thinking about it. Once you have learned to ride a bike, you do not forget. The autonomous phase is more like an open-loop model of feedback in which the action, once started, is completed without conscious feedback. The learner is not concentrating on "how to succeed." It is possible to make changes in one's performance during this stage, but they come much more slowly because there is less attention to detail. Once the autonomous stage is reached, the performer can direct attention to other higher-order cognitive activities.

Open and Closed Tasks

Movement results when an interaction exists among the mover, the task, and the environment. We have discussed the mover and the environment, but the task to be learned can be classified as either open or closed. Open skills are those done in environments that change over time, such as playing softball, walking on different uneven surfaces, and driving a car. Closed skills are skills that have set parameters and stay the same, such as walking on carpet, holding an object, or reaching for a target. These skills appear to be processed differently. Which type involves more perceptual information? Open skills require the mover to

update constantly and to pay attention to incoming information about the softball, movement of traffic, or the support surface. Would a person have fewer motor problems with open or closed skills? Closed skills with set parameters pose fewer problems. Remember that open and closed skills are different from open-loop and closed-loop processing for motor control or motor learning.

Theories of Motor Learning

Adams' Closed-Loop Theory

The closed-loop theory of motor learning was generated based on computer models in which feedback plays a role in either triggering or modifying an initial movement (Adams, 1971). A closed-loop model of feedback was presented earlier as part of motor control theories. This concept can also affect a mover's ability to learn new movements. Sensory feedback helps us to learn the "feel" of new movements. Intrinsic feedback comes from the feel of the movement; for example, a good shot in tennis feels right. Present performance is compared with an internal reference of correctness, according to Adams. How this internal reference of correctness develops is unclear, but the cerebellum is probably involved. Is the ability of the nervous system to recognize "normal movement" genetically programmed? We do not know. Some children appear to be able to recognize and repeat motor actions only after having them guided by the therapist. Intrinsic and extrinsic feedback plays an important role in motor learning.

The sound of the ball when it hits the "sweet spot" on the racquet is a form of extrinsic feedback. Feedback that comes from the learner is intrinsic. If feedback comes from an external source such as the sound of the ball hitting the racquet, it is extrinsic or external. Seeing where the ball lands—cross court or down the line—and the verbal encouragement of your doubles partner are examples of extrinsic feedback. External feedback is called knowledge of results in motor learning. Adams views knowledge of results as not merely supplying the learner with feedback to reinforce correct performance but also assisting the learner to solve the movement problem. Intrinsic and extrinsic feedback is needed for both motor control and motor learning. Adams' theory provides a good explanation for how slow movements are learned, but it does not explain how fast movements are controlled and learned.

Schmidt's Schema Theory

Schmidt (1975) developed his schema theory to address the limitations of Adams' theory. Once a movement, such as walking, is learned, it is called a motor program and can be called up with little cognitive or cortical involvement. The rules and relationships for a movement are stored in memory. Feedback is not needed when a motor program is performed unless the external or internal conditions pertaining to the movement change. The open-loop theory proposes that muscle commands are preprogrammed and, once triggered, proceed to completion with no sensory interference or feedback, as seen in the closed-loop control model. Open-loop control is helpful when one is performing fast movements in which one may have no time for feedback (see Fig. 3–8B). Most actions after they are learned are combinations of open-loop and closed-loop control.

Schmidt (1988) describes three types of feedback that may occur when a movement takes place. One type of feedback comes from the muscles as they contract during the movement, one type comes from the parts of the body moving in space, and one type comes from the environment in which the movement occurs. All this information is briefly stored when a person moves, along with the knowledge of the results, in the form of a schema. Schemas are used to adjust and evaluate the performance of a motor program. Researchers do not know how these motor programs are formed.

How much knowledge of results is good for optimal learning of a motor task? Unlike in many situations in which more is usually considered better, such is not the case in motor learning. Although continuous feedback may improve present performance, some researchers have found immediate knowledge of results to be detrimental to learning (Shumway-Cook and Woollacott, 1995). When knowledge of results was given on only half the trials, performance was poorer initially but improved later, with findings showing a greater retention of the motor task than would have been expected (Schmidt, 1991). Common sense dictates that as the learner becomes better at the task, feedback should be able to be withdrawn. Such a withdrawal of feedback is called "fading" and has been shown to have a positive effect on learning (Nicholson and Schmidt, 1989).

Effects of Practice

Motor learning theorists have also studied the effects of practice on learning a motor task and whether different types of practice make initial learning easier. Some types of practice make initial learning easier but make transferring that learning to another task more difficult. The more closely the practice environment resembles the actual environment where the task will take place, the better the transfer of learning will be. Therefore, if you are going to teach a person to walk

in the physical therapy gym, this learning may not transfer to walking at home, where the floor is carpeted. Many facilities use an Easy Street (a mock or mini home, work, and community environment) to help simulate actual conditions the patient may encounter at home. Of course, providing therapy in the home is an excellent opportunity for motor learning.

Part-Whole Training

Part-whole training is another facet of the practice issue in motor learning. Should a person practice the entire task, or is it easier to learn if it is broken down into its components? Research has shown that if the parts are truly subunits of the task, then working on them individually does enhance learning of the entire task. However, if the parts are not specific to the task, such as in weight shifting prior to walking, then breaking the task down may not make a difference to the performance of the task as a whole. However, working on weight shifting prior to walking may improve the quality of the task, something that clinicians are also interested in as an end result of therapeutic intervention. Again, it may not be possible for persons who have cognitive difficulties to understand all the steps involved in the task because of memory deficits or an inability to plan or execute movement sequences. In such a case, the entire task may need to be tackled at once.

RELATIONSHIP OF MOTOR LEARNING WITH MOTOR DEVELOPMENT

Motor learning is the functional connection between motor control and motor development. Motor learning is an essential part of motor development. The ability of the body to generate and control movement depends on a genetic blueprint for species-specific movement and on the adaptation of those movements to meet ever-changing demands from the mover and the environment. Infants have not previously moved against gravity even though they have practiced some motor patterns in utero (Milani-Comparetti, 1981). Without the ability to learn how to move against gravity, they would not acquire the ability to walk. Further refinement of bipedal locomotion leads to learning to ride a bike and to skip in childhood. Think of the developmental sequence as a road trip that in its early time course has an established route from point A to point B. During the first year, few side trips or detours are possible; after childhood, different routes are more possible. Most children learn fundamental motor skills such as running, jumping, hopping, skipping, throwing, catching, and striking during childhood. Sports-related skills usually build on these fundamental motor patterns, but in some instances, a child's participation in sports teaches the child these abilities. After childhood, the level of performance of motor skills varies greatly from person to person. Few people are able to perform at the level of an elite athlete.

Constraints to Motor Development, Motor Control, and Motor Learning

Our movements are constrained or limited by the biomechanical properties of our bones, joints, and muscles. No matter how sophisticated the neural message is or how motivated the person is, if the part of the body involved in the movement is limited in strength or range, the movement may occur incorrectly or not at all. If the control directions are misinterpreted, the intended movement may not occur. A person is only as good a mover as the weakest part. For some, that weakest part is a specific system, such as the muscular or nervous system, and for others, it is a function of a system, such as cognition.

Development of motor control and the acquisition of motor abilities occur while both the muscular and skeletal systems are growing and the nervous system is maturing. Changes in all the body's physical systems provide a constant challenge to the development of motor control. Thelen and Fisher (1982) showed that some changes in motor behavior, such as an infant's inability to step reflexively after a certain age, probably occur because the infant's legs become too heavy to move, not because some reflex is no longer exhibited by the nervous system. We have already discussed that the difficulty an infant encounters in learning to control the head during infancy can be attributed to the head's being too big for the body. With growth, the body catches up to the head. As a linked system, the skeleton has to be controlled by the tension in the muscles and the amount of force generated by those muscles. Learning which muscles work well together and in what order is a monumental task.

Adolescence is another time of rapidly changing body relationships. As children become adolescents, movement coordination can be disrupted because of rapid and uneven changes in body dimensions. The most coordinated 10- or 12-year-old can turn into a gawky, gangly, and uncoordinated 14- or 16-year-old. The teenager makes major adjustments in motor control during the adolescent growth spurt.

Age-Related Systems Changes Affecting Motor Control

As the muscular system matures, it becomes stronger and adapts to changes in growth of the skeletal system spurred by weight bearing. The cardiopulmonary system provides the basic energy for musculoskeletal growth, neuromuscular maturation, and muscular work. All systems of the body support movement. Movement responses can be limited by the size and weight of the whole body or the relationship of the size and weight of various parts. An infant may be able to crawl up the stairs in her home before she can walk up them because of the biomechanical limitations of her size relative to the size of the stairs. Typically, the inability of an infant to perform this activity is attributed to a lack of trunk control. Changes seen during motor development are a result of neuromuscular maturation and learning.

The brain does not function in a rigid top-down manner during motor development but instead is flexible in allowing other parts of the nervous system to initiate and direct movement. This concept of flexibility when it is applied to motor control is called distributed control. Control of movement is distributed to the part or parts of the nervous system that can best direct and regulate the motor task. What we do not know is whether the central nervous system works in a top-down manner as it is learning movement and then switches to a more distributed control at some age or level of nervous system maturation. Once movement patterns are learned, the body can then call up a motor program, providing us with yet another perspective on motor control. "A motor program is a memory structure that provides instructions for the control of actions" (VanSant, 1995). These motor programs can be initiated with little conscious effort. The systems of the body involved in movement always seem to be seeking the most efficient way to move and ways that do not require a lot of thought, thus leaving the brain free to do other, more important things such as think.

Relationship of Motor Control with Therapeutic Exercise

Physical therapists evaluate whether a child's development is typical or atypical based on the acquisition of movement. Results of developmental testing are used to plan treatment interventions. The developmental sequence is more closely followed when intervening with infants and children than with adults. Most standardized tests of motor development evaluate a child's performance of certain skills relative to chronologic age. Therefore, age has always been seen as a natural way to gauge a child's progress in acquiring motor skills. Assessing an adult's ability to perform certain skills has always been part of a physical therapy evaluation. Use of standardized functional tools is becoming more prevalent. The physical therapist assistant's view of motor development, motor control, and motor learning influences the choice of approach to therapy with children and adults with neuromuscular problems. Some physical therapists may approach patient care from a number of neurophysiologic perspectives such as proprioceptive neuromuscular facilitation, neurodevelopmental treatment (see Chapters 5 and 11), Rood's approach (see Chapter 4), and Brunnstrom's approach (see Chapter 5). These therapists may or may not incorporate recent knowledge of motor control and motor learning principles into their clinical practice. The foundation of many neurophysiologic approaches has been a top-down hierarchy of motor control, with emphasis on controlling spasticity, inhibiting primitive and tonic reflexes, and facilitating higher-level movements. Many therapists who have used any of the neurophysiologic approaches have begun incorporating more and more ideas from the motor control and motor learning literature into patient treatment plans. The techniques from the neurophysiologic approaches are still valid, but the rationale for their use has been tempered by new knowledge of motor control and learning.

If a hierarchic model is applied therapeutically, treatment will be focused on inhibiting reflexes and facilitating higher-level postural reactions in an effort to gain the highest level or cortical control of movement. Although attainment of postural reactions is beneficial to persons with movement dysfunction, these responses should always be practiced within the context of functional movement. Children with neuromotor problems need to learn these responses, and adults with neurologic deficits need to relearn them.

Many developmental techniques used in treating children with neurologic dysfunction focus only on developing normal protective, righting, and equilibrium reactions. Children need to be safe within any posture that they are placed in or attain on their own. Use of movable equipment, such as a therapy ball, may give the child added sensory cues for movement but should not be the entire focus of treatment. It may not always be necessary to spend the majority of a treatment session eliciting postural responses in a situation (such as on a ball) that the child may never find himself in during normal, everyday life. Movement experiences should be made as close to reality as possible. Using a variety of movement sequences to assist the infant or child to change and maintain postures is of the utmost importance during therapy and at home. Setting up situations in which the child has to try out different moves to solve a movement problem is ideal and sometimes is the best therapy.

Motor control and motor learning theorists recognize that the developing nervous system may function in a top-down manner. They also know that the developed or mature nervous system is probably controlled by many different neuroanatomic centers, with the actual control center determined by the type of task to be accomplished. Early on, an infant's movements seem to be under the control of spinal or supraspinal reflexes such as the crossed extension or asymmetric tonic neck reflex. Once the nervous system matures, the cortex can direct movement, or it can delegate more automatic tasks, such as walking, to subcortical structures. However, when a person is walking and carrying a tray of food in a crowded galley on a rolling ship, the cerebellum, visual system, and somatosensory system all have to work together to convey the person and the contents of the tray safely to a seat. The cortex does not always give up control, but it can engage in distributing the control to other areas of the nervous system. Anytime a familiar task is performed in a new environment, attention must be directed to how the execution of the task has to be changed to accommodate different information.

How a therapy session is designed depends on the type of motor control theory espoused. Theories guide clinicians' thinking about what may be the reason that the patient has a problem moving and about what treatments may remediate the problem. Therapists who embrace a systems approach may have the patient perform a functional task in an appropriate setting, rather than just practice a component of the movement thought to be needed for that task. Rather than having the child practice weight shifting on a ball, the assistant has the child sit on a bench and shift weight to take off a shoe. Therapists who use a systems approach in treatment may be more concerned about the amount of practice and the schedule for when feedback is given than about the degree or normality of tone in the trunk or extremity used for the movement. Using a systems approach, an assistant would keep track of whether the task was accomplished (knowledge of results), as well as how well it was done (knowledge of performance). Knowledge of results is important for learning motor tasks. The goal of every therapeutic approach, regardless of its theoretic basis, is to teach the patient how to produce functional movements in the clinic, at home, and in the community.

Treatment activities must be developmentally appropriate regardless of the age of the person. Although it may not be appropriate to have an 80-year-old creeping on the floor or mat table, it would be an ideal activity for an infant. All of us learn movement skills better within the context of a functional activity. Play provides a perfect functional setting for an infant and child to learn how to move. The physical therapist assistant working with an extremely young child should strive for the most typical movement possible in this age group while realizing that the amount and extent of the neurologic damage incurred will set the boundaries for what movement patterns are possible. Remember that it is also during play that a child learns valuable cause-and-effect lessons when observing how her actions result in moving herself or moving an object. Movement through the environment is an important part of learning spatial concepts.

When one is working with an extremely young child, normal motor development is an appropriate therapeutic goal within the limits of the child's disorder. Progression of therapy can follow the typical developmental sequence, with emphasis on establishing head control, attaining trunk control in rolling, attaining sitting, attaining trunk control in sitting, attaining a hands and knees position, moving on hands and knees, attaining upright standing, and finally, walking. Early in the treatment process, quality of movement should be stressed when one is trying to promote achievement of general developmental milestones. As a child grows older, more and more treatment emphasis should be placed on functional movement, with less emphasis placed on quality. This does not imply that abnormal movement patterns should be encouraged, because they can certainly increase a child's likelihood of developing contractures. It does mean, however, that it is more important for the child to be able to perform an activity and to function within an appropriate environment than to look perfect when doing it. Therapists are just beginning to realize that in all but the mildest neuromuscular problems, motor patterns may not be able to be changed, but motor behaviors can be changed. The child with a specific neuromotor disability may have only certain patterns of movement available to her but may be able to learn to use those patterns to move more effectively and efficiently. An example is a child with cerebral palsy who walks with a bilateral Trendelenburg gait. The gait pattern is abnormal, but it may be efficient. If the focus in therapy is to teach the child to walk without the Trendelenburg gait because it may improve the quality of the gait, but the therapist does not consider or recognize that in doing so the overall gait efficiency decreases, no positive functional change has occurred. If, however, by changing the gait pattern, the efficiency of the task is improved, then a positive functional outcome has occurred, and the treatment was warranted. Judgments about appropriate therapeutic goals cannot and should not always be made solely on the basis of quality of movement.

By stressing normal movement, the therapist encourages normal motor learning. Normal movement is what results when all body systems interact together during the process of overall human development. Motor learning must always occur within the context of function. It would not be an appropriate context for learning about walking to teach a child to walk on a movable surface, for example, because this task is typically performed on a nonmovable surface. The way a task is first learned is usually the way it is remembered best. When stressed or in an unsafe situation, we often revert to this way of moving. For example, I had on many occasions observed the daughter of a friend go up and down the long staircase in her parents' home foot over foot, without using a railing. While I filmed the motor skills of the same child in a studio in which the only stairs available were ones that had no back, she reverted to stepping up with one foot and bringing the other foot up to the same step (marking time) to ascend and descend. She perceived the stairs to be less safe and chose a less risky way to move. Infants and young children should be given every opportunity to learn to move correctly from the start. This is one of the major reasons for intervening early when an infant exhibits motor dysfunction. Motor learning requires practice and feedback. Remember what had to be done to learn to ride a bicycle without training wheels. Many times, through trial and error, you tried to get to the end of the block. After falls and scrapes, you finally mastered the task, and even though you may not have ridden a bike in a while, you still remember how. That memory of the movement is the result of motor learning.

Therapeutic exercise techniques based on older neurophysiologic approaches can be valuable adjuncts to treatment for patients with neurologic dysfunction. However, they must be combined with new knowledge of how to provide feedback, so the person will have the best chance of learning or relearning a motor skill. How much practice is enough to learn a new skill as compared with an already learned skill? The answer is unknown; therefore, the patient continues to practice until no changes occur and a plateau is recognized. Typically developing infants repeat seemingly non–task-oriented movements over and over again before moving on to some new skill. In fact, Thelen's research (1979) suggests that repetitive flexion and extension movements of the extremities and trunk, observed in typically developing infants, appear to be a prerequisite for attaining postural control within a position or as a precursor to moving on to a more demanding posture or developmental task. For example, infants may rock repetitively on their hands and knees prior to moving in the hands and knees position. Once upright posture and movement are attained, less practice may be needed in this position because most complex movements are variations of simpler movements, differing only in timing, sequencing, and force production. An adolescent or young adult may need less practice to learn a motor skill than an older adult. Learning any new skill as an older adult is more difficult but still possible. However, when nervous system disorders impair cognitive function, learning is more difficult. The amount of nervous system recovery possible after nervous system injury plays a large role in determining functional movement outcomes in any person who has a movement impairment.

Assessing functional movement status is a routine part of the physical therapist's evaluation. Functional status may provide cues for planning treatment activities within the context of the functional task to be achieved. Therapeutic outcomes must be documented based on the changing functional abilities of the patient. When the physical therapist reevaluates a patient with movement dysfunction, the physical therapist assistant can participate by gathering objective data about the number of times the person can perform an activity, what types of cues (verbal, tactile, pressure) result in better or worse performance, and whether the task can be successfully performed in more than one setting, such as the physical therapy gym or the patient's dining room. Additionally, the physical therapist assistant may comment on the consistency of the patient's motor behavior. For instance, does the infant roll consistently from prone to supine or roll only occasionally, when something or someone extremely interesting is enticing the infant to engage in the activity?

CHAPTER SUMMARY

Motor control is ever-present. It directs posture and movement. Without motor control, no motor development or motor learning could occur. Motor learning provides a mechanism for the body to attain new skills regardless of the age of the individual. Motor learning requires feedback in the form of sensory information about whether the movement occurred and how successful it was. Practice and experience play major roles in motor learning. Motor development is the age-related process of change in motor behavior. Motor development is also the tasks acquired and learned during the process. A neurologic deficit can affect an individual's ability to engage in age-appropriate motor tasks (motor development), to learn or relearn motor skills (motor learning), or to perform the required movements with sufficient quality and efficiency to be effective (motor control). Purposeful movement requires that all three processes be used continually and contingently across the life span.

REVIEW QUESTIONS

1. Define motor control and motor learning.
2. How does sensation contribute to motor control and motor learning?
3. How can the stages of motor control be used in treatment?
4. How do the components of the postural control system affect balance?
5. How is a postural response determined when visual and somatosensory input conflict?
6. When in the life span can "adult" sway strategies be consistently demonstrated?
7. How much attention to a task is needed in the various phases of motor learning?
8. Give an example of an open task and of a closed task.
9. Which type of feedback loop is used to learn movement? To perform a fast movement?
10. How much and what type of practice are needed for motor learning?

REFERENCES

Adams JA. A closed-loop theory of motor learning. J Motor Behav 3: 110–150, 1971.

Barnes MR, Crutchfield CA, Heriza CB. The Neurophysiological Basis of Patient Treatment, vol 2: Reflexes in Motor Development. Morgantown, WV, Stokesville Publishing Company, 1978.

Cech D, Martin S (eds). Functional Movement Development Across the Life Span. Philadelphia, WB Saunders, 1995.

Fitts PM, Posner MI. Human Performance. Belmont, CA, Brooks/Cole, 1967.

Forssberg H, Nashner L. Ontogenetic development of postural control in man: adaptation to altered support and visual conditions during stance. J Neurosci 2:545–552, 1982.

Maki BE, McIllroy WE. Postural control in the older adult. Clin Geriatr Med 12:635–658, 1996.

Milani-Comparetti A. The neurophysiological and clinical implications of studies on fetal motor behavior. Semin Perinatol 5:183–189, 1981.

Nashner LM. Sensory, neuromuscular and biomechanical contributions to human balance. In Duncan P (ed). Balance: Proceedings of the APTA Forum. Alexandria, VA, American Physical Therapy Association, 1990, pp 5–12.

Nicholson DE, Schmidt RA. Scheduling information feedback: fading, spacing and relative frequency of knowledge of results. In Proceedings of the North American Society for the Psychology of Sport and Physical Activity: June 1–4, 1989. Kent, OH, Kent State University, 1989, p 47.

Schmidt RA. A schema theory of discrete motor skill learning. Psychol Rev 82:225–260, 1975.

Schmidt RA. Motor Control and Learning, 2nd ed. Champaign, IL, Human Kinetics, 1988.

Schmidt RA. Motor learning principles for physical therapy. In Lister M (ed). Contemporary Concepts of Motor Control Problems. Proceedings of the II Step Conference. Alexandria, VA, Foundation for Physical Therapy, 1991, pp 49–63.

Shumway-Cook A, Woollacott M. The growth of stability: postural control from a developmental perspective. J Motor Behav 17:131–147, 1985.

Shumway-Cook A, Woollacott M. Motor Control: Theory and Practical Applications. Baltimore, Williams & Wilkins, 1995.

Stengel TJ, Attermeier SM, Bly L, et al. Evaluation of sensorimotor dysfunction. In Campbell SK (ed). Pediatric Neurologic Physical Therapy. New York, Churchill Livingstone, 1984, pp 13–87.

Sullivan PE, Markos PD, Minor MA. An Integrated Approach to Therapeutic Exercise: Theory and Clinical Application. Reston, VA, Reston Publishing Company, 1982.

Thelen E. Rhythmical stereotypies in infants. Anim Behav 27:699–715, 1979.

Thelen E, Fisher DM. Newborn stepping: an explanation for a "disappearing" reflex. Dev Psychobiol 16:29–46, 1982.

VanSant AF. Motor control and motor learning. In Cech D, Martin S (eds). Functional Movement Development Across the Life Span. Philadelphia, WB Saunders, 1995, pp 47–70.

CHAPTER 4

Motor Development

After reading this chapter, the student will be able to

1. Define the life span concept of development.
2. Understand the relationship of cognition and motivation to motor development.
3. Identify important motor accomplishments of the first 3 years of life.
4. Describe the acquisition and refinement of fundamental movement patterns during childhood.
5. Describe age-related changes in functional movement patterns across the life span.
6. Describe how age-related systems changes affect posture, balance, and gait in older adults.

INTRODUCTION

The Life Span Concept

Normal developmental change is typically presumed to occur in a positive direction; that is, abilities are gained with the passage of time. For the infant and child, aging means being able to do more. The older infant can sit alone, and the older child can run. With increasing age, a teenager can jump higher and throw farther than a school-age child. Developmental change can also occur in a negative direction. Speed and accuracy of movement decline after maturity. When one looks at the ages of the gold medal winners in the last Olympics, it is apparent that motor performance peaks in early adolescence and adulthood. Older adults perform motor activities more slowly and take longer to learn new motor skills. Traditional views of motor development are based on the positive changes that lead to maturity and the negative changes that occur after maturity. This view of development can be visualized as a triangle, as in Figure 4–1. Others have described a leveling off of abilities during adulthood prior to the decline at old age, which can be defined as beginning at 65 years. This view is depicted in Figure 4–2.

A true life span perspective of motor development includes all motor changes occurring as part of the continuous process of life. This continuous process is not a linear one, as depicted in the previous figures, but rather is a circular process. Although the cycle of life is most often represented as a circle (Fig. 4–3) because it is continuous, a circle can represent only two dimensions and does not adequately depict Erikson's view of life as an experience that is folded back on itself (Erikson, 1968). He sees the beginning and end of development as more closely related to each other than they are to the years that come in between. We offer a multidimensional representation of this concept of life's being folded back on itself, not like an accordion folded back on itself, but as a three-dimensional Möbius strip. This folding back places older adulthood closer to infancy rather than farther away. If one takes a strip of paper and merely puts the two ends together to make a circle, the circle will have an inner surface and an outer surface. However, by giving the strip a twist before attaching the ends, one produces something that looks like an infinity sign (∞) (Fig. 4–4). By placing the periods of development along the surface of the strip, one can visualize this new relationship of the periods of development. When one traces along the surface of the strip, it has no break—the design represents one continuous surface,

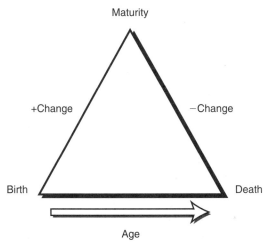

FIGURE 4-1 ■ Graphic depiction of development as a triangle with positive change as the up slope and negative change as the down slope.

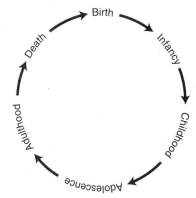

FIGURE 4-3 ■ Life as a circle or life cycle.

just the way one should think about life span development. Continuity occurs from beginning to end. The three-dimensional Möbius strip is more reflective of the finding that movement occurs within three domains—physical, psychologic, and social.

The Five Characteristics of a Life Span Approach

Baltes (1987) recognized five characteristics that identify a theoretic approach as having a life span perspective:

- Development is lifelong.
- Development is multidimensional.
- Development is plastic and flexible.
- Development is contextual.
- Development is embedded in history.

Although motor development meets all these criteria, not all developmental theories exhibit a life span approach. We have stated that motor skills change throughout a person's lifetime, not just during the early years. Movement fosters and supports the devel-

opment of intelligence and social interaction and is therefore multidimensional. Motor skills are flexible and can change in response to cognitive and social requirements. Although early development usually follows a set sequence of skill acquisition, not every child learns to creep before learning to walk. The surroundings in which a person develops can make a difference in how the person develops. Context can refer to the psychologic, social, or physical surroundings. The time in which a person lives and the person's life experiences and those of the family, friends, and teachers influence the person's view of life and may affect the acquisition of motor skills. Cultural and child-rearing practices can also affect the developmental sequence.

Life Span View of Motor Development

The concept of motor development has been broadened to encompass any change in movement abilities that occurs across the span of life, so changes in the way a person moves after childhood are included. Motor development continues to elicit change from conception to death. Think of the classic riddle of the pharaohs: what creeps in the morning and walks on two legs in the afternoon and on three in the evening?

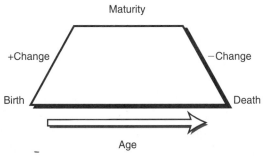

FIGURE 4-2 ■ Graphic depiction of development with a plateau between positive and negative changes.

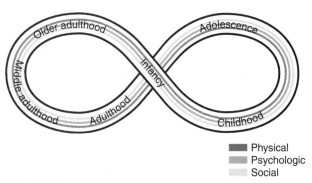

FIGURE 4-4 ■ A three-dimensional view of development including physical, psychologic, and social domains.

The answer is a human in various stages as an infant who creeps, a toddler who walks alone throughout adulthood, and an older adult who walks with a cane at the end of life.

DEVELOPMENTAL TIME PERIODS

Age is the most useful way to measure change in development because it is a universally recognized marker of biologic, psychologic, and social progression. Infants become children, then adolescents, and finally adults at certain ages. Aging is a developmental phenomenon. Stages of cognitive development are associated with age, as are societal expectations regarding the ability of an individual to accept certain roles and functions. Defining these time periods gives everyone a common language when talking about motor development and allows comparison across developmental domains (physical, psychologic, and social). Everyone knows that a 3-year-old child is not an adult, but when does childhood stop and adolescence begin? When does an adult become an older adult? A list of commonly defined time periods that are used throughout the text is found in Table 4–1.

Infancy

Infancy is the first period of development and spans the initial 2 years of life following birth. During this time, the infant establishes trust with caregivers and learns to be autonomous. The world is full of sensory experiences that can be sampled and used to learn about actions and the infant's own movement system. The infant uses sensory information to cue movement and uses movement to explore and learn about the environment. Therefore, home must be baby-proofed from the extremely curious and mobile infant or toddler.

Table 4–1 ▌ DEVELOPMENTAL TIME PERIODS

PERIOD	TIME SPAN
Infancy	Birth to 2 years
Childhood	2 years to 10 years (females)
	2 years to 12 years (males)
Adolescence	10 years to 18 years (females)
	12 years to 20 years (males)
Early adulthood	18 to 20 years to 40 years
Middle adulthood	40 years to 65 years
Older adulthood	65 years to death
Young-old	65 years to 74 years
Middle-old	75 years to 84 years
Old-old	85 years and older

Childhood

Childhood begins at 2 years and continues until adolescence. Childhood fosters initiative to plan and execute movement strategies and to solve daily problems. The child is extremely aware of the surrounding environment, at least one dimension at a time. During this time, she begins to use symbols such as language or uses objects to represent things that can be thought of but are not physically present. The blanket draped over a table becomes a fort, or pillows become chairs for a tea party. Thinking is *preoperational*, with reasoning centered around the self. Self-regulation is learned with help from parents regarding appropriate play behavior and toileting. Self-image begins to be established during this time. By 3 to 5 years of age, the preschooler has mastered many tasks such as sharing, taking turns, and repeating the plot to a story. The school-age child continues to work industriously for recognition on school projects or a special school fund-raising assignment. Now the child is able to classify objects according to certain characteristics, such as roundness, squareness, color, and texture. This furtherance of thinking abilities is called *concrete operations*. The student can experiment with which container holds more water—the tall, thin one or the short, fat one, or which string is longer. Confidence in one's abilities strengthens an already established positive self-image.

Adolescence

Adolescence covers the period right before, during, and after puberty, encompassing different age spans for boys and girls because of the time difference in the onset of puberty. Puberty and, therefore, adolescence begins at age 10 for girls and age 12 for boys. Adolescence is 8 years in length regardless of when it begins. Because of the age difference in the onset of adolescence, girls may exhibit more advanced social emotional behavior than their male counterparts. In a classroom of 13-year-olds, many girls are completing puberty, whereas most boys are just entering it.

Adolescence is a time of change. The identity of the individual is forged, and the values by which the person will live life are embraced. Physical and social-emotional changes abound. The end result of a successful adolescence is the ability to know who one is, where one is going, and how one is going to get there. The pursuit of a career or vocation assists the teenager in moving away from the egocentrism of childhood (Erikson, 1968). Cognitively, the teenager has moved into the *formal operations stage* in which abstract problems can be solved by inductive and deductive reasoning. These cognitive abilities help one to weather the adolescent identity crisis. Practicing logical decision making during this period of life prepares the adolescent for the rigors of adulthood, in which decisions become more and more complex.

Adulthood

Adulthood is achieved by 20 years of age biologically, but psychologically it may be marked by as much as a 5-year transition period from late adolescence (17 years) to early adulthood (22 years). Levinson (1986) called this period the *early adulthood transition* because it takes time for the adolescent to mature into an adult. Research supports the existence of this and other transition periods. Although most of adulthood has been considered one long period of development, some researchers such as Levinson identify age-related stages. *Middle adulthood* begins at 40 years, with a 5-year transition from early adulthood, and it ends with a 5-year transition into *older adulthood* (age 60). Gerontologists, those researchers who study aging, use age 65 as the beginning of *old age* and further divide older adulthood into three periods: *young-old* (65 to 74 years); *middle-old* (75 to 84 years); and *old-old* (85 years and older) (Atchley, 1991).

INFLUENCE OF COGNITION AND MOTIVATION

The three processes—motor development, motor control, and motor learning, which were discussed at length in the last chapter—are influenced to varying degrees by a person's intellectual ability. Impairments in cognitive ability can affect an individual's ability to learn to move. A child with mental retardation may not have the ability to learn movement skills at the same rate as a child of normal intelligence. The rate at which developmental change can be expected to occur is decreased in all domains—physical, psychologic, and social. The acquisition of motor skills is often as delayed as the acquisition of other knowledge.

Motivation to move comes from intellectual curiosity. Typically developing children are innately curious about the movement potential of their bodies. Children move to be involved in some sports-related activities such as tee-ball or soccer. Adolescents often define themselves by their level of performance on the playing field, so a large part of their identity is connected to their athletic prowess. Adults may routinely participate in sports-related activities as part of their leisure time. One hopes that activity is part of a commitment to fitness developed early in life.

Motor control is needed for motor learning, for the execution of motor programs, and for progression through the developmental sequence. The areas of the brain involved in idea formation can be active in triggering movement. Movement is affected by the ability of the mind to understand the rules of moving. Movement is also a way of exerting control over the environment. Remember the old sayings "mind over matter" and "I think I can." Learning to control the environment begins with controlling one's own body. To interact with objects and people within the environment, the child must be oriented within space. We learn spatial relationships by first orienting to our own bodies, then using ourselves as a reference point to map our movements within the environment. Physical educators and coaches have used the ability of the athlete to know where he or she is on the playing field or the court to better anticipate the athlete's own or the ball's movement.

The role of visualizing movement as a way to improve motor performance is documented in the literature (Epstein, 1980; Wang and Morgan, 1992). Sports psychologists have extensively studied cognitive behavioral strategies, including motivation, and recognize how powerful these strategies can be in improving motor performance (Meyers et al, 1996). We have all had experience with trying to learn a motor skill that we were interested in as opposed to one in which we had no interest. Think of the look on an infant's face as she attempts that first step; one little distraction and down she goes. Think also of how hard you may have to concentrate to master in-line skating; would you dare to think of other things while careening down a sidewalk for the first time? Because development takes place in more than one dimension, not just in the motor area, the following psychologic theories, with which you may already be familiar, are used to demonstrate what a life span perspective is and is not. These psychologic theories can also reflect the role movement may play in the development of intelligence, personality, and perception.

Piaget

Piaget (1952) developed a theory of intelligence based on the behavioral responses of his children. He designated the first 2 years of life the *sensorimotor stage of intelligence*. During this stage, the infant learns to understand the world by associating sensory experiences with physical actions. Piaget called these associations *schemas*. The infant develops schemas for looking, eating, and reaching, to name just a few examples. From 2 to 7 years is the *preoperational stage of intelligence*, during which the child is able to represent the world by symbols, such as words for people and objects. The increased use of language is the beginning of symbolic thought. During the next stage, *concrete operations*, logical thought occurs. Between 7 and 11 years of age, children can mentally reverse information. For example, if they learned that 6 plus 4 equals 10, then 4 plus 6 would also equal 10. The last stage is that of *formal operations*, which Piaget thought began at

12 years of age. Although research has not completely supported the specific chronologic years to which Piaget attributed these stages, the stages do occur in this order. Formal operations begins in adolescence, which, according to our time periods, begins at 10 years in girls and at 12 years in boys. Piaget's stages are related to developmental age in Table 4–2.

Piaget studied the development of intelligence up until adolescence, when *abstract thought* becomes possible. Because abstract thought is the highest level of cognition, he did not continue to look at what happened to intelligence after maturity. Because Piaget's theory does not cover the entire life span, his theory does not represent a life span approach to intellectual development. However, he does offer useful information about how an infant can and should interact with the environment during the first 2 years of life. These first two years are critical to the development of intelligence. Regardless of the age of the child, the cognitive level must always be taken into account when one plans therapeutic intervention.

Maslow and Erikson

In contrast, Maslow (1954) and Erikson (1968) looked at the entire spectrum of development from beginning to end. Maslow identified the needs of the individual and how those needs change in relation to a person's social and psychologic development. Rather than describing stages, Maslow developed a hierarchy in which each higher level depends on mastering the one before. The last level mastered is not forgotten or lost but is built on by the next. Maslow stressed that an individual must first meet basic physiologic needs to survive, and then and only then can the individual meet the needs of others. The individual fulfills *physiologic needs, safety needs, needs for loving and belonging, needs for esteem,* and finally *self-actualization.* Maslow's theory is visually depicted in Figure 4–5. A self-actualized person is self-assured, autonomous, and independent; is oriented to solving problems; and is not self-absorbed. Although Maslow's theory may not appear to be embedded in history, it tends to transcend any one particular time in history by being universally applicable.

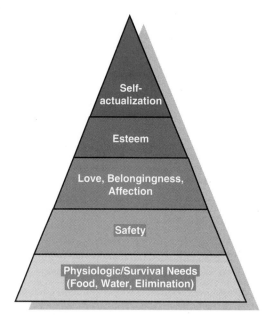

FIGURE 4–5 ❚ Maslow's hierarchy. (From Cech D, Martin S [eds]. Functional Movement Development Across the Life Span. Philadelphia, WB Saunders, 1995.)

Erikson described stages that a person goes through to establish personality. These stages are linked to ages in the person's life, with each stage representing a struggle between two opposing traits. For example, the struggle in infancy is between trust and mistrust. The struggle in adolescence is ego identity. Erikson's theory as shown in Table 4–3 is an excellent example of a life span approach to development.

Table 4–2 ❚ PIAGET'S STAGES OF COGNITIVE DEVELOPMENT

LIFE SPAN PERIOD	STAGE	CHARACTERISTICS
Infancy	Sensorimotor	Pairing of sensory and motor reflexes leads to purposeful activity
Preschool	Preoperational	Unidimensional awareness of environment
		Begins use of symbols
School age	Concrete operational	Solves problems with real objects
		Classification, conservation
Pubescence	Formal operational	Solves abstract problems
		Induction, deduction

Data from Piaget J. Origins of Intelligence. New York, International University Press, 1952.

Table 4–3 ❚ ERIKSON'S EIGHT STAGES OF DEVELOPMENT

LIFE SPAN PERIOD	STAGE	CHARACTERISTICS
Infancy	Trust versus mistrust	Self-trust, attachment
Late infancy	Autonomy versus shame or doubt	Independence, self-control
Childhood (preschool)	Initiative versus guilt	Initiation of own activity
School age	Industry versus inferiority	Working on projects for recognition
Adolescence	Identity versus role confusion	Sense of self: physically, socially, sexually
Early adulthood	Intimacy versus isolation	Relationship with significant other
Middle adulthood	Generativity versus stagnation	Guiding the next generation
Late adulthood	Ego integrity versus despair	Sense of wholeness, vitality, wisdom

Adapted from IDENTITY: Youth and Crisis by Erik H. Erikson. Copyright © 1968 by W. W. Norton & Company, Inc. Used by permission of W. W. Norton & Company, Inc.

Although all three of these psychologists present important information that will be helpful to you when you work with people of different ages, it is beyond the scope of this text to go into further detail. The reader is urged to pursue more information on any of these theorists to add to an understanding of people of different ages and at different stages of psychologic development. A life span perspective can assist in an understanding of motor development by acknowledging and taking into consideration the level of intellectual development the person has attained or is likely to attain.

DEVELOPMENTAL CONCEPTS

Many concepts apply to human motor development, but we are going to present only a few of the more widely recognized ones here. These are not laws of development but merely guiding thoughts about how to organize information on motor development. Those to be explored include concepts related to the direction of change in the pattern of skill acquisition and concepts related to the type of movement displayed during different stages of development. The one overriding concept about which all developmentalists agree is the concept that development is *sequential* (Gesell et al, 1974). The developmental sequence is recognized by most developmental authorities. Areas of disagreement involve the composition of the sequence. Which specific skills are always part of the sequence is debated, and whether one skill in the sequence is a prerequisite for the next skill in the sequence has been questioned.

Epigenesis

Motor development is *epigenetic. Epigenesis* is a theory of development that states that a human being grows and develops from a simple organism to a more complex one through progressive differentiation. An example from the plant world is the description of how a simple, round seed becomes a beautiful marigold. Motor development occurs in an orderly sequence, based on what has come before; not like a tower of blocks, built one on top of the other, but like a pyramid, with a foundation on which the next layer overlaps the preceding one. This pyramid allows for growth and change to occur in more than one direction at the same time (Fig. 4–6). The developmental sequence is generally recognized to consist of the orderly development of head control, rolling, sitting, creeping, and walking. This sequence is known as the *gross-motor milestones*. The rate of change in acquiring each skill may vary from child to child within a family, among families, and among families of different cultures. Se-

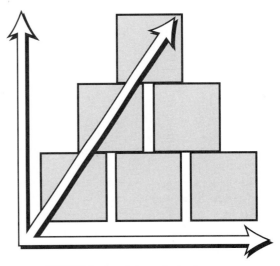

FIGURE 4–6 ■ Epigenetic development.

quences may overlap as the child works on several levels of skills at the same time. For example, a child can be perfecting rolling while learning to balance in sitting. The lower-level skill does not need to be perfect before the child goes on to try something new. Some children even bypass a stage such as creeping and go on to another higher-level skill such as walking without doing themselves any harm developmentally (Long and Cintas, 1995).

Directional Concepts of Development

Development tends to proceed from cephalic to caudal, proximal to distal, mass to specific, and gross to fine.

Cephalic to Caudal

The concept of *cephalocaudal* development relates to the finding that head control is developed before control of the trunk and that, in general, upper extremity usage is mastered before skillful use of the lower extremities. However, this concept does not imply that head movements are perfected before body or trunk movements, because the infant develops as a linked structure, so when one part moves, other parts are affected by that movement. Cephalocaudal development is seen in the postnatal development of posture. Head control in infants begins with neck movements and is followed by development of trunk control. Postnatal postural development mirrors what happens in the embryo when the primitive spinal cord closes. Closure occurs first in the cervical area and then progresses in two directions at once, toward the head and the tail of the embryo (Martin, 1989). The infant develops head and neck and then trunk control. Overlap exists between the development of head and trunk control: think of a spiral beginning around the mouth and spreading outward in all directions encompassing more and more of the body (Fig. 4–7).

Proximal to Distal

The second directional concept is that development occurs from *proximal to distal* in reference to the midline of the body. Because the body is a linked structure, the axis or midline of the body must provide a stable base for head, eye, and extremity movements to occur with any degree of control. The trunk is the stable base for head movement above and for limb movement distally. Imagine what would happen if you could not maintain an erect sitting posture without the use of your arms and you tried to use your arms to catch a ball thrown to you. You would have to use your arms for support, and if you tried to catch the ball, you would probably fall. Or imagine not being able to hold your head up. What chance would you have of being able to follow a moving object with your eyes? Early in development, the infant works to establish midline neck control by lifting the head from the prone position, then establishes midline trunk control by extending the spine against gravity, followed by establishing proximal shoulder and pelvic girdle stability through weight bearing. In some positions, the infant uses the external environment to support the head and trunk to move the arms and legs. Reaching with the upper extremities is possible early in development but only with external trunk support, as when placed in an infant seat in which the trunk is supported. Once again, the infant first controls the midline of the neck, then the trunk, followed by the shoulders and pelvis before she controls the arms, legs, hands, and feet.

Mass to Specific

The third directional concept to be presented here is that development proceeds from *mass movements to specific movements* or from simple movements to complex movements. This concept can be interpreted in several different ways. *Mass* can refer to the whole body, and *specific* can refer to smaller parts of the body. For example, when an infant moves, the entire body moves; movement is not isolated to a specific body part. Infant movement is characterized by the mass movements of the trunk and limbs. The infant learns to move the body as one unit, as in log rolling, before she is able to move separate parts. The ability to separate movement in one body part from movement in another body part is called *dissociation.* Mature movements are characterized by *dissociation,* and typical motor development provides many examples. When an infant learns to turn her head in all directions without trunk movement, the head can be said to be dissociated from the trunk. Reaching with one arm from a prone on elbows position is an example of limb dissociation from the trunk. While the infant creeps on hands and knees, her limb movements are dissociated from trunk movement. Additionally, when the upper trunk rotates in one direction and the lower trunk rotates in the opposite direction during creeping (counterrotation), the upper trunk is dissociated from the lower trunk and vice versa.

Gross to Fine

This last directional concept involves the direction of overall change in movement skill acquisition, which is from *gross,* large muscle movement to *fine,* more discrete movement. Although this concept is similar to the previous one of mass movements' coming before specific movements, it has relevance for the differentiation between gross-motor and fine-motor developmental sequences. Arm and leg thrusts occur in play before the infant reaches with a single limb. Mass grasp is possible before individual finger movements. Remember that the infant learns to move and respond on many levels at the same time. Not all gross-motor skills come before fine-motor skills.

Reciprocal Interweaving

Periods of stability and instability of motor patterns have been observed by many developmentalists. Gesell

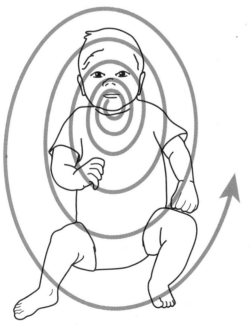

FIGURE 4–7 ■ Infant and spiral.

and colleagues (1974) presented the concept of reciprocal interweaving to describe the cyclic changes they observed in the motor control of children over the course of early development. Periods of equilibrium were balanced by periods of disequilibrium. Head control, which appears to be fairly good at one age, may seem to lessen at an older age, only to recover as the infant develops further. At each stage of development, abilities emerge, merge, regress, or are replaced. During periods of disequilibrium, movement patterns regress to what was present at an earlier time, but after a while, new patterns emerge with newfound control. At other times, motor abilities learned in one context, such as control of the head in the prone position, may need to be relearned when the postural context is changed, for example, when the child is placed in sitting. Some patterns of movement appear at different periods depending on need. The reappearance of certain patterns of movement at different times during development can also be referred to as *reciprocal interweaving.* One of the better examples of this reappearance of a pattern of movement is seen with the use of scapular adduction. Initially, this pattern of movement is used by the infant to reinforce upper trunk extension in the prone position. Later in development, the toddler uses the pattern again to maintain upper trunk extension as she begins to walk. This use in walking is described as a high guard position of the arms.

Kinesiologic Concepts

Physiologic Flexion to Antigravity Extension to Antigravity Flexion

The next concepts to be discussed are related to changes in the types of movement displayed during different stages of development. Some movements are easier to perform at certain times during development. Factors affecting movement include the biomechanics of the situation, muscle strength, and the level of neuromuscular maturation and control. Full-term babies are born with predominant flexor muscle tone *(physiologic flexion).* The limbs and trunk naturally assume a flexed position (Fig. 4–8). If you try to straighten or uncoil any extremity, it will return to its original position easily. It is only with the influence of gravity, the infant's body weight, and probably some of the early reflexes that the infant begins to extend and lose the predisposition toward flexion. As development progresses, active movement toward extension occurs. This is an example of the concept of flexion moving toward extension. *Antigravity extension* is easiest to achieve early on because the extensors are in lengthened position from the effect of the newborn's physio-

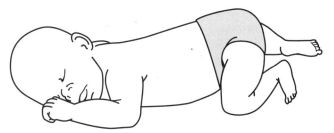

FIGURE 4–8 ■ Physiologic flexion in a newborn.

logic flexed posture. The extensors are ready to begin functioning before the shortened flexors. The infant progresses from being curled up in a fetal position, dominated by gravity, to exhibiting the ability to extend against gravity actively. *Antigravity flexion* is exhibited from the supine position and occurs later than antigravity extension.

Kinesiologic Types of Movements

Bly (1983) described the developmental process as a trend from random movements of the entire body to asymmetric movements to bilateral symmetric movements of the head and trunk against gravity in the prone, supine, and side lying positions. Next she described alternating reciprocal movements of the limbs followed by unilateral symmetric movements of the head and trunk that result in lateral bending, with the final accomplishment of bilateral diagonal movements as in trunk rotation or limb action in creeping or walking. Once antigravity control of the head and trunk is accomplished, lateral trunk flexion and rotation can occur. Lateral flexion of the head and trunk is possible only if the extensor and flexor muscles of the head and trunk are equally strong and balanced. If either muscle group is stronger, pure lateral flexion will not be possible. Voluntary lateral trunk flexion is present developmentally before voluntary trunk rotation. The entire progression of change in movement patterns for the head and trunk is from physiologic flexion to antigravity extension to antigravity flexion to lateral flexion and, finally, to rotation. Movement patterns of the extremities change from flexion and adduction to extension and abduction.

DEVELOPMENTAL PROCESSES

Motor development is a result of three processes—growth, maturation, and adaptation.

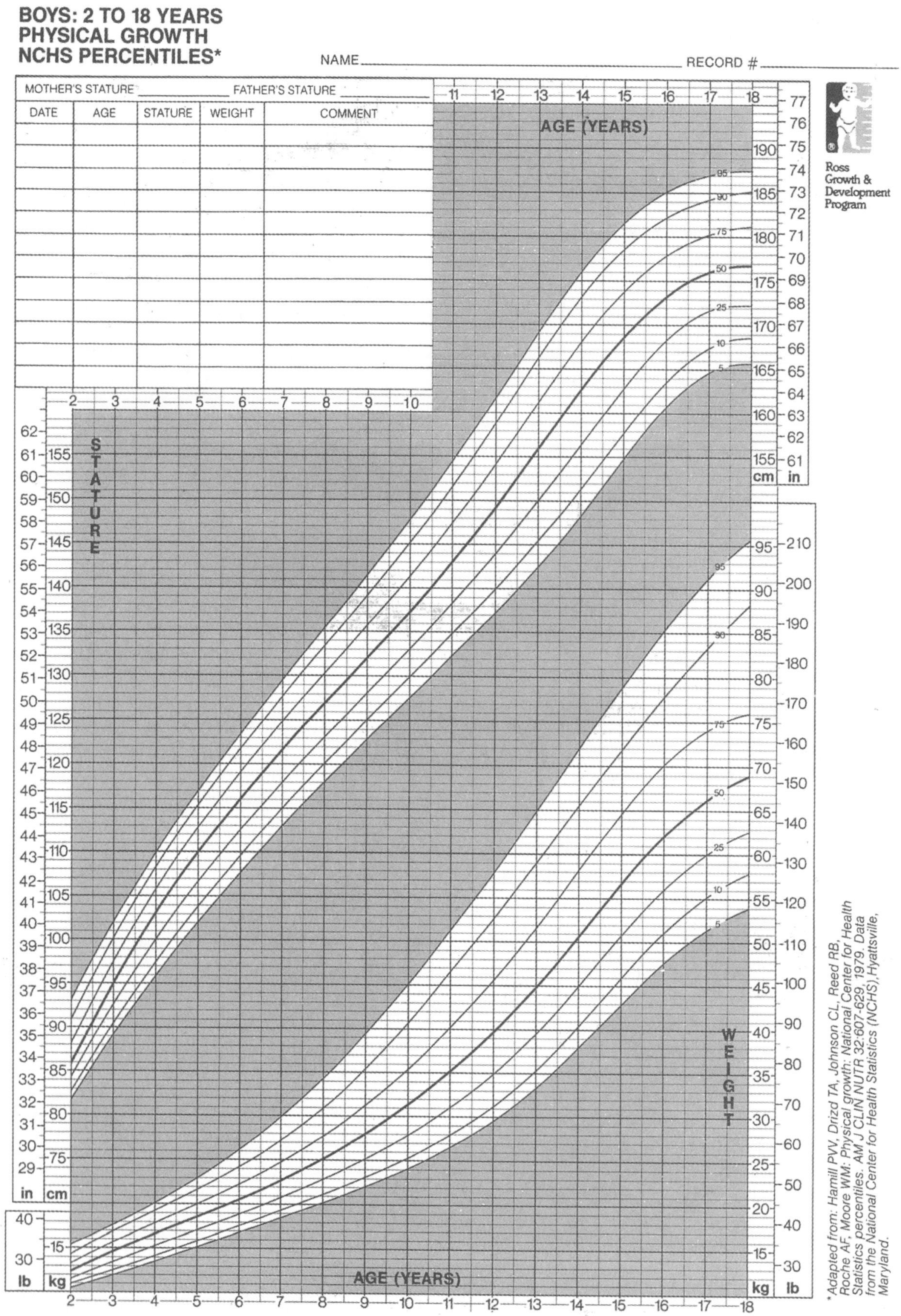

**BOYS: 2 TO 18 YEARS
PHYSICAL GROWTH
NCHS PERCENTILES***

NAME_____ RECORD #_____

FIGURE 4–9 ■ Growth chart. (Used with permission of Ross Products Division, Abbott Laboratories Inc., Columbus, OH 43216. From NCHS Growth Charts ©1982, Ross Products Division, Abbott Laboratories Inc.)

Growth

Growth is any increase in dimension or proportion. Examples of ways that growth is typically measured include size, height, weight, and head circumference. Infants' and children's growth is routinely tracked at the pediatrician's office by use of growth charts (Fig. 4–9). Growth is an important parameter of change during development because some changes in motor performance can be linked to changes in body size. Typically, the taller a child grows, the farther she can throw a ball. Strength gains with age have been linked to increases in a child's height and weight (Malina and Bouchard, 1991). Failure to grow or discrepancies between two growth measures can be an early indicator of a developmental problem.

Maturation

Maturation is the result of physical changes that are due to preprogrammed internal body processes. Maturational changes are those that are genetically guided, such as myelination of nerve fibers, the appearance of primary and secondary bone growth centers (ossification centers), increasing complexity of internal organs, and the appearance of secondary sexual characteristics. Some growth changes, such as those that occur at the ends of long bones *(epiphyses),* occur as a result of maturation; when the bone growth centers, which are under genetic control, are active, length increases. After these centers close, growth is stopped, and no more change in length is possible.

Adaptation

Adaptation is the process by which environmental influences guide growth and development. Adaptation occurs when physical changes are the result of external stimulation. An infant adapts to being exposed to a contagion such as chickenpox by developing antibodies. The skeleton is remodeled during development in response to weight bearing and the muscular forces *(Wolfe's law)* exerted on it during functional activities. As muscles pull on bone, the skeleton adapts to maintain the appropriate musculotendinous relationships with the bony skeleton for efficient movement. This same adaptability can cause skeletal problems if musculotendinous forces are abnormal (unbalanced) or misaligned and may thus produce a deformity.

GROSS- AND FINE-MOTOR MILESTONES

The motor milestones and the ages at which these skills can be expected to occur can be found in Tables

Table 4–4 ▌ GROSS-MOTOR MILESTONES

MILESTONE	AGE
Head control	4 months
Rolling	6 to 8 months
Sitting	8 months
Creeping	9 months
Cruising	10 months
Walking	12 months

4–4 and 4–5. Remember the wide variation in time frames during which milestones are normally achieved. *Gross motor* refers to large muscle movements, and *fine motor* refers to small muscle movements.

Gross-Motor Milestones

Head Control

An infant should exhibit good head control by 4 months of age. The infant should be able to keep the head in line with the body (ear in line with the acromion) when he or she is pulled to sit from the supine position (Fig. 4–10). When the infant is held upright in a vertical position and is tilted in any direction, the head should tilt in the opposite direction. A 4-month-old infant, when placed in a prone position, should be able to lift the head up against gravity past 45 degrees (Fig. 4–11). The infant acquires an additional component of antigravity head control, the ability to flex the head from supine position, at 5 months.

Segmental Rolling

Rolling is the next milestone. Infants log roll (at 4 to 6 months) before they are able to demonstrate segmental rotation (at 6 to 8 months). When log rolling, the head and trunk move as one unit without any trunk rotation. Segmental rolling or rolling with separate upper and lower trunk rotation should be accomplished by 6 to 8 months of age. Rolling from prone to supine precedes rolling from supine to prone because extensor control precedes flexor control. The prone position provides some mechanical advantage

Table 4–5 ▌ FINE-MOTOR MILESTONES

MILESTONE	AGE
Palmar grasp reflex	Birth
Raking	5 months
Voluntary palmar grasp	6 months
Radial palmar grasp	7 months
Radial digital grasp	9 months
Inferior pincer grasp	9 to 12 months
Superior pincer grasp	12 months
Three-jaw chuck	12 months

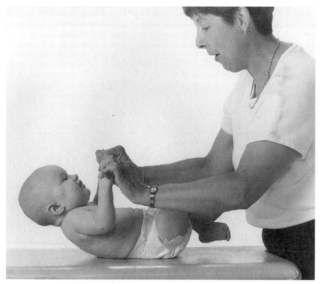

FIGURE 4–10 ■ Head in line with the body when pulled to sit.

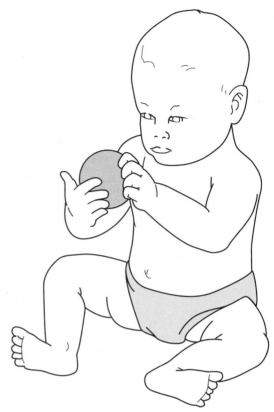

FIGURE 4–12 ■ Sitting independently.

because the infant's arms are under the body and can push against the support surface. If the head, the heaviest part of the infant, moves laterally, gravity will assist in bringing it toward the support surface and will cause a change of position.

Sitting

This next milestone represents a change in functional orientation for the infant. Independent sitting is typically achieved by 8 months of age (Fig. 4–12). *Sitting independently* is defined as sitting alone when placed. The back should be straight, without any kyphosis. No hand support is needed when an infant sits independently. The infant does not have to assume a sitting position but does have to exhibit trunk rotation

while in the position. The ability to turn the head and trunk is important for interacting with the environment and for dynamic balance.

Cruising and Creeping

By 9 months of age, most infants are pulling up to stand and are cruising around furniture. *Cruising* is walking sideways while being supported by hands or tummy on a surface (Fig. 4–13). The coffee table and couch are perfect for this activity because they are usually the correct height to provide sufficient support to the infant. At the same time or within a month (by 10 months), infants begin to reciprocally creep forward on their hands and knees (Fig. 4–14). *Reciprocal* means that the opposite arm and leg move together and leave the other opposite pair of limbs to support the weight of the body.

Walking

The last major gross motor milestone is walking (Fig. 4–15). The new walker assumes a wide base of support, with legs abducted and externally rotated; exhibits lumbar lordosis; and holds the arms in high guard with scapular adduction. The traditional age range for this skill has been 12 to 18 months; however, an infant as young as 7 months may demonstrate this ability. As with any guidelines, these milestones are

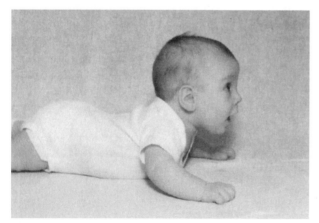

FIGURE 4–11 ■ Head lifting in prone. A 4-month-old infant lifts and maintains head past 45 degrees in prone. (From Wong DL. Whaley and Wong's Essentials of Pediatric Nursing, 5th ed. St. Louis, CV Mosby, 1997.)

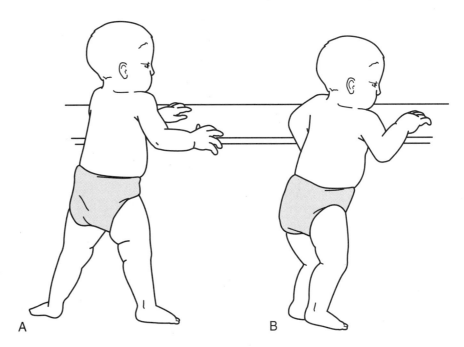

FIGURE 4-13 ■ *A* and *B*, Cruising around furniture.

suggested times. The most important milestones are probably head control and sitting because if an infant is unable to achieve control of the head and trunk, control of extremity movements will be difficult if not impossible. It is acceptable for a child to be ahead of typical developmental guidelines; however, delays in achieving these milestones are cause for concern.

Fine-Motor Milestones

Fine-motor milestones of development, as presented here, give the ages that major changes occur in the

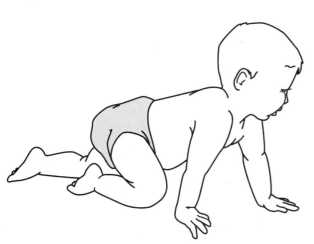

FIGURE 4-14 ■ Reciprocal creeping.

development of prehension. These are listed in Table 4–5. *Prehension* is the act of grasping. To prehend or grasp an object, one must reach for it. Reaching patterns depend on the position of the shoulder. Reaching patterns influence the ability of the hand to grasp objects. Take a moment to try the following reaching pattern. Elevate your scapula and internally rotate your shoulder before reaching for the pencil on your desk. Do not compensate with forearm supination, but allow your forearm to move naturally into pronation. Although it is possible for you to obtain the pencil using this reaching pattern, it would be much easier to reach with the scapula depressed and the shoulder externally rotated.

Hand Regard

The infant first recognizes the hands at 2 months of age, when they enter the field of vision (Fig. 4–16). The asymmetric tonic neck reflex, triggered by head turning, allows the arm on the face side of the infant to extend and therefore is in a perfect place to be seen or regarded. Because of the predominance of physiologic flexor tone in the newborn, the hands are initially loosely fisted.

Reflexive and Palmar Grasp

The first type of grasp seen in the infant is *reflexive,* meaning that it happens in response to a stimulus, in this case, touch. In a newborn, touch to the palm of the hand once it opens, especially on the ulnar side, produces a reflexive palmar grasp. Reflexive grasp is

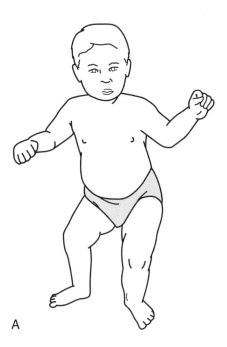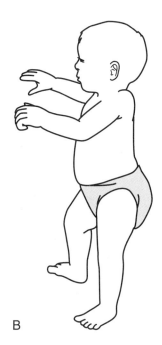

FIGURE 4–15 ▪ *A* and *B*, Early walking: wide stance, pronated feet, arms in high guard, "potbelly," and lordotic back.

replaced by a voluntary palmar grasp by 6 months of age. The infant is no longer compelled by the touch of an object to grasp but may grasp voluntarily. *Palmar grasp* involves just the fingers coming into the palm of the hand; the thumb does not participate.

Evolution of Voluntary Grasp

Once grasp is voluntary at 6 months, a progressive change occurs in the form of the grasp. At 7 months, the thumb begins to adduct, and this allows for a radial palmar grasp. The radial side of the hand is used along with the thumb to pick up small objects such as 1-inch cubes. Radial palmar grasp is replaced by radial digital grasp as the thumbs begin to oppose (Figs. 4–17 and 4–18). Objects can then be grasped by the ends of the fingers, rather than having to be brought into the palm of the hand. The next two types of grasp involve the thumb and index finger only and are called *pincer grasps*. In the inferior pincer grasp, the thumb is on the lateral side of the index finger, as if you were to pinch someone (Fig. 4–19). In the superior pincer grasp, the thumb and index finger are tip to tip, as in picking up a raisin or a piece of lint (Fig. 4–20). An inferior pincer grasp is seen between 9 and 12 months of age, and a superior pincer grasp is evident by 1 year. Another type of grasp that may be seen in a 1-year-old infant is called a *three-jaw chuck grasp* (Fig. 4–21). The wrist is extended, and the middle and index fingers and the thumb are used to grasp blocks and containers.

Release

As voluntary control of the wrist, finger, and thumb extensors develops, the infant is able to demonstrate

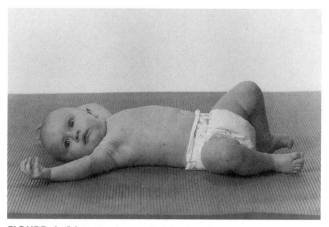

FIGURE 4–16 ▪ Hand regard aided by an asymmetric tonic neck reflex.

FIGURE 4–17 ▪ Age 7 months: radial palmar grasp (thumb adduction begins); mouthing of objects. (From Cech D, Martin S [eds]. Functional Movement Development Across the Life Span. Philadelphia, WB Saunders, 1995.)

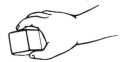

FIGURE 4–18 ■ Age 9 months: radial digital grasp (beginning opposition). (From Cech D, Martin S [eds]. Functional Movement Development Across the Life Span. Philadelphia, WB Saunders, 1995.)

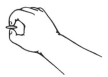

FIGURE 4–20 ■ Age 1 year: superior pincer grasp (tip to tip). (From Cech D, Martin S [eds]. Functional Movement Development Across the Life Span. Philadelphia, WB Saunders, 1995.)

the ability to release a grasped object (Duff, 1995). Transferring objects from hand to hand is possible at 5 to 6 months because one hand can be stabilized by the other. True voluntary release is seen around 7 to 9 months and is usually assisted by the infant's being externally stabilized by another person's hand or by the tray of a highchair. Mature control is exhibited by the infant's being able to release an object into a container without any external support (12 months) or by putting a pellet into a bottle (15 months) (Boehme, 1988; Erhardt, 1982). Release continues to be refined and accuracy improved with ball throwing in childhood (Cliff, 1979).

TYPICAL MOTOR DEVELOPMENT

The important stages of motor development in the first year of life are those associated with even months 4, 6, 8, 10, and 12 (Table 4–6). Typical motor behavior of a 4-month-old infant is characterized by head control, support on arms and hands, and midline orientation. Symmetric extension and abduction of the limbs against gravity and the ability to extend the trunk against gravity characterize the 6-month-old infant. An 8-month-old infant demonstrates controlled rotation around the long axis of the trunk that allows segmental rolling, counterrotation of the trunk in crawling, and creeping. The 8-month-old sits alone. A 10-month-old balances in standing, and a 12-month-old walks independently. Although the even months are important because they mark the attainment of these skills, the other months are crucial because they prepare the infant for the achievement of the control necessary to attain these milestones.

Infant

Birth to Three Months

Newborns assume a flexed posture regardless of their position because physiologic flexor tone dominates at birth. Initially, the newborn is unable to lift the head from a prone position. The newborn's legs are flexed under the pelvis and prevent contact of the pelvis with the supporting surface. If you put yourself into that position and try to lift your head, even as an adult, you will immediately recognize that the biomechanics of the situation are against you. With your hips in the air, your weight is shifted forward, thus making it more difficult to lift your head even though you have more muscular strength and control than a newborn. Although you are strong enough to overcome this mechanical disadvantage, the infant is not. The infant must wait for gravity to help lower the pelvis to the support surface and for the neck muscles to strengthen to be able to lift the head when in the prone position. The infant will be able to lift the head first unilaterally (Fig. 4–22), then bilaterally.

Over the next several months, neck and spinal extension develop and allow the infant to lift the head to one side, to lift and turn the head, and then to lift and hold the head in the midline. As the pelvis lowers to the support surface, neck and trunk extensors become stronger. Extension proceeds from the neck down the back in a cephalocaudal direction, so the infant is able to raise the head up higher and higher in the prone position. By 3 months of age, the infant can lift the head to 45 degrees from the supporting surface. Spinal extension also allows the infant to bring the arms from under the body into a position to

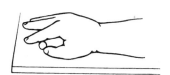

FIGURE 4–19 ■ Age 9 to 12 months: inferior pincer grasp (isolated index pointing). (From Cech D, Martin S [eds]. Functional Movement Development Across the Life Span. Philadelphia, WB Saunders, 1995.)

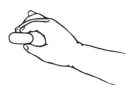

FIGURE 4–21 ■ Age 1 year: three-jaw chuck grasp (wrist extended with ulnar deviation); maturing release. (From Cech D, Martin S [eds]. Functional Movement Development Across the Life Span. Philadelphia, WB Saunders, 1995.)

Table 4–6 ▌ IMPORTANT STAGES OF DEVELOPMENT

AGE	STAGE
1–2 months	Internal body processes stabilize
	Basic biologic rhythms are established
	Spontaneous grasp and release are established
3–4 months	Forearm support develops
	Head control is established
	Midline orientation is present
4–5 months	Antigravity control of extensors and flexors begins
	Bottom lifting is present
6 months	Strong extension-abduction of limbs is present
	Complete trunk extension is present
	Pivots on tummy
7–8 months	Spontaneous trunk rotation begins
	Trunk control develops along with sitting balance
9–10 months	Movement progression is seen in crawling, creeping, creeping, pulling to stand, and cruising
11–12 months	Independent ambulation occurs
16–17 months	Carries or pulls an object while walking
	Walks sideways and backward
20–22 months	Easily squats and recovers toy
24 months	Arm swing is present during ambulation

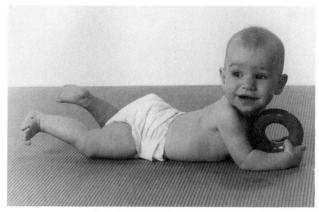

FIGURE 4–23 ■ Prone on elbows.

support himself on the forearms (Fig. 4–23). This position also makes it easier to extend the trunk. Weight bearing through the arms and shoulders provides greater sensory awareness to those structures and allows the infant to view the hands while in a prone position.

When in the supine position, the infant exhibits random arm and leg movements. The limbs remain flexed, and they never extend completely. In supine, the head is kept to one side or the other because the neck muscles are not yet strong enough to maintain a midline position. If you wish to make eye contact, approach the infant from the side because asymmetry is present. An asymmetric tonic neck reflex may be seen when the baby turns the head to one side (Fig. 4–24). The arm on the side to which the head is turned may extend and may allow the infant to see the hand while the other arm, closer to the skull, is flexed. This "fencing" position does not dominate the infant's posture, but it may provide the beginning of the functional connection between the eyes and the hand that is necessary for visually guided reaching. Initially the baby's hands are normally fisted, but in

the first month they open. By 2 to 3 months, eyes and hands are sufficiently linked to allow for reaching, grasping, and shaking a rattle. As the eyes begin to track ever-widening distances, the infant will watch the hands explore the body.

When an infant is pulled to sit from a supine position before the age of 4 months, the head lags behind the body. Postural control of the head has not been established. The baby lacks sufficient strength in the neck muscles to overcome the force of gravity. Primitive rolling may be seen as the infant turns the head strongly to one side. The body may rotate as a unit in the same direction as the head moves. The baby can turn to the side or may turn all the way over from supine to prone or from prone to supine (Fig. 4–25). This turning as a unit is the result of a primitive neck righting reflex. A complete discussion of reflexes and reactions is presented following this section. In this stage of primitive rolling, separation of upper and lower trunk segments around the long axis of the body is missing.

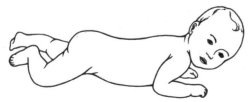

FIGURE 4–22 ■ Unilateral head lifting in a newborn. (From Cech D, Martin S [eds]. Functional Movement Development Across the Life Span. Philadelphia, WB Saunders, 1995.)

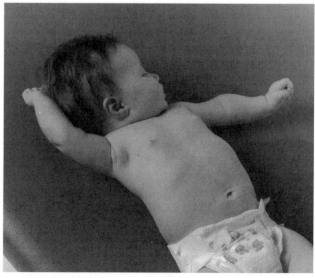

FIGURE 4–24 ■ Asymmetric tonic neck reflex in an infant.

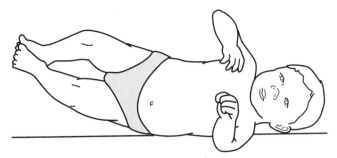

FIGURE 4–25 ■ Primitive rolling without rotation.

Four Months

Four months is a critical time in motor development because posture and movement change from asymmetric to more symmetric. The infant is now able to lift the head in midline past 90 degrees in the prone position. When the infant is pulled to sit from a supine position, the head is in line with the body. Midline orientation of the head is present when the infant is at rest in the supine position (Fig. 4–26). The infant is able to bring her hands together in the midline and to watch them. In fact, the first time the baby gets both hands to the midline and realizes that her hands, to this point only viewed wiggling in the periphery, are part of her body, a real "aha" occurs. Initially, this discovery may result in hours of midline hand play. The infant can now bring objects to the mouth with both hands. Bimanual hand play is seen in all possible developmental positions. The hallmark motor behaviors of the 4-month-old infant are head control and midline orientation.

Head control in the 4-month-old infant is characterized by being able to lift the head past 90 degrees in the prone position, to keep the head in line with the body when the infant is pulled to sit, and to maintain the head in midline with the trunk when the infant is held upright in the vertical position (see Fig. 4–10) and is tilted in any direction (Fig. 4–27). Midline orientation refers to the infant's ability to bring the limbs to the midline of the body, as well as to maintain a symmetric posture regardless of position. When held in supported sitting, the infant attempts to assist in trunk control. The positions in which the infant can independently move are still limited to supine and prone at this age. Lower extremity movements begin to produce pelvic movements. Pelvic mobility begins in the supine position when, from a hooklying position, the infant produces anterior pelvic tilts by pushing on her legs and increasing hip extension, as in bridging (Bly, 1983). Active hip flexion in supine produces posterior tilting. Random pushing of the lower extremities against the support surface provides further practice of pelvic mobility that will be used later in development, especially in gait.

Five Months

Even though head control as defined earlier is considered to be achieved by 4 months of age, control of the head against gravity in a supine position is not

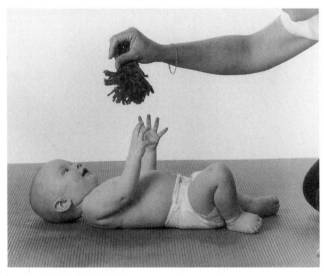

FIGURE 4–26 ■ Midline head position in supine.

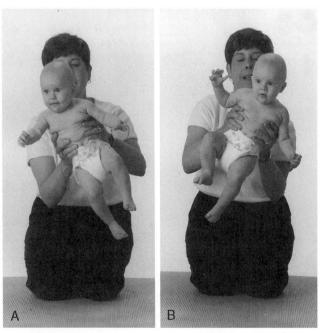

FIGURE 4–27 ■ *A* and *B*, Head control while held upright in vertical and tilted. The head either remains in midline or tilts as a compensation.

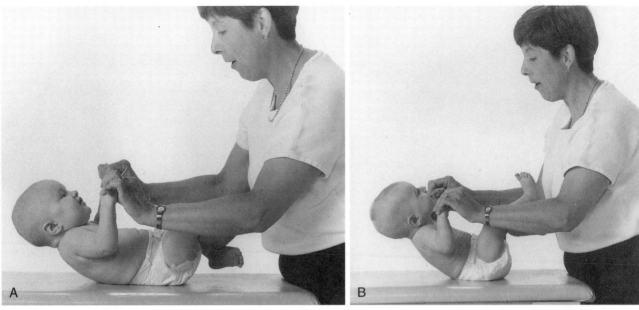

FIGURE 4-28 ▪ *A*, Use of trunk flexion to reinforce neck flexion as the head leads during a pull-to-sit maneuver. *B*, Use of leg elevation to counterbalance neck flexion during a pull-to-sit maneuver.

achieved until 5 months of age. At 5 months, the infant exhibits the ability to lift the head off the support surface *(antigravity neck flexion)*. Antigravity neck flexion may first be noted by the caregiver when putting the child down in the crib for a nap. The infant works to keep the head from falling backward as she is lowered toward the supporting surface. This is also the time when infants look as though they are trying to climb out of their car or infant seat by straining to bring the head forward. When the infant is pulled to sit from a supine position, the head now leads the movement with a chin tuck. The head is in front of the body. In fact, the infant often uses forward trunk

flexion to reinforce neck flexion and to lift the legs to counterbalance the pulling force (Fig. 4-28).

As extension develops in the prone position, the infant may occasionally demonstrate a "swimming" posture (Fig. 4-29). In this position, most of the weight is on the tummy, and the arms and legs are able to be stretched out and held up off the floor or mattress. This posture is a further manifestation of extensor control against gravity. The infant plays between this swimming posture and a prone on elbows or prone on extended arms posture (Fig. 4-30). The infant makes subtle weight shifts while in the prone on elbows position and may attempt reaching. Movements at this

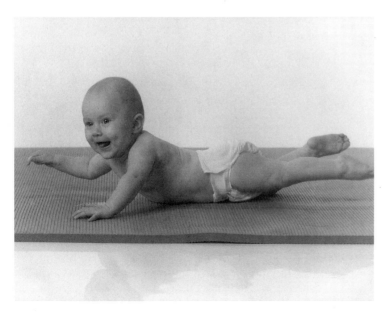

FIGURE 4-29 ▪ "Swimming" posture, antigravity extension of the body.

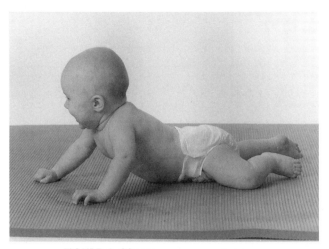

FIGURE 4–30 ■ Prone on extended arms.

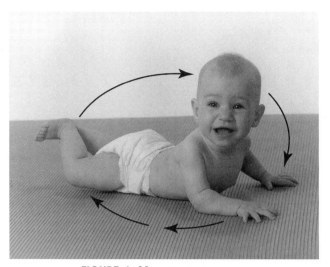

FIGURE 4–32 ■ Pivoting in prone.

stage show *dissociation* of head and limbs, as exemplified by the following movement sequences:

1. Bilateral arm and leg movements are present as compared with previous unilateral movements. The proximal joints, such as the shoulder and pelvic girdles, direct reaching and kicking movements. Just as the pattern of reaching is influenced by shoulder position, kicking can be changed by the position of the pelvis prior to and during the movement.

2. Pedaling is seen in the lower extremities. Starting with both hips flexed, the infant extends one leg, then the other, and then returns both legs to the original starting position. This leads to reciprocal kicking in which both legs continue to perform reciprocal alternating movements.

3. From a froglike position, the infant is able to lift her bottom off the support surface and to bring her feet into her visual field. This "bottom lifting"

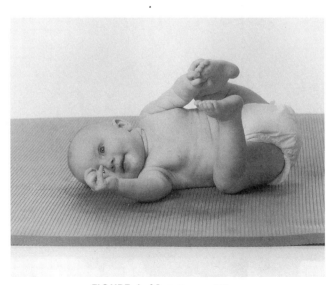

FIGURE 4–31 ■ Bottom lifting.

allows her to play with her feet and even to put them into her mouth for sensory awareness (Fig. 4–31). This play provides lengthening for the hamstrings and prepares the baby for long sitting. The lower abdominals also have a chance to work while the trunk is supported (Connor et al, 1978).

Six Months

A 6-month-old infant becomes mobile in the prone position by pivoting in a circle (Fig. 4–32). The infant is also able to shift weight onto one extended arm and to reach forward with the other hand to grasp an object. The reaching movement is counterbalanced by a lateral weight shift of the trunk that produces lateral head and trunk bending away from the side of the weight shift (Fig. 4–33). This lateral bending in response to a weight shift is called a *righting reaction*. Righting reactions of the head and trunk are more thoroughly discussed in the next section. Maximum extension of the head and trunk is possible in the prone position along with extension and abduction of the limbs away from the body. This extended posture is called the *Landau reflex* and represents total body righting against gravity. It is mature when the infant can demonstrate hip extension when held away from the support surface supported only under the tummy. The infant appears to be flying (Fig. 4–34). This final stage in the development of extension can occur only if the hips are relatively adducted. Too much hip abduction puts the gluteus maximus at a biomechanical disadvantage and makes it more difficult to execute hip extension. Excessive abduction is often seen in children with low muscle tone and increased range of motion such as in Down syndrome. These children have difficulty performing antigravity hip extension.

Segmental rolling is now present and becomes the preferred mobility pattern when rolling, first from

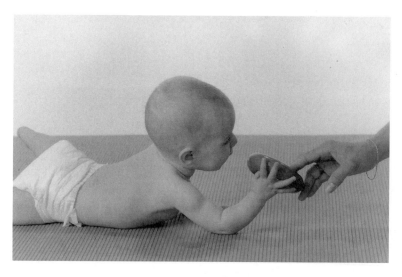

FIGURE 4-33 ▪ Lateral righting reaction.

prone to supine, which is less challenging, and then from supine to prone. Antigravity flexion control is needed to roll from supine to prone. The movement usually begins with flexion of some body part, depending on the infant and the circumstances. If enticed with a toy, the infant may reach up and over the body for the toy with the upper extremity. Another infant may lift one leg up and over the body and may allow the weight of the pelvis to initiate trunk rotation. Still another infant may begin the roll with head and neck flexion. Regardless of the body part used, segmental rotation is essential for developing transitional control (Fig. 4-35). *Transitional movements* are those that allow

a change of position such as moving from prone to sitting, from the four-point position to kneeling, and from sitting to standing. Only a few movement transitions take place without segmental trunk rotation, such as moving from the four-point position to kneeling and from sitting to standing. Individuals with movement dysfunction often have problems making the transition from one position to another smoothly and efficiently. The quality of movement affects the individual's ability to perform transitional movements.

The 6-month-old infant can sit up if placed and supported at the low back or pelvis. The typically developing infant can sit in the corner of a couch or on

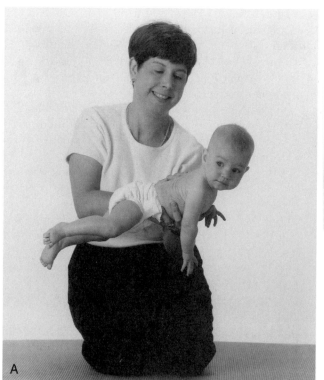

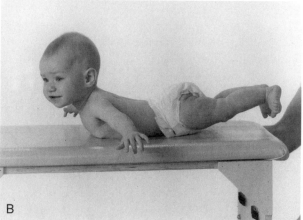

FIGURE 4-34 ▪ *A*, Eliciting a Landau reflex. *B*, Spontaneous Landau reflex.

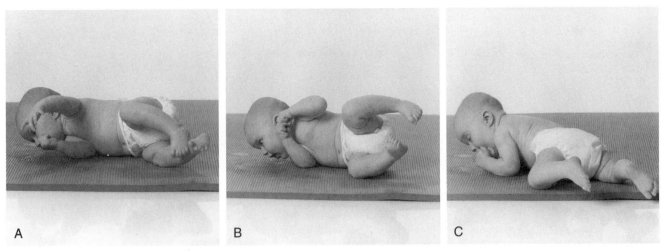

FIGURE 4–35 ■ *A* to *C*, Segmental rolling from supine to prone.

the floor if propped on extended arms. A 6-month-old cannot purposefully move into sitting from a prone position but may incidentally push herself backward along the floor. Coincidentally, while pushing, her abdomen may be lifted off the support surface, allowing the pelvis to move over the hips, with the end result of sitting between the feet. Sitting between the feet is called *W sitting* and should be avoided in infants with developmental movement problems because it can make it difficult to learn to use trunk muscles for balance. The posture provides positional stability, but it does not require active use of the trunk muscles. Concern also exists about the abnormal stress this position places on growing joints. Concern about this

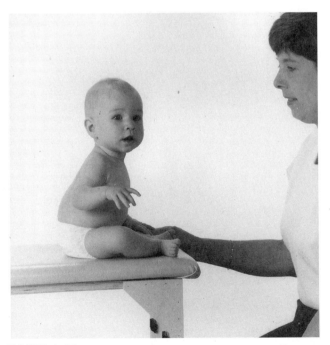

FIGURE 4–36 ■ Early sitting with a relatively straight back except for forward flexion in the lumbar spine.

sitting posture in typically developing children is less because these children move in and out of the position more easily, rather than remaining in it for long periods of time.

Having developed trunk extension in the prone position, the infant can sit with a relatively straight back with the exception of the lumbar spine (Fig. 4–36). The upper and middle back are not rounded as in previous months, but the lumbar area may still demonstrate forward flexion. Although the infant's arms are needed for support initially, with improving trunk control, first one hand and then both hands will be freed from providing postural support to explore objects and to engage in more sophisticated play. When balance is lost during sitting, the infant extends the arms for protection while falling forward. In successive months, this same upper extremity protective response will be seen in additional directions such as laterally and backward.

The pull-to-sit maneuver with a 6-month-old often causes the infant to pull all the way up to standing (Fig. 4–37). The infant will most likely reach forward for the caregiver's hands as part of the task. A 6-month-old likes to bear weight on the feet and will bounce in this position if she is held. Back and forth rocking and bouncing in a position seem to be prerequisites for achieving postural control in a new posture (Thelen, 1979). Repetition of rhythmic upper extremity activities is also seen in the banging and shaking of objects during this period. Reaching becomes less dependent on visual cues as the infant uses other senses to become more aware of body relationships. The infant may hear a noise and may reach unilaterally toward the toy that made the sound (Connor et al, 1978; Duff, 1995).

Although complete elbow extension is lacking, the 6-month-old's arm movements are maturing such that a mid–pronation-supination reaching pattern is seen.

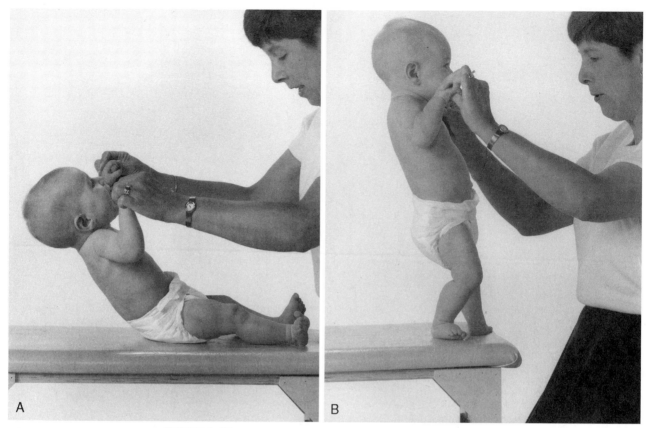

FIGURE 4–37 ■ *A* and *B*, Pull-to-sit maneuver becomes pull-to-stand.

A position halfway between supination and pronation is considered neutral. Pronated reaching is the least mature reaching pattern and is seen early in development. Supinated reaching is the most mature pattern because it allows the hand to be visually oriented toward the thumb side, thereby increasing grasp precision (Fig. 4–38). Reaching patterns originate from the shoulder because early in upper extremity development, the arm functions as a whole unit. Reaching patterns are different from grasping patterns, which involve movements of the fingers.

Seven Months

Trunk control improves in sitting and allows the infant to free one hand for playing with objects. The infant can narrow her base of support in sitting by adducting the lower extremities as the trunk begins to be able to compensate for small losses of balance. Dynamic stability develops from muscular work of the trunk. An active trunk supports dynamic balance and complements the positional stability derived from the configuration of the base of support. The different types of sitting postures such as ring sitting, wide abducted sitting, and long sitting provide the infant with different amounts of support. Figure 4–39 shows examples of sitting postures in typically developing in-

fants with and without hand support. Lateral protective reactions begin to emerge in sitting at this time (Fig. 4–40). Unilateral reach is displayed by the 7-month-old infant (Fig. 4–41), as is an ability to transfer objects from hand to hand.

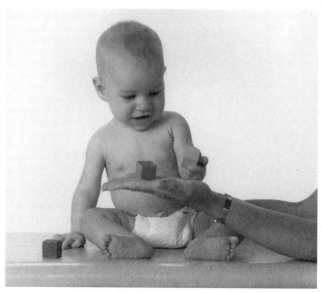

FIGURE 4–38 ■ Supinated reaching.

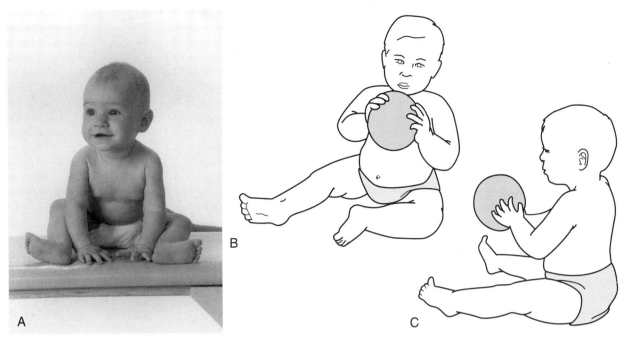

FIGURE 4–39 ■ Sitting postures. *A*, Ring sitting propped forward on hands. *B*, Half-long sitting. *C*, Long sitting.

Eight Months

Sitting is the most functional and favorite position of an 8-month-old infant. Because the infant's back is straight, the hands are free to play with objects or extend and abduct to catch the infant if a loss of balance occurs, as happens less frequently at this age. Upper trunk rotation is demonstrated during play in sitting as the child reaches in all directions for toys (see Fig. 4–39*C*). If a toy is out of reach, the infant can prop on one arm and reach across the body to extend the reach using trunk rotation and reverse the

rotation to return to upright sitting. With increased control of trunk rotation, the body moves more segmentally and less as a whole. This trend of dissociating upper trunk rotation from lower trunk movement began at 6 months with the beginning of segmental rotation. Dissociation of the arms from the trunk is seen as the arms move across the midline of the body. More external rotation is evident at the shoulder (turning the entire arm from palm down, to neutral, to palm up) and allows supinated reaching to be

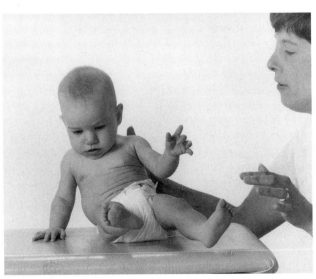

FIGURE 4–40 ■ Lateral upper extremity protective reaction in response to loss of sitting balance.

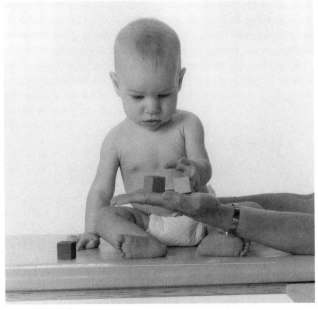

FIGURE 4–41 ■ Unilateral reach.

achieved. By 8 to 10 months, the infant's two hands are able to perform different functions such as holding a bottle in one hand while reaching for a toy with the other (Duff, 1995).

Now the infant can move into and out of sitting by deliberately pushing up from side lying. She may bear weight on her hands and feet and may attempt to "walk" in this position *(bear walking)* after pushing herself backward while belly crawling. Some type of prewalking progression, such as belly crawling (Fig. 4–42), creeping on hands and knees (see Fig. 4–14), or sitting and hitching, is usually present by 8 months. Hitching in a sitting position is an alternative way for some children to move across the floor. The infant scoots on her bottom with or without hand support. We have already noted how pushing up on extended arms can be continued into pushing into sitting. Pushing can also be used for locomotion. Because pushing is easier than pulling, the first type of straight plane locomotion achieved by the infant in a prone position may be backward propulsion. Pulling is seen as strength increases in the upper back and shoulders. All this upper extremity work in a prone position is accompanied by random leg movements. These random leg movements may accidentally cause the legs to be pushed into extension with the toes flexed and may thus provide an extra boost forward. In trying to reproduce the accident, the infant begins to learn to belly crawl or creep forward.

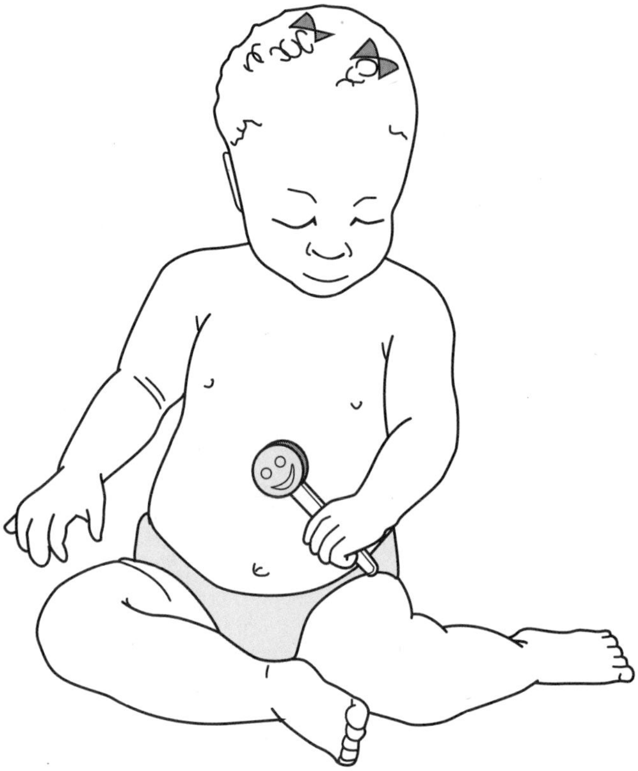

Nine Months

A 9-month-old is constantly changing positions, moving in and out of sitting, including side sitting (Fig. 4–43), and into the four-point position. As the infant experiments more and more with the four-point position, she rhythmically rocks back and forth and alternately puts her weight on her arms and legs. In this endeavor, the infant is aided by a new capacity for hip extension and flexion, other examples of the ability to dissociate movements of the pelvis from movements of the trunk. The hands and knees position, or

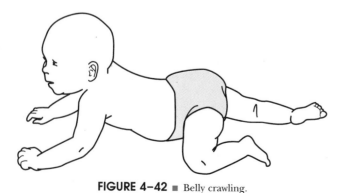

FIGURE 4–42 ▪ Belly crawling.

FIGURE 4–43 ▪ Side sitting.

quadruped position, is a less supported position requiring greater balance and trunk control. As trunk stability increases, simultaneous movement of an opposite arm and leg is possible while the infant maintains weight on the remaining two extremities. This form of reciprocal locomotion is called *creeping*. Creeping is often the primary means of locomotion for several months, even after the infant starts pulling to stand and cruising around furniture. Creeping provides fast and stable travel for the infant and allows for exploration of the environment.

Reciprocal movements used in creeping require counterrotation of trunk segments; the shoulders rotate in one direction while the pelvis rotates in the opposite direction. Counterrotation is an important element of erect forward progression (walking), which comes later. Other major components needed for successful creeping are extension of the head, neck, back, and arms, and dissociation of arm and leg movements from the trunk. Extremity dissociation depends on the stability of the shoulder and pelvic girdles, respectively, and on their ability to control rotation in opposite directions.

When playing in the quadruped position, the infant may reach out to the crib rail or furniture and may pull up to a kneeling position. Balance is maintained by holding on with the arms rather than by fully bearing weight through the hips. The infant at this age

is such control possible for the toddler. Pulling to stand is a rapid movement transition with little time spent in either true knee standing or half-kneeling. Early standing consists of leaning against a support surface, such as the coffee table or couch, so the hands can be free to play. Legs tend to be abducted for a wider base of support, much like the struts of a tower. Knee position may vary between flexion and extension, and toes alternately claw the floor and flare upward in an attempt to assist balance. These foot responses are considered equilibrium reactions of the feet (Connor et al, 1978) (Fig. 4–44).

Once the infant has achieved an upright posture at furniture, she practices weight shifting by moving from side to side. While in upright standing and before cruising begins in earnest, the infant practices dissociating arm and leg movements from the trunk by reaching out or backward with an arm while the leg is swung in the opposite direction. When side to side weight shift progresses to actual movement sideways, the baby is cruising. Cruising is done around furniture and between close pieces of furniture. This sideways "walking" is done with arm support and may be a means of working the hip abductors to ensure a level pelvis when forward ambulation is attempted. These maneuvers always make us think of a ballet dancer warming up at the barre before dancing. In this case, the infant is warming up, practicing counterrotation in a newly acquired posture, upright, before attempting

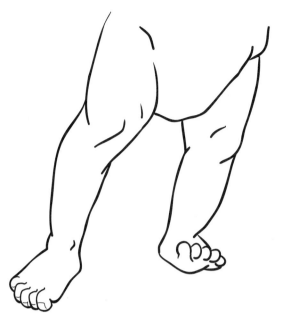

FIGURE 4–44 ■ Equilibrium reactions of the feet. Baby learns balance in standing by delicate movements of the feet—"fanning" and "clawing." (Redrawn by permission of the publisher from Connor FP, Williamson GG, Siepp JM [eds]. Program Guide for Infants and Toddlers with Neuromotor and Other Developmental Disabilities. [New York, Teachers College Press, ©1978 by Teachers College, Columbia University], p. 117. All rights reserved.)

does not have the control necessary to balance in a kneeling or half-kneeling (one foot forward) position. Even though kneeling and half-kneeling are used as transitions to pull to stand, only after learning to walk

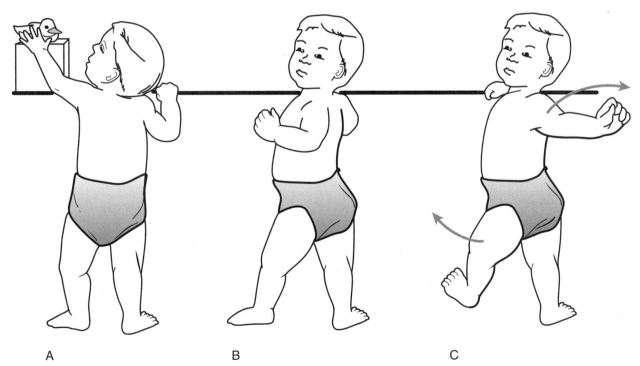

A   B   C

FIGURE 4–45 ■ Cruising maneuvers. *A,* Cruising sideways, reaching out. *B,* Standing, rotating upper trunk backward. *C,* Standing, reaching out backward, elaborating with swinging movements of the same-side leg, thus producing counterrotation. (Redrawn by permission of the publisher from Connor FP, Williamson GG, Siepp JM [eds]. Program Guide for Infants and Toddlers with Neuromotor and Other Developmental Disabilities. [New York, Teachers College Press, ©1978 by Teachers College, Columbia University], p. 121. All rights reserved.)

to walk (Fig. 4–45). Over the next several months, the infant will develop better pelvic and hip control, to perfect upright standing before attempting independent ambulation.

Toddler

Twelve Months

The infant becomes a toddler at 1 year. Most infants attempt forward locomotion by this age. The caregiver has probably already been holding the infant's hands and encouraging walking, if not placing the infant in a walker. Use of walkers has raised some safety issues (Walker et al, 1996); also, use of walkers too early does not allow the infant to sufficiently develop upper body and trunk strength needed for the progression of skills seen in the prone position. Typical first attempts at walking are lateral weight shifts from one widely abducted leg to the other (Fig. 4–46). Arms are held in *high guard* (arms held high with the scapula adducted, shoulders in external rotation and abducted, elbows flexed, and wrist and fingers extended). This position results in strong extension of the upper back that makes up for the lack of hip extension (Bobath and Bobath, 1962). As an upright trunk is more easily maintained against gravity, the arms are lowered to *midguard* (hands at waist level,

shoulders still externally rotated), to *low guard* (shoulders more neutral, elbows extended), and finally to no guard.

The beginning walker keeps hips and knees slightly flexed to bring the center of mass closer to the ground. Weight shifts are from side to side as the toddler moves forward by total lower extremity flexion, with the hip joints remaining externally rotated during the gait cycle. Ankle movements are minimal, with the foot pronated as the whole foot contacts the ground. Toddlers take many small steps and walk slowly. The instability of their gait is seen in the short amount of time they spend in single-limb stance (Martin, 1989). As trunk stability improves, the legs come farther under the pelvis. As the hips and knees become more extended, the feet develop the plantar flexion needed for the pushoff phase of the gait cycle.

Sixteen to Eighteen Months

By 16 to 17 months, the toddler is so much at ease with walking that a toy can be carried or pulled at the same time. With help, the toddler goes up and down stairs, one step at a time. Without help, the toddler creeps up the stairs and may creep or scoot down on her buttocks. Most children will be able to walk sideways and backward at this age if they started walking at 12 months or earlier. The typically developing toddler

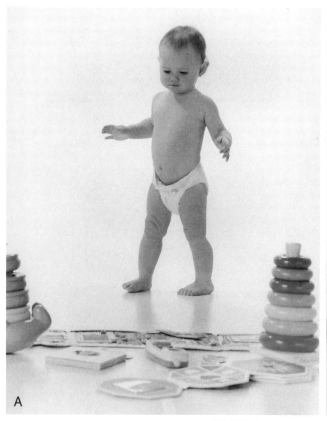

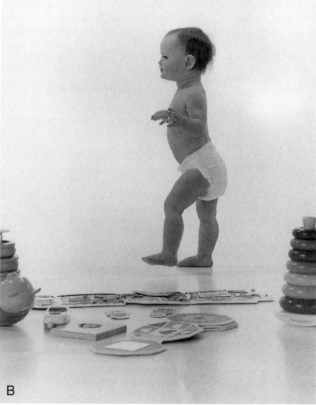

FIGURE 4–46 ▪ *A* and *B*, Independent walking.

comes to stand from a supine position by rolling to prone, pushing up on hands and knees or hands and feet, assuming a squat, and rising to standing (Fig. 4–47).

Most toddlers exhibit a reciprocal arm swing and heelstrike by 18 months of age, with other adult gait characteristics manifested later. They walk well and demonstrate a "running-like" walk. Although the toddler may still occasionally fall or trip over objects in her path because eye-foot coordination is not completely developed, the decline in falls appears to be the result of improved balance reactions in standing and the ability to monitor trunk and lower extremity movements kinesthetically and visually. The first signs

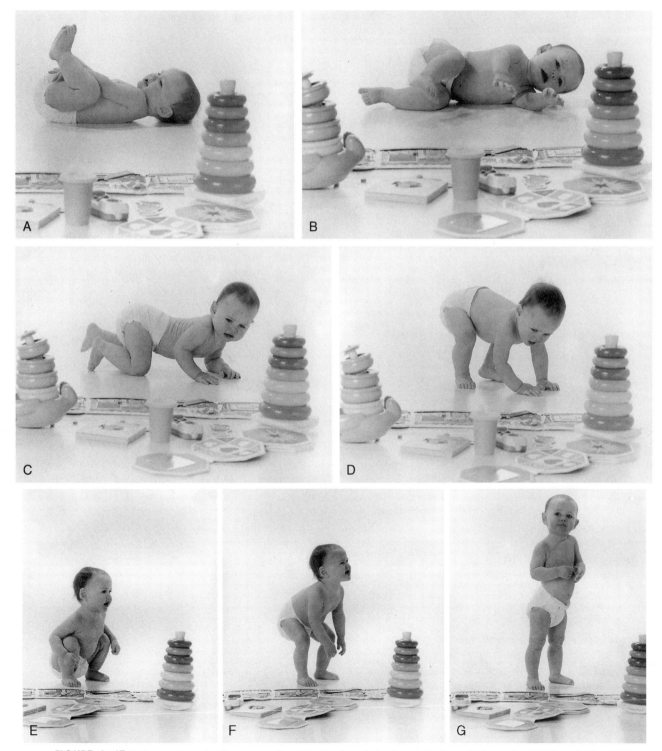

FIGURE 4–47 ■ Progression of rising to standing from supine. *A*, Supine. *B*, Rolling. *C*, Four-point position. *D*, Plantigrade. *E*, Squat. *F*, Semi-squat. *G*, Standing.

of jumping appear as a stepping off "jump" from a low object such as the bottom step of a set of stairs. Children are ready for this first step-down jump after being able to walk down a step while they hold the hand of an adult (Wickstrom, 1983). Momentary balance on one foot is also possible.

Two Years

The 2-year-old's gait becomes faster, arms swing reciprocally, steps are bigger, and time spent in single-limb stance increases. Many additional motor skills emerge during this year. A 2-year-old can go up and down stairs one step at a time, jump off a step with a two-foot takeoff, stand on one foot for 1 to 3 seconds, kick a large ball, and throw a small one. Stair climbing and kicking indicate improved stability during shifting of body weight from one leg to the other (Connor et al, 1978). Stepping over low objects is also part of the child's movement capabilities within the environment. True running, characterized by a "flight" phase when both feet are off the ground, emerges at the same time. Quickly starting to run and stopping from a run are still difficult, and directional changes by making a turn require a large area. As the child first attempts to jump off the ground, one foot leaves the ground, followed by the other foot, as if the child were stepping in air.

Fundamental Movement Patterns (Three to Six Years)

Fundamental movement patterns such as running and jumping are beginning to be perfected at 2 years, but it takes several years in some instances for these abilities to mature completely. Other fundamental motor skills such as hopping, skipping, throwing, catching, and striking develop over the next 4 years of life. Before discussing these skills, it is important to understand the development of postural control within the context of the two prevailing models of motor control. The reader may want to review Chapter 3. These theories affect how we view the development of postural control in the first 2 years of life and interpret the emergence of new motor skills and fundamental motor patterns in childhood.

Fundamental movement patterns are learned in early childhood and were defined by Wickstrom (1983) as basic motor skills with specific patterns. Running, jumping, galloping, skipping, throwing, catching, kicking, and striking are typically included in the category of fundamental skills. Each fundamental skill can be identified by a minimum standard of performance. The form used to meet the minimum standard of the movement is considered immature and can be improved on to acquire a mature form. Once walking, the child begins to try to walk faster and faster until

running develops by the age of 2 years. The minimum standard for running mandates that the feet move forward alternately and that a brief period of nonsupport occurs after the support foot pushes off. The mature form of running is that of a sprint.

Three Years

The following gait characteristics indicate mature gait, which is usually developed by age 3 or 4 years: both arms and legs move reciprocally in synchrony with each other; out-toeing has been reduced; pelvic rotation and a double knee-lock pattern are present. This pattern refers to the two periods of knee extension in gait, one just before heelstrike and another as the body moves over the foot during stance phase. In between, at the moment of heelstrike, the knee is flexed to help absorb the impact of the body's weight. A 3-year-old should exhibit heelstrike. By 4 years, 98% of toddlers exhibit mature gait characteristics according to Sutherland and coworkers (1988). However, Stout (1994) stated that gait is not mature until a child is 7 years of age.

Other reciprocal actions mastered by 3-year-olds are pedaling a tricycle and climbing a jungle gym or ladder. Locomotion can be started and stopped based on the demands of the environment or those of a task such as playing dodge ball on a crowded playground. A 3-year-old can make sharp turns while running and can balance on toes and heels in standing. Standing with one foot in front of the other, known as *tandem standing*, is possible, as is standing on one foot for up to 3 seconds. A reciprocal gait is used to ascend stairs; the child places one foot on each step in an alternating fashion but marks time (one step at a time) when descending.

Jumping begins with a step-down jump at 18 months of age and progresses to jumping off the floor with both feet at the same time when the child is 2 (Fig. 4–48). By the time a child is 3 years of age, jumping has continued to change, so the child can jump over an obstacle on the floor by leading with one foot. Types of jumps achieved by children in terms of progressive difficulty can be found in Table 4–7. One-foot jumps come before two-foot jumps, and one-foot landings come before two-foot landings. The time span between achieving various jumps varies greatly. Some possible ages of acquisition are also found in Table 4–7, but these ages vary for different individuals. Jumping skills progress, as evidenced by the ability of a 3½-year-old to jump over an obstacle by taking off with two feet and landing with two feet.

Once jumping off the floor with two feet is mastered, many other types of jumps become possible. At 3 years of age, a child may perform a running broad jump. The child runs and at some point jumps forward. The jump is from one foot, but the landing is

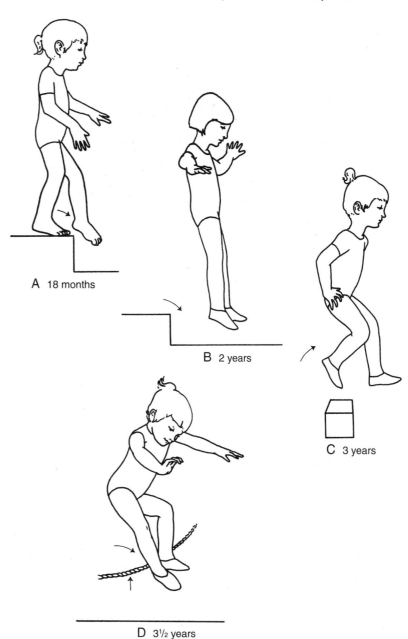

FIGURE 4–48 ■ Types of jumps. *A*, First attempts at jumping involve a one-foot step-down. Then the child engages in a two-foot takeoff (*B*) and later becomes able to jump over obstacles with a one-foot (*C*) and later a two-foot takeoff and landing (*D*). (From Cratty BJ. Perceptual and Motor Development in Infants and Children, 2nd ed. Copyright © 1979 by Allyn & Bacon. Reprinted by permission.)

A 18 months

B 2 years

C 3 years

D 3½ years

on two feet. Vertical jumps are possible, and the height of the jump increases with age (Fig. 4–49). Hopping on one foot is a special type of jump requiring balance on one foot and pushoff. It does not require a maximum effort. "Repeated vertical jumps from two feet can be done before true hopping can occur" (Wickstrom, 1983). Neither type of jump is seen at an early age. Hopping once or twice on the preferred foot may also be accomplished by 3½ years of age.

Four Years

A 4-year-old has better static and dynamic balance, as evidenced by an ability to stand on either foot for a longer period (4 to 6 seconds) than a 3-year-old. A child of 4 years can hop on one foot four to six times. Improved hopping ability is seen when the child learns to use the nonstance leg to help propel the body forward. Previously, all the work had been done by pushing off with the support foot. A similar pattern is observed in the arms, which are inactive at first, but then are used opposite the action of the moving leg. Gender differences for hopping are documented in the literature; girls perform better than boys (Wickstrom, 1983). This difference may be related to the finding that girls appear to have better balance than boys in childhood. Rhythmic relaxed galloping is possible for a 4-year-old. Galloping consists of a walk on the leading leg followed by a running step on the rear leg. Galloping is considered by some to be the first asymmetric gait seen in a young child and subsequently is

Table 4-7 ▌ **TYPES OF JUMPS ACHIEVED BY CHILDREN IN TERMS OF PROGRESSIVE DIFFICULTY**

APPROXIMATE AGE	TYPE OF JUMP
18 months	Jump down from one foot, land on the other foot
24 months	Jump up from two feet, land on two feet
26–28 months	Jump down from one foot, land on two feet
26–28 months	Jump down from two feet, land on two feet
29–31 months	Run and jump forward from one foot, land on the other foot
29–31 months	Jump forward from two feet, land on two feet
29–31 months	Run and jump forward from one foot, land on two feet
38–42 months	Jump over object from two feet, land on two feet
42 months	Jump from one foot to same foot rhythmically

Adapted from Wickstrom RL. Fundamental Movement Patterns, 3rd ed. Philadelphia, Lea & Febiger, 1983, p 69.

also called *unilateral skipping*. Think of a child riding a stick horse as a visual example of galloping. Toddlers have been documented to gallop as early as 20 months after learning to walk (Whitall, 1989), but the movement is stiff, with arms held in high guard, as seen during beginning walking.

Four-year-olds can catch a small ball with outstretched arms if it is thrown to them, and they can throw a ball overhand for some distance. Throwing begins with an accidental letting go of an object at about 18 months of age. From 2 to 4 years of age, throwing is extremely variable, with underhand and overhand throwing observed. Gender differences are seen. A child of 2½ years can throw a large or small ball 5 feet (Fig. 4–50 and Table 4–8) (Wellman, 1937). The ball is not thrown more than 10 feet until the child is more than 4 years of age. The distance a child is able to propel an object has been related to a child's height, as seen in Figure 4–51 (Cratty, 1979).

Development of more mature throwing is related to using the force of the body and combining leg and shoulder movements to improve performance.

"Although throwing and catching have a close functional relationship, throwing is learned a lot more quickly than catching" (Wickstrom, 1977). Catching ability depends on many variables, the least of which is ball size, speed, arm position of the catcher, skill of the thrower, and age-related sensory and perceptual factors. Some of these perceptual factors involve the use of visual cues, depth perception, eye-hand coordination, and the amount of experience the catcher has had with playing with balls. Closing the eyes when an object is thrown toward one is a fear response common in children (Wickstrom, 1977) and has to be overcome to learn to catch or strike an object.

Precatching requires the child to interact with a rolling ball. Such interaction typically occurs while the child sits with legs outstretched and tries to trap the ball with legs or hands. Learning about time and spatial relationships of a moving object proceeds from this seated position to standing and chasing after a rolling or bouncing ball. The child tries to stop, intercept, and otherwise control his movements and to anticipate the movement of the object in space. Next, the child attempts to "catch" an object moving through the air. Before the age of 3 years, most children must have their arms prepositioned to have any chance of catching a ball thrown to them. Most of the time, the thrower, who is an adult, bounces the ball to the child, so the burden is on the thrower to calculate where the ball must bounce to land in the child's outstretched arms. Figures 4–52 and 4–53 show two immature catchers, one 33 months old and the other 48 months old. As catching matures, the hands are used more, with less dependence on the arms and the body. The 4-year-old still has maturing to do in perfecting the skill of catching.

Striking, according to Wickstrom (1983), is the act of swinging and hitting an object. Developmentally, the earliest form of striking is for the child to use arm

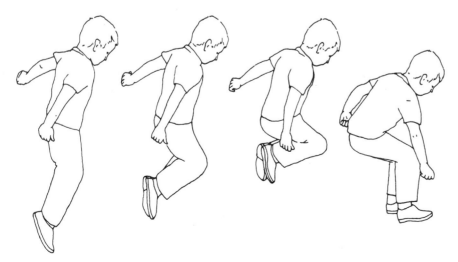

FIGURE 4–49 ■ Vertical jump. Immature form in the vertical jump showing "winging" arm action, incomplete extension, quick flexion of the legs, and slight forward jump. (From Wickstrom RL. Fundamental Movement Patterns, 3rd ed. Philadelphia, Lea & Febiger, 1983.)

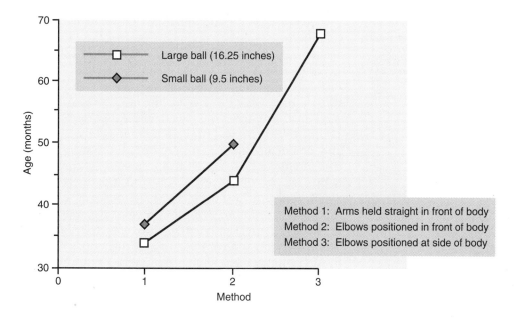

BALL-CATCHING ACHIEVEMENTS OF PRESCHOOL CHILDREN

Large ball (16.25 inches)
Small ball (9.5 inches)

Method 1: Arms held straight in front of body
Method 2: Elbows positioned in front of body
Method 3: Elbows positioned at side of body

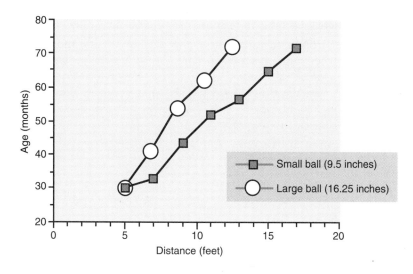

BALL-THROWING ACHIEVEMENTS OF PRESCHOOL CHILDREN

Small ball (9.5 inches)
Large ball (16.25 inches)

FIGURE 4–50 ■ Wellman graphs. *A,* Ball-catching skill is attained at a certain level of performance with the large ball before the same level of skill is achieved with the small ball. *B,* At 30 months, a small or large ball can be thrown 5 feet. It will take 10 more months for the child to be able to throw the large ball the same distance as the small ball. (Redrawn from Espanschade AS, Eckert HM. Motor Development. Columbus, OH, Charles E. Merrill, 1967.)

extension to hit something with her hand. When the child is holding an implement such as a stick or bat, this form results in striking down on the object. Two- to 4-year-olds demonstrate this immature striking behavior. Without any special help, the child will progress slowly to striking more horizontally.

Five Years

At 5 years of age, a child can stand on either foot for 8 to 10 seconds, walk forward on a balance beam, hop 8 to 10 times on one foot, make a 2- to 3-foot standing broad jump, and skip on alternating feet. One motor test expects a 5-year-old to be able to hop

50 feet in 11 seconds (Stott et al, 1984). Skipping is a skill that requires coordination of both sides of the body. A 5-year-old should be able to hit a 2-foot square target from a distance of 5 feet, first by throwing underhand, then progressing to overhand, and finally by bouncing the ball to the target (Folio and Fewell, 1983). Half of all 5½-year-olds are able to catch a ball when their hands are initially at their sides. Different motor skills can be expected, depending on the child's experiences and amount of practice.

Kicking is a special type of striking and one in which the arms play no direct role. Children most frequently kick a ball in spontaneous play and in organized games. A 2-year-old is able to kick a ball on the

Table 4–8 ▌ **BALL THROWING ACHIEVEMENTS OF PRESCHOOL CHILDREN**

DISTANCE OF THROW (Feet)	MOTOR AGE IN MONTHS	
	Small Ball (9½ inch)	Large Ball (16¼ inch)
4 to 5	30	30
6 to 7	33	43
8 to 9	44	43
10 to 11	52	63
12 to 13	57	above 72
14 to 15	65	
16 to 17	above 72	

From Wellman BL. Motor achievements of preschool children. Child Educ 13:311–316, 1937. Reprinted by permission of the Association for Childhood Education International, 3615 Wisconsin Avenue, NW, Washington, DC.

ground. The Peabody Developmental Motor Scales (Folio and Fewell, 1983) expect a child of 5 years to kick a ball rolled toward him 12 feet in the air and a child of 6 years to run and kick a rolling ball 4 feet (Folio and Fewell, 1983). Gesell (1940) expected a 5-year-old to kick a soccer ball 8 to 11½ feet and a 6-year-old to be able to kick a ball 10 to 18 feet. Measuring performance in kicking is difficult before the age of 4 years. Annual improvements begin to be seen at the age of 5 years (Gesell, 1940). Kicking requires good static balance on the stance foot and counterbalancing the force of the kick with arm positioning.

Hand preference, the tendency to use one particular hand, may be noted as early as a few days after birth to 4 months of age when the infant prefers to swipe or grasp objects with a particular hand. As the child learns to use more and more implements or tools, she experiments with using them in either hand. Hand preference develops because preschoolers practice skilled tasks such as eating with utensils and coloring. According to Levine (1987), hand preference is well established by 4 to 6 years of age. *Hand dominance* is the *consistent* use of one hand for tasks such as throwing a ball, writing with a pencil, and eating with a fork (Duff, 1995). Because the definitions of preference and dominance are often confused, the age at which true dominance is established remains controversial. Some sources say as early as 12 to 13 months (Fagard, 1990), others as late as 7 years. Five years of age is a time when confusion regarding dominance appears to be normal, even in a child who may have already shown a strong preference. The driving force behind hand dominance has always been considered to be the specialization of the cerebral hemispheres for specific purposes. This specialization process is complete by age 6 or 7 and results in laterality of brain functions. Laterality in hand usage means that one hand is consistently used to write with and is much better at the task than the other hand (Ayres, 1972; Murray, 1991). The majority of us are right-handed, meaning that the left cerebral hemisphere controls our hand movements.

Six Years

A 6-year-old is well coordinated in her movements. She can stand on either foot for 10 seconds or more with eyes open and with eyes closed. This ability is important to note because it indicates that vision can

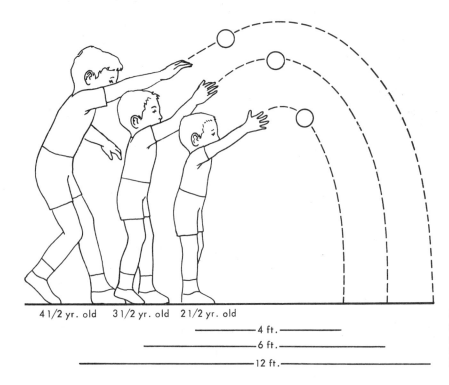

4 1/2 yr. old   3 1/2 yr. old   2 1/2 yr. old

—————— 4 ft. ——————
————————— 6 ft. —————————
———————————— 12 ft. ————————————

FIGURE 4–51 ▌ Throwing distances increase with increasing age. (From Cratty BJ. Perceptual and Motor Development in Infants and Children, 2nd ed. Copyright © 1979 by Allyn & Bacon. Reprinted by permission.)

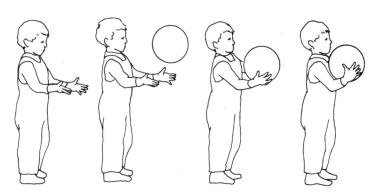

FIGURE 4–52 ■ Immature catching. A 33-month-old boy extends his arms before the ball is tossed. He waits for the ball without moving, responds after the ball has touched his hands, and then gently traps the ball against his chest. It is essentially a robot-like performance. (From Wickstrom RL. Fundamental Movement Patterns, 3rd ed. Philadelphia, Lea & Febiger, 1983.)

be ignored and balance maintained. A 6-year-old can throw and catch a small ball from 10 feet away. She walks on a balance beam forward, backward, and sideways without stepping off the beam. The child is able to use alternative forms of locomotion such as riding a bicycle or roller skating.

Between 6 and 10 years of age, children master the adult forms of running, throwing, and catching (Porter, 1989). Mature form in striking is usually not demonstrated until at least 6 years of age (Malina and Bouchard, 1991). Most of the studies on striking an object have been done with school-age children. Common patterns of striking are overhand, sidearm, and underhand. As the child progresses from striking down to a more horizontal striking (sidearm), more and more trunk rotation is seen as the child's swing matures (Roberton and Halverson, 1977). A mature pattern of striking consists of taking a step, turning away, and then swinging (step-turn-swing) (Wickstrom, 1983).

tion. Knowledge of normal motor development provides insights into movement dysfunction. The components of movement, the actual ways in which head, trunk, and limbs can move, are present by 6 months of age. It takes another 6 months for the infant to gain the postural control to attain and maintain upright standing needed for ambulation. Over the next year, movement in the upright position is refined, speeded up, and better controlled during stopping and starting. Three- to 6-year-olds develop fundamental patterns of movement that form the basis for later sports skills. Between 6 and 10 years of age, a child masters the adult forms of running, throwing, and catching (Porter, 1989). Throughout the process of changing motor activities and skills, the nervous and musculoskeletal systems are maturing, and the body is growing in height and weight. Although motor development continues to change throughout the life span, this section focuses on some of the significant changes that occur during the first 6 years.

Importance of Motor Skill Acquisition in Childhood

Understanding typical motor behavior is critical to understanding why and how we intervene therapeutically with individuals who exhibit movement dysfunc-

Age-Related Differences in Movement Patterns Beyond Childhood

Many developmentalists have chosen to look only at the earliest ages of life when motor abilities and skills are being acquired. The belief that mature motor be-

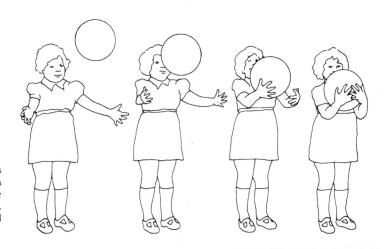

FIGURE 4–53 ■ A 4-year-old girl waits for the ball with arms straight and hands spread. Her initial response to the ball is a clapping motion. When one hands contacts the ball, she grasps at it and gains control by clutching it against her chest. (From Wickstrom RL. Fundamental Movement Patterns, 3rd ed. Philadelphia, Lea & Febiger, 1983.)

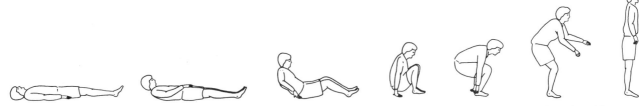

FIGURE 4-54 ∎ Most common form of rising to a standing position: upper extremity component, symmetric push; axial component, symmetric; lower extremity component, symmetric squat. (Reprinted from VanSant AF. Rising from a supine position to erect stance: description of adult movement and a developmental hypothesis. Phys Ther 68:185–192, 1988, with permission of the APTA.)

havior is achieved by childhood led researchers to overlook the possibility that movement could change as a result of factors other than nervous system maturation. Although the nervous system is generally thought to be mature by the age of 10 years, changes in movement patterns do occur in adolescence and adulthood (VanSant, 1995). VanSant and her students studied the movement patterns used by people of different ages to accomplish a simple motor task.

VanSant and others studied the task of rising from supine to standing by describing the movement components for different regions of the body. Although an explanation of the method used in the many studies is beyond the scope of this text, a summary of the results is most appropriate.

Research shows a developmental order of movement patterns across childhood and adolescence with trends toward increasing symmetry with increasing age (Sabourin, 1989; VanSant, 1988). VanSant (1988b) identified three common ways in which adults came to stand. These are shown in Figures 4–54 to 4–56. In this study, the most common way was to use upper extremity reach, symmetric push, forward head, neck and trunk flexion, and symmetric squat (see Fig. 4–54). The second most common way was identical, up to an asymmetric squat (see Fig. 4–55). The next most common way involved an asymmetric push and reach, followed by a half-kneel (see Fig. 4–56). In a separate study of adults in the third through fifth decades of life, the trend was toward increasing asymmetry with age (Ford-Smith and VanSant, 1993). Older adults were more likely to demonstrate the asymmetric patterns of movement seen in young children (VanSant,

1991). The asymmetry of movement in the older adult may reflect less trunk rotation resulting from stiffening of joints or lessening of muscle strength, factors that make it more difficult to come straight forward to sitting from a supine position.

Most recently, movement from supine to standing in elderly persons was studied by Thomas and colleagues (1998), who used VanSant's component approach to movement analysis. In a group of community-dwelling elders with a mean age of 74.6 years, shorter time to rise was related to younger age, greater knee extension strength, and greater hip and ankle range of motion (flexion and dorsiflexion, respectively). "It appears that elderly persons who maintain their strength and flexibility may rise to standing faster and more symmetrically" (Thomas et al, 1998). The 70- and 80-year-old persons in the study were more likely to use asymmetric patterns in the upper extremity and axial (trunk) regions, whereas the younger elderly persons demonstrated more symmetric patterns in the same body regions.

Although the structures of the body are mature at the end of puberty, changes in movement patterns continue throughout a person's entire life. Mature movement patterns have always been associated with efficiency and symmetry. Early in motor development, patterns of movement appear to be more homogenous and follow a fairly prescribed developmental sequence. As a person matures, movement patterns become more symmetric. With aging, movement patterns become more asymmetric. Less active middle-aged and older adults differ in movements used to come to stand (Green, 1989; Luehring, 1989). Because older

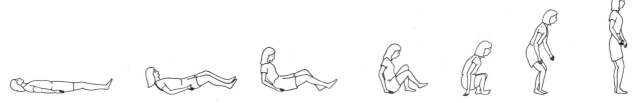

FIGURE 4-55 ∎ Second most common form of rising to a standing position: upper extremity component, symmetric push; axial component, symmetric; lower extremity component, asymmetric squat. (Reprinted from VanSant AF. Rising from a supine position to erect stance: description of adult movement and a developmental hypothesis. Phys Ther 68:185–192, 1988, with permission of the APTA.)

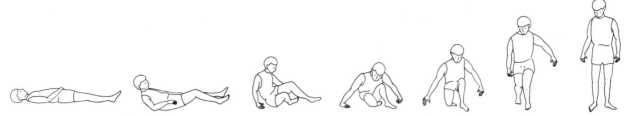

FIGURE 4-56 ■ Third most common form of rising to a standing position: upper extremity component, asymmetric push and reach; axial component, partial rotation; lower extremity component, half-kneel. (Reprinted from VanSant AF. Rising from a supine position to erect stance: description of adult movement and a developmental hypothesis. Phys Ther 68:185–192, 1988, with permission of the APTA.)

persons may exhibit different ways of moving and require more time to make the transition from one position to another, it is important to match our teaching to the individual's usual patterns of movement.

POSTURE, BALANCE, AND GAIT CHANGES WITH AGING

Posture

The ability to maintain an erect aligned posture declines with advanced age. Figure 4–57 shows the difference in posture anticipated with aging. Humans have two primary spinal curves at birth, a forwardly flexed thoracic curve and a forwardly flexed sacral curve. During infancy, secondary cervical and lumbar curves develop with movement. These curves are convex forward. The emergence of secondary curves depends on the development of the intervertebral discs (Lowrey, 1986). With advanced age, the two secondary curves decrease and result in kyphosis and accentuated lordosis. The discs are known to lose water, become stiffer, and flatten with age (Moncur, 1993). In contrast, some older individuals demonstrate a flatter back as they age, rather than an increase in lordosis, if they sit for long periods during the day (Lewis, 1990). This may be a result of lack of movement rather than a pure aging effect. A forward-positioned head is often thought to be part of an older adult's posture; however, it may be present before age 65 and may be further accentuated with aging as a compensation for thoracic kyphosis. Lack of cervical range may also be due to degenerative changes in the neck. Postural changes in the elderly can be a result of aging or may be additionally related to a lack of movement from a sedentary lifestyle. Decreased activity can accentuate age-related postural changes (Moncur, 1993).

Balance

Elderly patients can have major problems with balance and falling. However, whether an older person's ability to balance while standing and walking always declines with age is still undecided. Sensory information is needed to respond quickly to changes within the internal and external environments that signal the need for a postural response to maintain balance. Structural changes in the sensory receptors that provide information about the support surface, position of the arms and legs, and head movement are reported with age. A decline in structural integrity of these sensory receptors decreases the quality of the information relayed. The actual number of receptors also decreases. Awareness of vibration is lessened in the elderly and has been related to an increase in postural sway during quiet stance. Because vision is a strong source of information for balance, any decline in this sensory system may be detrimental to balance. Age-related declines in visual acuity, depth perception, peripheral vision, and the ability to adapt to changes in light or dark environments can significantly affect an older person's ability to detect threats to balance. Removal of visual information during balance testing in the elderly has been shown to increase postural sway (Sheldon, 1963; Woollacott, 1990).

A dynamic postural response depends on the strength and range of motion available at a joint. The ankle has to have enough range to allow some sway. Loss of passive range of motion is seen with advancing age. Women seem to lose less range in the ankles than men, and the upper extremities remain more flexible than the lower extremities in both men and women (Bell and Hoshizaki, 1981). Isometric strength decreases by 30 to 40% over time, but because isometric strength does not relate highly to the ability to perform functional skills, this decrease may not be problematic. The ability to produce a concentric contraction also declines with age, but interestingly, the production of an eccentric or lengthening contraction is not as greatly affected by age and may even remain normal. Muscle strength declines with age beginning around the age of 50 years (Larsson, 1982). The reduction does not become functionally important until the age of 60 years (Vandervoort, 1995). By the age of 80 years, the decline in muscle strength accelerates (Vandervoort et al, 1990). The decline in strength can be related to the finding that older adults have less muscle mass. Another explanation could be that the ability of the nervous system to produce muscle excitation is impaired. This hypothesis has not yet been proven.

Gait

Numerous changes in gait can be expected to occur in an older population. Generally, the older adult is more cautious while walking. Cadence and velocity are decreased, as is stride length. Stride width increases to provide a wider base of support for better balance. Increasing the base of support and taking shorter steps means that an older adult spends more time in double limb support than a young adult. Walking velocity slows as stride length decreases, and double-support time increases. Double-support time reflects how much time is spent with both feet on the ground. Winter and colleagues (1990) attributed these differences in gait to age alone. Those gait changes that cannot be linked to compensations for age-related musculoskeletal changes may be the result of the deterioration of the sensorimotor system (Olney and Culham, 1995).

Age-related changes in gait can create difficulties in other aspects of functional movement, such as stepping over objects and going up and down stairs. Chen and coworkers (1991) found that healthy older adults had more difficulty than healthy young adults in stepping over obstacles of increasing heights. Everyone slowed down and increased foot clearance as the height of the objects increased. However, the older adults used a significantly slower speed than the young adults and had less margin of error when clearing the obstacle. The decreased step length made it more likely for the older adult to step on the object and thereby increase her chance of falling. Stair climbing requires a period of single-limb stance while the swing leg is lifted up to the next step. Given the changes in gait with age already described, it is no surprise that older adults go up and down stairs more slowly.

Implications for Treatment

Age-related losses of range of motion, strength, and balance can be compounded in the older adult by a lack of habitual physical activity and can be intensified in the presence of neurologic deficits resulting from a stroke, spinal cord injury, or traumatic brain injury. The good news is that the decline in muscular strength and endurance can be partially reversed with an appropriate amount of resistive and endurance exercise. Precautions must always be considered in light of other preexisting disorders that would require modification of therapeutic intervention. The physical therapist is responsible for accurately documenting the patient's present level of abilities, recognizing mitigating

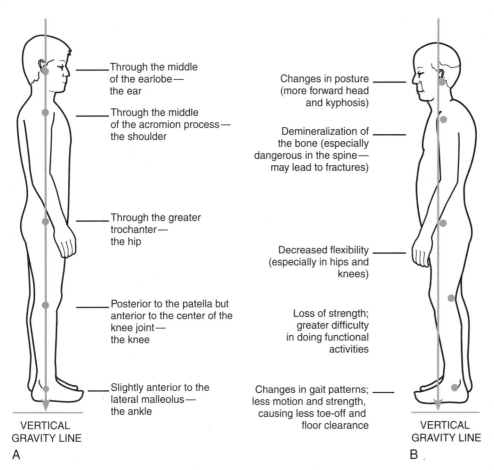

Through the middle of the earlobe—the ear

Through the middle of the acromion process—the shoulder

Through the greater trochanter—the hip

Posterior to the patella but anterior to the center of the knee joint—the knee

Slightly anterior to the lateral malleolus—the ankle

VERTICAL GRAVITY LINE

A

Changes in posture (more forward head and kyphosis)

Demineralization of the bone (especially dangerous in the spine—may lead to fractures)

Decreased flexibility (especially in hips and knees)

Loss of strength; greater difficulty in doing functional activities

Changes in gait patterns; less motion and strength, causing less toe-off and floor clearance

VERTICAL GRAVITY LINE

B

FIGURE 4–57 ❚ Comparison of standing posture: changes associated with age. *A*, Younger person; *B*, older person. (From Lewis C [ed]. Aging: The Health Care Challenge, 2nd ed. Philadelphia, FA Davis, 1990.)

circumstances, and planning appropriate therapeutic interventions. The therapist should instruct the physical therapist assistant in how the patient's exercise response should be monitored during treatment. If this information is not provided, the physical therapist assistant should request the information before treatment is initiated.

When the patient with a neurologic insult also has pulmonary or cardiac conditions, the physical therapist assistant should monitor the patient's vital signs during exercise. Decline in cardiopulmonary reserve capacity resulting from age can be compounded by a loss of fitness and loss of conditioning. Probably no more deconditioned patient exists than one who is in the hospital. As the patient is being mobilized and acclimated to the upright position in preparation for discharge, the decline in reserve can affect the patient's ability to perform normal activities of daily living. Walking can require up to 40% of the oxygen taken in by an individual. Therefore, an older person may need to slow down the speed of walking depending on how much oxygen is available. Measurements of heart rate, blood pressure, and respiratory rate are important, providing the supervising therapist with information about the patient's response to exercise. More specific monitoring of oxygen saturation, rate of perceived exertion, level of dyspnea (shortness of breath), or angina may be indicated by the supervising physical therapist, but further discussion of these methods is beyond the scope of this text. The complexity of the patient's condition may warrant limiting the involvement of the physical therapist assistant.

CHAPTER SUMMARY

Age and age-related changes in the structure and function of different body systems can significantly alter the functional movement expectations for any given individual. Functional tasks are defined by the age of the individual. An infant's function is to overcome gravity and learn to move into the upright position. The toddler explores the world in the upright position and adds fundamental movement patterns of running, hopping, and skipping during childhood. Manipulation of objects is continually refined from finger feeding Cheerios to learning to write. Self-care skills are mastered by the time a child enters school. Sport skills build on the fundamental movement patterns and are important in childhood and adolescence. Work and leisure skills become important during late adolescence and adulthood. Every period of the life span has different functional movement expectations. The movement expectations are driven by the mover, the task, and the social and physical environments.

REVIEW QUESTIONS

1. What are the characteristics that identify a developmental theory as being life span in approach?
2. What theorist described a pyramid of needs that the individual strives to fulfill?
3. What is an example of a directional concept of development?
4. What three processes guide motor development?
5. When does a child typically achieve gross- and fine-motor milestones?
6. What are the typical postures and movements of a 4-month-old and a 6-month-old?
7. What motor abilities constitute fundamental motor patterns?
8. Why do motor patterns continue to change throughout the life span?
9. What role does decreased activity play in an older adult's posture?
10. What gait changes can have an impact on functional abilities in older adults?

REFERENCES

Atchley RC. Social Forces and Aging, 6th ed. Belmont, CA, Wadsworth, 1991.

Ayres AJ. Sensory Integration and Learning Disorders. Los Angeles, Western Psychological Services, 1972, pp 25–234.

Baltes P. Theoretical propositions of life-span developmental psychology: on the dynamics between growth and decline. Dev Psychol 23:611–626, 1987.

Bell RD, Hoshizaki TB. Relationships of age and sex with range of motion of seventeen joint actions in humans. Can J Appl Sport Sci 6:202–206, 1981.

Bly L. Components of Normal Movement during the First Year of Life and Abnormal Development. Chicago, Neurodevelopmental Treatment Association, 1983.

Bobath B, Bobath K. An analysis of the development of standing and walking patterns in patient with cerebral palsy. Physiotherapy 48:144–153, 1962.

Boehme R. Improving Upper Body Control. Tucson, Therapy Skill Builders, 1988.

Chen H-C, Ashton-Miller JA, Alexander NB, et al. Stepping over obstacles: gait patterns of healthy young and old adults. J Gerontol 46:M196–M203, 1991.

Cliff S. The Development of Reach and Grasp. El Paso, TX, Guynes Printing, 1979.

Connor FP, Williamson GG, Siepp JM. Program Guide for Infants and Toddlers with Neuromotor and Other Developmental Disabilities. New York, Teacher's College Press, 1978.

Cratty BJ. Perceptual and Motor Development in Infants and Children, 2nd ed. Englewood Cliffs, NJ, Prentice-Hall, 1979.

Duff SV. Prehension. In Cech D, Martin S (eds). Functional Movement Development Across the Life Span. Philadelphia, WB Saunders, 1995, pp 313–353.

Epstein ML. The relationship of mental imagery and mental rehearsal to performance of a motor task. J Sport Psychol 2:211–220, 1980.

Erhardt RP. Developmental Hand Dysfunction: Theory, Assessment, and Treatment. Laurel, MD, RAMSCO, 1982.

Erikson EH. Identity, Youth, and Crisis. New York, WW Norton, 1968.

Fagard J. Development of bi-manual coordination. In Bard C, Fleury M, Hays L (eds). Development of Eye-Hand Coordination Across the Life Span. Columbia, SC, University of South Carolina Press, 1990, pp 262–282.

Folio M, Fewell R. Peabody Developmental Motor Scales and Activity Cards. Allen, TX, DLM Teaching Resources, 1983.

Ford-Smith CD, VanSant AF. Age differences in movement patterns used to rise from a bed in the third through fifth decades of age. Phys Ther 73:300–307, 1993.

Gesell A. The First Five Years of Life. New York, Harper & Brothers, 1940.

Gesell A, Ilg FL, Ames LB, et al. Infant and Child in the Culture of Today, rev. New York, Harper & Row, 1974.

Green LN. The relationship between activity level and the movement pattern of supine to standing. Unpublished masters' thesis, Kansas State University, 1989.

Larsson L. Aging in mammalian skeletal muscle. In Mortimer JA (ed). The Aging Motor System. New York, Praeger, 1982, pp 60–97.

Levine MD. Developmental Variation and Learning Disorders. Toronto, Educators Publishing Service, 1987, pp 68–136, 208–345, 472.

Levinson DJ. A conception of adult development. Am Psychol 41:3–13, 1986.

Lewis CB. Aging: The Health Care Challenge, 2nd ed. Philadelphia, FA Davis, 1990.

Long TM, Cintas HL. Handbook of Pediatric Therapy. Baltimore, Williams & Wilkins, 1995.

Lowrey GH. Growth and Development of Children, 8th ed. Chicago, Year Book, 1986.

Luehring SK. Component movement patterns of two groups of older adults in the task of rising to standing from the floor. Unpublished masters' thesis, Virginia Commonwealth University, 1989.

Malina RM, Bouchard C. Growth, Maturation and Physical Activity. Champaign, IL, Human Kinetics Books, 1991.

Martin, T. Normal development of movement and function: neonate, infant, and toddler. In Scully RM, Barnes MR (eds). Physical Therapy. Philadelphia, JB Lippincott, 1989, pp 63–82.

Maslow A. Motivation and Personality. New York, Harper & Row, 1954.

Meyers AW, Whelan JP, Murphy SM. Cognitive behavioral strategies in athletic performance enhancement. Prog Behav Modif 30:137–164, 1996.

Moncur C. Posture in the older adult. In Guccione AA (ed). Geriatric Physical Therapy. St. Louis, Mosby, 1993, pp 219–236.

Murray EA. Hemispheric specialization. In Fisher A, Murray EA, Bundy AC (eds). Sensory Integration Theory and Practice. Philadelphia, FA Davis, 1991.

Olney SJ, Culham EG. Changes in posture and gait. In Pickles B, Compton A, Cott C, et al (eds). Physiotherapy with Older People. London, WB Saunders, 1995, pp 81–94.

Piaget J. Origins of Intelligence. New York, International University Press, 1952.

Porter RE. Normal development of movement and function: child and adolescent. In Scully RM, Barnes ML (eds). Physical Therapy. Philadelphia, JB Lippincott, 1989, pp 83–98.

Roberton M, Halverson L. The developing child: his changing movement. In Logsdon BJ (ed). Physical Education for Children: A Focus on the Teaching Process. Philadelphia, Lea & Febiger, 1977.

Sabourin P. Rising from supine to standing: a study of adolescents. Unpublished masters' thesis, Virginia Commonwealth University, 1989.

Sheldon JH. The effect of age on the control of sway. Gerontol Clin 5:129–138, 1963.

Stott DH, Moyes FA, Henderson SE. The Henderson Revision of The Test of Motor Impairment. San Antonio, TX, Psychological Corporation, 1984.

Stout JL. Gait: Development and analysis. In Campbell SK (ed). Physical Therapy for Children. Philadelphia, WB Saunders, 1994, pp 79–104.

Sutherland DH, Olshen RA, Biden EN, Wyatt MP. The Development of Mature Walking. London, MacKeith Press, 1988.

Thelen E. Rhythmical stereotypies in infants. Anim Behav 27:699–715, 1979.

Thomas RL, Williams AK, Lundy-Ekman L. Supine to stand in elderly persons: relationship to age, activity level, strength, and range of motion. Issues Aging 21:9–18, 1998.

Vandervoort AA. Biological and physiological changes. In Pickles B, Compton A, Cott, C, et al (eds). Physiotherapy with Older People. London, WB Saunders, 1995, pp 67–80.

Vandervoort AA, Vramer JF, Wharram ER. Eccentric knee strength of elderly females. J Gerontol 45:B125–B128, 1990.

VanSant AF. Age differences in movement patterns used by children to rise from a supine position to erect stance. Phys Ther 68:1130–1138, 1988a.

VanSant AF. Rising from a supine position to erect stance: description of adult movement and a developmental hypothesis. Phys Ther 68:185–192, 1988b.

VanSant AF. Life-span motor development. In Lister MJ (ed). Contemporary Management of Motor Control Problems: Proceedings of the II Step Conference. Alexandria, VA, American Physical Therapy Association, 1991, pp 77–84.

VanSant AF. Development of posture. In Cech D, Martin S (eds). Functional Movement Development Across the Life Span. Philadelphia, WB Saunders, 1995, pp 275–294.

Walker JM, Breau L, McNeill D, et al. Hazardous baby walkers: a survey of use. Pediatr Phys Ther 8:25–30, 1996.

Wang Y, Morgan WP. The effect of imagery perspectives on the psychophysiological responses to imagined exercise. Behav Brain Res 52:1667–1674, 1992.

Wellman BL. Motor achievements of preschool children. Child Educ 13:311–316, 1937. In Espanschade AS, Eckert HM (eds). Motor Development. Columbus, OH, Charles E. Merrill, 1967.

Whitall J. A developmental study of the inter-limb coordination in running and galloping. J Motor Behav 21:409–428, 1989.

Wickstrom RL. Fundamental Movement Patterns, 2nd ed. Philadelphia, Lea & Febiger, 1977.

Wickstrom RL. Fundamental Movement Patterns, 3rd ed. Philadelphia, Lea & Febiger, 1983.

Winter DA, Patla AE, Frank JS et al. Biomechanical walking pattern changes in the fit and healthy elderly. Phys Ther 70:340–348, 1990.

Woollacott M. Postural control mechanisms in the young and old. In Duncan P (ed). Balance: Proceedings of the APTA Forum. Alexandria, VA, American Physical Therapy Association, 1990, pp 23–28.

SECTION 2

ADULTS

CHAPTER 5

Cerebrovascular Accidents

OBJECTIVES

After reading this chapter, the student will be able to

1. Understand the etiology and clinical manifestations of stroke.
2. Identify common complications seen in patients who have sustained cerebrovascular accidents.
3. Understand the role of the physical therapist assistant in the treatment of patients with stroke.
4. Describe appropriate treatment interventions for patients who have experienced strokes.
5. Recognize the importance of functional training for patients who have had strokes.

INTRODUCTION

Cerebrovascular accidents (CVAs), or *strokes* as they are more commonly called, are the most common and disabling neurologic condition of adult life. The National Stroke Association estimates that 4 million Americans are living with the effects of stroke, and 700,000 new CVAs occur annually. CVAs continue to be the third leading cause of death in the United States. The mortality rate for individuals with acute CVA in the United States is 26.7%, or approximately 160,000 patients. With improvements in medical management and reductions in predisposing risk factors, mortality rates for this condition had declined. Unfortunately, in 1993, the mortality rate following CVA increased for the first time in 40 years. Although no clear explanation exists for this increase, one possible hypothesis suggests that improved diagnostic tools are allowing physicians to more accurately identify stroke as a contributing factor in patients' deaths. In addition, a higher rate of noncompliance associated with antihypertensive medications may explain the increase (National Stroke Association, 1998).

Definition. A *cerebrovascular accident* may be defined as the sudden onset of neurologic signs and symptoms resulting from a disturbance of blood supply to the brain. The onset of the symptoms provides the physician with information regarding the vascular origin of the condition. The individual who sustains a CVA may have temporary or permanent loss of function as a result of injury to brain tissue.

ETIOLOGY

The two major types of CVAs are ischemic and hemorrhagic. Approximately 70% of all CVAs are due to ischemia, 20% are due to hemorrhage, and the remaining 10% have an unspecified origin (Ryerson, 1995).

Ischemic Cerebrovascular Accidents

Ischemia implies hypoxia or decreased oxygenation to the brain tissue as a result of poor blood supply. Ischemic strokes can be subdivided into two major categories, those that result from thrombosis and those that result from an embolus.

Thrombotic CVAs are most frequently a consequence of atherosclerosis. In atherosclerosis, the lumen (opening) of the artery decreases in size as plaque is deposited within the vessel walls. As a result, blood flow through the vessel is reduced, thereby limiting the amount of oxygen that is able to reach cerebral tissues. If an atherosclerotic deposit completely occludes the vessel, the tissue supplied by the artery will undergo death or cerebral infarction. A *cerebral infarct* is defined as the actual death of a portion of the brain.

CVAs of *embolic* origin are frequently associated with cardiovascular disease, specifically atrial fibrillation, myocardial infarction, or valvular disease. In embolic CVAs, a blood clot breaks away from the intima, or inner lining of the artery, and is carried to the brain. The embolus can lodge in a cerebral blood vessel, occlude it, and consequently cause death or infarction of cerebral tissue. Cell death occurs when blood flow remains below 12 mL/100 g of tissue per minute (Fuller, 1998). Once neuronal death has occurred, the cells that comprise the tissue have no opportunity to regenerate or replace themselves.

The area surrounding the infarcted cerebral tissue is called the *ischemic penumbra*. Neurons in this area are vulnerable to injury because cerebral blood flow is estimated to be approximately 20 to 50% of normal. Changes to neurotransmitters are believed to cause further injury after the ischemic insult. *Glutamate,* is a neurotransmitter present throughout the central nervous system (CNS) and stored at synaptic terminals. The amount released at the synapse is regulated so that the level of glutamate is minimal. However, following an ischemic injury, the cells that control glutamate levels are compromised, a condition that leads to overstimulation of postsynaptic receptors. Calcium ions are able to enter brain cells and to propagate cellular destruction. Various destructive enzymes and free radicals (neurotoxic byproducts) are activated by these calcium ions, and this process leads to additional damage. As a consequence of these events, brain injury may extend beyond the initial site of infarction (Fuller, 1998; National Stroke Association, 1998).

Hemorrhagic Cerebrovascular Accidents

Hemorrhagic strokes, including those that are caused by intracerebral and subarachnoid hemorrhage, arteriovenous malformation, and lacunar infarcts, result from abnormal bleeding from rupture of a cerebral vessel. The incidence of *intracerebral hemorrhage* is low among persons less than 45 years old and increases after age 65. Common causes of spontaneous intracerebral hemorrhage include vessel malformation and changes in the integrity of cerebral vessels brought on by the effects of hypertension and aging (Fuller, 1998).

Subarachnoid hemorrhages are a consequence of bleeding into the subarachnoid space. The subarachnoid space is located under the arachnoid membrane and above the pia mater. *Aneurysm,* a ballooning or outpouching of a vessel wall, and vascular malformations are the primary causes of subarachnoid hemorrhages. These types of conditions tend to weaken the vasculature and can lead to rupture. Approximately 90% of subarachnoid hemorrhages are due to berry aneurysms. A *berry aneurysm* is a congenital defect of a cerebral artery in which the vessel is abnormally dilated at a bifurcation (Fuller, 1998).

Arteriovenous malformations are congenital anomalies that affect the circulation in the brain. In arteriovenous malformations, the arteries and veins communicate directly (Fuller, 1998). Blood vessels become dilated and form masses within the brain (Ryerson, 1995). These defects weaken the blood vessels, which, in time, can rupture and cause a CVA.

Transient Ischemic Attacks

CVAs are not to be confused with *transient ischemic attacks* (TIAs), which also occur in many individuals. A TIA indicates that a patient has atherosclerosis or plaque formation within the cerebral vasculature. When a patient experiences a TIA, the blood supply to the brain is temporarily interrupted. The patient complains of neurologic dysfunction, including loss of motor, sensory, or speech function. These deficits, however, completely resolve within 24 hours. The patient does not experience any residual brain damage or neurologic dysfunction. Recurrent TIAs indicate thrombotic disease and may suggest that an individual is at increased risk for stroke (Roth and Harvey, 1996).

MEDICAL INTERVENTION

Diagnosis

Medical management of a patient who has had a stroke includes hospitalization to determine the cause of the infarct. The physician completes a physical examination to evaluate motor, sensory, speech, and reflex function. Subjective information received from the patient or a family member regarding the onset of symptoms is also important. Neuroimaging by either a computed tomographic scan or a magnetic resonance image is performed to determine whether the CVA is the result of ischemic or hemorrhagic injury. However, computed tomographic scans that are performed initially do not always show small lesions and may not be able to detect an acute embolic CVA (Fuller, 1998; Levine, 1987). The damaged cerebral tissue may not be apparent until 7 days after the insult. Surgical management by means of hematoma evacuation may be appropriate for those patients who are diagnosed with a blood clot or hemorrhage (Levine, 1987).

Acute Medical Management

Acute care management consists of monitoring the patient's neurologic function and preventing the development of secondary complications. Regulation of the patient's blood pressure, intracranial pressure, and blood glucose levels is recommended. Pharmacologic interventions may also be prescribed. Heparin, calcium channel blockers, and thrombolytic and neuroprotective agents can be administered to improve blood flow and to minimize tissue damage (Roth and Harvey, 1996). Thrombolytic medications such as tissue plasminogen activator (tPA) can decrease the effects of neurologic damage when these agents are administered to patients within 3 hours of the event. Neuroprotective agents minimize tissue damage when adequate blood supply does not exist. Medications that modify glutamate release or enhance recovery from calcium overload may show promise. Clinical trials will continue to determine whether these drugs will be effective for patients with acute CVA (Fuller, 1998; National Stroke Association, 1998).

RECOVERY FROM STROKE

Many survivors of CVA sustain permanent neurologic disability and are unable to resume previous social roles and functions (Roth and Harvey, 1996). Interventions administered during the first 6 to 18 months after the insult are believed to be the most beneficial (Fuller, 1998). General recovery guidelines estimate that 10% of the individuals who have a CVA recover almost completely, 25% have mild impairments, 40% experience moderate to severe impairments, 10% require placement in an extended care facility, and 15% die shortly after the incident (National Stroke Association, 1998). Specific data regarding functional outcome following CVA vary. Data obtained from the Framingham Heart Study indicated that 69% of individuals who had a stroke were independent in activities of daily living, 80% were independent in functional mobility tasks, and 84% had returned home. Despite independence in self-care and functional mobility skills, 71% of the study subjects had decreased vocational function, 62% had reduced opportunities for socialization in the community, and 16% were institutionalized (Ross and Harvey, 1996; National Stroke Association, 1998). Data obtained from the Functional Independence Measure suggest that patients who receive rehabilitation for approximately 28 days after their stroke exhibit the greatest improvements in walking, transfers, self-care, and sphincter control. Less dramatic improvements are noted in the areas of communication and social skills (Granger and Hamilton, 1992).

PREVENTION OF CEREBROVASCULAR ACCIDENTS

Although progress has been made in the medical management of patients after CVA, more attention has been given to the area of prevention. Individuals can reduce their risk of stroke by recognizing the risk factors associated with the condition. The two primary preventable risk factors for the development of CVA are hypertension and heart disease. Hypertension increases the risk of stoke four- to sixfold. Other risk factors that have been discussed in the literature include hyperlipidemia, cigarette smoking, a history of prior CVAs or TIAs, gender (males have a slightly higher risk), race (African Americans have a higher risk for stroke than most other racial groups), family history, alcohol consumption, physical inactivity, obesity, the use of oral contraceptives, and age (Kelly-Hayes, 1991). The risk of stroke doubles with each decade after age 55 (National Stroke Association, 1998). A review of these risk factors reveals that many of them are directly related to an individual's lifestyle and are potentially preventable or modifiable.

Unfortunately, most individuals do not recognize that strokes are preventable and that treatment interventions are available. The average person who experiences a CVA waits more than 12 hours before seeking medical treatment. The window of opportunity for some medications that enhance patient outcome is exceeded within this time frame. In an effort to reeducate the public, support to rename CVA as a *brain attack* is growing. Individuals are being encouraged to activate the emergency medical system once they recognize the onset of symptoms. It is hoped that this view (similar to that used following myocardial infarction) will lead to earlier entry to the medical system and improved outcomes for individuals who have had a CVA (National Stroke Association, 1998).

STROKE SYNDROMES

To understand the clinical manifestations seen in an individual who has sustained a stroke, it is necessary to know the structure and function of the various parts of the brain, as well as the circulation. A review of this information can be found in Chapter 2. Because of the distribution of the cerebral circulation to various parts of the cortex and brain stem, a blockage or hemorrhage in one of the vessels results in predictable clinical findings. Individual differences do occur, however. Table 5–1 provides a review of common stroke syndromes.

Anterior Cerebral Artery Occlusion

A blockage in the anterior cerebral artery is uncommon and is most frequently caused by an embolus (Fuller, 1998). The anterior cerebral artery supplies the superior border of the frontal and parietal lobes of the brain. A CVA in this distribution results in contralateral weakness and sensory loss, primarily in the lower extremity; aphasia; incontinence; and, in patients with severe infarcts, significant memory and behavioral deficits.

Table 5-1 ❚ CEREBRAL CIRCULATION AND
RESULTANT STROKE SYNDROMES

ARTERY	DISTRIBUTION	PATIENT DEFICITS
Anterior cerebral	Supplies the superior border of the frontal and parietal lobes	Contralateral weakness and sensory loss primarily in the lower extremity, incontinence, aphasia, memory and behavioral deficits
Middle cerebral	Supplies the surface of the cerebral hemispheres and the deep frontal and parietal lobes	Contralateral sensory loss and weakness in the face and upper extremity, less involvement in the lower extremity, homonymous hemianopia
Vertebrobasilar	Supplies the brain stem and cerebellum	Cranial nerve involvement (diplopia, dysphagia, dysarthria, deafness, vertigo) ataxia, equilibrium disturbances, headaches, and dizziness
Posterior cerebral	Supplies the occipital and temporal lobes, thalamus, and upper brain stem	Contralateral sensory loss, thalamic pain syndrome, homonymous hemianopia, visual agnosia, and cortical blindness

Middle Cerebral Artery Occlusion

Middle cerebral artery infarcts, which are the most common type of CVAs, can result in contralateral sensory loss and weakness in the face and upper extremity. Patients with middle cerebral artery infarcts often present with less involvement in the lower extremity. Infarction of the dominant hemisphere can lead to global aphasia. *Homonymous hemianopia,* which is a defect or a loss of vision in the temporal half of one visual field and the nasal portion of the other, may be evident. A patient may also experience a loss of *conjugate eye gaze,* which is the movement of the eyes in parallel.

Vertebrobasilar Artery Occlusion

Complete occlusion of the vertebrobasilar artery is often fatal. Cranial nerve involvement including *diplopia* (double vision), *dysphagia* (difficulty in swallowing), *dysarthria* (difficulty in forming words secondary to weakness in the tongue and muscles of the face), *deafness,* and *vertigo* (dizziness) may be present. In addition, infarcts to areas supplied by this vascular distribution may lead to *ataxia,* which is characterized by uncoordinated movement, equilibrium deficits, and headaches.

Blockage of the basilar artery can cause the patient to experience a *locked-in syndrome.* Patients with this type of stroke are severely involved. The patient is alert and oriented but is unable to move or speak because of weakness in all muscle groups. Vertical eye movements are the only type of active movement possible and thus become the patient's primary means of communication (Roth and Harvey, 1996).

Posterior Artery Occlusion

The posterior cerebral artery supplies the occipital and temporal lobes. Occlusion in this artery can lead to contralateral sensory loss; pain; memory deficits; homonymous hemianopia; *visual agnosia,* which is an inability to recognize familiar objects or individuals; and *cortical blindness,* which is the inability to process incoming visual information even though the optic nerve remains intact.

Lacunar Infarcts

Lacunar infarcts are most often encountered in the deep regions of the brain, including the internal capsule, thalamus, basal ganglia, and pons. The term *lacuna* is used because a cystic cavity remains after the infarcted tissue is removed. These infarcts are common in individuals with diabetes and hypertension and result from small vessel arteriolar disease. Clinical findings can include contralateral weakness and sensory loss, ataxia, and dysarthria.

Other Stroke Syndromes

Other stroke syndromes occur in patients. The neurologic impairments are closely related to the area of the brain affected. For example, a CVA within the parietal lobe can cause inattention or *neglect,* which is manifested as a disregard for the involved side of the body; an impaired perception of vertical, visual, spatial, and topographic relationships; and motor perseveration. *Perseveration* is the involuntary persistence of the same verbal or motor response regardless of the stimulus or its duration. Patients who demonstrate perseveration may repeat the same word or movement over and over. It is often difficult to redirect these patients to a new idea or activity.

The resultant patient findings also depend on the hemisphere of the brain affected. To review information covered in Chapter 2, the left hemisphere of the brain is the verbal and analytic side. The left hemisphere allows individuals to process information sequentially and to observe detail. Speech and reading comprehension are also functions of the left hemisphere. The right hemisphere of the brain tends to be the more artistic hemisphere. The ability to look at information holistically, to process nonverbal information, to perceive emotions, and to be aware of body image are all functions of the right hemisphere (O'Sullivan, 1994b).

Thalamic Pain Syndrome

Thalamic pain syndrome can occur following an infarction or hemorrhage in the lateral thalamus, the posterior limb of the internal capsule, or the parietal lobe. The patient experiences intolerable burning pain and sensory perseveration. The sensation of the stimulus remains long after the stimulus has been removed or terminated. The patient also perceives the sensation as noxious and exaggerated.

Pusher Syndrome

Patients with right CVAs and resultant left hemiplegia may demonstrate the *pusher syndrome*. This syndrome is characterized by uniform problems, including (1) cervical rotation and lateral flexion to the right, (2) absent or significantly impaired tactile and kinesthetic awareness, (3) visual deficits, (4) truncal asymmetries, (5) increased weight bearing on the left during sitting activities with resistance encountered when attempts are made to achieve an equal weight-bearing position, and (6) difficulties with transfers as the patient pushes backward and away with the right (uninvolved) extremities (Davies, 1985). Specific treatment interventions for patients with this syndrome are discussed later in the chapter.

In summary, although a description of the different stroke syndromes and a classification system for right and left hemisphere disorders have been provided, each patient may present with different clinical signs and symptoms. Patients should be viewed and treated as individuals and should not be classified on the basis of which side of the body is exhibiting difficulties. The information presented regarding the functional differences between the right and left hemispheres is meant only to serve as a guide or framework in which treatment interventions may be selected.

CLINICAL FINDINGS: PATIENT IMPAIRMENTS

A patient who has sustained a CVA may present with a number of different impairments. The extent to which these impairments interfere with the patient's functional abilities depends on the nature of the stroke and the amount of nervous tissue damaged. In addition, any preexisting medical conditions, the amount of family support available, and financial resources may ultimately affect the patient's outcome.

Motor Impairments

One of the primary clinical manifestations in patients following stroke is the spectrum of motor problems resulting from damage to the motor cortex. Initially, a patient may present with a state of low muscle tone or flaccidity. *Flaccid* muscles lack the ability to generate muscle contractions and to initiate movement. This condition of relative low muscle tone is usually transient, and the patient soon develops characteristic patterns of hypertonicity or spasticity. *Spasticity* is a motor disorder characterized by exaggerated deep tendon reflexes and increased muscle tone. Clinically, the patient with spasticity presents with increased resistance to passive stretching of the involved muscle, hyperreflexia of deep tendon reflexes, posturing of the extremities in flexion or extension, co-contraction of muscles, and stereotypical movement patterns called *synergies*.

Spasticity

Theories on the development of spasticity have been evolving as research in the area of motor behavior has increased. The classic theory of spasticity development centers around the idea that spasticity develops in response to an upper motor neuron injury. This view of spasticity incorporates a hierarchic view of the nervous system and the development of motor control and movement. Investigators had previously postulated that spasticity develops from hyperexcitability of the monosynaptic stretch reflex. This theory is based on muscle spindle physiology. Increased output from the muscle spindle afferents or sensory receptors controls alpha motor neuron activity in the gray matter of the spinal cord. Uninterrupted activity of the gamma efferent or motor system is believed to account for continuous activation of the afferent system by maintaining the muscle spindle's sensitivity to stretch (Craik, 1991).

Research raises questions regarding the validity of this theory. Investigators have postulated that the stretch reflex is not strong enough to control all alpha motor neuron activity. In today's view of spasticity, hypertonicity or increased muscle tone is believed to develop from abnormal processing of the afferent (sensory) input after the stimulus reaches the spinal cord. In addition, investigators have proposed that a defect in inhibitory modulation from higher cortical centers and spinal interneuron pathways leads to the presence of spasticity in many patients (Craik, 1991).

Assessment of Tone

The Modified Ashworth scale is a clinical tool used to assess the presence of abnormal tone. A 0 to 4 ordinal scale is used. A score of 0 equates to no increase in muscle tone, whereas a score of 4 indicates that the affected area is fixed in either flexion or extension (Bohannon and Smith, 1987). Table 5–2 describes each of the grades.

Brunnstrom Stages of Motor Recovery

Signe Brunnstrom did much to describe the characteristic stages of motor recovery following stroke. Brunnstrom observed many patients who had sustained CVAs and noted a characteristic pattern of muscle tone development and recovery (Sawner and LaVigne, 1992). Table 5–3 gives a description of each of the Brunnstrom stages of recovery.

Brunnstrom reported that, initially, the patient experienced flaccidity in involved muscle groups. As the patient recovered, flaccidity was replaced by the development of spasticity. Spasticity increased and reached its peak in stage 3. At this time, the patient's attempts at voluntary movements were limited to the flexion and extension synergies (Sawner and LaVigne, 1992).

A *synergy* is defined as a group of muscles that work together to provide patterns of movements. These patterns initially occur in flexion and extension combinations. The movements produced are stereotypical and primitive and can be elicited either reflexively or as a volitional movement response. Flexion and extension synergies have been described for both the upper and lower extremities (Sawner and LaVigne, 1992). Table 5–4 provides a description of the upper and lower extremity flexion and extension patterns.

In the later stages of Brunnstrom's recovery patterns, spasticity begins to decline, and the patient's movements are dominated to a lesser degree by the

Table 5–3 ▌ BRUNNSTROM STAGES OF RECOVERY

STAGE	DESCRIPTION
I. Flaccidity	No voluntary or reflex activity is present in the involved extremity.
II. Spasticity begins to develop	Synergy patterns begin to develop. Some of the synergy components may appear as associated reactions.
III. Spasticity increases and reaches its peak	Movement synergies of the involved upper or lower extremity can be performed voluntarily.
IV. Spasticity begins to decrease	Deviation from the movement synergies is possible. Limited combinations of movement may be evident.
V. Spasticity continues to decrease	Movement synergies are less dominant. More complex combinations of movements are possible.
VI. Spasticity is essentially absent	Isolated movements and combinations of movements are evident. Coordination deficits may be present with rapid activities.
VII. Return to normal function	Return of fine motor skills.

Modified from Sawner KA, LaVigne JM. Brunnstrom's Movement Therapy in Hemiplegia, 2nd ed. Philadelphia, JB Lippincott, 1992, pp 41–42.

synergy patterns. An individual may be able to combine movements in both the flexion and extension patterns and may have more voluntary control of movement components. In the final stages of recovery, spasticity continues to decrease, and isolated movement is possible. The patient is able to control speed and direction of movement with increased ease, and fine motor skills improve. Brunnstrom reported that a patient would pass through all these stages and would not skip a stage. However, variability in a patient's clinical presentation at any stage is possible. The patient may, in fact, move through a stage quickly, and thus observation of its typical characteristics may be difficult. Brunnstrom also postulated that a patient could experience a plateau at any stage, and consequently full recovery would not be possible (Sawner and LaVigne, 1992). As mentioned previously, each patient is unique and progresses through the stages at different rates. Therefore, a patient's long-term prognosis and functional outcome are difficult to predict in the early stages of rehabilitation.

Development of Spasticity in Proximal Muscle Groups

Spasticity often initially develops in the shoulder and pelvic girdles. At the shoulder, one can see adduction and downward rotation of the scapula. The scapular depressors, as well as the shoulder adductors and internal rotators, can develop muscle stiffness. As upper extremity muscle tone increases, tone in the biceps, forearm pronators, and wrist and finger flexors may become evident. This pattern of tone produces

Table 5–2 ▌ MODIFIED ASHWORTH SCALE FOR GRADING SPASTICITY

GRADE	DESCRIPTION
0	No increase in muscle tone
1	Slight increase in muscle tone, manifested by a catch and release or by minimal resistance at the end of the range of motion when the affected part is moved in flexion or extension
1+	Slight increase in muscle tone, manifested by a catch, followed by minimal resistance throughout the remainder (less than half) of the range of motion
2	More marked increase in muscle tone through most of the range of motion, but affected part easily moved
3	Considerable increase in muscle tone, passive movement difficult
4	Affected part rigid in flexion or extension

From Bohannon RW, Smith MB. Interrater reliability of a modified Ashworth scale of muscle spasticity. Phys Ther 67:207, 1987, with permission of the APTA.

Table 5–4 ▌ COMPONENTS OF THE BRUNNSTROM SYNERGY PATTERNS

	FLEXION	EXTENSION
Upper extremity	Scapular retraction and/or elevation, shoulder external rotation, shoulder abduction to 90 degrees, elbow flexion, forearm supination, wrist and finger flexion	Scapular protraction, shoulder internal rotation, shoulder adduction, full elbow extension, forearm pronation, wrist extension with finger flexion
Lower extremity	Hip flexion, abduction and external rotation, knee flexion to approximately 90 degrees, ankle dorsiflexion and inversion, toe extension	Hip extension, adduction, and internal rotation, knee extension, ankle plantar flexion and inversion, toe flexion

the characteristic upper extremity posturing seen in patients who have sustained CVAs. Figure 5–1 illustrates this positioning.

Anterior tilting or hiking is common at the pelvis. The pelvic retractors, hip adductors, and hip internal rotators can develop spasticity. Additionally, the knee extensors or quadriceps, the ankle plantar flexors and supinators, and the toe flexors can become hypertonic. This pattern of abnormal tone development produces the characteristic lower extremity extensor posturing seen in many patients. As the patient attempts to initiate movement, the presence of abnormal tone and synergies can lead to the characteristic flexion and extension movement patterns.

Other Motor Impairments

Additional motor problems can become evident in this patient population. The impact of muscle weakness or *paresis* is beginning to receive new emphasis in the literature. Patients who have sustained a stroke are often unable to generate normal levels of muscular force, tension, or torque to initiate and control movements or to maintain a posture. After a stroke, patients may have difficulty in maintaining a constant

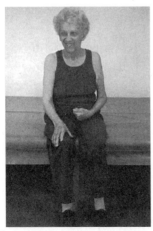

Figure 5–1 ■ Characteristic upper extremity posturing seen in patients following cerebrovascular accident. The patient presents with increased tone in the shoulder adductors and internal rotators, biceps, forearm pronators, and wrist and finger flexors. (From Ryerson S, Levit K. Functional Movement Reeducation: A Contemporary Model for Stroke Rehabilitation. New York, Churchill Livingstone, 1997.)

level of force production to control movements of the extremities. Atrophy of remaining muscle fibers on the involved side and motor units that are more easily fatigued are two common findings (Craik, 1991; Light, 1991). Research has suggested that the muscles controlling grip strength and the wrist and finger flexors are the most severely affected muscle groups following a stroke. This finding does not support what many investigators believed previously, that upper extremity extensors and lower extremity flexors were the weakest muscle groups following a stroke. Actually, the elbow extensors and the shoulder abductors and adductors are the least severely affected muscles in patients who have sustained CVAs. One additional point that must be made is that a stroke does not affect only one side of the body. The muscles on the uninvolved side can also exhibit weakness following the injury (Craik, 1991).

Motor Planning Deficits

Motor problems may be present in patients who have sustained a stroke. These problems are most frequently noted in patients with involvement of the left hemisphere because of its primary role in the sequencing of movements. Patients can exhibit difficulty in performing purposeful movements, although no sensory or motor impairments are noted. This condition is called *apraxia*. Patients with apraxia may have the motor capabilities to perform a specific movement combination such as a sit-to-stand transfer, but they are unable to determine or remember the steps necessary to achieve this movement goal. Apraxia may also be evident when the patient performs self-care activities. For example, the patient may not remember how to put on a piece of clothing or what to do with an item such as a comb or brush.

Sensory Impairments

Sensory deficits can also cause the patient many difficulties. Patients who sustain strokes of the parietal lobe may demonstrate sensory dysfunction. Individuals may lose their tactile (touch) or proprioceptive capabilities. *Proprioception* is defined as the patient's ability to perceive position sense. The way in which the physical therapist evaluates a patient's proprioception is to move a patient's joint quickly in a certain direction. Up-and-down movement is most frequently used. With eyes closed, the patient is asked to identify the position of the joint. Accuracy and speed of response are used to determine whether proprioception is intact, impaired, or absent. Many patients with CVAs tend to present with partial impairments, as opposed to total loss of sensory perception. A patient who experiences impaired sensation or sensory feedback can also lose the ability to control and coordinate movement. These sensory problems can affect the patient's perception of being upright while sitting and standing and can lead to difficulties in weight shifting, sequencing motor responses, and eye-hand coordination.

Communication Impairments

Infarcts in the frontal and temporal lobes of the brain can lead to specific communication deficits. *Aphasia* is an acquired communication disorder caused by brain damage and is characterized by impairment of language comprehension, oral expression, and the use of symbols to communicate ideas (Roth and Harvey, 1996). Several different types of aphasia are recognized. Patients can present with an expressive disorder called *Broca's aphasia,* a receptive aphasia called *Wernicke's aphasia,* or a combination of both expressive and receptive deficits termed *global aphasia.* Patients with expressive aphasia have difficulty in speaking. These patients know what they want to say but are unable to form the words to communicate their ideas or needs. Individuals with expressive aphasia frequently become frustrated when they are unable to articulate their wants and needs verbally. Patients with receptive aphasia do not understand the spoken word. When you are talking with a patient with receptive aphasia, the patient will not understand what you are trying to say or may misinterpret your remarks. Working with these patients can be challenging because you will not be able to rely on verbal instructions to direct activity performance. Patients with global aphasia have severe expressive and receptive dysfunction. Individuals with global aphasia do not comprehend spoken words and are unable to verbalize their needs. Frequently, these individuals also have difficulties in understanding gestures that may have communicative meaning. Developing a rapport with the patient and trying to establish some method of communicating basic needs can be challenging. Time and patience are needed so the patient will begin to trust the physical therapist assistant and a relationship can develop. The assistant should also seek advice from the speech-language pathologist to implement an effective communication system for the patient.

Other Communication Deficits

Other communicative deficits include dysarthria and emotional lability. *Dysarthria* is a condition in which the patient has difficulty in articulating words as a result of weakness and inability to control the muscles associated with speech production. *Emotional lability* may be evident in patients who have sustained right hemispheric infarcts. These patients exhibit difficulties in controlling emotions. A patient who is emotionally labile may cry or laugh inappropriately without cause. The patient is often unable to inhibit the emergence of these spontaneous emotions.

Orofacial Deficits

A patient's orofacial function may also be affected by the CVA. These deficits are often associated with cranial nerve involvement, which can occur with CVAs of the brain stem or midbrain region. Frequent findings include facial asymmetries resulting from weakness in the facial muscles, muscles of the eye, and muscles around the mouth. Weakness of the facial muscles can affect the patient's ability to interact with individuals in the environment. The inability to smile, frown, or initiate other facial expressions such as anger or displeasure affects a person's ability to use body language as an adjunct to verbal communication. Inadequate lip closure can lead to problems with control of saliva and fluids during drinking. Weakness of the muscles that innervate the eye can lead to drooping or ptosis of the eyelid. The patient may also be unable to close the eye to assist with lubrication.

Orofacial dysfunction can be manifested in a patient's difficulty or inability to swallow foods and liquids, also known as *dysphagia.* Dysphagia can result from muscle weakness, inadequate motor planning capabilities, and poor tongue control. Patients with dysphagia may be unable to move food from the front of the mouth to the sides for chewing and back to the midline for swallowing. Many of these patients present with pocketing of food within their oral cavities.

A final problem seen in patients with orofacial dysfunction is poor coordination between eating and breathing. Such difficulty can lead to poor nutrition and possible aspiration of food into the lungs. Aspiration frequently leads to pneumonia and other respiratory complications including *atelectasis* (collapse of a part of the lung tissue).

Respiratory Impairments

Lung expansion may be decreased following a CVA because of decreased control of the muscles of respiration, specifically the diaphragm. A stroke can affect the diaphragm just as it can affect any other muscle in the body. Hemiparesis of the diaphragm or external intercostal muscles may be apparent and can affect the individual's ability to expand the lungs. Poor lung expansion leads to a decrease in an individual's vital capacity. Therefore, to meet the oxygen demands of the body, the patient is forced to increase the respiration rate. Pulmonary complications including pneumonia and atelectasis may develop if shallow breathing continues. Lack of lateral basilar expansion can also lead to the foregoing pulmonary complications. Cough effectiveness may be impaired secondary to weakness in the abdominal muscles.

Lung volumes are decreased by approximately 30 to 40% in patients who have had a stroke (Watchie, 1994). Patient inactivity also reduces cardiopulmonary conditioning and adversely affects the oxygen transport system (Dean, 1996). Oxygen consumption is increased, leading to muscle and cardiopulmonary fatigue. Fatigue is a major complaint among these patients. Patients frequently ask to rest or stay in bed instead of participating in physical therapy. Although it is necessary to monitor the patient's cardiovascular and pulmonary responses, the patient and family should be advised that participation in exercise and functional activities will improve the patient's tolerance for activity.

Reflex Activity

Primitive spinal and brain stem reflexes may appear following a stroke. Both types of reflexes are present at birth or during infancy and become integrated by the CNS as the child ages, usually within the first 4 months of life. Once integrated, these reflexes are not present in their pure forms. They do, however, continue to exist as underlying components of volitional movement patterns. In adults, it is possible for these primitive reflexes to be seen again when the CNS is damaged or an individual is experiencing extreme fatigue or stress.

Spinal Reflexes

Spinal level reflexes occur at the spinal cord level and result in overt movement of a limb. Frequently, these reflexes are facilitated by a noxious stimulus applied to the patient. Table 5–5 provides a list of the most common spinal level reflexes seen in patients with CNS dysfunction. Family members must be instructed about the true meaning of these reflexes. The presence of a spinal level reflex such as a flexor withdrawal does not indicate that the patient is demonstrating volitional (voluntary) movement. These reflexive movements often occur when a patient is relatively unresponsive. For example, if a caregiver inadvertently stimulates the patient's foot, the patient may flex the involved lower extremity. This does not, however, mean that the patient is demonstrating conscious control of the leg.

Deep Tendon Reflexes

Patients who have experienced a stroke may also present with altered deep tendon reflexes. *Deep tendon reflexes* are stretch reflexes that can be elicited by striking the muscle tendon with a reflex hammer or the examiner's fingers. Common reflexes assessed include the biceps, brachioradialis, triceps, quadriceps/patellar, and gastrocnemius-soleus/Achilles. The patient's response to the tendon tap is assessed on a 0 to 4 scale: 0, no response; 1, minimal response; 2, normal response; 3, hyperactive response; and 4, clonus. Evaluation of the patient's deep tendon reflexes by the physical therapist gives valuable information about the presence of abnormal muscle tone. Flaccidity or hypotonia may cause the reflexes to be hypoactive or absent. Spasticity or hypertonia may cause deep tendon reflexes to be exaggerated or hyperactive. *Clonus* may also be present when the muscle tendon is tapped or stretched and is described as alternating periods of muscle contractions and relaxation. Clonus is frequently seen in the ankle or wrist in response to a quick stretch.

Brain Stem Reflexes

Brain stem reflexes occur and are integrated at the level of the midbrain. As with all primitive reflexes, these reflexes may initially be present in infants but become integrated during the first year of life. In adult patients with CNS disorders, brain stem level

Table 5–5 ▌ SPINAL REFLEXES

REFLEX	STIMULUS	RESPONSE
Flexor withdrawal	Noxious stimulus applied to the bottom of the foot	Toe extension, ankle dorsiflexion, hip and knee flexion
Cross extension	Noxious stimulus applied to the ball of the foot with the lower extremity prepositioned in extension	Flexion and then extension of the opposite lower extremity
Startle	Sudden loud noise	Extension and abduction of the upper extremities
Grasp	Pressure applied to the ball of the foot or the palm of the hand	Flexion of the toes or fingers, respectively

reflexes may become apparent during times of significant stress or fatigue. Brain stem reflexes are primitive reflexes that alter the posture or position of a part of the body. These reflexes frequently serve to alter or affect muscle tone. Table 5–6 lists examples of common brain stem level reflexes.

Associated Reactions

Associated reactions are automatic movements that occur as a result of active or resisted movement in another part of the body. Table 5–7 describes common associated reactions seen in patients with hemiplegia. As stated previously, associated reactions can be misinterpreted as voluntary movement by either the patient or a family member. All parties should recognize the meaning of a patient's involuntary movements.

Bowel and Bladder Dysfunction

Patients who have had a CVA may also present with bowel and bladder dysfunction. *Incontinence* or the inability to control urination may be present initially secondary to muscle paralysis or inadequate sensory stimulation to the bladder. For adult patients, incontinence can be problematic and embarrassing. Early weight bearing through either bridging or standing activities can assist the patient with regaining bladder control. Movement and activity help patients who are experiencing difficulties in regulating bowel function. Attention to the patient's bowel and bladder program by all members of the rehabilitation team can be beneficial in assisting the patient to relearn these activities of daily living.

Table 5–6 ❚ BRAIN STEM REFLEXES

REFLEX	RESPONSE
Symmetric tonic neck reflex	Flexion of the neck results in flexion of the arms and extension of the legs. Extension of the neck results in extension of the arms and flexion of the legs.
Asymmetric tonic neck reflex	Rotation of the head to the left causes extension of the left arm and leg and flexion of the right arm and leg. Rotation of the head to the right causes extension of the right arm and leg and flexion of the left arm and leg.
Tonic labyrinthine reflex	Prone position facilitates flexion. Supine position facilitates extension.
Tonic thumb reflex	When the involved extremity is elevated above the horizontal, thumb extension is facilitated with forearm supination.

Table 5–7 ❚ ASSOCIATED REACTIONS

REACTION	RESPONSE
Souques' phenomenon	Flexion of the involved arm above 150 degrees facilitates extension and abduction of the fingers.
Raimiste's phenomenon	Resistance applied to hip abduction or adduction of the uninvolved lower extremity causes a similar response in the involved lower extremity.
Homolateral limb synkinesis	Flexion of the involved upper extremity elicits flexion of the involved lower extremity.

Functional Limitations

Patients often exhibit functional impairments after CVA. Individuals may lose the ability to perform activities of daily living such as feeding or bathing or may be unable to roll over in bed, sit up, or walk. Functional limitations are the result of motor or sensory deficits caused by the stroke. Patients may lack the volitional movement in the involved arm needed to wash their faces or comb their hair. The presence of spasticity in the involved lower extremity may limit patients' ability to ambulate.

Great emphasis is placed on function in current physical therapy practice. The purpose of physical therapy is to help patients to achieve their optimal level of physical functioning and to improve their quality of life. Treatment goals and intervention plans must be functionally relevant. For example, if a patient who has had a CVA has decreased active dorsiflexion in the involved ankle, an appropriate goal would be for the patient to demonstrate dorsiflexion during the heelstrike phase of the gait cycle 50% of the time with verbal cueing. The goal of improving active dorsiflexion has been put into the context of a functional activity.

TREATMENT PLANNING

When the primary physical therapist develops the patient's treatment goals and plan, he or she must do so in consultation with the patient and family. The patient must be actively involved in the planning and delivery of care. Information must be gathered regarding the patient's previous level of function and the patient's goals for resuming those activities. If a patient did not, for example, perform housework or gardening before the stroke, it would not be realistic to expect that the patient would perform those tasks after such an event. The physical therapist should select treatment activities that are meaningful to the patient, to assist the patient in returning to his prior level of function.

Functional Assessments

With more and more attention placed on the achievement of functional outcomes, many assessment tools have been developed that quantify a patient's recovery or progress and the effectiveness of therapeutic interventions. Although a detailed description of all the functional assessment tools available is outside the scope of this text, several of those tools that are most frequently used in the evaluation and treatment of patients with neurologic deficits are discussed.

The Functional Independence Measure (FIM) was developed in the early 1980s in response to the need for a national data system that could be used to differentiate among various clinical services and to establish the efficacy of services provided. The FIM measures a patient's ability to perform self-care and sphincter control activities and also assesses mobility, locomotion, communication, social adjustment and cooperation, and cognition. A seven-point ordinal scale is used to score the various categories. A score of 1 equates to complete dependence, and a score of 7 indicates that a patient is completely independent during performance of the activity (Baldrige, 1993). The primary physical therapist is responsible for completing the FIM at the time of the patient's initial evaluation and also at discharge. The physical therapist assistant may use the FIM to provide the rehabilitation team with updates regarding the patient's progress.

The Fugl-Meyer Assessment is an assessment instrument used to quantify motor functioning following a stroke. In addition, the tool can be used to analyze the efficacy of treatment interventions provided. The Fugl-Meyer evaluates passive joint range of motion, pain, light touch, proprioception, motor function, and balance. The tool is easy to administer and can be completed in 20 to 30 minutes (Baldrige, 1993; Duncan and Badke, 1987).

If a facility is not using a standardized functional assessment, it is still imperative that the physical therapist develop functional goals and expectations for the patient. Treatment activities that address bed mobility, transfers, ambulation, stair negotiation, wheelchair propulsion (if appropriate), and safety issues should all be included in the plan of care. Patient and family education is also necessary. If it appears that the patient may not be able to resume his previous level of function, instruction of the family will become even more important. A more detailed discussion occurs in the section of this chapter on discharge planning.

COMPLICATIONS SEEN FOLLOWING STROKE

Abnormal Posturing and Positioning

Patients can develop certain complications following CVAs. As previously stated, spasticity often develops in certain muscle groups and can lead to the development of contractures and deformities. Patients may present with flexion contractures of the elbow, wrist, and fingers as a result of spasticity in the flexor muscle groups. This condition can lead to the characteristic upper extremity posturing often seen in patients who have had a stroke. Hygiene and other self-care activities can become extremely difficult in the presence of wrist and finger contractures. The patient may not be able to open the fist to wash the palm of the hand or to perform nail care.

Spasticity in the gastrocnemius-soleus complex can lead to plantar flexion contractures of the involved ankle. Ankle contractures make ambulation and transfers difficult by preventing the patient from bearing weight on a flat or plantigrade foot. Several oral medications are available for patients with significant spasticity including baclofen (Lioresil), diazepam (Valium), and dantrolene sodium (Dantrium). A major disadvantage with several of these medications is that they decrease CNS activity and promote lethargy (Katz, 1996). These are undesirable side effects for patients with neurologic dysfunction. Additionally, the medications do not cure the underlying problem. Instead, they provide a temporary change in the level of muscle tone.

Dantrolene sodium has become the preferred antispasticity medication for patients who have had a CVA. It is less likely to cause lethargy or cognitive changes. The drug intervenes at the muscular level and decreases the force production of muscle units. In approximately 1% of patients, it does cause hepatotoxicity, and therefore patients must be carefully monitored (Katz, 1996).

In some situations, the presence of spasticity is advantageous for the patient. Extensor tone in the lower extremity may assist a patient in ambulation attempts. Increased tone around the shoulder joint may limit the patient's predisposition for shoulder subluxation. Often, the extent and severity of the abnormal tone become most problematic for the patient.

Shoulder pain is extremely common in patients with hemiplegia. Of these patients, 70 to 80% experience shoulder discomfort (Roth and Harvey, 1996). Decreased muscle tone and muscle weakness can reduce the support provided by the rotator cuff muscles, specifically the supraspinatus. Consequently, the joint capsule and the ligaments of the shoulder become the sole supporting structures for the head of the humerus within the glenoid fossa. In time, the effects of this weakness combined with the effects of gravity can lead to shoulder subluxation.

Spasticity or increased muscle tone can also lead to shoulder dysfunction and pain. Spasticity within the scapular depressors, retractors, and downward rotators contributes to poor scapular position and joint alignment. Abnormal positioning of the scapula causes secondary tightness in the ligaments, tendons, and joint capsule of the shoulder and can lead to a decrease in the patient's ability to move the involved shoulder. Shoulder pain and loss of upper extremity function can develop as a consequence of changes in the orientation of anatomic structures within the shoulder girdle.

Reflex Sympathetic Dystrophy

Reflex sympathetic dystrophy can also develop in individuals who have sustained a CVA. Patients with reflex sympathetic dystrophy experience pain in the shoulder, as well as edema and tenderness in the involved hand and fingers. As the condition progresses, the patient exhibits temperature changes in the hand. In addition, the skin of the involved hand becomes red and shiny, and trophic changes occur in the nails. Because pain is a primary complaint, patients frequently limit their movement, thereby creating a continuous cycle of pain and immobility. Ultimately, the involved upper extremity becomes stiff from contracture formation and muscle atrophy. As with the other complications previously discussed, prevention of reflex sympathetic dystrophy through early range-of-motion exercises, positioning, and upper extremity weight-bearing activities is of significant benefit to the patient.

Additional Complications

Other complications seen after CVA include the following: (1) increased risk of trauma and falls because of impaired upper extremity and lower extremity protective reactions; (2) increased risk of thrombophlebitis secondary to decreased efficiency of the calf skeletal muscle pump; (3) pain in specific muscles and joints; and (4) psychologic problems including anxiety, depression, and denial. A review of the physical therapy interventions used to decrease the risk of these complications is provided later in this chapter.

ACUTE CARE SETTING

Depending on the severity of the individual's stroke, the physical therapist assistant may or may not be involved in the patient's treatment sessions in the acute care setting. Average lengths of hospitalization following a CVA are approximately 5 to 6 days. In certain geographic areas, patients may not be admitted to an acute care facility unless a strong medical need exists. Patients who have sustained uncomplicated CVAs may be evaluated by their physician and instructed to begin outpatient or home-based therapies. Once the patient is medically stable, the physician may determine that it is appropriate for the patient to begin rehabilitation.

DELEGATION OF A PATIENT TO A PHYSICAL THERAPIST ASSISTANT

Following the patient's initial evaluation, the supervising physical therapist may determine that a patient who has sustained a CVA is an appropriate candidate for delegation to the physical therapist assistant. The supervising physical therapist needs to evaluate the patient carefully for the appropriateness of sharing a patient with an assistant. Factors to be considered when delegating patients to physical therapist assistants as identified in Chapter 1 include acuteness of the patient's condition, special patient problems (including medical, cognitive, or emotional), and the patient's current response to physical therapy. Prior to the assistant's initial visit with the patient, the supervising physical therapist should review the patient's evaluative findings with the assistant. In addition, the physical therapist must also discuss with the assistant the patient's plan of care and the short- and long-term treatment goals. Any precautions, contraindications, or special instructions should also be provided (American Physical Therapy Association, 1998).

A discussion of the patient's discharge plans should begin at the time of the initial evaluation. As lengths of stay have decreased, it has become necessary to begin discharge planning the first time one sees the patient. The supervising physical therapist's responsibility is to begin the discharge planning process. Although state practice acts do not prohibit a physical therapist assistant from engaging in planning and preparing for the patient's discharge, the American Physical Therapy Association's guidelines regarding delegation and supervision of physical therapist assistants state that it is the responsibility of the supervising therapist to initiate and plan for the patient's discharge from the treatment facility. This includes performance of the discharge summary (American Physical Therapy Association, 1998).

With input from the supervising therapist, the assistant may find himself or herself responsible for the patient's daily treatment activities. Requirements for contact with the primary therapist differ from state to state. The assistant is advised to review the state practice act and to adhere to any specific requirements regarding therapist supervision or patient reevaluations that may be required by the state legislature.

EARLY PHYSICAL THERAPY INTERVENTION

Cardiopulmonary Retraining

An area of physical therapy care that often receives limited attention in patients who have sustained strokes is cardiopulmonary retraining. Individuals who have had strokes frequently have significant cardiac and pulmonary medical histories. Previous myocardial infarctions, hypertension, and chronic obstructive pulmonary disease are common medical findings in this patient population. In addition, diaphragmatic weakness and generalized deconditioning, decreased endurance, and fatigue affect the patient's ability to participate in rehabilitation by decreasing pulmonary capabilities.

Diaphragmatic Strengthening

The diaphragm is a muscle and may respond to therapeutic techniques designed to improve strength and endurance. Diaphragmatic strengthening is accomplished by having the assistant place one hand on the patient's upper abdomen. Initially, the patient is directed to try, during inspiration, to lift the weight of the clinician's hand. A semireclined position may be the easiest for the patient because the patient will not have to contract the diaphragm directly against gravity. A quick stretch applied to the diaphragm prior to an active inspiratory movement can facilitate a stronger contraction. As the patient performs these exercises with increased ease, the clinician can make the exercise more challenging by increasing manual resistance, changing the patient's position, or incorporating the performance of a functional task during the exercise. Expansion of the lateral lobes of the lungs should also be practiced. The assistant places his hands on the patient's lateral lower rib cage and encourages the patient to breathe out against the manual pressure. Initially, the weight of the assistant's hands may be sufficient resistance. As the patient progresses, the assistant can increase resistance during the activity.

Other Cardiopulmonary Activities

Other activities that can be performed to improve cardiopulmonary functioning include deep breathing exercises, the use of blow bottles or incentive spirometers, and stretching activities to the lateral trunk, especially in the presence of lateral chest wall tightness. Breathing exercises improve the efficiency of air intake. Breath support is important as the patient tries to perform activities and talk at the same time. The patient's speech-language pathologist can assist the patient in coordinating breathing during speaking and eating activities. As the patient progresses in rehabilitation, the assistant will need to be cognizant of the patient's cardiopulmonary function and medications. For patients with complicated medical histories, it may be necessary to monitor vital signs during activity performance. It is important to check with the primary physical therapist to determine whether this type of monitoring is appropriate. All patients should be instructed to avoid holding their breath during activity performance because this phenomenon is known to increase blood pressure.

Positioning

Initially, one of the most important aspects of physical therapy care is the proper positioning of the patient. Positioning should be started immediately following the patient's stroke and should continue throughout all phases of the patient's recovery. Positioning is the responsibility of the patient and all members of the rehabilitation team. Proper positioning out of the characteristic synergy patterns assists in stimulating motor function, increases sensory awareness, improves respiratory and oromotor function, and assists in maintaining normal range of motion in the neck, trunk, and extremities. Additionally, common musculoskeletal deformities and the potential for pressure ulcers can be minimized with proper patient positioning.

The patient should be alternately positioned on the back, the involved side, and the uninvolved side. Areas of the patient's body that require special attention and should be addressed first are the shoulder and pelvic girdles. The rhomboids and gluteus maximus muscles frequently become tight and contribute to retraction at the shoulder and pelvic girdles. Therefore, both the shoulder and pelvis should be positioned in slight protraction to minimize the effects of muscle spasticity and tightness.

Supine Positioning

When the patient is in the supine position, the assistant will want to place small towel rolls (approximately 1½ inches thick) underneath the patient's scapula and pelvis on the involved side to promote protraction. The towels should encompass approximately two thirds of the bony structures. (The rolls should not extend all the way to the vertebral column.) Care must be taken to avoid placing too much toweling under the scapula and pelvis because this will cause excessive rotation and asymmetry. The involved upper extremity should be externally rotated and extended with the forearm supinated. In addition, a neutral or slightly extended wrist position with finger extension and thumb abduction is desirable. Placement of a pillow under the involved upper extremity assists in maintaining this position and can help with venous return. Pelvic protraction, coupled with hip and knee flexion and ankle dorsiflexion, is the preferred position for the lower extremity. A pillow can be used under the patient's leg to help maintain this posture. Intervention 5-1 illustrates supine positioning for the patient with hemiplegia. Positioning the patient in the supine position as described earlier is beneficial because it counteracts the strong flexion and extension

Intervention 5–1 ❚ SUPINE POSITIONING

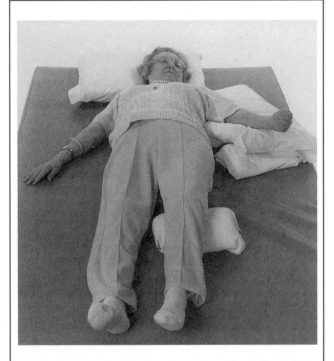

Protraction of the scapula, external rotation of the shoulder, and elbow extension are emphasized in the upper extremity. Pelvic protraction with slight hip and knee flexion is used to decrease extensor tone in the lower extremity.

synergies that develop in the upper and lower extremity, respectively.

In addition to the emphasis placed on the shoulder and hip, the clinician must also be aware of the patient's neck and head position. Often, in an effort to make the patient more comfortable, family members place extra pillows under the patient's head. This type of positioning promotes cervical flexion and can accentuate forward head posturing. A single pillow under the neck is sufficient unless a patient's medical condition warrants a more elevated neck and upper trunk position. The patient should also be encouraged to look toward the involved side to enhance visual awareness.

Side Lying Positioning

As stated previously, positioning the patient on either side should be employed. When the patient is lying on the uninvolved side, the patient's trunk should be straight, the involved upper extremity should be protracted on a pillow, the patient's elbow should be extended, and the forearm should be in a neutral position. The patient's wrist should also be in a neutral or slightly extended position, and the fingers should be relaxed. The lower extremity should be positioned with the pelvis protracted, the hip and knee flexed, and the ankle in dorsiflexion. Intervention 5–2 illustrates positioning of the patient in side lying on the uninvolved side.

Having the patient positioned on the involved side is also beneficial because it increases weight bearing and proprioceptive input into the involved extremities. When preparing the patient for this activity, one should ensure that the patient's involved shoulder is protracted and well forward. This positioning prevents the patient from lying directly on the shoulder and causing impingement. It is again optimal to have the elbow extended and the forearm supinated. The pelvis should be protracted, with the involved hip extended and the knee slightly flexed. The uninvolved limbs (both the upper and lower extremity) should be supported with pillows.

Intervention 5–2 ❚ SIDE LYING POSITIONING (UNINVOLVED SIDE)

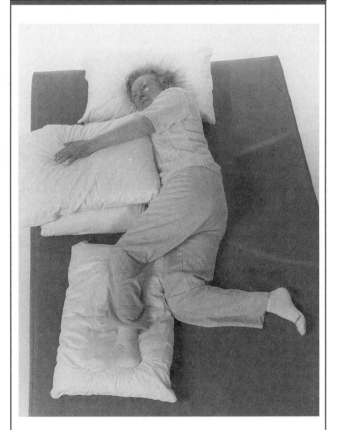

Scapular protraction with elbow extension is desired. Hip and knee flexion with ankle dorsiflexion is the preferred position for the lower extremity.

Minimizing the Development of Abnormal Tone and Patient Neglect

The positioning examples previously described have other variations. Many of the positioning alternatives are the results of clinicians' attempts to minimize the effects of abnormal tone or spasticity that develop in patients who have had CVAs. Positions need to be altered as the patient's mobility improves and as tightness develops in various muscle groups. Regardless of the specific positioning techniques used, special attention must be placed on the achievement of symmetry, midline orientation, and protraction of the scapula and pelvis. Care must also be taken to avoid the potential development of patient neglect of the involved extremities. *Neglect* of the involved side of the body and visual field is often present when the right cerebral hemisphere is damaged. This neglect may be described as an impairment in the patient's awareness of body image or body parts. In addition, if the sensory cortex has been damaged, the patient may be unable to perceive sensory stimulation in the involved extremities. Both these situations can lead to the patient's inability to attend to the involved side or may cause the patient to neglect the involved upper or lower extremity. Positioning the patient in side lying on the involved side decreases the effects of this neglect by increasing sensory input into the affected joints and muscles and by enhancing visual awareness of that side of the body.

Leaving Items Within Reach

When leaving the patient in any of the previously described positions, one should place needed items such as the nurse's call bell, the bedside table, and telephone within the patient's reach and visual field. Therapists often instruct families to place commonly used objects on the patient's involved side to increase awareness and attention given to that side of the body. This practice should not, however, be employed if it creates a safety concern for the patient or family members. Families and caregivers alike should be encouraged to interact with the patient on his involved side because it reinforces the importance of visually attending to the affected side.

Other Considerations

Family members frequently suggest placing a washcloth or soft, squeezable ball in the patient's palm. Many individuals believe that this activity improves hand control. On the contrary, squeezing a soft object often increases tightness (spasticity) in the wrist and finger flexors and facilitates the palmar grasp reflex. A resting hand splint for the involved hand may be ben-

eficial. A footboard placed at the end of the patient's bed can promote a similar type of unwanted response in the lower extremity. Instead of preventing the development of gastrocnemius-soleus tightness, the board provides a constant stimulus for the patient to push against and, in fact, can lead to increased spasticity at the ankle. Having family members bring in a pair of low-top tennis shoes for the patient to wear in bed provides improved positioning for the foot.

Early Functional Mobility Tasks

Early physical therapy treatment activities to facilitate movement should be initiated while the patient is still in bed. The hip and shoulder are the areas that should be targeted first because proximal control and stability are essential for distal movement.

Bridging and Bridging with Approximation

Examples of early activities that can be performed with the lower extremities include *bridging* and *bridging with approximation* applied through the knees. *Approximation* or *compression* occurs when joint surfaces are

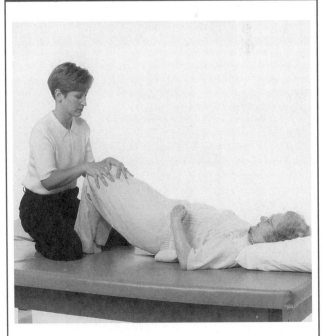

Intervention 5-3 ▍ PREPARATION FOR BRIDGING

Gentle approximation is applied downward through the patient's knees in preparation for bridging.

brought together. These compressive forces activate joint receptors and facilitate postural holding responses (O'Sullivan, 1994a). Approximation applied downward through the knee prior to the patient's attempt to lift the buttocks prepares the foot for early weight bearing. Intervention 5–3 illustrates this technique. Approximation can also be administered superiorly through the hip in preparation for bridging. The physical therapist assistant must observe the quality of the patient's bridge. Weakness in the gluteus maximus muscle and lack of lower extremity control may be evident. This condition can result in asymmetric lifting and lagging of the involved side. The assistant may need to provide more tactile assistance under the buttocks. Intervention 5–4 shows an assistant helping a patient with this exercise. Intervention 5–5 depicts an assistant helping a patient with bridging using a draw sheet. Holding on to the draw sheet, the assistant pulls up and back, thus shifting his weight posteriorly. This technique is extremely beneficial for patients who have low function or who are slightly larger and require greater physical assistance.

Other Bedside Activities

Other bedside exercises include hip extension over the edge of the bed and straight leg raising with the uninvolved lower extremity while the involved lower extremity is flexed. Interventions 5–6 and 5–7 illustrate these exercises. One of the benefits of these exercises is that they facilitate early activation of the gluteus maximus and hamstring muscles. Other early treatment techniques that promote movement and control of the hip musculature include lower trunk rotation, scooting from one side of the bed to the other, and retraining the hip flexors. Lower trunk rotation provides for separation of the trunk and pelvis, assists in promoting general relaxation, and also facilitates pelvic protraction, which is necessary for functional activities such as rolling, supine-to-sit transfers, and ambulation. Lower trunk rotation is depicted in Intervention 5–8. Facilitation of active hip flexion can be achieved by passively flexing the patient's hip and knee and then working on active hip flexion within various points in the range of motion (Intervention 5–9). As the patient is able to perform this exercise actively and as the quality of the lower extremity movement improves, the exercise can be advanced, and the patient can begin to work on active hip and knee flexion with voluntary ankle dorsiflexion. A final progression of this exercise is to have the patient reverse the movement and work on hip and knee extension with ankle dorsiflexion. The patient's ability to perform this movement combination demonstrates an ability to combine various components of the lower extremity flexion and extension synergy patterns. Intervention 5–10 shows the assistant using a more distal handhold at the toes to prevent excessive toe flexion

---

Intervention 5–4 ▌ USING TACTILE CUES TO ASSIST BRIDGING

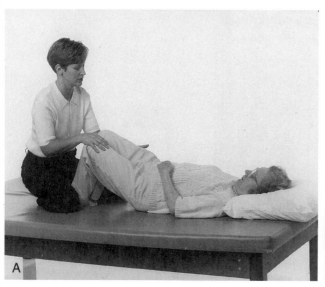 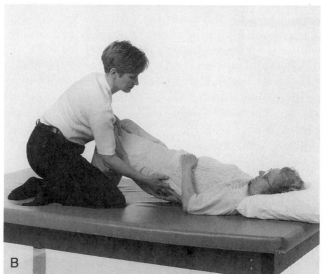

The assistant may need to help the patient with bridging. Tactile cues (tapping) performed to the patient's gluteal muscles will assist the patient with lifting her buttocks.

Intervention 5-5 ▌ USING A DRAW SHEET TO ASSIST BRIDGING

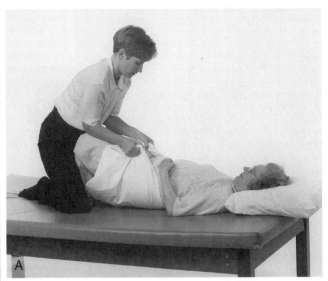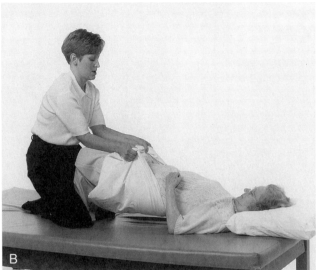

A draw sheet placed under the patient's hips can be used to assist the patient with bridging.

A. The assistant places her forearms along the patient's femurs to maintain positioning of the patient's lower extremities and to provide proprioceptive input.

B. The assistant uses a posterior weight shift of her body to help lift the patient's buttocks.

Intervention 5-6 ▌ HIP EXTENSION OVER THE EDGE OF A SURFACE

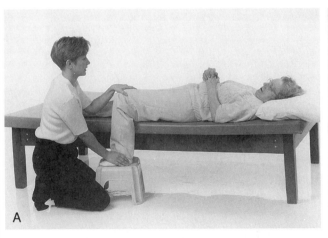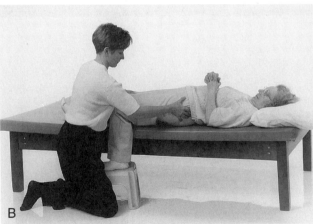

Hip extension can be accomplished over the edge of the bed or mat table. The patient must scoot to the edge of the mat.

A. The assistant may need to help the patient with moving the involved leg off the support surface. The plantar surface of the patient's foot must be supported. A small step stool, a garbage can, or the assistant's leg can be used. The patient pushes down with the involved lower extremity.

B. The assistant can palpate the gluteus maximus muscle to assess the strength of the patient's efforts.

Intervention 5-7 ■ STRAIGHT LEG RAISING (UNINVOLVED LOWER EXTREMITY)

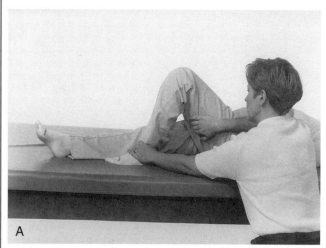

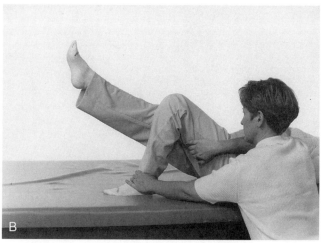

A. The patient is instructed to perform a straight leg raise with the uninvolved lower extremity.

B. As the patient lifts her leg, the assistant palpates the hamstring musculature on the involved side. Contraction of the involved hamstrings should be felt as the patient lifts the uninvolved leg.

and to promote ankle dorsiflexion. Whenever distal joints are used to guide the patient's movement, the patient must possess adequate control of the more proximal components.

Importance of Movement Assessment

Any time the patient moves, the physical therapist assistant should observe and monitor the quality of the

Intervention 5-8 ■ LOWER TRUNK ROTATION

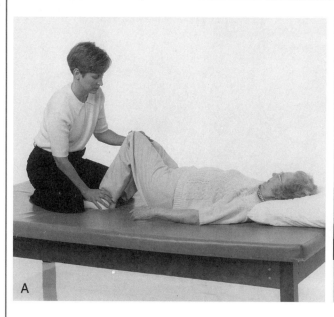

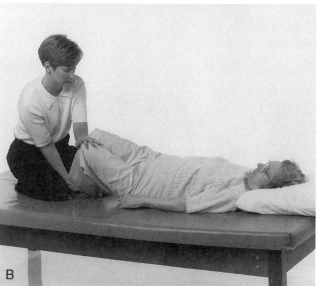

The assistant guides the patient's lower extremities as the patient performs lower trunk rotation in hooklying.

Intervention 5-9 ▌ HIP AND KNEE FLEXION

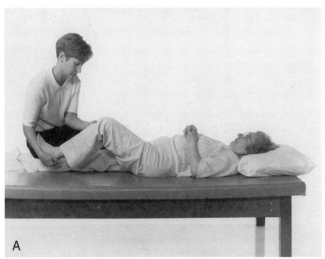

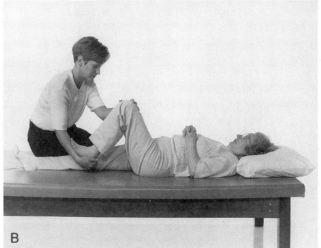

In the acute stages, facilitation of hip and knee flexion is performed with the patient in a supine position. The assistant supports the entire plantar surface of the patient's foot to avoid stimulating a plantar flexion response.

A. Initially, the assistant may need to support the patient's lower extremity.

B. As the patient is able to assume more active control of the movement, the assistant can use a more anterior handhold slightly above the patient's patella.

Intervention 5-10 ▌ INHIBITING TOE FLEXION AND PROMOTING ANKLE DORSIFLEXION

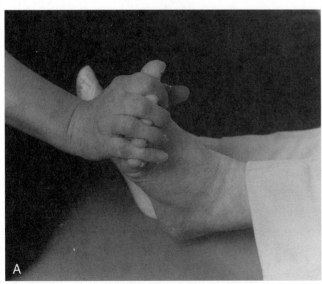

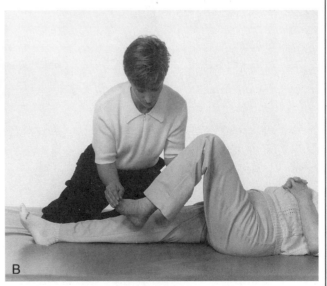

A. The assistant can use her fingers to abduct (separate) the patient's toes. This positioning combined with slight traction applied to the toes will inhibit toe clawing and facilitate ankle dorsiflexion.

B. A more distal handhold can be used to guide the patient's lower extremity movement.

patient's movement. Although no uniformly accepted quality indicators are available in the physical therapy literature to describe movement, the following characteristics should be considered: (1) timing of the movement, (2) sequencing of muscle responses, (3) amount of force generated by the muscle during the movement, and (4) reciprocal release of muscle activity. To address these areas in treatment, the physical therapist assistant should select motor tasks that demand the proper muscle response. For example, having a patient work on sit-to-stand movement transitions in which the timing of hip and knee extension is coordinated is beneficial. Flexion of the elbow followed by a controlled release of the biceps into elbow extension is another example of an activity that addresses the quality of the patient's motor response.

Scapular Mobilization

Treatment techniques for the upper extremity must be included at all times. Scapular mobilization when the patient is in a side lying position is extremely beneficial. This type of mobilization should not be confused with the orthopedic mobilization techniques described by Maitland (Maitland, 1977). Scapular mobilization of the patient with hemiplegia can be thought of as a range-of-motion or mobility exercise. The goal of the mobilization is to keep the scapula moving on the thorax so that upper extremity function is not lost. Intervention 5–11 demonstrates gentle protraction (abduction) of a patient's scapula performed by a physical therapist assistant. The assistant's hand is placed along the border of the patient's scapula. From that position, the assistant can guide the patient's scapular movement. The scapula can also be mobilized in the directions of the proprioceptive neuromuscular facilitation (PNF) diagonals including elevation, abduction, and upward rotation, which are the scapular components of the D1 flexion pattern, and elevation, adduction, and upward rotation, which are the scapular movements observed in the D2 flexion pattern. Care should be taken to stabilize the trunk properly in order to avoid compensatory motion. Scapular mobility is essential in maintaining the normal

---

Intervention 5–11 ▌ SCAPULAR MOBILIZATION

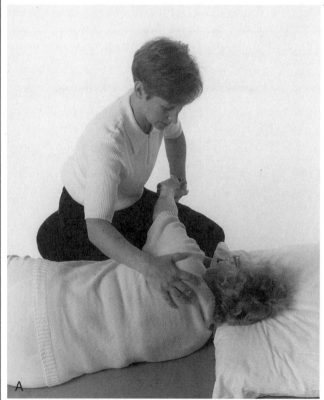 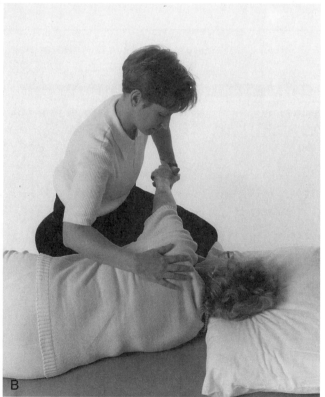

With her hand on the patient's scapula, the assistant gently protracts the involved scapula. The assistant uses a handshake grasp to support the patient's involved hand.

scapulohumeral rhythm necessary for upper extremity range of motion and functional reaching. If the scapula is unable to move on the rib cage, the upper extremity will become tightly fixed to the side of the body and thus will limit the patient's ability to use the arm. In addition, individuals who have had a stroke commonly develop tightness or increased tone in the scapular elevators and retractors (rhomboids, upper trapezius, and teres minor). This condition can lead to abnormal scapular positioning and upper extremity posturing.

Other Upper Extremity Activities

The patient should be instructed in the performance of self-directed upper extremity elevation with external rotation (double arm elevation), as illustrated in Intervention 5–12. This movement combination assists in maintaining function of the shoulder and can limit the development of spasticity in the latissimus dorsi muscle, which has been noted to contribute to abnormal posturing (Johnstone, 1995). Passive range-of-motion exercises performed to the patient's involved shoulder, elbow, wrist, and fingers should also be performed during this early stage of rehabilitation. These exercises are absolutely essential, especially in the absence of volitional upper extremity movement, because they prevent the development of upper extremity joint contractures.

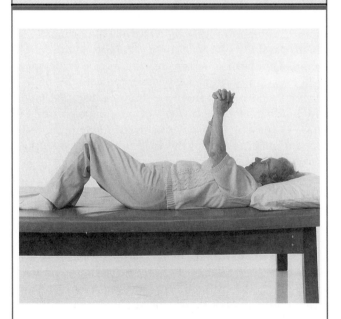

Intervention 5–12 ‖ DOUBLE ARM ELEVATION

The patient clasps her hands together. The involved thumb should be outermost to maintain the web space and to inhibit abnormal tone.

Facilitation and Inhibition Techniques

Depending on the patient's motor responses, the presence or absence of tone, and the quality of volitional movement present, it may be necessary to perform facilitation or inhibitory activities in preparation for the patient's attempts at functional activities.

Facilitation Techniques. The use of primitive (spinal) or tonic (brain stem) reflexes, quick stretching, tapping, vibration, approximation, and weight bearing may be required to prepare the patient for the performance of functional activities.

Primitive or Spinal Level Reflexes. Primitive or spinal level reflexes have limited usefulness in physical therapy practice. To establish the patient's level of responsiveness, it may be appropriate for the assistant to attempt to elicit a flexor withdrawal or a palmar or plantar grasp reflex. A noxious stimulus applied to the bottom of the patient's foot may elicit extension of the toes, with dorsiflexion of the ankle and flexion of the hip and knee. Maintained pressure applied to the palm of the hand or ball of the foot can cause the patient to flex the fingers or toes. Eliciting these spinal level reflexes should be avoided in treatment. More important, however, is the education that the patient and his family members receive regarding the correct meaning of these reflexes. Individuals often misinterpret this type of reflexive response as volitional movement and may develop false hopes regarding the patient's current status or eventual outcome.

Using Brain Stem or Tonic Reflexes. The use of brain stem reflexes such as the asymmetrical tonic neck reflex to elicit patient responses is also controversial. However, if a patient is not responding to conventional treatment interventions, then other avenues must be employed. The use of the asymmetrical tonic neck reflex, the symmetrical tonic neck reflex, and the tonic labyrinthine reflexes can affect the patient's muscle tone by increasing tone in otherwise flaccid or hypotonic extremities. Having the patient rotate the head to one side causes increased extension in the face arm and increased flexor tone in the skull arm. Flexing the patient's head may also elicit flexion in the upper extremities and increased extensor tone in the lower extremities. Positioning a patient supine or prone can increase extensor or flexor tone, respectively.

Other Facilitation Techniques. Additional facilitation techniques include quick stretching of the muscle that facilitates the muscle spindle to fire and consequently causes contraction of muscle fibers. A quick stretch followed by a request to the patient to perform an active movement may also facilitate a motor response. Once the patient is able to recruit a muscle actively, this technique should be discontinued. Tapping, vibration, approximation, and weight bearing are other facilitory treatment techniques. Gentle tapping over a muscle belly often assists in preparing the muscle for activation. Tapping and vibration can be performed to both the agonist and antagonist of a given muscle group. The sensory stimulus should be applied from the muscle's insertion to its origin. Effects of vibratory stimulation last only as long as the stimulus is applied. Vibration can be applied for 1 to 2 minutes, and then the stimulus should be removed. In the presence of significant muscle tone, tapping or vibration administered to the muscle's antagonist often provides insufficient muscle activation to overcome the increased tone. Approximation and weight bearing are two other commonly used facilitory techniques that provide the patient with proprioceptive input to the joint and muscle receptors. Approximation and early weight-bearing activities performed at the shoulder and hip often stimulate muscle activation around the joint and assist in the development of joint stability (O'Sullivan, 1994a).

Inhibition Techniques. For patients who present with increased tone, inhibitory techniques should be employed. Slow, rhythmic rotation can assist in reducing tone in spastic body parts. As stated previously, beginning these activities in proximal body segments is important if the desired outcome is to change the tone more distally. Weight bearing is another useful inhibitory technique. Prolonged ice applied with an ice pack or iced towels or static stretch applied in conjunction with pressure administered to a tendon of a spastic muscle can assist in normalizing tone in hypertonic muscle groups. Once the tone is at a more manageable level, the patient must then attempt a movement or functional task. Movement must be superimposed on the improved tonal state if carryover is to occur (Bobath, 1990).

A note of caution when using ice to inhibit abnormal tone is in order. Duration of the icing should not exceed 20 minutes. In addition, the patient's skin should be checked periodically. The use of ice is contraindicated in patients with autonomic nervous system instability, circulatory problems, and impaired sensation (O'Sullivan, 1994a).

Treatment Adjunct. Air (pressure) splints can be employed to assist with positioning, tone reduction, and sensory awareness. For some patients, air splints are used as an adjunct to the treatment they are receiving; for others, the therapist may recommend an air splint as a necessary piece of equipment for a patient's home exercise and positioning program.

Johnstone described the use of air splints in her book (Johnstone, 1995). Inflatable air splints are available for a number of different body part combinations, such as full-length arm and leg splints, splints for the elbow, forearm, and hand, and a splint for the foot and ankle. These splints can be applied to the involved joint or extremity and can assist with positioning and tone management. The dual-channeled air splints are inflated by the therapist. Warm air from the therapist's lungs allows the inner sleeve to contour to the patient and thus provides constant sensory feedback. The splint must be firmly applied, with the pressure reaching between 38 and 40 mm Hg. Numbness or tingling while wearing the splint may indicate over-inflation. Splints should not be worn for longer than 1 hour at a time. They can be reapplied several times throughout the day or during the course of a treatment session. A thin cotton sleeve can be applied under the splint to protect the patient's skin (Johnstone, 1995).

Long Arm Splint. The long arm splint is frequently used in patients who have sustained a CVA. The splint is applied to the patient's involved upper extremity. Maintaining the patient's hand in a handshake grasp during application of the splint assists in the process. Intervention 5–13 shows an assistant applying a long arm splint to a patient. As the patient's arm is placed through the splint, the patient's fifth finger should be on the side of the splint with the zipper. Positioning of the hand in this manner allows for ulnar weight bearing, which facilitates forearm pronation and radial opening of the patient's hand. Once the splint is on, the patient's fingers should rest securely within the confines of the splint. Initially, the assistant may want to use the splint for positioning. The splint is applied, the upper extremity is positioned in external rotation, and the patient wears the splint during supine positioning, as depicted in Figure 5–2. The splint allows the arm to be maintained in the antispasm or recovery position. The air splint can also be worn during treatment sessions. When the patient is in a side lying position, the assistant can work on protraction of the scapula. Intervention 5–14 illustrates this activity. The splint inhibits the development of abnormal tone, which develops as the patient attempts active movements of the arm. The patient can also wear the splint as he works on arm elevation exercises. As the patient develops control of shoulder movements, placement and holding of the arm at various points within the range of motion can be initiated. Intervention 5–15 shows a patient wearing the long arm splint for upper extremity treatment activities.

Elbow and Hand Splint. The elbow or hand splint may be used for patients who lack more distal control and movement. The elbow splint can be applied as the patient works on upper extremity weight-bearing activities. The splint holds the elbow passively in extension. The hand splint is especially useful for patients who experience increased flexor tone in the involved wrist and fingers during functional activities. As stated previously, these splints can also be used as static positioning devices when necessary. For example, a patient may be working on a high-level developmental sequence activity such as kneeling. A hand splint can be applied to the involved hand to decrease the effects of

Intervention 5–13 ▌ APPLYING A LONG ARM SPLINT

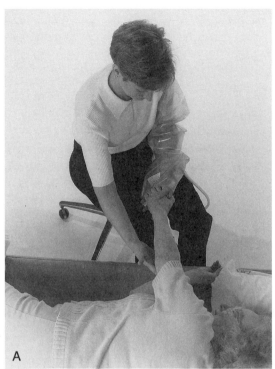

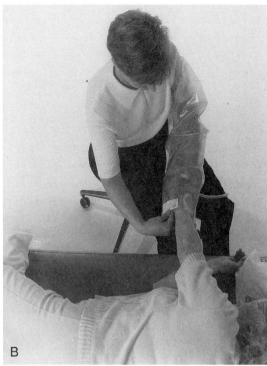

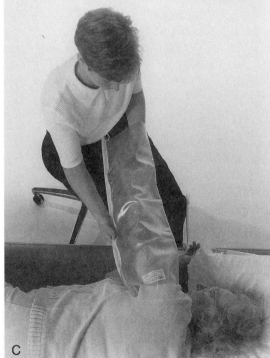

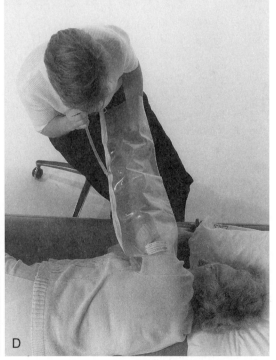

A. With the zipper of the splint closed, the assistant gathers the splint on her own arm. The assistant then supports the patient's involved hand with a handshake grasp.

B and C. The splint is applied to the patient's involved upper extremity. The zipper remains on the ulnar or little finger side of the forearm. The assistant maintains a handshake grasp or other inhibitory handhold to the wrist and fingers as the splint is applied.

D. Once in place, the splint is inflated.

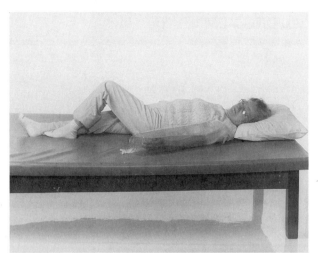

Figure 5-2 ▪ A patient wearing an air splint while lying in bed. The splint can be used as a static positioning device, or it can be applied prior to treatment to prepare the involved extremity for activity.

increased flexor tone in the wrist and fingers that may be present while the patient practices this activity.

Long Leg Splint. The lower extremity splint can be used during gait training activities early on for individuals who lack control or movement in their legs. When the splint is inflated, the patient does not have to be concerned that the involved lower extremity will give way (collapse) when weight is applied. The anterior and posterior chambers of the splint also provide the clinician with the ability to pre-position the patient's leg in slight knee flexion prior to beginning standing activities.

Foot Splint. The foot splint can be used for static positioning and the development of lower extremity control. When the patient is wearing the foot splint, the ankle is maintained in a neutral 90-degree position and the heel is able to accept weight. This can be beneficial for patients who have limited active ankle movement. The foot splint may also be used when

Intervention 5–14 ▌ **SCAPULAR PROTRACTION WITH A SPLINT**

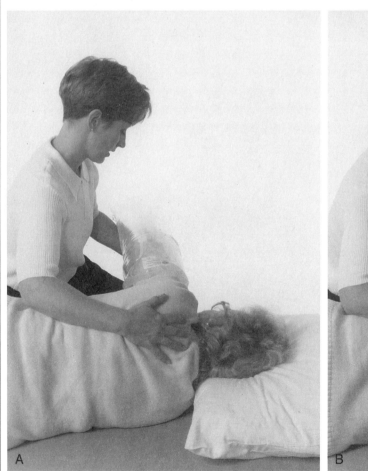

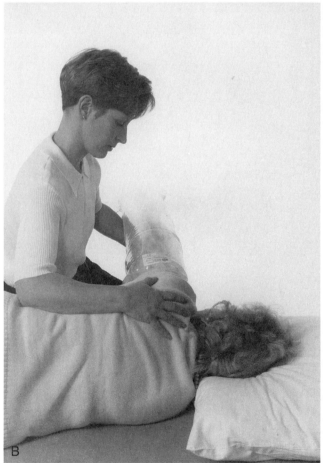

Scapular protraction exercises can be practiced with the patient wearing a long arm splint. The assistant guides the movement of the scapula.

Intervention 5–15 ▮ DOUBLE ARM ELEVATION WITH A SPLINT

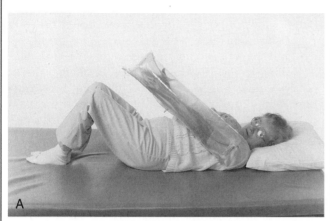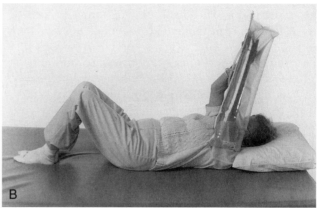

The patient is practicing double arm elevation exercises while wearing a long arm air splint.

working on activities within the developmental sequence such as four-point position, tall-kneeling, and half-kneeling. The splint prevents the gastrocnemius-soleus from exhibiting its strong plantar flexion action and limits excessive ankle inversion.

Neurodevelopmental Treatment Approach

The neurodevelopmental treatment approach, developed by Karl and Berta Bobath in the 1940s, is a common therapeutic intervention for individuals with hemiplegia. Initially, the Bobaths worked with children with cerebral palsy. They noted that these children presented with gross and fine motor delays, abnormal tone and movements, and primitive reflexes. The Bobaths proposed that the children's movements were elicited by peripheral stimuli and primitive reflexes that resulted in their abnormal movement patterns. Thus, the Bobaths believed that the goal of physical therapy was to inhibit abnormal postural reflex activity and movements and to facilitate normal motor patterns including head and trunk control, upper extremity support, and balance reactions (Bobath, 1971; Whiteside, 1997).

The theory of treatment developed by the Bobaths has changed over the years. Initially, treatment was centered around static positioning of children in reflex inhibiting postures. These static positions were directly opposite the tonal pattern exhibited by the child. From reflex inhibiting patterns, the Bobaths began to focus on the patient's performance of the developmental sequence. Physical therapists would assist patients into static developmental postures. The pa-

tients, however, were passive participants, and little carryover to functional activities occurred.

As the treatment approach continued its evolution, emphasis shifted to the patient's postural reflex mechanism. An intact postural reflex mechanism implies that the patient has normal muscle tone and is able to grade and regulate movements. Berta Bobath believed that an injury to the CNS would impair an individual's postural reflex mechanism. Consequently, righting and equilibrium reactions, as well as an individual's ability to hold a limb against gravity *(placing responses)*, would be impaired (Ostrosky, 1990). From these ideas came the philosophic principles on which neurodevelopmental treatment is based.

The goal of physical therapy treatment became to facilitate normal postural control mechanisms and to provide the patient with the sensation of normal movement by inhibiting abnormal postural reflex activity and muscle tone. The focus of treatment was to reestablish the basic components of movement, including (1) head and trunk control, (2) midline orientation, (3) the patient's ability to shift weight over the base of support, (4) static and dynamic balance, and (5) distal control of the extremities. In a clinical context, the therapist would control and guide the patient's motor performance through the use of sensory facilitation applied at key points of control. Thus, therapists could influence a patient's tone and abnormal movement patterns by using key points of control such as the head, shoulders, hips, or distal extremities.

Key points of control are still a primary emphasis within the neurodevelopmental treatment approach. Proximal key points such as the shoulder and pelvic girdles are the most important points from which to influence postural alignment and tone. Manual contacts applied to the shoulder and pelvis influence muscle tone distribution and distal movements. The use of distal key points such as elbows, hands, knees, and feet affects movements of the trunk (Bobath, 1990). The use of key points of control must be individualized to the patient and the patient's movement needs. Once the patient's tone is at a more normal or manageable state, the therapist superimposes normal movements and postures. This is always done within the context of a functional activity. Through the use of key points, therapists are able to give patients the necessary control and stability to initiate movement in other areas. For example, by providing a manual point of control at the pelvis, the patient may be able to improve trunk posturing. By controlling the patient's proximal shoulder, hand position for grasp may be easier. It is important to grade the manual assistance provided through these manual contacts and gradually withdraw assistance as the patient learns to control the movement (Ostrosky, 1990).

Many of the treatment interventions presented in the remaining portion of this chapter and the rest of the text are based on the work of Karl and Berta Bobath. However, current motor control and motor learning theories focus less on the actual techniques and more on the process used to maximize patient function. These theories emphasize the need for the patient to be an active participant in learning or relearning movement strategies. Patients must become active problem solvers of their own movement deficits. Patients must learn to perform movements in different environments and within multiple functional contexts (Whiteside, 1997).

Functional Activities

Rolling

During the period of early rehabilitation, the patient should begin functional movements. Rolling to the right and left should begin immediately. The patient must be instructed in methods to assist in active performance of this activity.

Rolling to the Involved Side. Rolling to the involved side is often easier because the patient initiates the movement with the uninvolved side of the body. The activity begins with the patient turning the head to the side toward which the patient is going to roll. Head and eye movements provide strong cues to the body to prepare for movement. Head turning also helps to unweight the opposite upper extremity and facilitates upper trunk rotation. The patient should be encouraged to use the uninvolved upper and lower extremities to assist with the transition from supine to side lying on the involved side. Patients often want to reach and hold on to the bed rails to assist with rolling. This practice should be discouraged by all members of the patient's rehabilitation team and by the patient's family members, because few patients return home with hospital beds. To roll over, the patient should reach across the body with the uninvolved upper extremity and should flex and adduct the uninvolved hip and knee. This maneuver provides the patient with the momentum needed to complete the roll.

Rolling to the Uninvolved Side. Rolling to the uninvolved side is usually more challenging for the patient. Again, the activity must be initiated with rotation of the head to the side toward which the patient is rolling. Patients with neglect often have a difficult time initiating cervical rotation for head turning. The patient should be encouraged to look in the direction in which she is moving. It is also important to note the position of the patient's eyes during this activity. If neglect is significant, it may be difficult for the patient to move her eyes past midline to focus on items, tasks, or individuals presented on the involved side. To initiate rolling to the uninvolved side, the patient is encouraged to assist as much as possible. If the patient is able to initiate any active movement in the involved extremities, the sequence will be similar to that presented for rolling to the involved side. If the patient's extremities are flaccid or essentially hypotonic, the following preparatory activities are often beneficial in assisting the patient. The patient should clasp both hands together with the involved thumb outermost, thus promoting abduction of the thumb. Thumb abduction is an inhibitory technique used to promote relaxation in the patient's hand. The clasping of the patient's hands facilitates finger abduction and extension. With the hands clasped, the patient flexes the shoulders to approximately 90 degrees. Slight shoulder adduction should also be present. The patient's lower extremities should then be positioned in hooklying. If the patient is unable to flex the involved lower extremity actively, the therapist can assist with positioning by unweighting the involved leg and encouraging the patient to flex the hip and the knee while the therapist approximates through the femur toward the hip. Intervention 5–16 illustrates a patient rolling in this manner. A compensatory strategy frequently used by patients involves hooking the uninvolved lower extremity under the involved leg and bringing the two legs up into hooklying together.

An alternative technique is to place the uninvolved lower extremity on top of the involved leg and bring both legs up into hooklying as a unit. The patient is encouraged to do this independently or is assisted by the therapist. The advantage of this technique over the one mentioned previously is that proprioceptive input is applied into the anterior shin of the involved lower extremity, and the patient is required to use the involved leg actively, as much as possible. The more sensory input that can be applied through the involved lower extremity, the better it is for the patient. Once

Intervention 5–16 ▌ROLLING TO THE UNINVOLVED SIDE

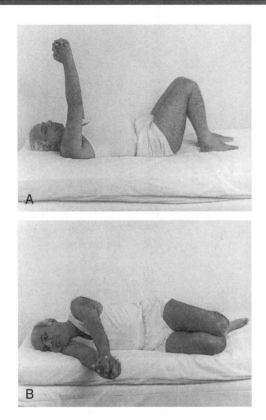

The patient is rolling to side lying with the upper extremities clasped and the lower extremities in hooklying.

From Bobath B. Adult Hemiplegia: Evaluation and Treatment, 3rd ed. Boston, Butterworth Heinemann, 1990.

the patient has the upper and lower extremities in flexion, the patient is asked to turn the head and eyes to the uninvolved side to initiate the roll. The physical therapist assistant must assess the patient's ability to perform the activity and assist the patient with verbal and tactile cues as needed. PNF techniques can also be used to assist the patient in his ability to roll. Techniques such as slow reversals and hold-relax active movement can be beneficial in improving lower extremity strength and movement control.

Scooting

Another bed mobility activity that should be practiced is scooting in the supine position. Patients who are able to move independently in bed possess greater freedom because they do not require assistance from health care personnel to reposition themselves in bed. The patient needs to be able to scoot the hips to both sides but must also be able to move the upper trunk

in the same direction as the hips. Having the patient flex the head and neck is the first step when trying to move the shoulders for scooting. The assistant can place his or her hands under the patient's scapulae to assist with moving the upper trunk to the side. Positioning the patient's lower extremities in a hooklying position assists with moving the patient's lower trunk in the desired direction. As the patient is able to initiate more of the movement, the assistant can decrease the tactile input.

Movement Transitions

Other early functional mobility tasks include movement transitions from supine to sitting and from sitting to supine. Because of shorter hospital and rehabilitation stays, the patient's physical therapy treatment plan must address the performance of functional activities from the first treatment session.

Supine-to-Sit Transfer. Transitions from supine to sitting should be practiced from both the patient's involved and uninvolved sides. Too often, patients are taught to perform activities in a single, structured way and then find it difficult to generalize the task to other environmental conditions. Based on a patient's living arrangements, it may not always be possible for the patient to transfer to the stronger, less involved side. Examples of ways to facilitate movement from supine to sitting include having the patient roll to the uninvolved side, as previously described, followed by moving the lower extremities off the bed. From that point, the patient can use the uninvolved upper extremity to push up into an upright sitting position. The physical therapist assistant provides appropriate manual assistance at the patient's shoulders and pelvis. As the patient is able to assume a greater degree of independence in the performance of this activity, the assistant decreases the manual assistance and allows the patient more control over the movement transition. Intervention 5–17 shows a patient performing a supine-to-sit transfer with assistance.

Care must be taken to ensure that distractional forces are not applied to the involved upper extremity during performance of this activity. Too often, one observes health care workers and family members using both the patient's upper extremities to assist with coming to sit and other movement transitions. Distraction applied to the shoulder joint can lead to subluxation and can promote the development of painful upper extremity conditions, including shoulder-hand syndrome and frozen shoulder. All family members and health care personnel should receive instruction in proper transfer techniques including care of the involved upper extremity.

Supine-to-sit transfers can also be facilitated in other ways. Patients can be taught to use diagonals versus straight plane movements to perform this transi-

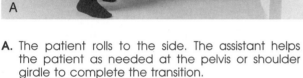

Intervention 5-17 ▌ **SUPINE-TO-SIT TRANSFER**

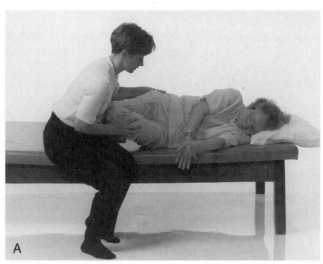

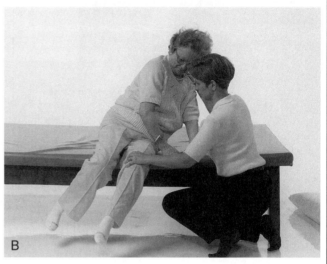

A. The patient rolls to the side. The assistant helps the patient as needed at the pelvis or shoulder girdle to complete the transition.

B. The patient pushes up with the upper extremity to a sitting position.

tion. Supine-to-sit transfers performed in a diagonal pattern can be practiced from either the involved or uninvolved side. Most able-bodied individuals perform functional activities in diagonal movement patterns. Diagonal movement patterns tend to be more functional and are also more energy efficient. To assist the patient with this type of movement, the physical therapist assistant needs to place the patient's lower extremities in a hooklying position. The legs are then brought off the bed or mat surface. The patient is asked to tuck the chin and, with the uninvolved upper extremity, reaches forward. This technique enables patients to activate their abdominal muscles to assist in the achievement of upright sitting. Intervention 5-18 demonstrates a patient performing this transition. The physical therapist assistant may raise the head of the bed or prop the patient on pillows or a wedge to make the task easier for individuals with weak abdominal muscles. This technique provides the patient with a mechanical advantage and decreases the work the abdominals need to perform. As the patient is able to complete the transition with increased ease, the degree of inclination can be decreased.

Some patients require increased physical assistance for supine-to-sit transfers. The technique is essentially the same when a second person is used. Often, it is easiest to divide the work and have one person control and assist at the patient's trunk and the other be responsible for the patient's lower extremities. Both individuals must be clear about who is leading the activity and who is responsible for providing the verbal directions.

Wheelchair-to-Bed/Mat Transfers. Once the patient has made the transition from supine to sitting, transfers to the wheelchair are attempted. A stand-pivot transfer is the most common. The patient must initially scoot forward in the wheelchair or on the mat table to ensure that both feet are flat on the floor. If the patient is sitting in a wheelchair, it is not uncommon for the patient to lean against the back of the chair to scoot the hips forward. Weight shifting from one side to the next is the preferred technique and should be encouraged. As the patient moves the left hip forward, she shifts her weight to the right. This weight shift should be accompanied by elongation of the trunk musculature on the right side. The patient repeats this sequence with movement of the right hip forward and a weight shift to the left. Once the patient's feet are flat on the floor, the gait belt is applied, and the involved upper extremity is pre-positioned. The patient performs an anterior weight shift and is instructed to stand. The assistant guards the patient closely and uses his or her knees to block the patient's hemiplegic knee if necessary. Weakness or spasticity in the involved lower extremity may cause the knee to buckle as weight is transferred to the limb. The patient steps with the uninvolved leg and pivots to the mat table or bed. The position of the involved ankle must be carefully monitored to avoid instability or inadvertent weight bearing on the lateral malleolus.

Intervention 5–18 ▌ SUPINE-TO-SIT TRANSFER ON A DIAGONAL PATTERN

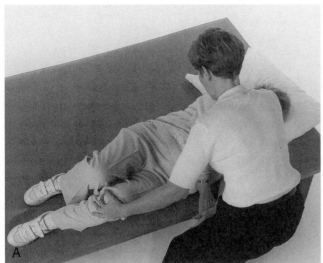

A

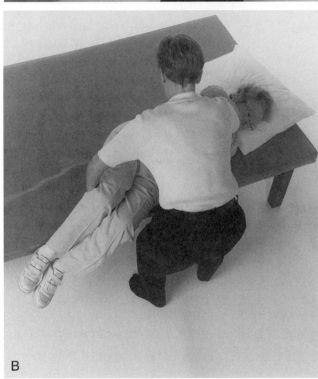

B

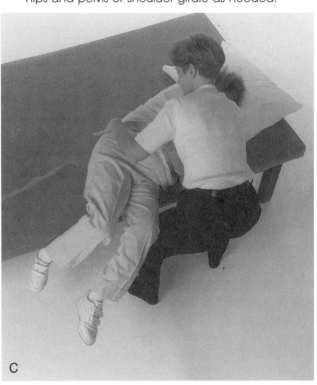

C

A. The patient scoots to the edge of the mat. This maneuver is accomplished by bridging and then moving the upper trunk and head.

B. The patient brings her lower extremities off the mat table or surface of the bed.

C. The patient is encouraged to tuck her chin and to reach forward with her uninvolved upper extremity. The assistant provides manual cues at the hips and pelvis or shoulder girdle as needed.

Intervention 5–19 depicts a patient performing a stand-pivot transfer from the wheelchair to the mat table.

Summary

Treatment interventions that can be performed by the patient in the early stages of rehabilitation have been presented. Before more advanced treatment interventions are discussed, a summarized list of techniques that may make up the initial treatment plan is provided.

Positioning
Bridging and bridging with approximation
Hip extension over the edge of the mat or bed
Hamstring co-contraction (modified straight leg raising)
Lower trunk rotation and lower trunk rotation with bridging

Intervention 5–19 | STAND-PIVOT TRANSFER

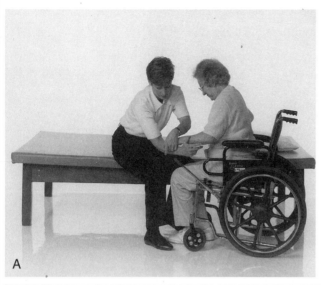

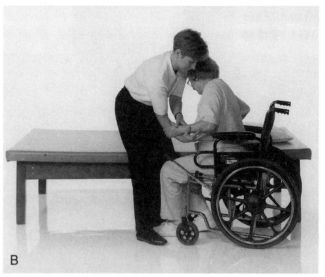

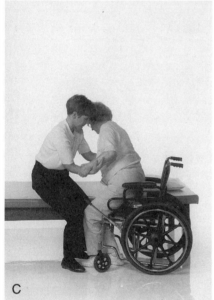

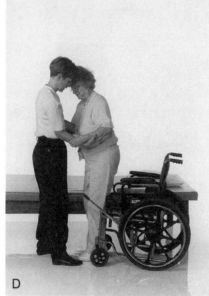

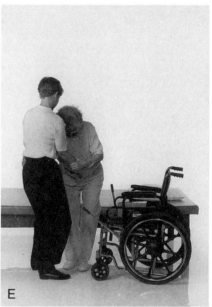

A. The patient shifts weight forward in the chair so her feet are supported and are in a plantigrade position on the floor.

B. The assistant pre-positions the patient's involved arm.

C. The patient is encouraged to perform an anterior weight shift to come to standing. The assistant guards the involved knee to prevent buckling.

D. The patient stands erect.

E. The patient pivots on her feet to sit down. Some patients may require continuous support of the involved lower extremity during performance of stand-pivot transfers.

Hip flexor retraining
Hip and knee extension with ankle dorsiflexion
Scapular mobilization
Upper extremity elevation

Functional activities including rolling, scooting, and supine-to-sit and wheelchair-to-bed transfers

Adjuncts to treatment at this phase include air

splints, the use of spinal and brain stem level reflexes, and various facilitation and inhibition techniques. The treatment of the patient in other functional positions will now be discussed. The inclusion of any of the following interventions into the plan of care depends on the cognitive and functional status of the patient.

Other Functional Positions

Sitting

Once the patient is able to achieve a *short-sitting position,* which is defined as sitting on a surface such as a bed or mat table with one's hips and knees flexed and one's feet supported on the floor, the physical therapist assistant may begin to work on sitting posture and balance activities with the patient. Figure 5–3 shows a patient who exhibits fair sitting posture and balance. It will become apparent that some patients with hemiplegia have poor or nonfunctional sitting balance. Patients with hemiplegia, because of their poor sense of midline and motor control deficits, often lose their balance. In this case, it may be necessary for the physical therapist assistant to seek help from another person. The second person can be positioned behind the patient and can assist with the patient's trunk. The physical therapist assistant may elect to be

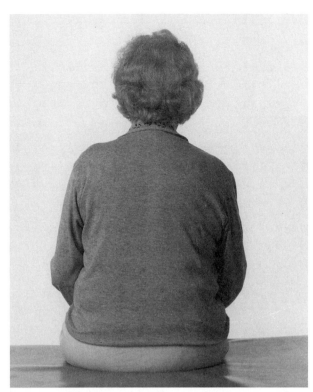

Figure 5–4 ■ A posterior view of a patient's sitting posture. The patient sits with a slight posterior pelvic tilt, increased weight bearing on the right without associated trunk elongation, and right shoulder depression.

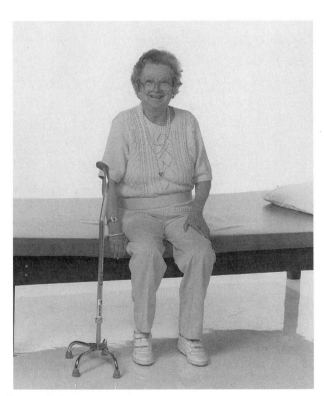

Figure 5–3 ■ A patient who exhibits fair sitting posture and balance. The assistant should observe the position of the patient's pelvis and trunk, the height of the shoulders, the symmetry of weight bearing on both hips, and the position of the patient's feet.

in front of the patient, to try to establish eye contact and to control the patient's head and trunk position. If not guarded correctly, the patient can fall off the support surface and be injured. Thus, patients functioning at a low level often benefit from treatment sessions with more than one individual.

Motor Control. The first problem area that must be addressed is the patient's sitting posture. A patient cannot progress to functional movements of the limbs without a stable upper and lower trunk from which to initiate movement and perform skilled activities of the extremities. *Stability* is defined as the ability to fix or maintain a position or posture in relation to gravity, and it is a prerequisite for the more advanced stages of motor development including controlled mobility and skill. *Controlled mobility* refers to the ability to maintain postural stability while moving. An example of this would be weight shifting in a quadruped (four-point) position with the hands fixed and the proximal joints, in this example the shoulders, moving. *Skilled activities* are described as coordinated, purposeful movements that are superimposed on a stable posture. The ability to perform skilled activities comprises the tasks that our patients often aspire to achieve. Ambulation and fine motor activities of the hand are two common examples of skill activities.

Sitting Posture: Positioning the Pelvis. The position of the patient's pelvis must be assessed initially. Figure

5–4 provides a posterior view of the patient's sitting posture. Clinicians often ignore the pelvis and try to correct deviations noted in the trunk. A patient will be unable to maintain adequate trunk and/or head control if unable to achieve a neutral position of the pelvis. A posteriorly tilted pelvis creates a bias toward thoracic kyphosis and a forward head position. This type of posturing is common in our everyday world, and as a consequence, many patients present with these premorbid postural deviations. By placing one's hands over the lumbar paraspinal musculature, one can gently guide the patient's pelvis in the direction of an anterior pelvic tilt. This technique provides the patient with tactile feedback for achieving a more neutral pelvic position. Intervention 5–20 depicts this activity. Care must be taken to avoid overly tilting the pelvis and locking the patient in an anterior pelvic tilt. An anterior tilt puts the spine in extension, thus creating

a closed-pack position and preventing movement. This closed-pack position limits the patient's abilities to perform functional movement transitions that require lateral weight shifts and rotation.

Achieving Pelvic Tilts in Supine. For individuals who are having difficulty in isolating pelvic movements, the assistant can have the patient work on achieving anterior and posterior pelvic tilts in the supine position. A large therapy ball can be placed under the patient's lower extremities. While stabilizing the patient's legs on the ball, the assistant can gently move the ball forward and backward. This technique allows the patient to feel the movement of the pelvis in a controlled and secure position.

Positioning the Trunk. Once the assistant has taught the patient to move the pelvis actively and the patient is able to maintain a neutral pelvic position in sitting, attention is then given to the trunk muscula-

---

Intervention 5–20 ▌ ACHIEVING A NEUTRAL PELVIS

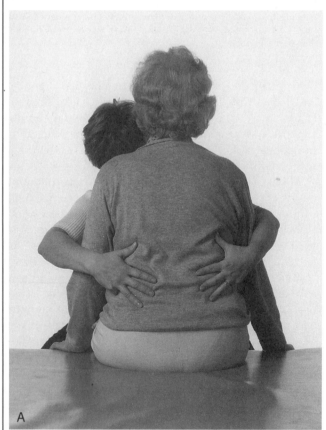 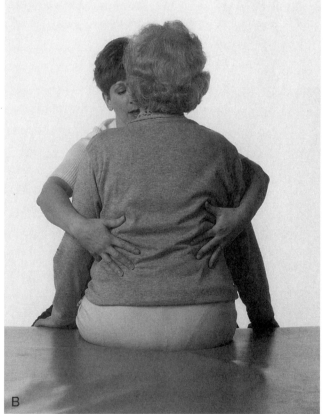

A. The assistant provides tactile cues to the patient's paraspinals to achieve a neutral pelvis.

B. Tension within the intrinsic finger musculature provides tactile feedback to the patient. Care is-

taken to avoid poking the patient with the assistant's fingertips. The little fingers are positioned on the patient's abdominals to facilitate movement back into a posterior pelvic tilt.

ture. Alignment of the shoulders over the hips is desired for good erect sitting posture. Gentle extension of the trunk should be encouraged by having the patient look up and bring the shoulders back. Initially, the patient may require tactile cues to be able to extend the trunk and contract the abdominal muscles. While maintaining a tactile cue in the patient's low back region, the assistant may place the other hand on the patient's sternum and move the patient's upper trunk into extension. Eventually, the patient must be taught to self-correct her own positioning in sitting. Recognizing when posture should be corrected facilitates motor learning of this task and enables the patient to assume this posture during other functional activities such as standing. If the patient has difficulty in maintaining an upright sitting posture, the assistant may try increasing the patient's visual input through the use of a mirror. It may be necessary to work jointly with another clinician to provide adequate manual contacts for equal weight bearing over both hips and to maintain the patient's trunk erect.

Positioning the Head. Poor pelvic positioning often contributes to misalignment of the patient's head. The patient must be able to hold the head erect to orient to the environment. An inability to maintain an upright position of the head causes visual and postural deficits through incorrect input into the vestibular system. Forward flexion of the cervical spine causes the patient's gaze to be directed toward the floor. This condition can affect arousal and the patient's ability to attend to persons or events within the environment. Excessive flexion of the head also biases the patient toward increased thoracic kyphosis and posterior tilting of the pelvis. If the patient is unable to maintain an upright position of the head and neck, facilitation techniques must be employed to correct the deficit. Quick icing or gentle tapping to the posterior cervical muscles produces cervical extension. At times, it is necessary for the assistant to provide manual cues to maintain the patient's head upright. A second person may be needed to achieve this outcome. Once the patient is able to maintain his head positioning independently, the assistant should decrease the manual support.

Additional Sitting Balance Activities: Weight Bearing on the Involved Hand. Once the patient is able to maintain an upright sitting posture with minimal to moderate assistance, progression to additional balance activities is warranted. An early sitting activity that promotes sitting balance and upper extremity function is weight bearing on the involved hand. The patient's upper extremity should be placed in neutral rotation and abducted approximately 30 degrees, the elbow should be extended, and the wrist and fingers should also be extended, as depicted in Intervention 5–21. Care must be taken to avoid excessive external rotation of the shoulder. Extreme external rotation of the

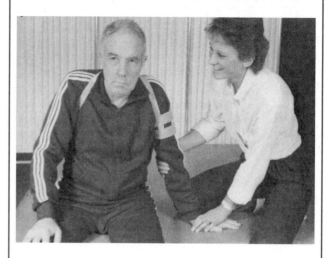

Intervention 5–21 ▎ WEIGHT BEARING ON THE INVOLVED HAND

Sitting with the involved upper extremity extended. The patient is wearing a Bobath arm sling with a humeral cuff to prevent subluxation of the shoulder. The clinician assists in stabilizing the patient's elbow and fingers in extension.

From O'Sullivan SB, Schmitz TJ (eds). Physical Rehabilitation Assessment and Treatment. Philadelphia, FA Davis, 1994.

shoulder causes the elbow to become anatomically locked, thus eliminating the need for the patient to use the triceps actively to maintain elbow extension. Extension of the wrist and fingers with thumb abduction assists in decreasing spasticity in the wrist and finger flexors. Some patients, however, find this position uncomfortable or painful secondary to tightness in the wrist and fingers or because of preexisting arthritis. Thus, modifications of this position can be used. Weight bearing on a flexed elbow with the forearm resting on a bolster or half-roll offers the same benefits. Weight bearing stimulates joint and muscle proprioceptors to contract and assists in development of muscle control around a joint. It is especially beneficial to patients who have flaccid or hypotonic upper extremity musculature and who demonstrate glenohumeral subluxation.

Shoulder Subluxations. A subluxation is the separation of the articular surfaces of bones from their normal position in a joint. Shoulder subluxation is relatively common in patients who have sustained strokes. If the upper extremity is flaccid, the scapula can assume a position of downward rotation. This orientation causes the glenoid fossa to become oriented posteriorly. Loss of muscle tone, stretch on the capsule, and this abnormal bony alignment results in an inferior shoulder subluxation. Strong hypertonicity in the scapular and shoulder musculature can predispose the patient to an anterior subluxation (Ryerson, 1995).

To determine whether a patient has a subluxation, place the patient's upper extremity in a non–weight-bearing position and palpate the acromion process. Moving distally from the border of the acromion, you should be able to palpate whether a separation exists between the process and the head of the humerus. Figure 5–5 depicts a shoulder subluxation. Compare the involved shoulder with the uninvolved joint. Measure the separation in terms of finger widths with the fingers oriented horizontally to the acromion. The extent of the separation can vary from a half-finger width up to a four or more finger widths of separation. In addition to the resulting bony malalignment, subluxations also lead to ligamentous laxity around the joint. Weight bearing temporarily moves the head of the humerus back up into the glenoid fossa and assists in realignment of the joint. Weight bearing offers only temporary remediation of the condition, however. Active control of the middle deltoid and rotator cuff muscles is necessary to bring the head of the humerus back into proper alignment permanently. Alternative treatments that assist in reducing subluxations include functional electric stimulation, biofeedback, and slings. The use of functional electric stimulation and biofeedback for the purposes of muscle reeducation is beyond the scope of this text. Slings can be prescribed for patients needing support of the shoulder joint. However, clinicians disagree regarding the use of slings in patients with hemiparesis. Many slings do not fit the patient properly and consequently do little to support the shoulder. In addition, slings promote neglect and disregard of the involved upper extremity and facilitate asymmetry within the trunk and upper extremities.

Weight-Shifting Activities. A gradual progression of sitting activities includes weight shifting in both anteroposterior and mediolateral directions. Weight-shifting activities are performed with the patient's arms in a weight-bearing position or with the arms resting in his lap. Initially, patients should relearn to shift their weight within their base of support. Patients with hemiplegia often exhibit difficulties with weight shifting, especially toward the involved side, because many patients lack the ability to control their trunk musculature actively. A lateral weight shift to the right requires the ability to elongate or lengthen the trunk muscles on the right and to shorten the trunk muscles on the left, thus maintaining the weight of the body within the base of support. In addition, the head rights in an attempt to keep the eyes vertical and the mouth horizontal. Patients with spasticity or hypotonia may not be able to activate their neck or trunk muscles in such a way. An attempt to shift weight to the right frequently results in a collapse of the head and trunk into right lateral flexion. As a consequence, the patient experiences increased weight bearing on the right side. This, however, is not a controlled weight-bearing condition. Figure 5–6 shows a patient performing a weight shift to the right side with trunk shortening on the weight-bearing side. A patient's inability to perform weight shifts while sitting may affect his ability to perform activities of daily living including self-care tasks, feeding, and dressing.

In an effort to assist the patient in relearning the appropriate trunk strategies, the assistant can provide tactile cues on the trunk musculature. Intervention 5–22 depicts an assistant who is facilitating trunk elonga-

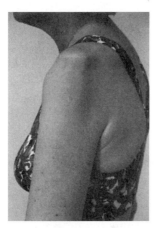

Figure 5–5 ■ Shoulder subluxation. (From Ryerson S, Levit K. Functional Movement Reeducation. New York, Churchill Livingstone, 1997.)

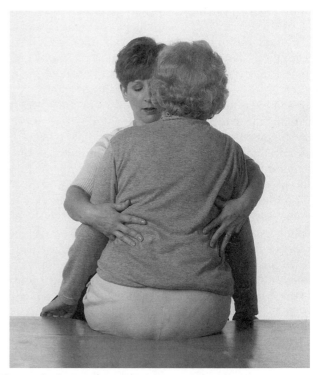

Figure 5–6 ■ Weight shifting to the right in sitting. The patient's trunk should elongate on the weight-bearing side.

Intervention 5–22 ▌ FACILITATING WEIGHT SHIFTS

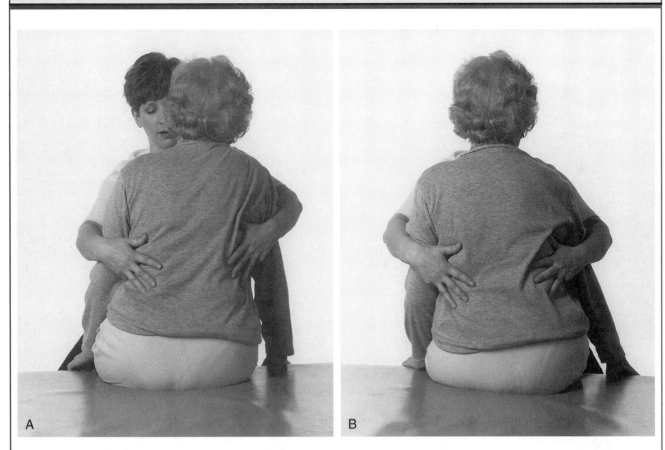

The assistant facilitates weight shifts to the right and left in sitting. The assistant provides tactile cues to the patient's paraspinals to facilitate the desired response.

tion on the patient's weight-bearing side. This activity should be practiced on both right and left sides.

Sitting Balance Activities to Improve Trunk Control. Once the patient is able to maintain a stable sitting position with proper alignment, additional static sitting balance activities can be practiced. The physical therapist assistant can apply manual resistance *(alternating isometrics)* at the shoulders or pelvis in an anteroposterior or mediolateral direction to promote co-contraction around the joints. Manual resistance with a rotational component *(rhythmic stabilization)* can also be performed to promote trunk stability.

Assessing Protective Reactions. While the patient is sitting, the physical therapist assistant may also want to observe the patient's protective reactions. Patients should demonstrate protective reactions laterally, anteriorly, and posteriorly. *Protective extension,* characterized by extension and abduction, is evident in the upper extremities when a patient's balance is quickly disturbed and the patient realizes that he may fall. Often, this protective reaction is absent or delayed in patients

who have had strokes. A patient with a flaccid or spastic upper extremity may not be able to elicit the motor components of the protective response. When testing this reaction, one should try to elicit an unanticipated response. Too often, clinicians inform the patient of what they are going to do, thus allowing the patient an opportunity to prepare a muscle response and react with co-contraction around the joint and thus eliminating any spontaneous movement.

Activities that can be performed to facilitate weight shifting in sitting include reaching to the right and left and to the floor and ceiling. Intervention 5–23A depicts a patient reaching to the left with her hands clasped. Incorporating these activities within the context of a functional activity is highly desirable and therapeutically beneficial. For example, to challenge a patient's ability to shift weight forward, the assistant can have the patient practice putting on shoes and socks or picking up an object off the floor. Other tasks that challenge a patient's sitting balance include the performance of activities of daily living such as sitting

Intervention 5–23 ▌ REACHING ACTIVITIES

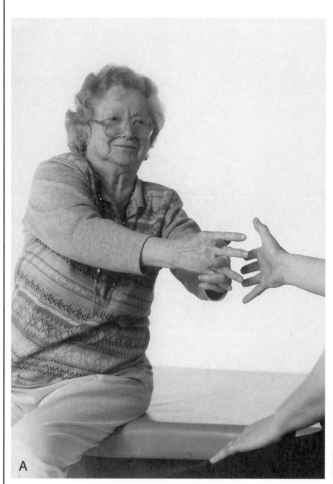

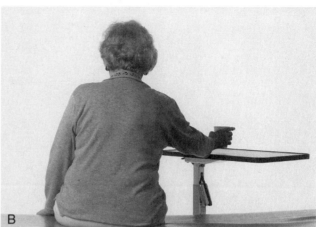

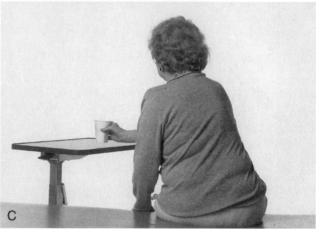

A. Reaching with the hands clasped. Patients should practice reaching to the right and left and at various heights.

B and C. Reaching with the uninvolved upper extremity to the right and left. The involved arm is in a weight-bearing position during performance of the activity. If the patient has active movement in the involved arm, she can perform reaching tasks with it.

on the edge of the bed or in a chair to don items of clothing or sitting in a chair to reach for a cup, as depicted in Intervention 5–23B and C. Reaching activities in sitting should also incorporate trunk rotation. Rotation is a frequently lost movement component in older patients. Passive or active assisted lower trunk rotation performed in the supine position assists the patient in maintaining the necessary flexibility in the trunk musculature to perform this movement component. Furthermore, maintaining separation of the upper and lower trunk assists the patient's ability to rotate and dissociate movements of the shoulder and pelvic girdles. As the patient progresses, performance of the bilateral PNF patterns (chops and lifts) can

be used to facilitate trunk rotation. These exercises are illustrated in Intervention 5–24.

Sitting Activities. A summary of techniques to be performed in sitting follows:

Pelvic positioning
Trunk positioning
Head positioning
Weight bearing on the involved upper extremity
Weight shifting in anteroposterior and mediolateral directions
Alternating isometrics
Rhythmic stabilization
Functional reaching

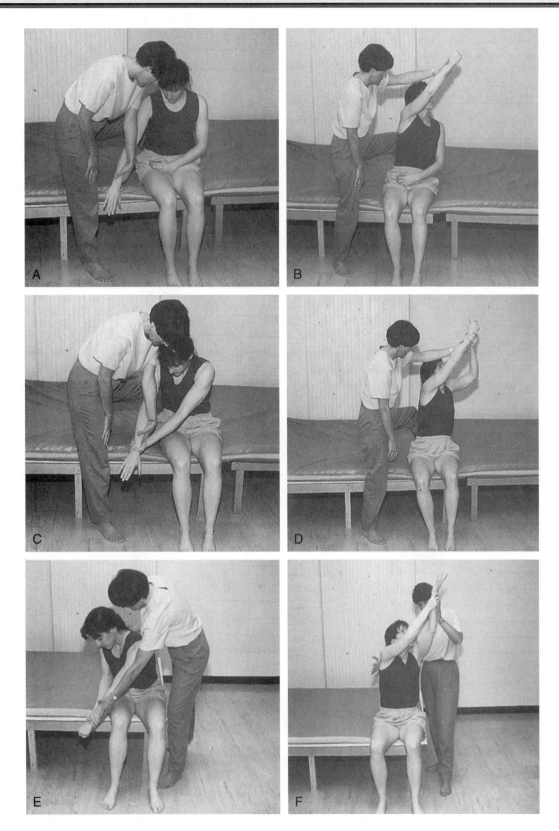

A and B Proprioceptive neuromuscular facilitation (PNF) upper extremity D1 flexion and extension patterns.

C and D. PNF chop and reverse-chop patterns.
E and F. PNF lift and reverse-lift patterns.

From O'Sullivan SB, Schmitz TJ. Physical Rehabilitation Laboratory Manual Focus on Functional Training. Philadelphia, FA Davis, 1999.

Standing

As the patient is able to tolerate more treatment activities during sitting, the patient should be progressed to upright standing. It is not necessary to perfect one posture or activity before advancing the patient to a more challenging one. Patients should work in all possible postures to reach the highest functional level. As the patient is working on sitting activities, he may also advance to supported standing. However, the physical therapist assistant must follow the plan of care developed for the patient by the supervising physical therapist. The primary physical therapist should evaluate the patient's standing abilities before the assistant stands the patient for the first time.

Position of the Physical Therapist Assistant in Relation to the Patient. A common question asked by students is where to position oneself when assisting the patient from sitting to standing. Much depends on the patient and the patient's current level of motor control and function. Sitting in front of the patient as she transfers to standing gives her space to move into and also offers the clinician the opportunity to assess the patient's posture in standing. This transition is depicted in Intervention 5–25. The assistant may also elect to start from a squat position in front of the patient and move to standing with her. If this method is employed, the assistant must allow the patient physical space to perform the forward weight shift that accompanies trunk flexion prior to lifting the buttocks off the support surface. Often, clinicians guard the patient so closely that it is nearly impossible for the patient to complete the necessary movement sequences and weight shifts. Standing on the patient's side should be avoided initially because it can promote excessive weight shift to that side. As the patient progresses and exhibits increased control, the assistant

---

Intervention 5–25 ▮ SIT-TO-STAND TRANSITION

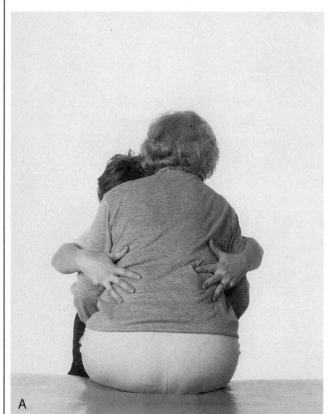 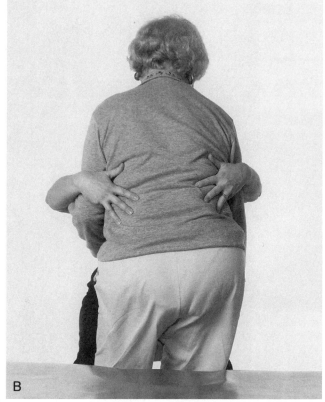

A. Patient pre-positioning is important before a sit-to-stand transition is performed. The patient must be able to shift weight to scoot forward on the mat so that only half of the femurs are supported. The patient's feet should be shoulder width apart.

B. The assistant sits in front of the patient with her hands on the patient's paraspinals to facilitate an anterior weight shift. The patient should be encouraged to push up with both lower extremities equally to promote symmetric weight bearing.

may be able to guard the patient from the side, as shown in Intervention 5–26. In addition to the assistant's position relative to the patient, a safety belt must always be used. Use of safety belts is standard in most facilities. Even if a patient insists that she does not need a safety belt, it is always in the patient's and the assistant's best interest to use one.

Sit-to-Stand Transition. The transition from sitting to standing is the first part of the standing progression. The patient must initially be able to maintain the lower extremities in flexion at the hips, knees, and ankles. In addition, the patient must be able to

achieve and maintain a neutral or slightly anterior tilt of the pelvis during a forward weight shift over the fixed feet. It therefore becomes essential that the patient be able to advance the tibias over the feet. Patients who present with plantar flexion contractures of the ankles or increased tone in the gastrocnemius-soleus complex may not be able to achieve the amount of passive ankle dorsiflexion necessary to complete this activity. In people without neurologic deficits the ascent to standing is accomplished by combining knee extension with hip extension. Frequently, patients are unable to perform this part of the move-

---

Intervention 5–26 ▌ GUARDING THE PATIENT FROM THE SIDE DURING A SIT-TO-STAND TRANSITION

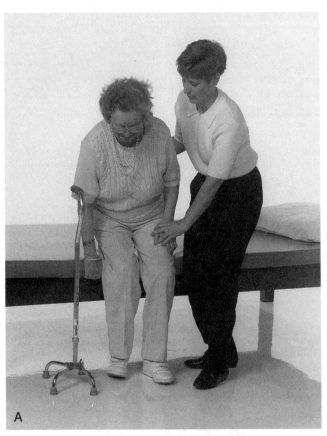
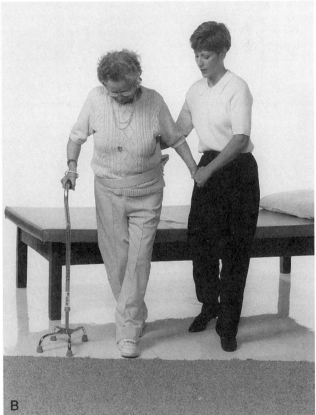

Patients with fair to good static and dynamic standing balance may be able to be guarded from their involved side.

A. The assistant provides a tactile cue to the patient's upper extremity to inhibit abnormal tone. Note the position of the patient's involved lower extremity during the transition. The left leg is positioned in front of the right leg. This position reinforces reliance on the uninvolved lower extremity to assume standing.

B. Once the patient is standing, an inhibitory hand-hold can be used to decrease flexor tone, which is present in the patient's elbow, wrist, and fingers.

ment smoothly and exhibit difficulty maintaining a neutral hip position once they are upright because of lack of strength in their hip extensors. These patients often appear to be in a crouched or flexed position, or they use strong knee hyperextension while coming to stand. Because of the lower extremity weakness and insecurity experienced by many patients, they often rely extensively on the uninvolved leg to perform sit-to-stand transfers. This reliance is evident by increased weight bearing on the uninvolved leg and truncal asymmetry. The problem can be accentuated if the patient is allowed to push up with the upper extremity. Intervention 5–27 shows a patient coming to stand with the use of the upper extremity. Continued performance of sit-to-stand transitions in this manner results in the patient's inability to bear weight on the involved leg and can accentuate the patient's insecurity about stability of the involved lower extremity. Patients with hemiplegia must be encouraged to perform sit-to-stand transitions with equal weight bearing on both lower extremities. Symmetric foot placement, with feet shoulder-width apart, and the patient's feet flat on the floor can assist in the achievement of equal weight bearing.

The patient's upper extremity must be carefully monitored during a sit-to-stand transfer. The involved arm should not be allowed to hang down at the patient's side. In this situation, gravity applies a distractional force that can accentuate shoulder subluxation. The upper extremity can be pre-positioned by placing the involved arm on the patient's knee or the assistant's arm, as shown in Intervention 5–28. In some instances, a sling may be necessary to give additional support, or the patient may be advised to place the involved hand in a pants pocket. By pre-positioning the upper extremity in these ways, one is supporting the shoulder and also applying a minimal amount of approximation to the shoulder joint and surrounding musculature.

During the sit-to-stand transition, the assistant needs to gauge carefully the amount of physical assistance required by the patient. The clinician can provide manual cues over the patient's gluteus maximus muscle to promote hip extension. As previously stated, if

---

Intervention 5–27 ❙ SIT-TO-STAND USING THE UNINVOLVED UPPER EXTREMITY

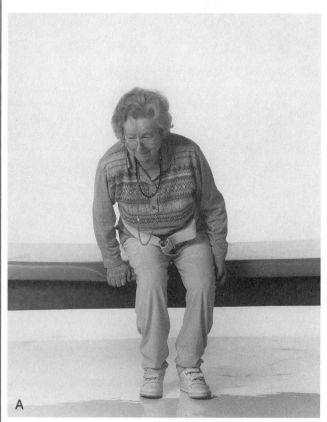 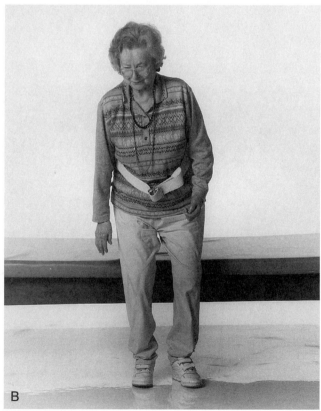

A   B

Using the uninvolved upper extremity to assist with coming to stand. Note the increased weight bearing on the uninvolved side and the associated asymmetry.

Intervention 5–28 ▌ PRE-POSITIONING THE PATIENT'S INVOLVED UPPER EXTREMITY

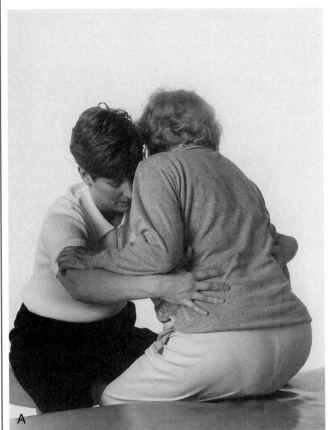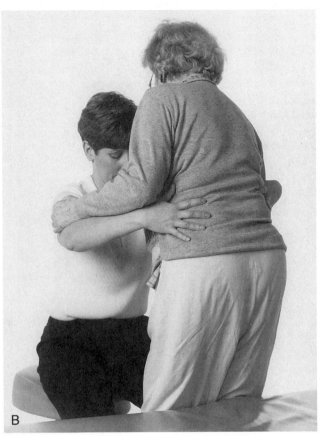

It is necessary to pre-position the patient's involved upper extremity during movement transitions to prevent injury to the shoulder.

the patient is unable to extend the hips, the patient will often assume a forward flexed posture. The assistant may find it physically necessary to move the patient's hips into extension to achieve an upright position. Intervention 5–29 illustrates an assistant who is providing manual contacts at the patient's gluteal muscles.

In addition to monitoring the position of the patient's hips, one must observe the alignment of the patient's involved knee and ankle for proper positioning. If the ankle musculature is flaccid and unstable, the patient may bear weight on his malleolus or the lateral aspect of his foot, with resulting long-lasting ligamentous disorders. To avoid this complication, the physical therapist assistant needs to pre-position the patient's foot or block the patient's ankle to keep it from turning inward. This can be accomplished by having the assistant place both his feet around the patient's involved ankle, thus providing additional support. This type of positioning also provides additional

support to the entire involved lower extremity. Intervention 5–30 shows an assistant blocking the patient's ankle to prevent instability.

Establishing Knee Control. Inadequate knee control impedes the patient's ability to stand and to ambulate. The patient's knee may buckle when the joint is required to accept weight. This condition is often due to weakness in the quadriceps. Clinically, when individuals with quadriceps weakness stand up, they immediately assume a crouched or flexed posture. Quadriceps weakness or inefficient gastrocnemius-soleus function can lead to strong knee hyperextension or genu recurvatum during standing. Patients who demonstrate this condition lock their knees into extension to maintain stability. Several explanations for this phenomenon have been suggested. Decreased proprioceptive input from the joint may cause the patient to hyperextend the knee joint in an attempt to find a stable point as maximum input is received at the joint's end range or closed-pack position. Overactive

Intervention 5–29 ▌ USING TACTILE CUES TO ASSIST THE SIT-TO-STAND TRANSITION

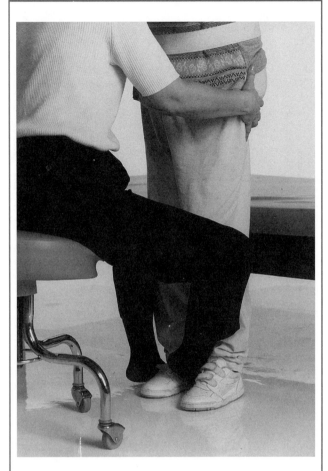

During sit-to-stand and standing activities, the assistant can apply tactile cues to the gluteals to help achieve hip extension and an upright posture.

Intervention 5–30 ▌ BLOCKING THE PATIENT'S ANKLE

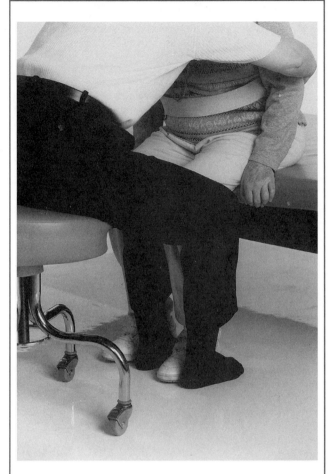

The assistant blocks the patient's involved ankle with both her feet to prevent weight bearing on the malleoli and possible injury.

or spastic quadriceps and a lack of balance between the hamstrings and quadriceps have also been cited as reasons for knee hyperextension. In both situations, knee instability results because the patient does not have active control over the thigh muscles. To control these deviations, appropriate manual (tactile) cues around the knee must be used. Pressure on the anterior shin may be needed when buckling is present. The physical therapist assistant may actually have to assist the knee joint into extension, as illustrated in Intervention 5–31. In contrast, manual cues applied to the posterior knee may be required in the presence of knee hyperextension. The assistant may need to prevent the knee from extending to a completely locked position. Continued knee hyperextension can cause long-term ligamentous and capsular problems and therefore should be avoided.

Positioning the Standing Patient. Once the patient

is standing, the goal is to achieve symmetry and midline orientation. Equal weight bearing on both lower extremities, an erect trunk, and midline orientation of the head are the desired postural outcomes. Patients who have extremely low function may require additional assistance. In some instances, it may initially be necessary to have the patient work on standing on the tilt table. The tilt table should be used only when the patient requires excessive assistance or when the patient is unable to tolerate upright standing because of medical complications.

For patients who do not need the tilt table but who have poor trunk and lower extremity control, the therapist may determine that a second person is needed to assist with positioning the patient's trunk and involved upper or lower extremity. The support person can be behind the patient providing tactile cues for trunk extension. The person may assist with positioning of the involved upper extremity. A bedside table is often

Intervention 5–31 ▍ USING TACTILE CUES TO PROMOTE KNEE EXTENSION

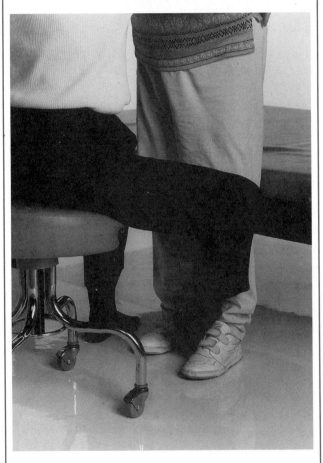

The assistant uses her leg to provide a tactile cue to the patient's shin. This cue is used to promote knee extension in the involved lower extremity.

Intervention 5–32 ▍ USING A BEDSIDE TABLE DURING STANDING ACTIVITIES

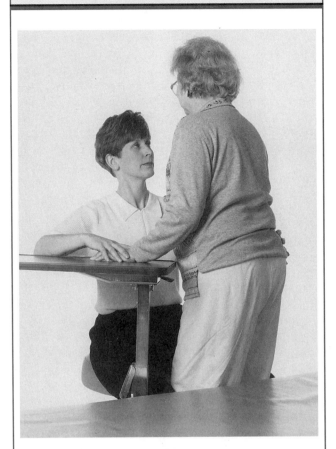

A bedside table can be used during standing activities to support the involved upper extremity. The assistant provides a tactile cue to maintain the wrist in a neutral to slightly extended position with the fingers extended.

used to provide the involved arm with a weight-bearing surface. Increased proprioceptive input is received through the involved upper extremity during weight bearing. The use of upper extremity support also assists in unloading the lower extremity and decreases the amount of control needed for the patient to stand and to bear weight. Intervention 5–32 illustrates a patient who is using a bedside table during standing activities. At times, it is helpful for the second person to be at the patient's side. Much depends on the individual patient and his response to standing and weight-bearing activities.

Early Standing Activities: Weight Shifting. The assistant can help the patient to practice standing activities from the patient's bed, from the mat table, or in the parallel bars. Early standing activities should include weight shifts (moving the patient's center of gravity) to the right and left and in anterior and poste-

rior directions. Small, controlled weights shifts are preferred to those that are extreme. Observation of the patient's responses to these early attempts at weight shifting are essential. Patients are often reluctant to shift weight onto the involved lower extremity. To avoid weight shifting, the patient laterally flexes the trunk toward the side of the weight shift instead of accepting weight onto the extremity and elongating the trunk.

The physical therapist assistant must monitor the position of the patient's hip, knee, and ankle during all standing weight-shifting activities. Achievement of hip extension with the patient's pelvis in a neutral or slightly anterior position is desired. As stated previously, tactile cues applied to the gluteus maximus may be necessary to assist the patient with hip extension. If the patient is experiencing difficulty with knee control, the assistant may elect to spend part of the treatment session working on this problem. Having the patient slowly bend and straighten the involved knee is the first step. The assistant may have to guide the knee into flexion and then extension manually. The patient should gauge the amount of muscle force generated during this task. Frequently, patients exaggerate knee extension by quickly snapping the knee back into an extended position. Once the patient is able to control this movement, the physical therapist assistant should have the patient relax the knee into flexion and then slowly extend it without producing knee hyperextension or genu recurvatum. Active achievement of the last 10 to 15 degrees of extension is often difficult for the patient. Clinicians often use terminal knee extension exercises to assist with this control. However, research has shown that little carryover of motor tasks occurs from sitting to standing. Therefore, if the patient needs to achieve the final few degrees of knee extension in standing or walking, then the patient should practice this component of the movement in an upright standing position.

Assessing Balance Responses. As the patient continues to perform weight-shifting activities, one should detect the presence of appropriate standing balance responses. Ankle dorsiflexion should be elicited as the patient's body mass is shifted backward. Figure 5-7 shows an ankle strategy. This motor response normally occurs as a balance strategy in standing. If the patient's balance is disrupted too much, the patient will exhibit a hip or stepping strategy. Movement of the hip occurs to realign the patient. A *stepping strategy* is used if the patient's balance is displaced too far, and a step is taken to prevent the patient from falling. Many patients who have sustained CVAs lack the ability to

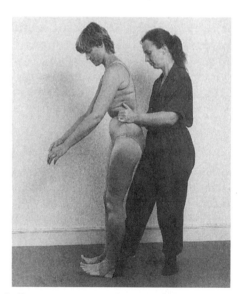

Figure 5-7 ■ A typical person moved backward. The patient exhibits an equilibrium response. Note the dorsiflexion of the ankles and toes; the arms move forward as well as the head. (From Bobath B. Adult Hemiplegia: Evaluation and Treatment, 3rd ed. Boston, Butterworth Heinemann, 1990.)

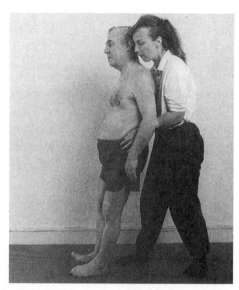

Figure 5-8 ■ Moving a patient backward. Note the active dorsiflexion of the uninvolved right foot (normal balance reaction) and its absence in the affected foot. (From Bobath B. Adult Hemiplegia: Evaluation and Treatment, 3rd ed. Boston, Butterworth Heinemann, 1990.)

elicit appropriate balance responses in standing secondary to muscle weakness and the inability to time muscle responses. This problem is depicted in Figure 5-8. The assistant should note the patient's ability to perform these strategies (ankle, hip, stepping), especially if the patient is working on ambulation skills.

Standing Progression (Walking): Position of the Physical Therapist Assistant in Relation to the Patient

Once the patient is able to maintain an upright position and to accept weight on both lower extremities, it is time to progress the patient to stepping. Because walking is a primary goal of many of our patients and it is the treatment activity in which patients most wish to participate, walking should be practiced and encouraged during therapy if the patient is an appropriate candidate. Although patients are eager to begin walking activities, they need to possess adequate trunk and lower extremity control for ambulation. It is not safe or functional to drag a patient down the parallel bars just to satisfy the patient's need to walk. On the other hand, it is not necessary to perfect the patient's sitting or standing posture prior to introducing ambulation activities. The assistant can position himself or herself in several different places during standing activities with a patient. The assistant can sit or stand in front of the patient and can control the patient at the hips. The assistant can also stand on the patient's hemiplegic side. This method of guarding can be of benefit if the patient requires tactile cues at the pelvis or posterior hip area. Standing on the patient's involved side can, in some patients, promote excessive weight shifting to that extremity and should be avoided. The therapist's presence on the involved side may also provide the patient with a false sense of security.

Advancing the Uninvolved Lower Extremity. Initially, patients should be taught to step forward with the uninvolved lower extremity, as shown in Intervention 5–33. The advantage to this sequence is that it causes the patient to bear weight exclusively on the involved leg, thus promoting single-limb support (weight bearing) on the involved lower extremity. Many patients take a small step with the uninvolved leg or simply slide the foot forward along the floor in an effort to make this task easier. Both situations decrease the amount of time spent in unilateral limb support on the involved lower extremity. Although patients are able to ambulate in such a fashion, the continuance of this pattern can lead to the development of postural deviations and increased lower ex-

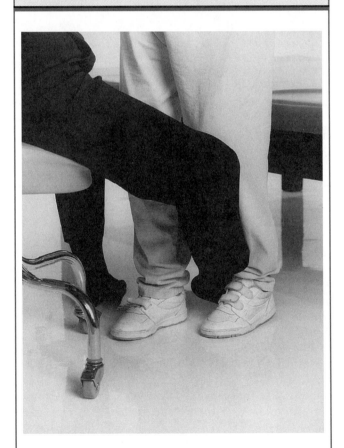

Intervention 5–33 ∎ PREGAIT ACTIVITIES

In standing, the patient initially steps forward with the uninvolved lower extremity. This maneuver facilitates single weight bearing on the involved leg as the patient steps. The assistant blocks the patient's involved lower extremity as needed to prevent knee buckling.

tremity tone. To achieve a more normal gait pattern, the patient must be able to maintain single-limb support on the involved side during stance, to allow the other leg to take a normal-sized step. Single-limb support is also required for other functional activities such as negotiating curbs and stairs.

Advancing the Involved Lower Extremity. Often, a portion of the patient's treatment session is devoted to practicing forward stepping. Once the patient is able to advance the uninvolved leg forward and to maintain weight on it, the patient is progressed to advancing the involved lower extremity. Patients often have difficulty in initiating hip flexion for lower extremity advancement. As previously stated, the extension synergy pattern is frequently present in the involved lower extremity and becomes evident as the patient tries to take a step forward. Instead of using hip flexion to advance the leg forward, the patient uses *hip circumduction* (hip abduction with internal rotation). Pelvic retraction frequently accompanies this movement pattern. Knee extension and ankle plantar flexion, also part of the extension synergy, can be evident. Consequently, as the patient moves the involved leg forward, the extremity advances as an extended unit. This extension limits the patient's ability to initiate knee flexion, which is needed for the swing phase of the gait cycle, and ankle dorsiflexion, which is necessary for heelstrike. Strong extension in the lower extremity results in decreased weight bearing on the involved lower extremity during stance. Because of the synergy patterns and the strong desires of many patients to walk, physical therapists and physical therapist assistants frequently see patients who ambulate in this fashion. Patients should be discouraged from walking like this if at all possible. Continued substitution of hip circumduction for true hip flexion can cause the patient to relearn an abnormal and inefficient movement pattern. Concomitantly, abnormal stresses are placed on the involved joints, and it becomes increasingly difficult to change or replace the abnormal pattern with a more normal gait. Ambulation performed in this way reinforces the patient's lower extremity spasticity.

Achieving a Normal Gait Pattern: Positioning the Pelvis. To assist the patient in initiating hip flexion, the following techniques can be used. Prior to providing any tactile cues, the assistant must determine the position of the patient's pelvis. The assistant should note the relative position of the patient's pelvis in terms of pelvic tilt and observe whether the pelvis is in a retracted position. If the patient's pelvis is retracted or in an elevated or hiked position, the assistant needs to provide a downward and slightly forward tactile cue on the patient's pelvis to restore proper pelvic alignment. It may be necessary for the assistant to also apply a tactile cue on the patient's posterior buttocks to assist the pelvis into a more neutral pelvic tilt. Of-

Intervention 5-34 ▌ ADVANCING THE INVOLVED LEG FORWARD

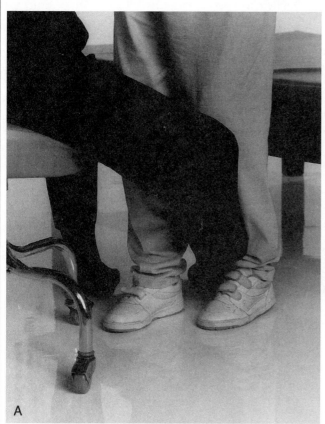 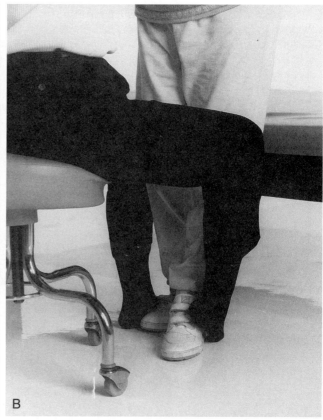

The patient may need assistance stepping forward with the involved leg.

A. The assistant can use her foot behind the patient's heel to advance the involved leg.

B. Repositioning the foot may be necessary.

---

ten, the patient can be asked to flex (bend) the involved knee to assist in bringing the pelvis into a better position.

Advancing the Involved Lower Extremity Forward. Once the pelvis is in proper alignment, the patient is asked to slide the involved foot forward. If the patient is unable to initiate this movement, the assistant may need to help the patient manually. This technique is demonstrated in Intervention 5–34. Sliding the foot forward is easier than having the patient attempt to lift the involved limb forward. Increased effort and possible patient frustration can increase abnormal tone. At times, it may be difficult to slide the involved foot forward because of the friction created between the patient's shoe and the floor. Patients can be requested to take their shoes off, or a pillowcase or small towel can be placed under the patient's foot to make it easier to advance. A stockinette can also be placed on the toe of the patient's shoe to reduce friction. The patient should practice bringing the foot forward and

backward several times. The assistant can make this activity easier for the patient by physically moving the towel or pillowcase for the patient. Again, tactile cues applied at the hip and pelvis are beneficial. Maintaining the involved knee in slight flexion decreases the likelihood that the patient will initiate lower extremity advancement with hip hiking or circumduction.

Backward Stepping. Stepping backward should also be practiced. When asking the patient to step backward, the assistant should note the position of the patient's hip and pelvis. Often, the patient performs hip extension with hiking and retraction. The patient should be encouraged to work toward isolated hip extension with knee flexion.

Putting It All Together. Once the patient is able to move the involved leg forward and back with fairly good success, the patient is progressed to putting several steps together. The patient is told to step forward first with the uninvolved lower extremity in preparation for toe-off and the swing phase of the gait cycle.

Intervention 5–35 ▐ ASSISTING AMBULATION

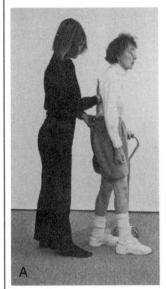
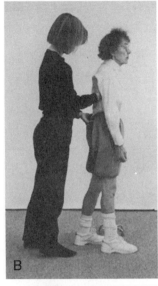
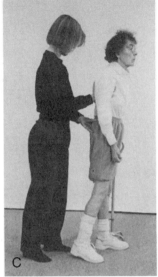
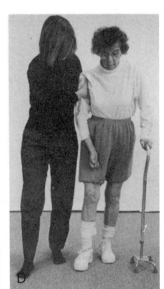
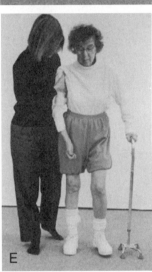
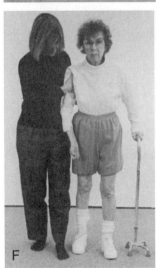

A. The clinician uses an axillary grip with her right arm and lifts the patient's upper trunk up and back. The patient was previously trained to use a quad cane. As the patient gains control, a straight cane can be introduced.

B. The clinician uses her left hand to assist the patient to initiate the movements from her legs in right step/stance. It is important to teach the patient how to shift weight over both legs without excessive leaning onto the quad cane.

C. As the patient practices the same movements in left step/stance, she cannot keep her right heel on the floor because of overshifting to the cane, insufficient hip extension range and control, or insufficient ankle dorsiflexion range. Forward and backward weight shifting movements are practiced repeatedly in the right and left step/stance positions.

D. The clinician's right hand uses an axillary grip to support the upper trunk while her left hand is on the posterolateral side of the patient's left rib cage.

E. The clinician reminds the patient to keep her upper trunk extended as she shifts her trunk and hip forward. Note how the clinician's feet step in parallel with the patient's.

F. The clinician must be careful to time her corrections and assistance to the patient's movement initiation patterns.

From Ryerson S, Levit K. Functional Movement Reeducation: A Contemporary Model for Stroke Rehabilitation. New York, Churchill Livingstone, 1997.

Intervention 5–35 illustrates a patient who is ambulating several steps. In addition, Table 5–8 provides a review of the normal gait training progression.

Normal Components of Gait. When assessing the patient's movements during the initial stages of ambulation training, the assistant should note the following movement components. A weight shift to the uninvolved side should occur during advancement of the involved lower extremity. This shift is accompanied by trunk elongation. The patient then needs to flex the involved knee and advance the hip forward. Many patients have a difficult time with this specific movement combination. The ability to flex the knee with the hip in a relatively neutral or extended position, coupled with adequate ankle dorsiflexion to prevent toe drag, is extremely difficult. If one thinks in terms of the Brunnstrom stages of recovery, the patient must be able to perform a stage 5 movement combination, which means combining different components of the various synergy patterns.

Patients who lack the ability to flex the knee and to dorsiflex the foot for swing tend to exaggerate the weight shift to the uninvolved side in an effort to shorten the extremity so that the foot can clear the floor. It may be necessary for the assistant to help the patient with lower extremity advancement. Again, the assistant can use a towel under the patient's foot or manual cues to the posterior leg to advance the patient's leg forward. The assistant may also need to guide the patient's weight shifts during this time. As stated previously, many patients are unable to gauge the degree of movement during early weight-shifting activities appropriately. The patient may need tactile cues at the hip or trunk to promote the proper postural response.

Turning Around. As the patient practices putting several steps together to walk forward, he should also learn to turn around. Turning toward the involved side is usually easier. Instead of having the patient think about picking up the involved foot and taking a step, the assistant should ask the patient to move the involved heel toward the midline. When the patient moves the heel inward, the toes are automatically moved outward and are ready for the directional change. From this position, the patient can easily step with the uninvolved lower extremity. It may be necessary for the patient to repeat this sequence several times to complete the turn. The assistant must carefully observe the patient performing this activity. Frequently, the patient attempts to turn by twisting the lower extremity, a movement that, if not prohibited, can result in injury to the knee and ankle.

Upper Extremity Positioning During Ambulation. Care must always be given to the position of the patient's upper extremity during gait activities. The involved arm can be pre-positioned on the assistant's upper extremity, on a bedside table, in the patient's pocket, or in a sling. The patient's arm should not be allowed to hang unsupported with gravity pulling down on it, especially in the presence of shoulder subluxation. Many patients experience an increase in the amount of tone present in the upper extremity during ambulation activities. This is the result of overflow of abnormal muscle tone, which often is exaggerated as patients attempt more challenging activities. Patients should be encouraged to consciously try to relax, therefore controlling the amount of tone present. Inhibiting handholds and armholds can be used for patients who do not require a great deal of physical assistance for ambulation. Intervention 5–36 demonstrates one of the most common inhibiting upper extremity positions. The handshake grasp and upper extremity abduction with wrist extension and thumb abduction can be used effectively in patients who experience an increase in flexor tone during ambulation. The handhold maintains the upper extremity in a position opposite that of the dominant flexor synergy pattern. For ambulatory patients with good upper extremity motor return, treatment should focus on the return of reciprocal arm swing.

Common Gait Deviations. As previously mentioned,

Table 5–8 ❚ AMBULATION PROGRESSION

1. Standing activities	The patient should practice weight shifting to the right and left, and forward and backward. Knee control activities should also be emphasized.
2. Advancing the uninvolved lower extremity	The patient should practice stepping forward and backward with the uninvolved lower extremity. Emphasis should be on weight bearing on the involved lower extremity and achievement of the proper step length.
3. Advancing the involved lower extremity	The patient should practice advancing the involved lower extremity forward. A tactile cue at the hip may be necessary to promote hip flexion and to decrease hip hiking and circumduction.
4. Stepping back with the involved lower extremity	Stepping backward with the involved lower extremity must also be practiced. The tendency again is for the patient to hike the hip. Patients must concentrate on releasing the extensor tone and allowing for hip and knee flexion.
5. Putting several steps together	Once the patient can step forward and backward with both the uninvolved and involved extremities, the patient must begin to put several steps together. Emphasis must be placed on advancing the involved lower extremity during swing and appropriate weight shifts during the stance phase of the gait cycle.

Intervention 5-36 ▌ INHIBITING THE PATIENT'S INVOLVED UPPER EXTREMITY WHILE AMBULATING

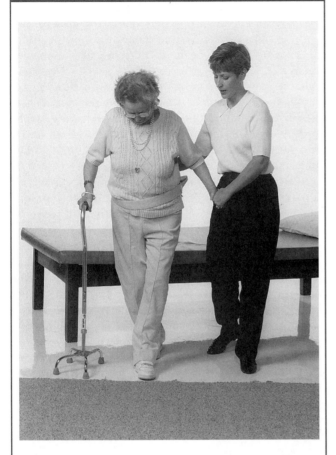

Ambulating the patient while inhibiting increased tone in the involved upper extremity. Shoulder abduction and external rotation combined with elbow extension and wrist and finger extension are desired.

given to the goals or activities the patient wishes to pursue. Physical therapists and physical therapist assistants no longer have the luxury of spending months working with patients. In the current managed care environment, the physical therapist must carefully design the patient's plan of care and choose activities that effectively address function and an optimal patient outcome. In addition, clinicians must use the patient's resources appropriately to achieve optimal benefit. Clinicians will continue to assist patients in the achievement of more normal movement patterns during performance of functional tasks; however, the emphasis of physical therapy intervention must be on the patient's ability to function in the home and community environment.

Selection of an Assistive Device

For the patient who is progressing well with ambulation activities, selection of the most appropriate assis-

Table 5-9 ▌ COMMON GAIT DEVIATIONS SEEN IN PATIENTS WITH STROKE

HIP	
Deviation	Possible Causes
Retraction	Increased lower extremity muscle tone
Hiking	Inadequate hip and knee flexion, increased tone in the trunk and lower extremity
Circumduction	Increased extensor tone, inadequate hip and knee flexion, increased plantar flexion in the ankle or footdrop
Inadequate hip flexion	Increased extensor tone, flaccid lower extremity

KNEE	
Deviation	Possible Causes
Decreased knee flexion during swing	Increased lower extremity extensor tone, weak hip flexion
Excessive flexion during stance	Weakness or flaccidity in the lower extremity, increased flexor tone in the lower extremity
Hyperextension during stance	Hip retraction, increased extensor tone in the lower extremity, weakness in the gluteus maximus, hamstrings, or quadriceps
Instability during stance	Increased lower extremity flexor tone, flaccidity

ANKLE	
Deviation	Possible Causes
Footdrop	Increased extensor tone, flaccidity
Ankle inversion or eversion	Increased tone in specific muscle groups, flaccidity
Toe clawing	Increased flexor tone in the toe muscles

several common gait deviations are seen in patients with hemiplegia. For the purposes of our discussion here, possible gait deviations that may develop are addressed by each individual joint and are summarized in Table 5-9.

Ambulation

Quality of Movement Versus Function

Clinicians often ask themselves whether they should allow the patient to walk even though the patient's gait pattern does not possess the desired quality of movement. In the present health care environment in which resources are limited, clinicians must work toward functional patient goals. Function must be considered at all times; however, consideration must be

tive device is the next step in the patient's rehabilitation. This decision should be discussed with the patient, the patient's family if appropriate, and the primary physical therapist. Individual differences and preferences do exist regarding which assistive device may be optimal for the patient.

Generally, walkers are not appropriate for patients who have sustained a CVA because these patients frequently lack the hand and upper extremity function needed to use the walker safely and effectively. Most often, clinicians recommend some type of cane for the patient. Hemiwalkers (walk-canes), wide-base and narrow-base quad canes, and straight canes are the most popular assistive devices. The wider the base of the cane, the more support it offers. Unfortunately, some of the wider-base canes are not as functional in the patient's home. For example, if a person lives in a small home or trailer, a hemiwalker may be difficult to maneuver in areas with limited space. In addition, hemiwalkers cannot be used on stairs. Wide-base quad canes are a little smaller than hemiwalkers, but they are still not as easy to use on steps because they often need to be turned sideways to fit on a step. Narrow-base quad canes and straight canes usually offer the most flexibility in the patient's home and can be easily used in the community.

Some physical therapists often suggest starting the patient with a more stable cane that provides greater support and then decreasing the support as the patient progresses. That is certainly an option, but one must recognize that once a patient has trained with a device, it is often difficult to advance the patient to the next, less stable one because of the patient's fear and overreliance. Many clinicians therefore challenge the patient early on by providing less support initially and moving to a different device if the patient requires additional support. Canes should be of adequate height to allow the patient's elbow to bend approximately 20 to 30 degrees when the patient has his hand on the handgrip. It is important to know whether a patient is going to purchase an assistive device for home use, because a physician's order is necessary for reimbursement.

Any equipment that may be needed for the patient at home should be ordered early enough so that when the patient is ready for discharge, the equipment will have been delivered and is properly adjusted. This need can create a dilemma for the physical therapist and physical therapist assistant because it is difficult to know how much the patient will progress and what his long-term needs will be.

Ambulation Training with Assistive Devices

The patient may need to work on assisted ambulation for some time. It is often difficult for patients to coordinate all parts of the body during walking. The patient needs to be able to maintain a stable postural base at the pelvis and trunk to initiate more distal movement. Frequently, a patient masters a more general skill, such as standing and weight shifting, but when asked to move from that position, the patient regresses and seems to lose the basic postural components. As the patient is able to assume more control, the assistant should begin to decrease his manual assistance.

If the patient is having difficulty with standing or gait activities or if the assistant finds it difficult to control the patient, additional assistive devices can be used. At times, having the patient stand with an object in front of him can be helpful. For example, some clinicians use a bedside table to the side of the patient to allow the patient to bear weight on the upper extremity during ambulation training. This technique can be especially beneficial if the patient requires more external trunk control or support or if he needs proper positioning of the involved upper extremity. Grocery carts offer the same benefits. The patient can position the upper extremities on the handle of the cart and then push it. The assistant can stand behind the patient and offer tactile cues and feedback to assist with lower extremity advancement and single-limb support. For some patients, ambulation training may be best practiced in the parallel bars or at the hemirail. Both these pieces of therapeutic equipment provide the patient with a railing to grasp. However, many patients do not just hold on to the bars; they actually pull themselves along, thus making the transition to an assistive device more difficult. The hand support of a cane is considerably less than that of the parallel bars, and if the patient pulls on the cane, he will lose his support. An additional criticism of the parallel bars is that patients lean against the bars to receive more tactile and physical assistance. The patient can rely on this cue to assist with balance correction.

Ambulation Progression with a Cane. The proper progression for a patient using an assistive device for ambulation is as follows: the patient advances the cane forward with the uninvolved hand, and the involved leg steps forward, followed by the uninvolved lower extremity. Manual assistance may be necessary to help the patient advance the involved lower extremity forward. Physical assistance can be given by having the assistant lift or slide the patient's leg forward. The assistant can also advance the patient's involved lower extremity with the assistant's own leg. The patient must be instructed to limit how far forward she advances the cane. On average, a distance of 18 inches in front of the lower extremities is adequate. The patient may need assistance with weight shifting to allow for the swing phase of the gait cycle. The patient is encouraged to maintain proper postural alignment during ambulation by actively contracting the trunk extensors and the abdominals.

As discussed previously, care must be exercised with the placement of the involved upper extremity during ambulation activities. A permanent sling or a temporary one made from Theraband, placement of the patient's hand in a pocket, the use of a bedside table, or tactile support provided by the therapist can support the patient's arm during upright activities.

The patient may have more difficulty with ambulation activities when the assistive device is introduced. This is not uncommon because the cane offers more of a challenge for the patient. Shifting weight during the stance phase of the gait cycle and maintaining the correct sequence with the device can be difficult. The ambulation progression with the cane is identical to the one the patient used when beginning ambulation activities from the mat or in the parallel bars. With repetition, the patient's abilities in this area should improve.

Cane Use and Asymmetry. A common concern expressed by therapists after issuing a cane to a patient is the tendency toward body asymmetry, which the cane promotes. Having the cane in the patient's uninvolved hand promotes weight bearing on that side and often makes it difficult for the patient to shift weight toward and elongate the trunk on the affected side adequately. Inadequate weight shifting, coupled with the patient's asymmetric performance of a sit-to-stand transition, will accentuate previously discussed problems with equal weight bearing on both lower extremities. This point is illustrated in Figure 5–9. The patient

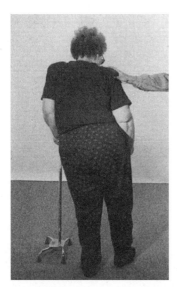

Figure 5–9 ■ Use of the quad cane during ambulation contributes to asymmetry in the trunk and poor weight shift to the hemiplegic side. The clinician's hand is guarding the patient. (From Ryerson S, Levit K. Functional Movement Reeducation: A Contemporary Model for Stroke Rehabilitation. New York, Churchill Livingstone, 1997.)

should achieve symmetry and bilateral weight bearing on both lower extremities during all upright movement transitions.

Walking on Different Surfaces

The patient should begin ambulation on standard flooring. This activity is most often accomplished in the physical therapy gym. The patient should, however, be quickly progressed to carpeting and other types of floor coverings because these are much more prevalent in home environments. Once the patient has fair dynamic ambulation balance and can advance the involved leg forward with good control, the patient should begin ambulation outside on different types of terrains. Walking on sidewalks, grass, and gravel is beneficial to the patient as the patient begins reentry into the community. Eventually, the patient will need to be able to walk in a crowded mall or to walk while negotiating environmental barriers.

Pusher Syndrome

As stated previously, some patients with left hemiplegia may exhibit pusher syndrome. The previously described treatment interventions are appropriate for patients with this condition. Specific activities that should be practiced include weight bearing on the involved lower extremity, provision of appropriate tactile and proprioceptive input, midline retraining in both sitting and standing positions, and incorporation of the hands during activity performance. The use of fixed resistance such as that given by the assistant's body or a table can provide the patient with the sensory feedback needed to allow her to correct her alignment and to relearn appropriate movement strategies (Davies, 1985).

Orthoses

The patient may reach a plateau at any stage and may be left with a variety of motor capabilities. Recovery usually begins proximally and then moves distally. Thus, for many patients, the hand and the ankle do not regain normal function. Decreased or absent ankle dorsiflexion can make ambulation activities difficult for the patient. Gait deviations emerge as the patient attempts to clear the foot and to prevent toe drag.

If the patient is not able to activate the anterior tibialis for heelstrike and to maintain the foot in relative dorsiflexion for the swing phase of the gait cycle, some type of orthosis may be needed.

Physical therapists may have varying views on the use of orthoses. Some physical therapists recommend orthoses for all patients, others may be more selective, and still others may not want to recommend orthoses at all for fear that a brace will interfere with the patient's ability to demonstrate normal movement patterns. The assistant and the supervising physical thera-pist should discuss the philosophy that is to be applied when recommending orthoses for patients.

Various types of custom-made orthoses and shoe in-serts are available. Many of these can be fabricated by physical therapists in the clinic. A discussion of the fabrication of these devices is outside the scope of this text. What is important to remember, however, is that orthoses can be beneficial pieces of equipment for many patients. The primary physical therapist and the assistant must discuss the patient's needs to determine whether an orthosis would be therapeutically benefi-cial. If the opportunity exists for the patient to use a training orthosis and for the assistant and supervising physical therapist to work together with the patient, a positive outcome may be expected. This approach al-lows for a thorough recommendation to be made to the physician about the best orthotic option for the patient.

Prefabricated Ankle-Foot Orthoses. For the patient who has sustained a CVA, the ankle-foot orthosis (AFO) is the orthosis or brace most frequently pre-scribed. Figure 5–10 shows an AFO. Patients may be-gin early ambulation tasks with a plastic prefabricated orthosis found in the clinic or physical therapy gym. These plastic training orthoses are relatively inexpen-sive and serve to maintain the patient's ankle and foot in a neutral or slightly dorsiflexed position. AFOs nor-mally come in small, medium, large, and extra-large sizes and are made for either the right or left lower

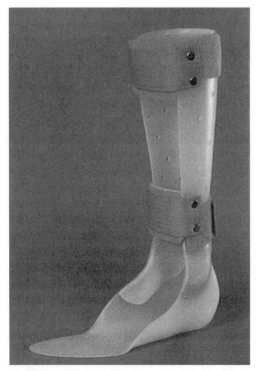

Figure 5–10 ■ The rigid polypropylene ankle-foot orthosis is capa-ble of providing tibial control in stance. (From Nawoczenski DA, Epler ME. Orthotics in Functional Rehabilitation of Lower Limb. Philadelphia, WB Saunders, 1997.)

extremity. The patient dons the orthosis, and then the shoe is applied. The positioning of the patient's foot in the orthosis allows the patient to ambulate without dragging the toes and allows the patient to have some degree of heelstrike. However, movement of the tibia over the fixed foot is difficult and may affect the pa-tient's ability to perform a sit-to-stand transfer. AFOs are excellent training tools for patients. Use of the orthosis during treatment provides the assistant with information on how the patient would be better able to ambulate if he had improved control of the ankle.

Posterior Leaf Splints. A posterior leaf splint is a plastic orthosis that controls ankle movement by limit-ing dorsiflexion and plantar flexion. During the stance phase of the gait cycle, the posterior portion of the orthosis becomes slightly bent. As the patient advances the lower limb forward, the orthosis recoils and helps to lift the foot to prevent footdrop.

Checking for Skin Irritation. Because some AFOs are prefabricated, they do not fit the unique bony and soft tissue structures of each patient's lower extremity. Thus, areas of redness may develop, and the potential for pressure areas must be considered. This problem can be compounded by a patient's decreased or absent sensation. It is recommended that when a patient first starts to use an orthosis or brace, wearing times should be limited. Initially, a patient may wear the orthosis for 10 to 15 minutes or for one walk with the clini-cian. The assistant should then remove the orthosis and should check the patient's skin for any areas of redness. As the patient begins to accommodate and tolerate the orthosis, wearing times can be increased. Patients should be instructed to check their feet fre-quently. Skin checks are extremely important for pa-tients with decreased sensation secondary to their stroke or who exhibit complications of diabetes or im-paired circulation. Patients must be advised to remove the AFO and to check their skin frequently to avoid the development of pressure ulcers. If the patient is unable to remove the orthosis himself, a caregiver should be instructed to assist.

Customized Ankle-Foot Orthoses. In addition to prefabricated plastic AFOs, custom-fabricated solid AFOs are also available. These types of orthoses must be made by an orthotist. An orthotist is a health care provider who specializes in the fabrication of orthoses and braces. The orthotist frequently makes a cast of the patient's foot and then fabricates the orthosis from this model. The orthoses are usually set in a neutral or slightly dorsiflexed position. Custom-fabricated ortho-ses usually fit the patient well. Several problems do exist. One obstacle to this type of orthosis is the cost. Custom-fabricated orthoses are expensive. In some sit-uations, the cost may be prohibitive. In addition, de-pending on the patient's stage in the recovery process, an orthosis ordered for a patient today may not be what the patient will need next week or when the patient is ready for discharge home. Therapists often wait to order a custom-made orthosis until later in the patient's rehabilitation stay, to ensure that the most appropriate device is fabricated. This is becoming more of a challenge, however, as lengths of stay in rehabilitation are becoming shorter.

Articulated Ankle-Foot Orthoses. Other custom-made orthoses do exist. Orthoses with articulated ankle joints may also be prescribed for the patient. These types of orthoses offer the clinician and the orthotist the opportunity to vary the degree of ankle joint motion available to the individual patient. The orthosis can be locked in a position of slight dorsiflexion for the patient who has difficulty initiating heelstrike. An orthosis positioned in dorsiflexion assists the patient who has a tendency to hyperextend the knee. The dorsiflexed position of the ankle causes the knee to move into slight flexion. Articulated orthoses also offer the clinician flexibility in choosing the position of the ankle. Figure 5–11 depicts an articulated AFO.

As stated previously, the ankle can be locked; however, most clinicians like to adjust the orthosis individually to the patient's needs. If the patient has weak or absent dorsiflexors, a posterior stop can be used to limit the patient's ability to plantar flex. Alternatively, an anterior stop may be used if the patient has marked weakness in the plantar flexors or if the anterior tibialis is hyperactive.

Articulated orthoses have several advantages. For example, the orthosis can be adjusted and changed at various times during the patient's recovery. Initially, when the involved ankle is weak, the ankle joint can be locked to provide the patient stability. As the patient progresses and more active movement becomes possible, the ankle joint can be adjusted to allow the patient greater opportunity to initiate as much dorsiflexion as possible. The orthosis could still be adjusted to limit plantar flexion, however. This type of positioning would encourage the patient's active attempts at dorsiflexion for heelstrike, but it would also provide passive positioning when the patient is fatigued. If a patient is placed in an orthosis that does not allow active movement, the patient may lose the opportunity to exercise and strengthen weak muscle groups.

An obvious disadvantage of an articulated AFO is the cost. Custom-fabricated orthoses are expensive and as a consequence may not be available to all patients.

Metal upright orthoses are a type of articulated AFO that can be attached to the patient's shoe. Figure 5–12 shows a metal upright orthosis. These types of orthoses are similar to the articulated plastic orthoses just discussed. Metal uprights were the orthoses of choice for many years. They have, however, been replaced in many settings because of the lightweight nature and cosmesis associated with plastic orthoses. Although this system offers advantages in progression of ankle motion similar to those of the articulated AFO,

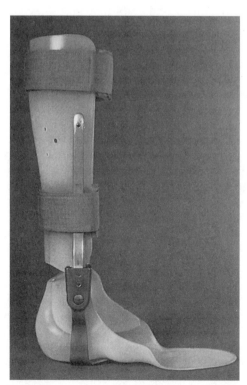

Figure 5–11 ■ A rigid polypropylene ankle-foot orthosis shell can be modified to incorporate a double-adjustable ankle joint for improved versatility in patient management. (From Nawoczenski DA, Epler ME. Orthotics in Functional Rehabilitation of Lower Limb. Philadelphia, WB Saunders, 1997.)

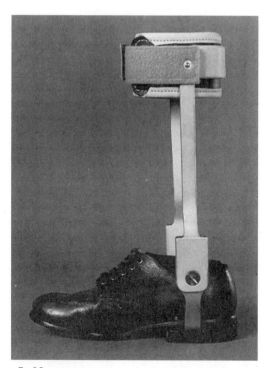

Figure 5–12 ■ The bichannel adjustable ankle-locking ankle-foot orthosis offers a wide range of adjustability options but lacks cosmetic appeal. (From Nawoczenski DA, Epler ME. Orthotics in Functional Rehabilitation of Lower Limb. Philadelphia, WB Saunders, 1997.)

the patient is limited to use of one pair of shoes for all occasions.

Knee-Ankle-Foot Orthoses. Knee-ankle-foot orthoses (KAFOs), or long leg braces as they are sometimes called, may be prescribed in special circumstances. Figure 5–13 shows a KAFO. This type of orthosis locks the patient's knee in extension. Thus, the patient is required to ambulate with the involved lower extremity in complete extension. These orthoses tend to be difficult to don and are heavy, and for the reasons cited are not appropriate for many of the patients with strokes. They are frequently used with patients with paraplegia. A discussion of this type of orthosis is included here because one may treat a patient for whom this type of orthosis would be appropriate.

Following the Developmental Sequence

Performance of postures and movement transitions that comprise the developmental sequence remains a popular choice among practicing clinicians. Having the patient practice transitional movements between postures is not only therapeutic but, also functional. Moving from a prone on elbows position to a four-point (quadruped) position, from quadruped to tall-kneeling, from tall-kneeling to half-kneeling, and from

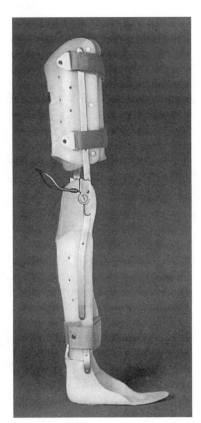

Figure 5–13 ■ Knee-ankle-foot orthosis. (From Nawoczenski DA, Epler ME. Orthotics in Functional Rehabilitation of Lower Limb. Philadelphia, WB Saunders, 1997.)

half-kneeling to standing is used in activities of daily living. Practicing these movement transitions independently or with assistance depends on the patient's motor control, balance, and cardiopulmonary function. Because adults do not perform all the postures within the sequence on a daily basis, it is not necessary for every patient to practice all components of the developmental sequence.

Kneeling and half-kneeling positions are important for the patient to practice in the clinic. They are the transition positions that the patient will need to perform if she falls and must get up from the floor. Often, anxiety and apprehension result when a patient falls at home. By practicing transfers to and from the floor, the patient and family should feel comfortable with the steps necessary should a fall occur once the patient is discharged from the health care facility.

Caution. The patient must be carefully monitored during the performance of the developmental sequence. During the more difficult and challenging positions, the patient must be observed for signs of fatigue or cardiac compromise. Shortness of breath, diaphoresis, and increased heart rate or blood pressure are signs that the activity may be too difficult for the patient. Thus, the selection of some of the more challenging positions such as the four-point position, tall-kneeling, and half-kneeling must be carefully considered. If a patient does not tolerate developmental sequence activities, the assistant, in consultation with the primary physical therapist, needs to select other treatment interventions that will address the patient's goals.

Prone Activities

Prone is an extremely difficult position for many older patients to achieve, especially in the presence of arthritic and cardiopulmonary changes. If the patient is able to tolerate the prone position, several activities can be practiced. In a completely prone position, the patient can work on knee flexion and hip extension with the knees bent. Many patients have difficulty in initiating antigravity knee flexion with the hip maintained in a neutral position secondary to decreased control of the hamstrings. The patient has the tendency to flex the hips at the same time the knees are flexed. Hip extension with the knee bent requires that the patient be able to activate the gluteus maximus with minimal assistance from the hamstrings. Careful monitoring of the patient's performance is necessary because substitution is extremely common.

If the patient can tolerate it, prone on elbows is another excellent position for treatment because the patient bears weight through the elbows and into the shoulders. Use of the PNF techniques of alternating isometrics and rhythmic stabilization applied to the shoulders aids in developing proximal control. If the patient has difficulty in maintaining the hand in a relaxed position, a hand or short arm air splint can be used to keep the wrist in a relatively neutral position with the fingers extended.

Transition from Prone on Elbows to Four-Point

The transition to a four-point or quadruped position from prone on elbows requires that the patient be able to maintain the involved upper extremity in extension and accept weight on it. Because the four-point position is more stressful, only those patients without medical complications and with moderately intact trunk control should attempt this position. Often it is easiest for the clinician to be behind the patient holding on to the patient's waist. The assistant can then direct the patient's weight back toward the feet. As the patient does this, he should be instructed to straighten the arms. If the patient lacks the necessary control in the triceps to maintain adequate elbow extension, a long arm air splint can be used. As stated

previously, it is desirable to have the patient bearing weight on extended arms with the wrists and fingers extended and the thumb abducted. If the patient is unable to achieve this resting posture actively or passively, the assistant should allow the patient's fingers to stay in a flexed position. The patient's fingers should not be pulled into extension as it may cause joint subluxation.

Four-Point Activities

Once in the quadruped position, the patient works on maintenance of the position. Forward, backward, medial, and lateral weight shifts are performed but should be practiced with control and should not be excessive. Alternating isometrics and rhythmic stabilization techniques can again be applied to the patient's shoulder or pelvic region, as depicted in Intervention 5–37A. For the advanced patient, unilateral upper and lower extremity lifting and reaching exercises can be attempted, as shown in Intervention 5–37B. The assist-

---

Intervention 5–37 ▌ QUADRUPED ACTIVITIES

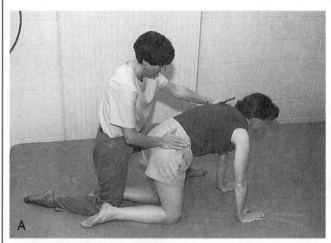

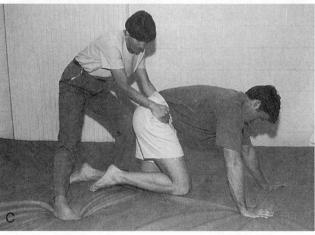

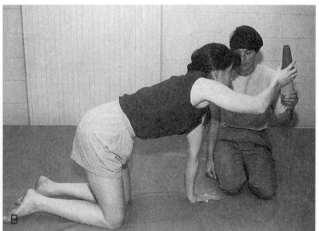

A. Holding—alternating isometric resistance applied in an anteroposterior direction.
B. Upper extremity reaching.
C. Creeping—resisted.

From O'Sullivan SB, Schmitz TJ. Physical Rehabilitation Laboratory Manual Focus on Functional Training. Philadelphia, FA Davis, 1999.

ant needs to monitor the patient's response carefully during performance of these activities. Exaggerated weight shifts to the involved or uninvolved sides may occur. Collapse of the involved upper extremity may occur if the patient has triceps weakness.

Creeping. *Creeping* on hands and knees, better known to much of the lay population as crawling, may also be practiced during the patient's treatment session. Creeping provides the patient with the opportunity to practice reciprocal upper and lower extremity activities while maintaining support on the opposite limbs. The patient should move one upper extremity, followed by the opposite lower extremity, then the contralateral upper extremity, followed by the remaining leg. Reciprocal movement of the extremities during creeping is closely related to the movement skills necessary for ambulation. Creeping is also a good activity to practice in the clinic because patients often need to be able to move in this fashion when they fall at home. The patient can creep to a piece of furniture to transfer back to the upright position. To make creeping more difficult, the assistant can provide resistance at the patient's pelvis or hips, as illustrated in Intervention 5–37C.

Transition from Four-Point to Tall-Kneeling

From a four-point position, the patient can make the transition to tall-kneeling. The patient should shift the weight posteriorly and then extend the trunk to assume the upright position. The assistant may need to provide the patient with assistance at the upper trunk (anterior shoulders) to achieve a complete upright position. Patients who have gluteal and back extensor weakness may push on their thighs in an effort to assist with knee extension. To achieve and maintain a tall-kneeling position, the patient must possess adequate muscular control of the trunk and balance. If the patient appears unstable in the tall-kneeling position, a small table or roll can be placed in front of the patient to assist with balance. By providing additional trunk support through upper extremity weight bearing, the assistant may make the patient may feel more secure, and balance may be improved.

Physical Observations. The assistant must diligently observe the patient's position in tall-kneeling. Patients often have difficulty in maintaining the pelvis in a neutral or slightly anterior position. As in sitting, the patient's hips should be in line with the shoulders. The patient should bear weight equally on both lower extremities. Frequently, patients present with an excessive anterior pelvic tilt and truncal asymmetries. It may be necessary to begin with posture correction prior to advancing the patient to specific exercises in the tall-kneeling position.

Tall-Kneeling Activities

Alternating isometrics and rhythmic stabilization techniques can be applied at the patient's shoulder

---

Intervention 5–38 ▐ TALL-KNEELING ACTIVITIES

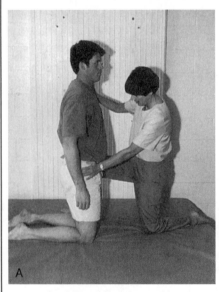 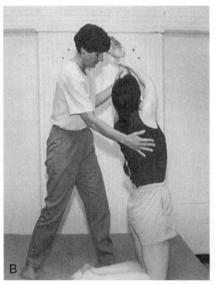 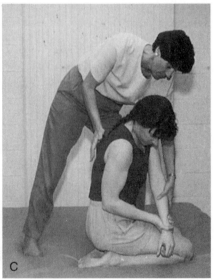

A. Alternating isometrics.
B and C. Kneeling to heel-sitting using proprioceptive neuromuscular facilitation lift and reverse-lift patterns.
From O'Sullivan SB, Schmitz TJ. Physical Rehabilitation Laboratory Manual Focus on Functional Training. Philadelphia, FA Davis, 1999.

and pelvic girdles while the patient is in the tall-kneeling position. Intervention 5–38A illustrates these techniques in the tall-kneeling position. These techniques assist in the development of proximal stability and aid the patient in improving balance and coordination. Upper extremity PNF patterns can be performed including the D1 and D2 diagonal patterns and lifts and chops, as seen in Intervention 5–38B and C. The benefit of performing the bilateral lifting and chopping patterns is that they incorporate a greater amount of trunk movement, specifically flexion and rotation. Functional activities such as gardening and house cleaning can be simulated in this position.

Another activity that can be performed in this position is tall-kneeling to heel sitting. In this exercise, the patient moves from a tall-kneeling position to one of sitting on the heels as illustrated in Intervention 5–38C. This exercise allows the patient to work on eccentric control of the quadriceps, a skill needed for many functional activities, including stand-to-sit transitions and stair negotiation. The patient can also perform forward and backward knee walking while in tall-kneeling. The assistant should observe the quality of the patient's lower extremity movement during knee walking. The lower extremity, specifically the hip, should advance in flexion. Hip hiking or circumduction should not be evident.

Helpful Tip. During the patient's performance of all these developmental postures, the assistant must guard the patient appropriately. Because the patient's balance is challenged, it is possible that the patient may experience a loss of balance and fall.

Transition from Tall-Kneeling to Half-Kneeling

The transition from kneeling to half-kneeling is difficult for many patients. To initiate the transition, the patient must be able to perform a controlled weight shift to one side. The trunk on the side that will move forward to assume the half-kneel, foot-flat position must shorten. The hip on the moving side must hike and slightly abduct. The moving knee must remain flexed as the patient brings the leg forward. The patient must also keep the foot in a neutral to slightly dorsiflexed position to clear the foot from the floor as the patient brings the leg forward. Adequate ankle range of motion is necessary to maintain the foot on the floor or mat with good contact. Often, patients need physical assistance in assuming this challenging position. Half-kneeling with the stronger, uninvolved leg forward is often easier for the patient to achieve.

Half-Kneeling Activities

Initially, the patient should work on maintaining the half-kneeling position. The patient may sway from side to side while attempting to maintain the center of

---

Intervention 5–39 ▎ HALF-KNEELING ACTIVITIES

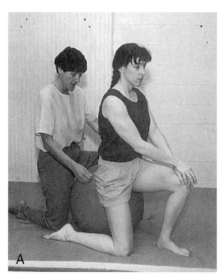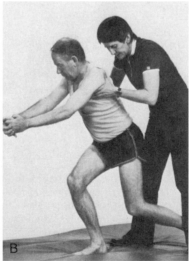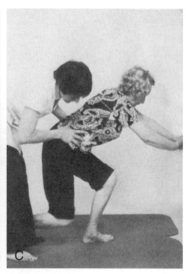

A. Half-kneeling on a Swiss ball: active-assistive movements.

Standing up from half-kneeling:

B. The therapist facilitates the transition with her hands in the patients' axillae (left hemiplegia).

C. Facilitation from the pelvis (right hemiplegia).

A, from O'Sullivan SB, Schmitz TJ. Physical Rehabilitation Laboratory Manual Focus on Functional Training. Philadelphia, FA Davis, 1999; B and C, from Davies PM. Steps to Follow: A Guide to Treatment of Adult Hemiplegia. New York, Springer Verlag, 1985.

gravity over the base of support. Asymmetric weight bearing may also be observed. If the patient is having difficulty in maintaining the position, a Swiss ball can be placed under the hips, as shown in Intervention 5–39*A*. Active control of hip extension can be practiced in the half-kneeling position. The patient can work on shifting the weight forward and backward over the fixed front foot while reaching for an object. As with the other developmental positions previously described, once the patient is in half-kneeling, the PNF techniques of alternating isometrics and rhythmic stabilization can be applied to promote stability and balance control. Active upper extremity exercises and PNF chops and lifts can be performed in this position. The patient should practice half-kneeling with both the uninvolved and involved lower extremities forward. The transition to and from the position is also important to master. Once the patient is able to maintain the position independently and to move in and out of the position, the patient should be progressed to standing. Initially, the patient may need help from the assistant or from a piece of equipment or the wall, as depicted in Intervention 5–39*B* and *C*. To complete the ascent to upright, the patient must be able to perform a forward weight shift over the fixed front foot. This prerequisite demands the necessary postural control and range of motion at the ankle. As the patient assumes more active control of the transition from half-kneeling to standing, the assistant should decrease support. For the more advanced patient, this activity can be manually resisted with pressure applied to the patient's hips and pelvis.

Modified Plantigrade Position

The final developmental position that we discuss in this section is modified plantigrade. In plantigrade, the patient is weight bearing on both the upper and lower extremities. Plantigrade is a position that children often experiment with as they attempt upright standing. It is not, however, a position that most adults achieve with much regularity. It does offer therapeutic benefits to patients because it allows for upper and lower extremity weight bearing in a modified standing position. Upper and lower extremity weight bearing will deliver proprioceptive input into the shoulder and hip joints, respectively, and will assist with tone reduction. The therapist may also want to approximate down through the shoulders or pelvis when the patient is in this position, to increase sensory awareness and motor recruitment.

In plantigrade, the patient can work on rocking forward, backward, and to the sides. These activities can be performed actively at first, and, with practice, the assistant can resist the exercise. Alternating isometrics can once again be used to promote stability. Intervention 5–40 illustrates this activity. Lower extremity progressions can be initiated when the patient is in

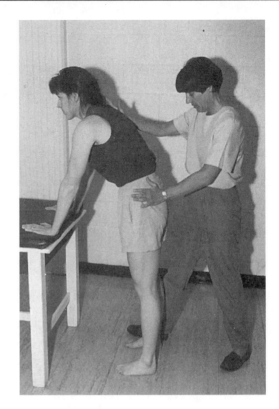

Intervention 5–40 ▌ MODIFIED PLANTIGRADE ACTIVITIES

Modified plantigrade position: alternating isometrics.

From O'Sullivan SB, Schmitz TJ. Physical Rehabilitation Laboratory Manual Focus on Functional Training. Philadelphia, FA Davis, 1999.

this position, including forward and backward stepping. Knee control activities such as knee flexion, extension, and squats can also be practiced. The patient can also perform functional activities in this position including self-care and homemaking activities.

MIDRECOVERY TO LATE RECOVERY

Depending on the patient's injury, recovery stage, age, and insurance status, the next phase of the patient's rehabilitation may be termed *midrecovery to late recovery*. The physical therapist assistant's involvement with the patient at this stage of recovery can occur in a number of different practice settings. The services may be provided in a skilled care or subacute unit, in a rehabilitation center, in the patient's home, or in an outpatient clinic. Regardless of the treatment setting, the primary goals for the patient still focus on the achievement of functional skills. Mat activities may continue, but the types of exercises selected should be more challenging. The assistant and primary physical therapist will want to discuss advancing the patient to exercises performed in sitting and standing positions. The amount of time spent performing exercises in the supine position should be limited.

The treatment activities for midrecovery to late recovery phases vary, based on the patient's motor and functional return. Through regular reevaluations by the primary physical therapist, the assistant will receive guidance and feedback regarding appropriate interventions for each phase of recovery. As the patient is able to assume more independence in the performance of functional activities, the physical therapy team will want to incorporate more challenging activities into the patient's plan of care.

Negotiation of Environmental Barriers

Activities that address the negotiation of environmental barriers including stairs, curbs, and ramps should be considered.

Stairs

Patients should be instructed in the following sequence when learning to negotiate stairs.

A patient who is using a handrail should lead with the stronger uninvolved foot when ascending the stairs. The involved foot follows. This sequence continues until the patient has negotiated all the steps. Intervention 5-41 illustrates a patient who is walking up the stairs. The assistant must guard the patient carefully to avoid loss of balance or a fall. The assistant may find it easier to guard the patient from behind during stair ascent.

When descending the stairs with a handrail, the patient needs to lead with the involved foot. Intervention 5-42 shows a patient going down the steps. The assistant observes the response of the involved lower extremity as it begins to accept weight. The patient must possess ample lower extremity control to maintain the leg in relative extension during lowering of the uninvolved lower extremity. As previously stated, the extension synergy pattern is common in many patients who sustained CVAs. This extension pattern may cause the involved lower extremity to stay extended during stair climbing. When the patient is descending the stairs, the assistant may find it easier to guard the patient from the front. Prevention of genu recurvatum on descent should be encouraged by maintaining the involved knee in slight flexion.

Caution. A safety belt should always be used during stair training.

Stair Climbing with a Cane. If the patient is going to use an assistive device on the stairs, the sequence will be the same. When going up the stairs, the patient leads with the uninvolved foot, followed by the involved leg, and then the cane. The sequence for going down the stairs is similar; the patient begins the descent with the cane, followed by the involved lower extremity, and finally the uninvolved leg.

Please Note. Depending on the type of cane selected for the patient, the cane may or may not fit on the step. Straight canes and narrow-base quad canes can be used without modification. A wide-base quad cane must be turned sideways to fit safely on the step. Hemiwalkers cannot be used on steps safely.

Curbs and Ramps

Negotiation of a curb is similar to that of a single step. Ramps can be a challenge, based on their degree of incline or grade.

Family Participation

Family members should practice the skills needed to assist the patient at home and should be responsible for return demonstrations in the clinic. Encourage family members to take an active roll in practicing these activities. Family members may tell you that they feel confident with the activity simply after observing it. It is optimal for both the patient and the family members to have had the opportunity to practice with a skilled practitioner present. These practice sessions allow the assistant to provide feedback on techniques and to identify potential problems that the patient and caregiver may experience in the home setting.

Working on Fine Motor Skills

Frequently, at this point in the recovery process, the patient is trying to gain full control of the distal joint components. Often the wrist, fingers, and ankle are unable to perform coordinated movements. Exercises or activities that stress these skills should be included in the patient's treatment plan. Depending on the level of motor return in the hand, the patient may be able to complete fine motor activities. Dressing, bathing, and grooming tasks are frequently used to improve hand coordination because of the large degree of fine motor control necessary to complete these activities. In addition, activities of daily living are functionally oriented. Finding out from the patient or a family member whether the patient has any hobbies or areas of interest helps in identifying treatment tasks. If the therapist can select tasks that have importance to the patient and have functional relevance, the assistant will usually find much better compliance with activity performance. Cooking, gardening, writing, computer programming, and crafts are just a few examples of the types of activities that may promote fine motor control and dexterity in the upper extremity. The patient should be encouraged to use the involved upper extremity as much as possible. If the involved arm lacks the necessary motor control to complete fine motor tasks, it should be positioned in weight bearing or be used as an assist.

Advanced Exercises for the Lower Extremity

Exercises designed to enhance lower extremity function can also be performed. Again, the selection of

---

Intervention 5–41 ▌ STAIR CLIMBING

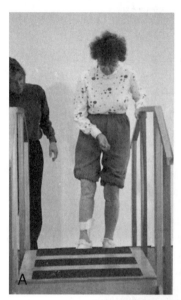
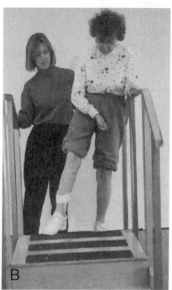
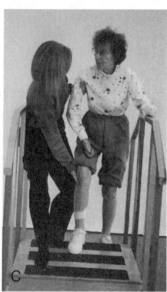
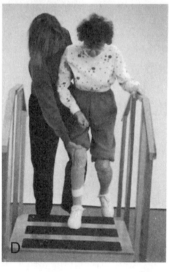
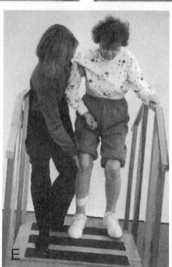

A and B. The patient with right hemiplegia initiates lifting the leg onto a step. She initiates the pattern with pelvic elevation and a strong overshift of her trunk to the left as she circumducts and lifts her leg with knee extension.

C. The clinician uses her left hand in an axillary grip to correct trunk alignment and uses her right hand to help the patient learn to lift her right leg with hip and knee flexion.

D and E. The clinician uses her right hand on the distal femur to teach the patient to move forward over her extending right leg. The clinician's left hand moves the trunk forward and upward as the leg extends and the patient lifts her left leg upward. The patient does not overshift and rely on her left arm as the clinician helps her to learn to use her right leg.

From Ryerson S, Levit K. Functional Movement Reeducation: A Contemporary Model for Stroke Rehabilitation. New York, Churchill Livingstone, 1997.

Intervention 5-42 ▌ DESCENDING STAIRS

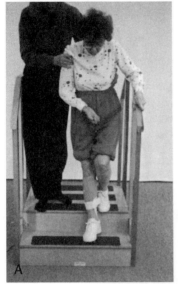 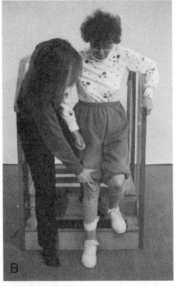 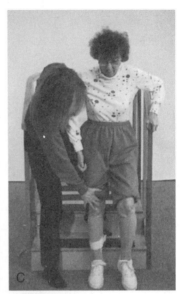

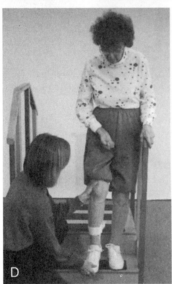 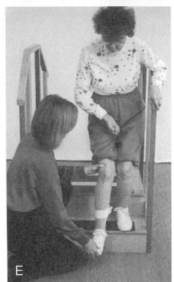

A. The patient leads with her right leg. The right leg is adducting as it reaches to the step. This leg adduction contributes to the feeling of "falling" to the hemiplegic side.

B and C. The clinician uses her left hand in an axillary grip to support the patient's trunk and pelvis. She reminds the patient to keep the

upper trunk extended over the pelvis as the right foot reaches to the floor and the left foot steps down.

D and E. The clinician lets the patient control the trunk as she reeducates the forward movement pattern of the right leg.

From Ryerson S, Levit K. Functional Movement Reeducation: A Contemporary Model for Stroke Rehabilitation. New York, Churchill Livingstone, 1997.

different treatment tasks depends on the patient's level of motor control. Once the patient is up and moving around, supine exercises should be limited, and more challenging positions should be used for exercising and training purposes. To continue to improve hip and knee control, the patient can transfer to

a high-low mat table. With the height of the table raised and the involved lower extremity weight bearing on the floor, the patient can work on straightening the knee and hip from this position. In a supported standing position, the patient can perform standing hip abduction on both the involved and uninvolved sides, hip extension with the knee straight, hip flexion or marching, and knee flexion with the hip in a neutral or slightly extended position. The benefits of these exercises are that they activate the lower extremity musculature in ways directly opposite the normal lower extremity synergy patterns, and they allow for unilateral weight bearing and promote balance and coordination skills.

Advanced Exercises for the Ankle

Exercises that address movement of the involved ankle should also be included. Patients who are experiencing difficulties in achieving active ankle dorsiflexion can place a rolling pin under the foot and work on moving the rolling pin back and forth. This maneuver can be performed when the patient is either sitting or standing. If the patient has relatively good active dorsiflexion and plantar flexion, she can work on tapping her foot, drawing a circle or alphabet on the floor, or kicking a small ball forward. Additional activities that can be performed include heel raises with the knee in slight flexion, active ankle eversion, or resistive exercises with Theraband.

Coordination Exercises

Exercises targeted at improving coordination of the upper and lower extremities should also be performed. Standard coordination tests performed when the patient is sitting include finger to nose, the patient's finger to the therapist's finger, alternating nose to finger, finger opposition, and bilateral pronation and supination activities. Lower extremity coordination exercises include alternating heel to knee and heel to toe, toe to examiner's finger, and heel to shin. The incorporation of these exercises into the patient's treatment plan depends on the degree of motor return in the upper and lower extremities.

Balance Exercises

Balance and coordination exercises can be performed with the patient in a standing position. Examples of exercises that can be performed to improve a patient's static balance include standing with both feet together with a narrow base of support; *tandem standing,* which is standing with one foot directly in front of the other; and standing on one foot. In addition, the patient's balance strategies should be observed by displacing the patient's center of gravity unexpectedly. As described previously, the assistant should observe the presence of appropriate ankle, hip, and stepping strategies. *Balance responses* are normal responses to perturbation or a sudden change in the patient's center of gravity as it relates to the patient's base of support.

Patients who do not possess adequate dorsiflexion may not be able to initiate or perform the ankle strategy. Patients with limited ability to activate lower extremity musculature may not be able to use hip and protective stepping responses to prevent falls when their balance is disturbed.

Dynamic Balance Activities

Other examples of activities that can be performed to challenge the patient's dynamic balance include walking on uneven surfaces, tandem walking, walking on a balance beam, side stepping, walking backward, braiding (walking sideways, crossing one foot over the other), throwing and catching a small ball, batting a balloon, and marching in place. All are useful activities for the patient to perform if the goal is to improve the patient's ability to maintain a balanced postural base while moving the lower extremities; in the case of throwing and catching, the upper extremities are moving also. Additional activities that can be performed include walking activities in which the patient is asked to change speed or direction. Abrupt stopping and starting, walking in a circle, or having the patient walk on heels or toes will challenge the patient's balance and coordination.

Advanced Balance Exercises

For patients who need even more challenging activities, the assistant can remove the patient's visual feedback and have the patient stand on a level surface with eyes closed. A patient who is able to do this can be progressed to standing on different types of surfaces with eyes open and then with eyes closed. It is extremely important to guard the patient closely during advanced balance activities. If the assistant provides too much physical help, the patient will rely on the assistance and will not make the necessary postural modifications to maintain balance.

Dynamic Balance Exercises Using Movable Surfaces

Movable surfaces provide another means of working on the patient's dynamic balance. Swiss (therapeutic) balls and tilt boards can be used effectively for the patient who needs to continue to work on dynamic balance.

Swiss Ball. When the Swiss ball is used, the right-size ball must be selected for the patient. The patient should be able to sit on the ball and have both feet touch the floor. In addition, the hips, knees, and ankles should be at a 90-90-90 position. Intervention 5–43 illustrates the use of the Swiss ball during treatment. The patient can be assisted to the ball and can work on the achievement of an upright erect posture. The ability to achieve proper posture requires that the

Intervention 5–43 ▍ SITTING ON A SWISS BALL

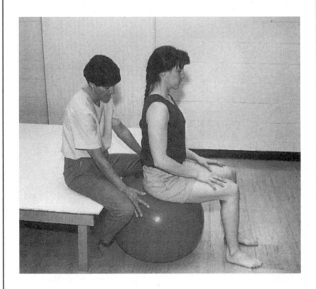

The patient should be able to sit on the ball and have both feet touch the floor. Hips, knees, and ankles should be at a 90-90-90 position. The patient should first work on maintaining an upright erect posture on the ball before progressing to other exercises such as pelvic mobility and movement of the limbs.

From O'Sullivan SB, Schmitz TJ. Physical Rehabilitation Laboratory Manual Focus on Functional Training. Philadelphia, FA Davis, 1999.

patient actively contract the abdominal muscles to keep the shoulders in line with the hips. In addition, the patient must keep the knees over the feet. Some of the first exercises that should be performed on the ball are those that address pelvic mobility. While sitting on the ball, the patient can isolate anterior and posterior pelvic tilts and lateral tilts to the right and left. The lateral shifts assist the patient with the ability to elongate the trunk on the weight-bearing side and shorten it on the opposite side. Once the patient is able to maintain balance on the ball while moving the pelvis, the patient can be progressed to adding movements of the limbs. While sitting on the ball, the patient can perform the following exercises: reciprocal arm movements of the upper extremities, marching in place, and unilateral knee extension. As the patient's balance improves, he can perform PNF chops and lifts or trunk rotation exercises. A discussion of placing the patient in the prone position over the ball occurs in Chapter 6.

The ball, as a movable surface, provides the patient with some uncertainty in terms of stability. A sudden movement of the ball requires the patient to be able to make a quick, unanticipated postural response, to realign the center of gravity in relation to the base of support. Many patients lack the ability to adjust their postural responses in this way. As stated previously, it is necessary to guard the patient carefully while on the ball. Only those patients who already exhibit a certain amount of trunk control should attempt these activities.

Tilt Boards. Tilt boards offer another type of movable surface for our patients. Therapists often use boards on which the adult patient can stand to work on postural reactions. As with the ball, selection of a tilt board as part of the treatment regimen requires that the patient possess a certain amount of trunk and extremity control in addition to fairly good dynamic balance. A patient who requires an assistive device for ambulation would not be an appropriate candidate for standing tilt board activities. It is often beneficial first to demonstrate for the patient what the clinician wants the patient to do on the board. The patient needs to be advised that the board will move as the patient tries to position herself on it. The patient should be assisted onto the board. Standing in front of the patient and allowing her to hold on to your hands is often easiest. At times, it may be necessary to have someone else hold the board as the patient steps up onto it. The first thing the patient should do once she has ascended onto the board is to accommodate to the movable surface, as illustrated in Figure 5–14. A slight shift in the patient's weight from one side to the next causes the board to move. Frequently, during this process, the patient may have difficulty in controlling the involved lower extremity. In an attempt to improve stability, the patient often locks her knees into extension so she does not have to concentrate on knee control in addition to maintaining her balance on the board. If the assistant should observe this phenomenon, it may indicate that the activity is too difficult for the patient. Discussion with the primary therapist is warranted.

During the patient's acclimation to the tilt board, the assistant should continue to hold on to the patient's arms for balance support. Once the assistant believes that the patient is relatively comfortable and safe on the board, the assistant can help the patient with small weight shifts to the right and left. The assistant, through manual contacts, is able to grade the excursion of the patient's weight shift.

Observations. When the patient shifts the weight to the right, the assistant will want to see the patient exhibit elongation of the trunk on the right with trunk and head righting. Intervention 5–44 shows a patient on a tilt board. The position of the patient's lower extremities should also be noted, in addition to the position of the upper extremities. On occasion, the patient will overcompensate with the upper extremities if he believes that his balance is being compromised.

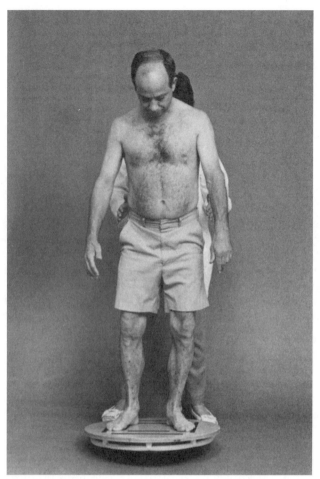

Figure 5–14 ■ A patient can increase speed amplitude and the type of balance responses on an adjustable tilt board. (From Duncan PW, Badke MB. Stroke Rehabilitation: Recovery of Motor Control. Chicago, Year Book, 1987.)

Extension and abduction of the upward side with protective extension on the opposite (downward) side may be evident. As the patient becomes more comfortable on the board, he can begin to shift his weight actively to the right and left. The patient needs to possess adequate control of the weight shift. Often, the patient limits the shift to the involved side because of anxiety associated with having all the weight on his involved lower extremity. The patient can also work on trying to maintain the board in a neutral position with equal weight on both lower extremities.

Anterior and Posterior Weight Shifts on the Tilt Board. The position of the board can also be changed to allow the patient to work on anterior and posterior weight shifts. The patient again needs to be assisted onto the board. The advantage of this board position is that it allows the patient to work on active ankle dorsiflexion and plantar flexion. As the board moves in a posterior direction, the patient is dorsiflexing both ankles. For patients who have difficulties with active dorsiflexion or performance of the ankle strategy for balance control, this exercise can be effective. Selection of a tilt board requires that the patient possess a fairly high level of motor function and is simply in need of refinement of ankle movements and postural responses.

Management of Abnormal Tone

The presence of abnormal tone may become apparent during the patient's recovery. Spasticity and the dominance of the synergy patterns can interfere with the patient's attempts at active movement. Although at present no medical or physical therapy interventions can permanently remediate the tone, physical therapists and physical therapist assistants can do several things to make the tone more manageable for a short period of time. Our goal is to decrease the abnormal tone long enough so that the patient can perform an active movement or a functional task while the tone is lessened. This allows the patient the opportunity to move with increased ease and to have the sensory experience of more normal movement. Patients who sustain neurologic injuries often lose the ability to perceive the sensory feedback associated with normal movement. Abnormal movement patterns develop in response to the abnormal sensory feedback that patients with strokes experience. Thus, abnormal movement patterns are reinforced each time the patient moves.

As mentioned earlier, positioning the patient in the antispasm patterns described can assist in decreasing the abnormal tone that may develop. Rhythmic rotation applied with steady passive movement, such as that applied with lower trunk rotation or rhythmic rotation of the extremities, is beneficial. Rotational exercises followed by activities that incorporate weight bearing can be extremely beneficial in providing the patient with a more normal postural base. Weight bearing through the upper or lower extremities is an excellent treatment modality for tone reduction. Other activities that can be administered to assist in managing the patient's abnormal tone include PNF diagonals including the chopping and lifting patterns, tapping and vibration to the weaker antagonist muscles, tendon pressure applied directly to the spastic tendon, air splints, prolonged ice application, functional electrical stimulation, and biofeedback. Any of these treatment interventions may be beneficial to the patient. Often, it is necessary to try one and then grade the patient's response to the sensory intervention applied. Again, it is not sufficient simply to apply a tone-reducing modality. The patient's tone should be decreased through a therapeutic modality, but the patient must then be provided with a movement transition or functional

Intervention 5–44 ▌ USING A TILT BOARD

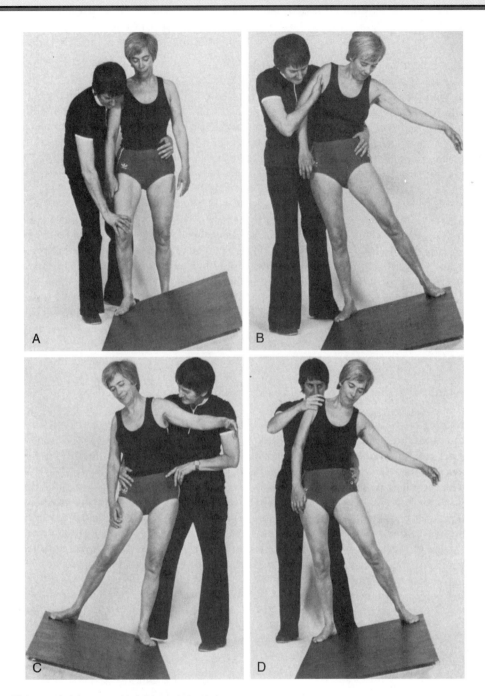

Moving the tilt board sideways (right hemiplegia).

A. Stepping onto the board with the hemiplegic foot first. The clinician guides the patient's knee forward.

B. Transferring weight to the hemiplegic side. The clinician lengthens the side of the trunk, and her hip maintains extension of the patient's hip.

C. Transferring the weight to the uninvolved leg. The clinician has changed her position so that the patient moves toward her.

D. The clinician reduces the amount of support.

From Davies PM. Steps to Follow: A Guide to Treatment of Adult Hemiplegia. New York, Springer Verlag, 1985.

task that allows the patient to experience more normal sensory feedback. This concept should ultimately reinforce the desired movement and, one hopes, should lead to improved function.

Preparation for Discharge

Depending on the patient's recovery and home situation including family support, the physical therapist and physical therapist assistant will need to plan for the patient's discharge to home or another type of health care facility.

Assessing the Patient's Home Environment

During the initial evaluation, the primary physical therapist needs to begin to ask questions regarding the patient's home environment. As mentioned previously, discharge planning must begin during the patient's first physical therapy visit. Factors that must be considered when addressing discharge include the type of dwelling in which the patient resides, whether it is an apartment (with steps or an elevator), a house, a trailer, or another type of structure. Asking patients or significant others whether they rent or own their home is also important because renting may preclude the family from making any permanent structural changes. The entrance to the home should also be assessed. The number, height, and condition of the steps, the presence or absence of a handrail or landing area, proximity to the driveway or parking lot, and the direction in which the front door opens will help to plan for the patient's safe return to the home environment.

The following is a list of general considerations for exterior accessibility. These guidelines are provided to assist clinicians in suggesting environmental modifications to their patients' existing dwellings.

1. Steps should not be higher than 7 inches (17.5 cm) or deeper than 11 inches (27.9 cm).
2. Handrails should measure 32 inches (81.3 cm) in height.
3. One handrail should extend 18 inches (45.7 cm) beyond the foot and top of the stairs.
4. If a ramp is needed, the recommended grade for wheelchairs is 12 inches of ramp for every inch of threshold height.
5. Ramps should be a minimum of 48 inches wide and should be covered with a nonslip surface.
6. A door width of 32 to 34 inches (81.3 to 86.3 cm) is acceptable and accommodates most wheelchairs (Schmitz, 1994).

Much of the information about the patient's home can be provided by the family. Many facilities use a checklist that a family member can complete regarding the home and its accessibility. In some cases, it may be necessary for the rehabilitation team to go out and perform a home assessment. This assessment may be conducted by the primary physical therapist, the physical therapist assistant, the occupational therapist, or a combination of these team members. Family members are often included in these assessments, so information regarding home modifications or equipment needs can be provided.

Other information that is needed regarding the patient's home includes interior accessibility, specifically in the areas of the bedroom and bathroom. The amount of space needed by the patient for negotiation depends on his ambulatory status. Wheelchairs require space for turning and also for positioning of the chair near furniture for transfers. In the patient's bedroom, the therapist will want to note the type of bed, whether space is adequate for transfers, the location of a night stand or bedside table, and the need for a bedside commode or urinal. The width of the bathroom door also needs to be assessed because frequently these entrances are narrower than other interior door frames. An elevated toilet seat and grab bars may be necessary to ensure the patient's safety. Talking with the patient and primary caregiver provides information on the bathing patterns of the patient. A tub bench or shower chair in addition to a hand spray attachment may be suggested.

Other considerations for interior accessibility include the type of carpeting. Low, dense-pile carpets are recommended because they tend to be the easiest on which to ambulate or over which to propel a wheelchair. All throw rugs should be discarded because they create a safety hazard for the patient who is ambulatory. The design of the kitchen should also be observed. Counter heights and handles on cabinets should be noted. Frequently used items should be moved to lower cabinets to allow for easier reach.

The assistant will also want to question the patient about the patient's primary means of transportation at discharge. This information helps in identifying the most appropriate car transfer to practice and aids in planning follow-up care for the patient. Car transfers with and without the patient's family should be practiced prior to discharge. In addition, family members should be instructed in safe techniques for loading and unloading the wheelchair from their vehicle.

Further recommendations for rehabilitation services should be made prior to the patient's discharge from the health care facility. The primary physical therapist needs to reevaluate the patient and, with input from the physical therapist assistant, to suggest equipment and additional physical therapy needs to the patient's physician. Properly planning for the patient's discharge facilitates the patient's transition from the rehabilitation setting to home and the community.

CHAPTER SUMMARY

Adults who have experienced a CVA comprise a significant number of the patients treated in physical therapy. Based on the type and extent of the initial insult, patients can present with a multitude of different problems, and the extent of these problems can be highly variable. Different treatment interventions are presented in this chapter to assist patients in improving their volitional motor control and functional abilities. As physical therapists and physical therapist assistants working with this patient population, the primary goal of our interventions is to improve patients' abilities to perform meaningful functional activities and thus improve their quality of life.

REVIEW QUESTIONS

1. Describe the major impairments seen in patients who have had CVAs.
2. What are risk factors for the development of a CVA?
3. Describe the upper and lower extremity flexion and extension synergy patterns.
4. Discuss the benefits of patient positioning.
5. The acute care physical therapy management of a patient who has had a CVA should include what?
6. The basic philosophical principles regarding the neurodevelopmental treatment approach include what?
7. What are appropriate physical therapy interventions to be performed with the patient in sitting?
8. Describe the gait training sequence for patients with postacute CVA.
9. Name four advanced dynamic standing balance exercises.
10. What environmental factors must be considered when preparing the patient for discharge to home?

REHABILITATION UNIT INITIAL EVALUATION: ALICE

Chart Review: Alice is a 65-year-old female who was admitted to St. John's Medical Center 7 days ago with complaints of aphasia, right-sided facial and arm weakness, and right hemisensory deficits. Initial CT scan was normal, repeat scan 5 days later showed decreased density in left middle cerebral artery distribution. Pertinent medical history includes hypertension partially controlled with medications, arthritis in both knees, and frequent TIAs (three in the last 6 months). PT order for evaluation and treatment received.

SUBJECTIVE

Alice is unable to communicate verbally. Social history was obtained from her husband, who was present at Alice's bedside during the initial evaluation. Husband states he and Alice have been married for 45 years. They live in a one-story home with three steps to enter. A handrail is present on the right. Alice has two grown children who live locally. Alice is unable to state goals secondary to communication deficits. Husband reports he would like for Alice to return to her previous level of function. Husband provided consent for Alice to participate in the evaluation.

OBJECTIVE

Appearance: Alice is supine in bed, right shoulder is internally rotated and adducted, right elbow is flexed to 60 degrees, right wrist and fingers are flexed. Right hip is extended, adducted, and internally rotated. Right knee is extended, right ankle is plantar flexed and slightly inverted. Drooping is noted at right corner of mouth. Alice has an IV in right forearm and Foley catheter.

Cognition: Alice is alert. Yes/no responses unreliable. Alice is unable to follow one-step verbal commands.

Visual: Pupils are reactive to light. Tracking is present to midline bilaterally.

Communication: Alice presents with receptive and expressive aphasia. Speaking with jargon.

Continued on following page

REHABILITATION UNIT INITIAL EVALUATION: ALICE *Continued*

OBJECTIVE *Continued*

Cardiopulmonary: Heart rate 72 bpm. BP 130/84 in supine. Respiration rate 12 breaths/minute. Patient exhibiting a two chest–two diaphragm breathing pattern. Vital capacity 1600 mL.

Range of Motion: PROM of the left UE and LE and the right UE is WFL. PROM of the right hip and knee is WFL. Right ankle passive dorsiflexion lacks 10 degrees from neutral. AROM of left UE and LE is WFL. No active movement noted at right shoulder, elbow, wrist, or fingers. Alice is able to actively move the right LE through one-half to three-fourths of the flexion and extension synergy patterns.

Tone: Right UE is flaccid throughout. Shoulder presents with one-half finger width subluxation. Right LE presents with a moderate increase in tone in the right gluteus maximus, hip adductors, quads, and gastrocnemius-soleus.

Neurologic Testing: Babinski (+) on right. No associated or primitive reflexes noted.

Deep Tendon Reflexes: Right biceps reflex 1+, triceps 1+, patellar and Achilles 3+. DTRs 2+ on left.

Sensation: Unable to assess sensation accurately secondary to Alice's inability to communicate and follow one-step commands. Perception of light touch and pain appears impaired in the right extremities.

Functional Mobility: Alice requires minimal assist with rolling to the right; rolling to the left requires moderate assist of one. Bridging requires moderate assist of one. Asymmetry noted with bridging. Supine-to-sit and sit-to-supine transfers require moderate-maximal assist of one. Alice's sitting balance is poor. Alice requires moderate assist of one and SBA of another to maintain sitting balance. Alice sits with a posterior pelvic tilt, increased weight bearing on the left hip, thoracic kyphosis, and forward head posturing. Alice uses left UE to help support self in sitting. No protective extension noted in the right UE. Alice performed a stand-pivot transfer from the bed to a wheelchair with moderate assist of two. Alice is able to bear weight on the right LE during standing and the transfer.

ASSESSMENT

Alice is a 65-year-old female who is status post left CVA of the middle cerebral artery distribution with right hemiparesis and sensory deficits. Alice's rehabilitation potential for stated goals is good secondary to her level of motor return, motivation, and family support. Alice is able to tolerate 45-minute evaluation without obvious signs of fatigue.

Problem List
1. Decreased volitional movement right extremities
2. Decreased functional abilities
3. Decreased passive ROM right ankle
4. Decreased communication abilities
5. Decreased balance in sitting and standing
6. Decreased sensory awareness
7. Dependent in ADLs

Short-Term Goals (1 week)
1. Alice will be able to roll to the right with SBA.
2. Alice will be able to roll to the left with minimal assist.
3. Alice will transfer supine to sit with minimal assist of one.

4. Alice will maintain sitting balance with left UE support with minimal assist of one for 5 minutes.
5. Alice will pre-position right upper extremity for transfers.

Long-Term Goals (4 weeks)
1. Alice will roll to the right and left independently.
2. Alice will transfer from supine to sitting independently.
3. Alice will perform a stand-pivot transfer independently to all surfaces.
4. Alice will perform HEP independently.
5. Alice will demonstrate right lower extremity AROM to assist with dressing and self-care from a seated position.
6. Alice will ambulate with a WBQC 50 feet with moderate assist on level surfaces.
7. Family will demonstrate understanding of correct techniques to assist Alice with transfers and gait.

REHABILITATION UNIT INITIAL EVALUATION: ALICE *Continued*

PLAN

Will see Alice BID Monday through Saturday for 45-minute treatment sessions for the next 4 weeks. Treatment sessions to include positioning, early hip and shoulder care, facilitation and inhibition techniques to improve volitional movement of right extremities, and functional mobility training. Will ask physician for ST consult. Will begin family instruction and discharge planning. May recommend home assessment. Will reassess Alice weekly.

Positioning
1. Side lying on involved side to increase proprioceptive input to right extremities.
2. Supine and side lying on uninvolved side in recovery patterns.

Early Hip and Shoulder Care
1. Scapular protraction to maintain scapular mobility.
2. Double arm elevation.
3. Bridging (agonist reversals, resistive bridging).
4. Hip extension over the edge of the mat.
5. Hip and knee flexion exercises.
6. SLRs of the uninvolved LE to promote hamstring co-contraction.

Facilitation and Inhibition Techniques
1. Use of Urias air splint to right UE during sitting weight-bearing activities to increase proprioceptive input.
2. Tapping and vibration applied to right biceps during hand-to-mouth activities to facilitate muscle response.
3. Approximation applied through right ankle and then into right hip during bridging.
4. Approximation applied through the right knee and into the right ankle during sitting.
5. Use of cross-facilitation to increase sensory awareness.

Functional Mobility Training
1. Rolling to the right and left.
2. Supine-to-sit movement transitions on diagonal patterns to facilitate abdominal control.
3. Sitting postural alignment with and without UE support:

    Achievement of a neutral pelvic tilt
    Equal weight bearing on both hips
    Erect trunk
4. Scooting forward on the mat in sitting.
5. Weight shifting and reaching in sitting position to facilitate lateral trunk righting.
6. Sit-to-stand movement transition, height of surface varied.
7. Standing balance activities:
    Upright static positioning
    Equal weight bearing on both LEs
    Hip and knee control, tactile cues applied to the gluteals to promote hip extension
    Unilateral weight bearing, stepping forward with left leg
8. Dynamic standing balance activities:
    Walking
    Reaching activities
    Mini squats
9. Wheelchair mobility: negotiation of wheelchair parts and wheelchair propulsion on level surfaces.

Family Training
1. Schedule family training days.
2. Work with family on wheelchair-to-bed transfers, car transfers, and ambulation.
3. Educate family regarding Alice's condition and potential complications.

Discharge Planning
1. Perform home assessment if needed.
2. Secure necessary medical equipment (elevated toilet seat, grab bars, wheelchair, cane).

QUESTIONS TO THINK ABOUT

- What type of facilitation and/or inhibition techniques may be appropriate for Alice at this time?
- As Alice's sitting posture and balance improve, how may more challenging activities be incorporated into the treatment plan?
- Identify some areas of possible patient education.

REFERENCES

American Physical Therapy Association. Direction, Delegation and Supervision in Physical Therapy Services, HOD 06-96-30-42. House of Delegates: Standards, Policies, Positions, and Guidelines. Alexandria, VA, American Physical Therapy Association, 1998.

Baldrige RB. Functional assessment of measurements. Neurol Rep 17:3–10, 1993.

Bobath B. Motor development, its effect on general development, and application to the treatment of cerebral palsy. Physiotherapy 57:526–532, 1971.

Bobath B. Adult Hemiplegia, 3rd ed. Boston, Butterworth Heinemann, 1990, pp 9–66.

Bohannon RW, Smith MB. Interrater reliability of a modified Ashworth scale of muscle spasticity. Phys Ther 67:206–207, 1987.

Craik RL. Abnormalities of motor behavior. In Contemporary Management of Motor Control Problems. Proceedings of the II STEP Conference. Alexandria, VA, Foundation for Physical Therapy, 1991, pp 155–164.

Davies PM. Steps to Follow: A Guide to the Treatment of Adult Hemiplegia. Berlin, Springer, 1985, pp 266–284.

Dean E. Cardiopulmonary manifestations of systemic conditions. In Frownfelter D, Dean E (eds). Principles and Practice of Cardiopulmonary Physical Therapy, 3rd ed. St. Louis, CV Mosby, 1996, pp 99–113.

Duncan PW, Badke MB. Measurement of motor performance and functional abilities following stroke. In Duncan PW, Badke MB (eds.). Stroke Rehabilitation: The Recovery of Motor Control. Chicago, Year Book, 1987, pp 199–221.

Fuller KS. Stroke. In Goodman CC, Boissonnault WG (eds). Implications for the Physical Therapist. Philadelphia, WB Saunders, 1998, pp 748–762.

Granger CV, Hamilton BB. The uniform data system for medical rehabilitation report of first admissions for 1992. Am J Phys Med Rehabil 73:51–55, 1994.

Johnstone M. Restoration of Normal Movement After Stroke. New York, Churchill Livingstone, 1995, pp 49–74.

Katz RT. Management of spasticity. In Braddom RL (ed). Physical Medicine and Rehabilitation. Philadephia, WB Saunders, 1996, pp 580–604.

Kelly-Hayes M. A preventive approach to stroke. Nurs Clin North Am 26:931–940, 1991.

Levine RL. Diagnostic, medical, and surgical aspects of stroke management. In Duncan PM, Badke MB (eds). Stroke Rehabilitation: The Recovery of Motor Control. Chicago, Year Book, 1987, pp 1–47.

Light KE. Clients with spasticity: to strengthen or not to strengthen. Neurol Rep 15:63–64, 1991.

Maitland GD. Peripheral manipulation, 2nd ed. Boston, Butterworths, 1977, pp 3–31.

National Stroke Association. Stroke Facts. Englewood, CO, National Stroke Association, 1998.

Ostrosky KM. Facilitation vs. motor control. Clin Manage 10:34–40, 1990.

O'Sullivan SB. Strategies to improve motor control and learning. In O'Sullivan SB, Schmitz TJ (eds). Physical Rehabilitation Assessment and Treatment, 3rd ed. Philadelphia, FA Davis, 1994a, pp 225–249.

O'Sullivan SB. Stroke. In O'Sullivan SB, Schmitz TJ (eds). Physical Rehabilitation Assessment and Treatment, 3rd ed. Philadelphia, FA Davis, 1994b, pp 327–360.

Roth EJ, Harvey RL. Rehabilitation of stroke syndromes. In Braddom RL (ed). Physical Medicine and Rehabilitation. Philadelphia, WB Saunders, 1996, pp 1053–1087.

Ryerson SD. Hemiplegia. In Umphred DA (ed). Neurological Rehabilitation, 3rd ed. St. Louis, CV Mosby, 1995, pp 681–721.

Sawner KA, LaVigne JM. Brunnstrom's Movement Therapy in Hemiplegia, 2nd ed. Philadelphia, JB Lippincott, 1992, pp 41–65.

Schmitz TJ. Environmental assessment. In O'Sullivan SB, Schmitz TJ (eds). Physical Rehabilitation Assessment and Treatment, 3rd ed. Philadelphia, FA Davis, 1994, pp 209–223.

Watchie J. Cardiolopulmonary implications of specific diseases. In Hillegass EA, Sadowsky HS (eds). Essentials of Cardiolpulmonary Physical Therapy. Philadelphia, WB Saunders, 1994, pp 285–323.

Whiteside A. Clinical goals and application of NDT facilitation. NDTA Network Sept/Oct:2–14, 1997.

CHAPTER 6

Traumatic Brain Injuries

INTRODUCTION

Approximately 520,000 new traumatic brain injuries (TBIs) occur each year. Of this number, 80% are classified as mild TBIs, and these patients have a survival rate of almost 100%. The remaining 20% of all cases are evenly divided between moderate and severe injuries. Patients with moderate TBI have a survival rate of 93% as compared with 42% for patients with severe TBI. Patients with severe TBI constitute a small portion of total survivors, but they also account for the majority of patients who receive intensive rehabilitation (Bontke and Boake, 1996). The rate of survival and improved outcomes for persons with brain injuries are the direct result of enhanced medical technology and the prevention of secondary brain damage (Van-Sant, 1990a).

The most common cause of TBI is motor vehicle accidents, followed by automobile-pedestrian accidents, falls, assaults and violent crimes, and sports and recreational incidents. Men are more frequently affected than women at a ratio of 2:1. The typical age of individuals injured is 15 to 24 years (Winkler, 1995). However, a high incidence of TBI is also seen in infants, children, and older adults. Falls, automobile accidents, and bicycle accidents are the primary causes of brain injury in these populations (Bontke and Boake, 1996). Although we primarily discuss injury to the brain and the resultant motor and cognitive deficits, individuals with TBI often experience secondary trauma to other areas or body systems along with the injury to the nervous system.

Three primary factors influence the patient's final outcome following TBI: (1) the amount of immediate damage from the impact or insult; (2) the cumulative effects of secondary brain damage; and (3) the patient's premorbid status and family support (Leahy, 1994).

Cognitive characteristics such as intellect, level of education, and memory are believed to affect the patient's outcome. Preinjury personality, interpersonal relationships, and emotional disturbances may also contribute to the patient's outcome after brain injury (Bontke and Boake, 1996; Winkler, 1995).

CLASSIFICATIONS OF BRAIN INJURIES

Open and Closed Injuries

The two major classifications of brain injuries are open and closed injuries. *Open injuries* result from penetrating types of wounds such as those received from a gunshot or stabbing. The damage to the brain appears to follow the path of the object's entry and exit, thus resulting in more focal deficits. A *closed or intracranial injury* is the second type of injury, and several subtypes are reconized. An individual is said to have sustained a closed injury when neural (brain) tissue is damaged without penetration or disruption of the skull by an object and the dura remains intact.

Types of Closed Head Injuries

Concussion

The first subtype of closed head injury is a concussion. A *concussion* is defined as a momentary loss of consciousness and reflexes. The patient can have retrograde (before the injury) or anterograde (post-traumatic) amnesia. *Retrograde amnesia* is characterized by a loss of memory of the events prior to the injury, whereas in *post-traumatic amnesia,* individuals are unable to remember or learn new information (Bontke and Boake, 1996). With a concussion, there is no structural damage to the brain tissue. However, the synapses are disrupted where the shearing forces occurred.

Contusion

A contusion is the second subtype of a closed or intracranial injury. With a *contusion,* bruising on the surface of the brain is sustained at the time of impact. Small blood vessels on the surface of the brain hemorrhage and lead to the condition. A contusion that occurs on the same side of the brain as the impact is called a *coup lesion.* Surface hemorrhages that occur on the opposite side of the trauma as a result of deceleration are called *contrecoup lesions.* The acceleration associated with contrecoup injuries can cause further vessel occlusion and edema formation. Figure 6–1 depicts both a coup injury and a contrecoup injury.

Damage to brain tissue can take several forms. The extent of the injury depends on the nature of the insult. In patients with open wounds, local brain damage occurs at the site of impact. Secondary brain damage can occur as a consequence of laceration to cerebral tissue, as is frequently seen with skull fractures. Acceleration and deceleration forces can produce coup or contrecoup injuries. Polar brain damage can occur as the brain moves forward within the skull. The frontal and parietal lobes are most frequently affected (Gelber, 1995; Leahy, 1994). High-velocity injuries can cause diffuse axonal injury because the brain tissue accelerates and decelerates within the skull. Subcortical axons can shear and become disrupted within the myelin sheath, and small punctate hemorrhages can appear (Leahy, 1994). This diffuse axonal injury can disconnect the brain stem activating centers from the cerebral hemispheres (Bontke et al, 1992). Areas most susceptible to this type of injury include the corpus callosum, basal ganglia, periventricular white matter, and superior cerebellar peduncles (Gelber, 1995). The cumulative effects of brain injury can include coma, autonomic dysfunction, and abnormal motor control (Leahy, 1994).

Hematomas

Vascular hemorrhage with *hematoma* formation is the third subcategory of closed head injuries. There are two specific types of hematomas worthy of notation. *Epidural hematomas* form between the dura mater and the skull (Fig. 6–2A). These types of injuries are frequently seen after a blow to the side of the head or severe trauma from a motor vehicle accident. Rupture

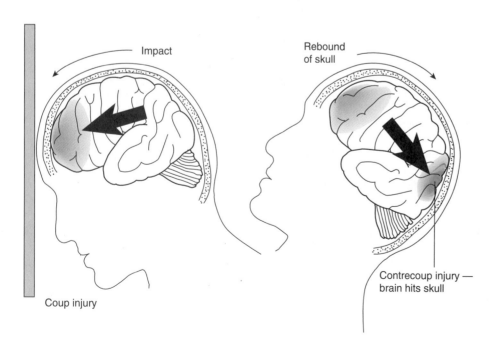

FIGURE 6–1 ■ Types of head injury—closed and open. (From Gould BE. Pathophysiology for the Health-Related Professions. Philadelphia, WB Saunders, 1997.)

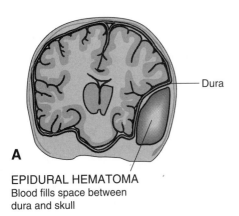

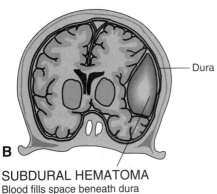

FIGURE 6-2 ■ Types of hematomas. (From Gould BE. Pathophysiology for the Health-Related Professions. Philadelphia, WB Saunders, 1997.)

of the middle meningeal artery within the temporal fossa can cause epidural hematomas. Clinically, the patient has a period of unconsciousness and then becomes alert and lucid. This is followed by rapid deterioration of the patient's condition if the hematoma enlarges. Immediate surgical intervention consisting of craniotomy and hematoma evacuation is necessary to save the patient's life or to prevent further deterioration of the patient's condition.

A *subdural hematoma,* on the other hand, is an acute venous hemorrhage that results because of rupture to the cortical bridging veins. This hematoma develops between the dura and the arachnoid. Blood accumulates more slowly, generally over a period of several hours to a week. An injury of this type is often seen in the elderly after a fall with a blow to the head. The symptoms fluctuate and can resemble those seen in patients with cerebrovascular accident. The patient can experience decreased consciousness, ipsilateral pupil dilation, and contralateral hemiparesis. Smaller clots may be able to be reabsorbed by the body, whereas larger hematomas may require surgical removal. Figure 6–2B shows the location of a subdural hematoma.

SECONDARY PROBLEMS

Individuals who sustain a TBI may also sustain secondary cerebral damage as a result of the brain's response to the initial injury. This damage can occur within an hour of the initial injury or as much as several months later. The following is a discussion of several secondary problems that may affect the patient's outcome.

Increased Intracranial Pressure

Increased intracranial pressure (ICP) is common after head injury. Approximately 80% of patients in coma admitted to an acute care facility have increased ICP (Jennett and Teasdale, 1981). The adult skull is rigid and does not expand to accommodate increasing volumes of fluid secondary to edema formation or hemorrhage. The result is an increase in pressure that can lead to compression of brain tissue and possible herniation. Normal ICP is approximately 10 mm Hg. Pressures greater than 20 mm Hg are considered abnormal and can result in neurologic and cardiovascular changes. Signs and symptoms of increased ICP include (1) decreased responsiveness, (2) impaired consciousness, (3) severe headache, (4) vomiting, (5) irritability, (6) papilledema, and (7) changes in vital signs including increased blood pressure and decreased heart rate (Gould, 1997; Jennett and Teasdale, 1981). If a patient is going to develop increased ICP, it will normally occur within the first week after the injury. However, it is important for all clinicians to recognize the signs and symptoms of this condition because patients can develop it months or weeks after their initial injuries. Treatment of increased ICP includes careful monitoring and ventricular peritoneal shunting if permanent correction is needed. Positioning the patient in an inverted (head-down) position is contraindicated in patients with increased ICP or unstable blood pressure (O'Sullivan, 1994).

Damage from head trauma results in secondary complications including hypoxia or decreased oxygen to brain tissue, anoxia, intracranial hematoma, infection as a consequence of open head injuries, and posttraumatic epilepsy or seizure activity.

Anoxic Injuries

Brain tissue demands 20% of the body's oxygen intake to maintain proper oxygen saturation levels and metabolic functions (Fitzgerald, 1992). Anoxic injuries are most frequently caused by cardiac arrest. These types of injuries typically cause diffuse damage. However, some areas have been shown to be more vulnerable to local damage such as neurons in the hippocampus (an area involved in memory storage), the cerebellum, and the basal ganglia. This may explain the prevalence of amnesia and movement disorders in this patient population (Bontke and Boake, 1996; Jennett and Teasdale, 1981).

Post-traumatic Epilepsy

Individuals have an increased risk of seizure activity after TBI. Approximately 5% of all patients develop post-traumatic epilepsy (Bontke and Boake, 1996). It is possible for seizure activity to develop several years after the injury. Post-traumatic epilepsy is more common in patients with open head injuries (Davies, 1994). If a patient should have a grand mal seizure during treatment, the assistant should transfer the patient to the floor to avoid possible injury. Notification of the patient's physician and primary nurse is necessary. Patients who remain unconscious after the seizure should be positioned on their side to prevent possible aspiration (Davies, 1994).

Numerous medications are prescribed for patients with seizure activity. Common medications given to control seizure activity include phenytoin (Dilantin) and phenobarbital. Both these medications have sedative effects that can decrease a patient's arousal, memory, and cognition. Carbamazepine (Tegretol) is another antiseizure medication that is well tolerated and has fewer adverse side effects (Naritoku and Hernandez, 1995). An important consideration for physical therapists and physical therapist assistants is that relatively small changes in a patient's level of arousal or awareness may affect his ability to respond to his environment (Bontke et al, 1992).

PATIENT EVALUATION

Glasgow Coma Scale

A patient who is brought to the emergency room following TBI is evaluated to determine the extent of injury. The Glasgow Coma Scale (GCS) is used to assess the individual's level of arousal and function of the cerebral cortex. The scale specifically evaluates pupillary response, motor activity, and the patient's ability to verbalize (VanSant, 1990a) (Table 6–1). Scores for this assessment can range from 3 to 15, with higher scores indicating less severe brain damage and a better chance of survival. Individuals who are admitted through the emergency room with scores of 3 or 4 often do not survive. A score of 8 or less indicates that the patient is in a coma and has sustained a severe brain injury (Leahy, 1994). "It has been repeatedly demonstrated that the depth and duration of unconsciousness, as indexed by the GCS score, is the single

Table 6–1 ▌ GLASGOW COMA SCALE*

EYE OPENING	SCORE
Spontaneous	4
To speech	3
To pain	2
No response	1

MOTOR RESPONSE	SCORE
Obeys verbal command	6
Localized	5
Withdraws to pain	4
Decorticate posturing	3
Decerebrate posturing	2
No response	1

VERBAL RESPONSE	SCORE
Oriented	5
Conversation confused	4
Use of inappropriate words	3
Incomprehensible sounds	2
No response	1

* Overall score = sum of eye opening and motor response and verbal response.

Modified from Jennett B, Teasdale G. Management of Head Injuries. Philadelphia, FA Davis, 1981, p 78.

most powerful predictor of outcome from TBI" (Bontke and Boake, 1996).

Classifying the Severity of Traumatic Brain Injury

TBIs are classified as mild, moderate, or severe. A patient with mild TBI has a GCS of 13 or higher, a loss of consciousness lasting less than 20 minutes, and a normal computed tomography scan. Patients with mild TBI are awake on their arrival to the acute care facility. A patient with moderate TBI has a GCS score of 9 to 12. On admission to the hospital, the patient is unable to answer questions appropriately. Many patients with moderate TBIs have permanent deficits. A severe TBI corresponds to a score of 3 to 8 and indicates that the individual is in a coma. Most patients with severe TBIs have permanent functional and cognitive impairments (Bontke and Boake, 1996).

PATIENT PROBLEM AREAS

The clinical manifestations of TBI are varied, secondary to diffuse damage. Common problems seen in this patient population include (1) decreased level of consciousness, (2) cognitive impairments, (3) motor or movement disorders, (4) sensory problems, (5) communication deficits, (6) behavioral changes, and (7) associated problems.

Decreased Level of Consciousness

A decreased or altered level of arousal or consciousness is frequently seen in patients who have sustained a TBI. Arousal is a primitive state of being awake or alert. The reticular activating system is responsible for an individual's level of arousal. To be aware means that an individual is conscious of internal and external environmental stimuli. *Consciousness* is the state of being aware. The term *coma* is used to describe individuals with a decreased level of awareness. A coma is a state of unconsciousness in which the patient is neither aroused nor responsive to what is going on internally or within the external environment (Rappaport et al, 1992). When patients are in a coma, their eyes remain closed, and one cannot distinguish between sleep and wake cycles on the electroencephalogram. True comas do not last longer than 3 to 4 weeks. Patients who demonstrate a return of brain stem reflexes and sleep-wake cycles yet remain unconscious are said to be in a *vegetative state.* Vegetative functions such as respiration, digestion, and blood pressure control resume when brain stem function is restored (Lehmkuhl and Krawczyk, 1993). The patient at this stage may experience periods of arousal and may demonstrate spontaneous eye opening without tracking. The patient does, however, remain unaware of the external environment or his internal needs (Rappaport et al, 1992). An individual who remains in a vegetative state for a year or longer is classified as being in a *persistent vegetative state.* A persistent vegetative state is the prognosis given to a patient when no improvement in neurologic status is seen and the patient is anticipated to remain at the current level (Lehmkuhl and Krawczyk, 1993).

Cognitive Deficits

In addition to deficits in patient arousal and responsiveness, many individuals with TBIs also experience cognitive deficits. Cognitive dysfunction can include disorientation, poor attention span, loss of memory, and inability to control emotional responses. The severity of the patient's cognitive deficits greatly affects the ability to learn new skills, an ability that is an integral part of the rehabilitation process (VanSant, 1990a; VanSant, 1990b). The following is a case example that illustrates this point. A patient receiving physical therapy services in an inpatient rehabilitation center was able to ambulate independently without an assistive device, to negotiate environmental barriers, and to perform complex fine motor tasks. The patient was not, however, able to remember his name, he could not identify family members, and he was not oriented to time or place. The patient would often become confused by the external environment and would confabulate stories. This patient's cognitive defi-

cits were much more problematic to his functional independence than were his physical limitations. Treatment strategies to address these problems are discussed later in this chapter.

Motor Deficits

A second major area affected in patients with TBI is motor function. When a patient is unconscious, mobility is impaired. The patient is not able to initiate active movements. Abnormal postures are frequently seen as a consequence of brain stem injury. The two most prevalent abnormal postures are decerebrate rigidity and decorticate rigidity. In *decerebrate rigidity,* the patient's lower extremities are in extension. The hips are adducted and internally rotated, the knees are extended, the ankles are plantar flexed, and the feet are supinated. The upper extremities are internally rotated and extended at the shoulders, extended at the elbows, pronated at the forearms, and flexed at the wrists and fingers. Thumb entrapment within the palm of the hand may be present. Injury to the brain between the red nucleus and the vestibular nucleus results in this type of posturing because the vestibular nucleus provides the source for the abnormal tone with no regulation. *Decorticate rigidity* appears as upper extremity flexion with adduction and internal rotation of the shoulders, flexion of the elbows, pronation of the forearms, flexion of the wrists, and extension of the lower extremities. Decorticate posturing results from dysfunction above the level of the red nucleus, specifically between the basal nuclei and the thalamus. Patients with significant injuries can be dominated by either abnormal posture. Difficulties arise when the patient is unable to deviate from the posture, and voluntary active movement is not possible (VanSant, 1990a).

In addition to abnormal postures, individuals who have sustained a TBI can present with other types of motor disorders. Patients can demonstrate generalized weakness and difficulty initiating movement, as well as disorders of muscle tone. The reemergence of primitive and tonic reflexes without voluntary motor control can also affect the patient's ability to move into and out of different positions. The presence of the tonic labyrinthine reflex, asymmetric tonic neck reflex, symmetric tonic neck reflex, positive support reflex, and flexor withdrawal reflex can inhibit the patient's ability to initiate active movement. Motor sequencing, ataxia, incoordination, and decreased balance abilities may also interfere with the patient's ability to perform functional movements.

Sensory Deficits

Sensory deficits are also apparent in patients with TBI. Patients' perceptions of cutaneous sensations can be impaired or absent. Additionally, visual, perceptual, and proprioceptive deficits may be noted, depending on the area of the brain that was affected.

Communication Deficits

The ability to communicate is often initially lost or severely impaired in the patient with TBI. A decreased awareness of one's environment can limit opportunities for interaction. Patients with severe motor deficits may not be able to initiate communication because of abnormal tone or posturing. Mechanisms other than verbal communication must be explored. Eye blinks, head nods, or finger movements may be the only available options to establish yes/no responses. Physical therapists and physical therapist assistants often discover that the patient's first successful attempts at communication occur during the physical therapy treatment session. The inhibitory techniques used to manage abnormal tone and the facilitation of normal movement patterns may allow the patient to initiate a motion or verbal response that can serve as a means of communication.

Behavioral Deficits

Behavioral problems can also become evident after TBI. These deficits are frequently the most enduring and socially disabling. Patients can be debilitated by changes in their personalities and temperaments. Patients can exhibit neuroses, psychoses, sexual disinhibition, apathy, aggression, and low frustration tolerance. These personality changes can be challenging for the rehabilitation professionals, as well as for caregivers and family members. The physical therapist and physical therapist assistant should consult with a psychologist who is knowledgeable about and experienced with behavioral interventions to develop and implement appropriate strategies that address the patient's behavioral issues.

Associated Problems

A final area that must be mentioned in this patient population is that of associated problems the patient can experience. Serious medical complications, as well as orthopedic injuries, can occur during the traumatic event leading to the actual brain injury. A patient who has sustained a TBI may also present with fractures, lacerations, and even spinal cord injury. These associated problems affect the patient's care and can make rehabilitation more challenging.

PHYSICAL THERAPY INTERVENTION: ACUTE CARE

The physical therapy care of the patient with a TBI should begin in the acute care setting as soon as the patient is medically stable. Early goals of treatment should include (1) increasing the patient's level of arousal, (2) preventing the development of secondary complications, (3) improving patient function, and (4) providing the patient and family with education regarding the injury. The patient's length of stay in the acute care facility may be short, especially if the patient does not experience any medical complications. Average lengths of stay may be less than 2 weeks.

Positioning

One of the most important early treatment activities that must be addressed is patient positioning. This is imperative because of the abnormal tone and postures patients with TBI can exhibit. Supine is the position in which many of these patients are placed because it facilitates performance of both nursing and self-care tasks. Supine is also the position in which one sees the greatest impact of the tonic labyrinthine reflexes. Interventions 6–1 and 6–2 provide positioning examples. Side lying and semiprone positions are more desirable. Care must be taken when one is repositioning these patients because of respiratory concerns. Often, these patients may be receiving mechanical ventilation or may have tracheostomies. Patients can be positioned in prone by placement of a pillow under the chest and forehead. This position maintains the patient's airway. Positioning the upper extremities in slight abduction and external rotation while the patient is in the prone or supine position also exerts an inhibitory influence on abnormal muscle tone (Davies, 1994).

The therapist or assistant should position the patient out of the decerebrate or decorticate posture. Nursing staff members and the patient's family must be educated on the ways in which the patient should be positioned. Firm towels, small bolsters, or half-rolls should be used to assist the patient in maintaining the optimal position. Pillows and other soft objects should be avoided because they provide the patient with something to push against, which can elicit a stretch reflex and may exacerbate abnormal posturing.

The abnormal muscle tone present in these patients can be significant. Contractures can develop quickly, especially in the elbow and ankle. Proper positioning, accompanied by range-of-motion exercises, can alleviate these potentially limiting complications.

Intervention 6–1 ‖ **SIDE LYING POSITIONING**

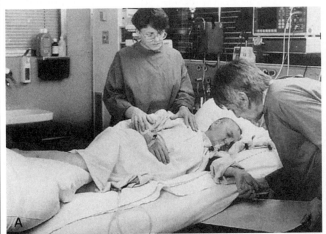

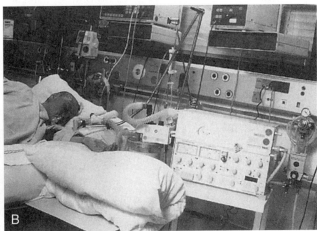

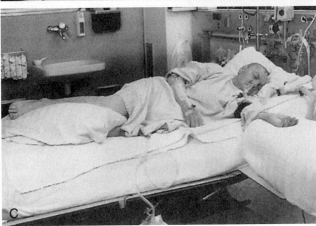

A. One end of the footboard is beneath the mattress.

B. A rolled pillow supports the extended arm.

C. The arm is well supported in the corrected position.

From Davies PM. Starting Again: Early Rehabilitation after Traumatic Brain Injury or Other Severe Brain Lesion. New York, Springer-Verlag, 1994.

Intervention 6–2 ‖ **PRONE POSITIONING**

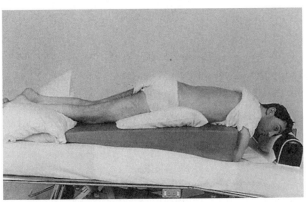

Despite severe contractures, this patient is able to lie prone with the help of different supports.

From Davies PM. Starting Again: Early Rehabilitation after Traumatic Brain Injury or Other Severe Brain Lesion. New York, Springer-Verlag, 1994.

Heterotopic Ossification

Heterotopic ossification is abnormal bone formation in soft tissues and muscles surrounding joints that can occur after TBI. The origin of this problem is unknown; however, this condition is noted after injury to the brain and spinal cord. A common denominator in all cases of heterotopic ossification is prolonged immobilization. The incidence of this condition in patients with TBI is between 11 and 76% (Varghese, 1992). Patients can present with loss of range of motion, pain on movement, localized swelling, and erythema (Davies, 1994). A definitive diagnosis is made with a bone scan (Varghese, 1992). Common joints affected include the hips, knees, shoulders, and elbows. In patients with TBI, the hip is the most common joint affected. That there is no effective method available to treat heterotopic ossification once it has developed leads to some controversy regarding the continuation of physical therapy after diagnosis of the condition. Most experts do agree that range-of-motion exercises should continue to prevent possible ankylosis and that positioning, splinting, and managing abnormal muscle tone can be helpful (Varghese, 1992). Pharmacologic interventions include etidronate disodium, nonsteroidal anti-inflammatory drugs, and salicylates (Bontke et al, 1992; Varghese, 1992).

Reflex Inhibiting Postures

Reflex inhibiting postures were first discussed by Karl and Berta Bobath. After observing children with cerebral palsy and the abnormal postures these children assumed, the Bobaths believed that one could reverse the influence of abnormal tone from the tonic reflexes by positioning a patient in the opposite pattern. Reflex inhibiting postures were developed for the tonic labyrinthine reflexes, the asymmetric tonic neck reflex, and the symmetric tonic neck reflex. Initially, the Bobaths used these postures as static positions; however, with evolution of their treatment approach, active movement was superimposed on the reflex inhibiting postures. These postures are now used to inhibit abnormal tone, and once a more manageable degree of muscle tone is achieved, the clinician facilitates normal movement patterns (Bobath and Bobath, 1984).

Activities Aimed at Increasing Patient Awareness

Also during this acute stage, activities aimed at increasing the patient's level of awareness are employed. These activities are important even for those patients who are said to be in a coma. Even though a patient may not be able to respond verbally or by moving, one cannot assume that the patient is unable to understand or is not hearing the information provided. That is why it is important for the patient to be informed about what is happening to him at all times. All members of the rehabilitation team are orienting the patient to his name, the facility in which he is currently residing, and why the patient is receiving medical intervention. The rehabilitation team often develops a script outlining pertinent orientation information about the patient. Referring to subjects that are familiar to the patient within treatment sessions and conversations is beneficial. As clinicians work with the patient, it is imperative that they explain what they are doing at all times. Communicating with the patient on a personal level also demonstrates to the patient and family that physical therapists and physical therapist assistants are caring, respectful professionals who are attempting to develop a rapport with the patient.

Sensory Stimulation

The use of sensory stimulation for patients in coma is currently under review. Initially, the rationale for the use of sensory modalities was to increase the patient's level of arousal and responsiveness and to facilitate the patient's emergence from coma (Bontke et al, 1992). Research studies have not supported the value of sensory stimulation in improving the patient's level of arousal, however. Sensory stimulation does play a significant role in assisting the rehabilitation team in the assessment of the patient's level of arousal and ability to perceive and attend to stimuli in the environment (Bontke et al, 1992). Auditory, olfactory, tactile, kinesthetic, and oral stimuli can be administered for assessment and treatment purposes.

When administering sensory stimulation to the patient who is unresponsive, it is best to limit the time. Brief periods of stimulation are best. Overstimulation can agitate the patient and may cause increased fatigue. It is also important to attempt stimulation when the patient is most alert. Therapists are more likely to see a response when the patient is in an alert or aroused state. Only one sensory stimulus should be administered at a time. If the therapist is using tactile stimuli, no other sensory input should be provided. When multiple inputs are administered, it is not possible to determine what stimuli elicited the patient's response. Patients must also be given adequate time to respond once the stimulus has been presented. Response time can be greatly increased in patients who have sustained a TBI (Krus, 1988).

Patients' responses to the different sensory modalities administered must be observed. The rehabilitation team hopes that one type of stimulus will be effective in eliciting a patient response. Once that has been determined, the team can use this stimulus during patient interactions. Small vials of different scents such as coffee, peppermint, or ammonia are passed under the patient's nose. Tactile stimuli such as different textures (cotton, paintbrushes, sandpaper) can be applied to areas of the patient's skin. Noxious stimuli can be used if the patient is not responding to other forms of stimulation. Pressure on the patient's nail bed, sticking the patient with a pin, or pinching the patient's skin slightly may elicit a pain response. Brightly colored objects, familiar pictures, or objects presented to the patient can provide visual stimulation. Ice, mouth swabs, and tongue depressors can provide oral stimulation. Finally, range-of-motion exercises and position changes can be performed to assess the patient's response to kinesthetic input (Krus, 1988).

The voice of a therapist or assistant can also be used as a tool to influence the patient's response. For those patients who are in a heightened state of awareness, the use of a soft tone of voice may calm the patient. On the contrary, for those patients who need to be stimulated, the use of the patient's name followed by a brief, concise command in a loud voice may be needed to arouse the patient.

Cognitive Functioning

The Rancho Los Amigos Scale of Cognitive Functioning is a tool that can be used to measure the patient's level of cognitive function. Table 6–2 highlights major patient responses in each of the categories. The levels start with the patient at level 1. Patients at this level do not respond to any type of stimuli, whereas individuals at level VIII are alert, oriented, and able to function independently within the community. Although this scale would appear to be an easy way to classify patients and their recoveries, some individuals may exhibit behaviors or responses from more than one category as they make the transition between stages. In addition, not all patients progress through each of the stages. Other assessment tools have also been developed to assist health care providers in the classification of patients with TBIs.

Patient responses may be generalized or localized. Generalized responses are inconsistent and nonpurposeful. They can be physiologic changes including fluctuations in respiration rates, sweating, skin color changes, or goose bumps. Generalized responses may also present as gross body movements including changes in extremity movement, increased abnormal posturing, or withdrawal from the stimulus. Vocalizations or increased oral movements also are characteristic of generalized patient responses. Patients exhibiting generalized responses frequently respond in the same way regardless of the stimulus (VanSant, 1990a).

Patients able to localize sensory responses will react specifically to the stimulus applied. Patients demonstrating this type of sensory processing may be able to follow simple one-step commands; however, responses are frequently delayed and are not consistently completed (VanSant, 1990a). An example of this is when the therapist touches the patient's right shoulder and asks the patient to do the same; after a short delay, the patient reaches and touches his right upper arm.

Patient and Family Education

Patient and family education is an important component of treatment. TBI is devastating to the family and friends as well as to the patient. Most families are overwhelmed initially and may not know how to react to the patient. It is important for physical therapists and physical therapist assistants to provide the family with support and accurate information. Family mem-

Table 6–2 ▌ LEVELS OF COGNITIVE FUNCTIONING

LEVEL	BEHAVIORS TYPICALLY DEMONSTRATED
I	No responses: Patient appears to be in a deep sleep and is completely unresponsive to any stimuli.
II	Generalized response: Patient reacts inconsistently and nonpurposefully to stimuli in a nonspecific manner. Responses are limited and often the same regardless of stimulus presented. Responses may be physiologic changes, gross body movements, and/or vocalization.
III	Localized response: Patient reacts specifically but inconsistently to stimuli. Responses are directly related to the type of a stimulus presented. May follow simple commands in an inconsistent, delayed manner, such as closing eyes or squeezing hand.
IV	Confused-agitated: Patient is in heightened state of activity. Behavior is bizarre and nonpurposeful relative to immediate environment. Does not discriminate among persons or objects; is unable to cooperate directly with treatment efforts. Verbalizations frequently are incoherent and/or inappropriate to the environment; confabulation may be present. Gross attention to environment is very brief; selective attention is often nonexistent. Patient lacks short-term and long-term recall.
V	Confused-inappropriate: Patient is able to respond to simple commands fairly consistently. However, with increased complexity of commands or lack of any external structure, responses are nonpurposeful, random, or fragmented. Demonstrates gross attention to the environment, but is highly distractible and lacks ability to focus attention to a specific task. With structure, may be able to converse on a social-automatic level for short periods of time. Verbalization is often inappropriate and confabulatory. Memory is severely impaired; often shows inappropriate use of objects; may perform previously learned tasks with structure but is unable to learn new information.
VI	Confused-appropriate: Patient shows goal-directed behavior, but is dependent on external input for direction. Follows simple directions consistently and shows carry-over for relearned tasks with little or no carry-over for new tasks. Responses may be incorrect due to memory problems but appropriate to the situation; past memories show more depth and detail than recent memory.
VII	Automatic-appropriate: Patient appears appropriate and oriented within hospital and home settings; goes through daily routine automatically, frequently robotlike with minimal-to-absent confusion, but has shallow recall of activities. Shows carry-over for new learning, but at a decreased rate. With structure is able to initiate social or recreational activities; judgment remains impaired.
VIII	Purposeful and appropriate: Patient is able to recall and integrate past and recent events and is aware of and responsive to environment. Shows carry-over for new learning and needs no supervision once activities are learned. May continue to show a decreased ability relative to premorbid abilities, abstract reasoning, tolerance for stress, and judgment in emergencies or unusual circumstances.

Reprinted from Malkmus D: Integrating cognitive strategies into the physical therapy setting. Phys Ther 63:1958, 1983; with permission of the ATPA.

bers must be educated about changes in the patient's appearance and cognitive and physical functioning. Although this information may be initially shared with the family in the acute care setting, it will need to be repeated and updated as the patient makes the transition to new facilities and progresses in recovery. As soon as possible, family members should be encouraged to participate in the patient's care (VanSant, 1990a).

PHYSICAL THERAPY INTERVENTIONS DURING INPATIENT REHABILITATION

Once the patient is medically stable, the patient will most likely be transferred to an inpatient rehabilitation setting if further intensive intervention is required. Primary patient problems at this stage are as follows: (1) decreased range of motion and the potential for contractures; (2) increased muscle tone and abnormal posturing; (3) decreased awareness and responsiveness to the environment; (4) the presence of primitive tonic reflexes; (5) decreased functional mobility and tolerance to upright; (6) decreased endurance; (7) decreased sensory awareness; (8) an impaired or absent communication system; and (9) decreased knowledge of his condition.

Positioning

Proper positioning continues to be an important aspect of care during rehabilitation. As discussed in the section on acute care treatment, positioning warrants much attention by all health care providers. Proper positioning depends on the patient's resting posture, abnormal muscle tone, and the presence of any primitive reflexes. Side lying and prone are the two most desirable positions. As the patient becomes medically stable, sitting in a wheelchair and acclimation to the upright position become important. Sitting orients the patient to a different position and assists with endurance and bronchial hygiene. For patients who have a low functioning level and who lack head and trunk control, a tilt-in-space wheelchair may be necessary. A tilt-in-space wheelchair differs from a reclining wheelchair by allowing the trunk to recline while 90-degree angles are maintained at the hips, knees, and ankles. The tilt-in-space feature is beneficial because it assists in positioning the trunk and in maintaining proper alignment. The only drawback to this type of wheelchair and seating system is that it changes the patient's visual field. Gaze is directed upward, thus making it difficult for the patient to visualize individuals and objects in his environment.

Standard wheelchairs may be satisfactory. Lap trays securely fastened to the chair support the patient's upper extremities and help to maintain proper sitting alignment. Intervention 6–3 provides an example of a patient positioned in a standard wheelchair. The patient must be carefully monitored when sitting activities are initiated. Complications that result from immobility and prolonged supine positioning can become evident, including orthostatic hypotension and fatigue. In addition, the patient's skin condition must be carefully monitored to avoid any chance of pressure areas or skin breakdown. When attempting to position the patient, the therapist must remember the basic positioning concepts discussed in Chapter 5. One must begin by positioning the patient's proximal body areas including the pelvis and the shoulder girdle. From there, the therapist can work more distally. It is necessary to decrease muscle tone proximally to influence the tone more distally. Poor positioning in the wheelchair or bed can lead to the development of contractures and an increase in abnormal muscle tone.

Wheelchair Propulsion

Once the patient is able to tolerate sitting in the wheelchair, self-propulsion activities can be initiated.

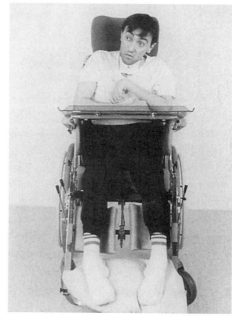

Intervention 6–3 ▌ WHEELCHAIR POSITIONING

It is important for a patient with severe contractures to sit out of bed and to lie prone.

From Davies PM. Starting Again: Early Rehabilitation after Traumatic Brain Injury or Other Severe Brain Lesion. New York, Springer-Verlag, 1994.

Initially, the therapist or assistant may need to help the patient with hand-over-hand or guided practice. As the patient becomes more proficient, the goal will be for the patient to propel the wheelchair independently and to negotiate safely around the facility.

Range of Motion

Range-of-motion exercises are also important at this stage to minimize the likelihood of contracture formation. Because of the many problems these patients have, it is necessary to be efficient with our treatment. Stretching of each individual joint can be time-consuming and may have short-term benefits. Instead, it is often more efficient to maintain or increase a patient's flexibility through the use of different postures and positions. For example, prone positioning and tall-kneeling can be used to stretch the hip flexors, quadruped positioning and sitting can be used to stretch the gluteals and quadriceps, and standing on a tilt table or approximation directed down through the knee during sitting can assist with stretching the gastrocnemius and soleus. Dedicated treatment time, however, may need to be spent to manually stretch the hamstrings and the heel cords more aggressively.

Whenever functional positions or developmental postures will meet the same goal as static stretching, they should be used. Patients who have developed deformities or contractures as a result of abnormal tone and posturing may require more intensive stretching. A more effective intervention for these individuals may be serial casting or splinting. A plaster cast is applied to the joint with the range-of-motion limitation or contracture and is left on for 7 to 10 days. Thus, a prolonged stretch is applied to the joint and soft tissues. The goal is to decrease the contracture through subsequent castings and stretching. Three to four casts may need to be applied to achieve the desired results (Booth et al, 1983). Ultimately, the final cast should be bivalved as it is removed so it can become a permanent splint for the patient. Areas that respond well to serial casting include the ankle, knee, elbow, and wrist. Clinicians working with patients who have been casted need to monitor the patient's response to the cast. Skin discoloration of the toes or fingers may indicate that the cast is too tight. Casts that are applied too loosely may slip down. It is not uncommon to find that a patient may have worked the cast off completely. A detailed description of the application of serial casts is beyond the scope of this text (Davies, 1994).

Improving Awareness

Increasing awareness of self and the environment is another important aspect of the patient's treatment plan. Enhancing a patient's awareness is most often accomplished through the administration of various sensory stimuli. An assessment tool that can be administered to the patient and that assists in identifying or categorizing the patient's responses to stimuli is the Rappaport Coma/Near-Coma Scale (CNC). This tool was developed to measure small changes in awareness and responsivity in patients with severe brain injuries who function at levels characteristic of vegetative status. The CNC looks at the patient's responses to auditory, visual, olfactory, tactile, and painful stimuli. In addition, the patient's attempts at vocalizations, the ability to respond to a threat, and the ability to follow a one-step command are assessed. This assessment tool is used at admission to the facility and is repeated at regular intervals to document the patient's progress. Multiple disciplines can administer the test. Scores for the test items are determined, and the patient's level of awareness or responsivity is categorized as no coma (level 1) to extreme coma (level 4). Once the patient has progressed to a level 1 or near-coma category, the administration of the CNC can be discontinued and the Multisensory Assessment can be used. Research suggests that patients with CNC scores less than 2.0 and who are involved in intensive rehabilitation are most likely to improve (Rappaport et al, 1992).

The Multisensory Assessment is a tool used to measure the patient's response to different sensory modalities. Movement, various auditory stimuli, tactile sensations, and visual stimuli are used to identify the sensory systems that may be functioning for the patient. This tool identifies possible patient responses, which include generalized body movements such as voluntary and involuntary movements, changes in facial expressions, autonomic changes including changes in the skin or respiration patterns, oral movements, or movements of the eyes. By administering different sensory modalities and noting the patient's response, the rehabilitation team is able to identify which sensory systems are functioning. In addition, the assessment allows therapists to isolate a sensory system that may be used by the patient for communication purposes. For example, the Multisensory Assessment may indicate that the patient is able to use eye blinks successfully to communicate yes/no responses. The Multisensory Assessment, like the CNC, can be used at the time of the patient's admission to the facility and can then be repeated at different intervals to document the patient's progress.

As stated earlier, it is important to explain to the patient what is being done even if the patient appears to be unresponsive. Orienting the patient to his surroundings and the circumstances regarding admission to the facility may be beneficial in increasing awareness levels. Many brain injury rehabilitation teams develop patient scripts that assist in orienting the patient to the environment. Strategies to manage some of the other cognitive concerns are discussed later in this chapter.

Family Education

Educating the patient's family about ways in which they can assist the patient with orientation and awareness is important. Encouraging the family to bring in favorite pictures, music, or other items can be of assistance. Family members should be cautioned against overstimulating the patient, however. In an effort to arouse the patient, families often play music or leave the patient's television on for extended periods. Few of us listen to music or watch television 24 hours a day. It is important to vary the amounts and intensities of the stimuli provided so the patient does not accommodate to the sensory modality.

Functional Mobility Training

Functional mobility tasks are another important aspect of treatment. Often, patients are dependent in all aspects of mobility. Early on, it may be necessary for the physical therapist or physical therapist assistant to co-treat the patient with another rehabilitation provider. When patients have an extremely low functioning level, it can be helpful to have two sets of hands available. However, in this current climate of cost containment, clinicians must use resources efficiently. For example, it may be more cost-effective for the assistant and the rehabilitation aide rather than the assistant and the occupational therapist to see the patient. The patient's needs and the acuteness of those needs must be assessed before these types of decisions can be made. Frequently, therapists need to spend some time inhibiting abnormal tone or postures so functional activities can be attempted. Methods to inhibit abnormal tone are discussed in Chapter 5 and include prolonged stretch, weight bearing, approximation, slow rhythmic rotation, and tendon pressure. These techniques work effectively with this patient population as well. Total body postures and positions such as upper and lower trunk rotation, sitting, prone, and standing are also effective in decreasing abnormal tone. As stated in Chapter 5, once the abnormal muscle tone has been decreased, normal movement patterns must be facilitated to promote motor relearning.

Individuals who have sustained a severe TBI lack postural and motor control. They are unable to initiate voluntary movement, are dominated by abnormal muscle tone and reflex activity, and exhibit difficulty in dissociating extremity movements from the trunk. In addition, these patients often are unable to perform automatic postural adjustments (VanSant, 1990a). Consequently, an early emphasis in the patient's physical therapy treatment plan must be on the development of postural control. Head and trunk control must be developed before the patient can hope to have control over the distal extremities. The principles discussed in Chapter 5 regarding the neurodevelopmental treatment approach are also applicable to this patient population. Therapeutic activities performed with the patient in prone or prone over a wedge or bolster may provide excellent opportunities to address head and trunk control. These positions require that the patient work the cervical extensors against gravity and also provide inhibition to the supine symmetric tonic labyrinthine reflex. The prone position facilitates increased flexor tone in patients with the presence of this reflex. Patients who have extreme extensor tone can also be positioned in prone over a ball. Although transferring and maintaining the patient's position on the ball is challenging, the activity has a profound effect on reducing abnormal tone. Once the patient is on the ball, one can perform gentle rocking to decrease the effects of abnormal tone even further. This position is contraindicated in patients with seizure disorders and increased ICP. Additionally, all patients should be carefully monitored during prone activities to ensure adequacy of respiration.

Practicing through repetition of well-learned and automatic activities is beneficial and promotes motor learning. Often, patients have difficulty in learning new motor tasks, but they respond well to activities they have performed thousands of times before. Selection of common, daily activities such as washing the face, brushing the teeth, and combing the hair is often successful because they are meaningful to the patient. During the performance of these types of tasks, the therapist or assistant may see active movement attempts by the patient. Hand-over-hand or therapeutic guiding techniques, in which the therapist guides the patient's own extremity or body movements, are effective. The patient receives proprioceptive and kinesthetic feedback as he or she performs a functional movement pattern (Davies, 1994). Intervention 6–4 shows examples of a family member assisting a patient with hand-over-hand techniques.

Vision is a valuable sensory modality that can be used during treatment. Activities that incorporate visual tracking or maintained visual contact with an object assist with the development of head control. For example, if the patient is in a sitting position and is unable to maintain the head in an erect position, the patient can be encouraged to maintain eye contact with the therapist or to look at a specific object. Vision can also be used to guide a patient's movement, as with rolling or turning the body.

Intervention 6–4 ▌ HAND-OVER-HAND GUIDING (FACE WASHING)

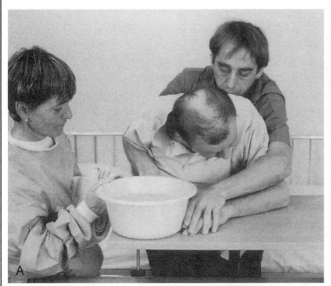
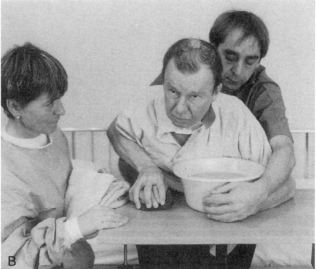
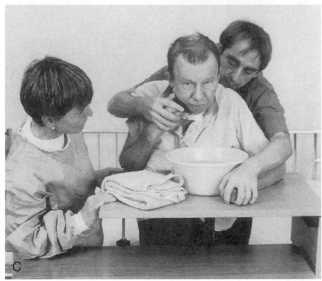

A. A task is presented as the patient's wife watches.

B. During hand-over-hand guiding, the patient lifts his head.

C. Active neck and trunk extension are achieved as he washes his face.

From Davies PM. Starting Again: Early Rehabilitation after Traumatic Brain Injury or Other Severe Brain Lesion. New York, Springer-Verlag, 1994.

Sitting Activities

Sitting is an important position to emphasize during treatment. Sitting can increase arousal and also provides a challenge to the patient's postural alignment and righting and equilibrium responses (VanSant, 1990b). Transferring the patient from supine to sitting can be accomplished in the same ways as discussed in Chapter 5. Intervention 6–5 shows a progression to sitting. Patients with a low functioning level may require assistance from two individuals, one who is responsible for the head and upper trunk and one who transfers the lower trunk and legs. Changes in the patient's level of awareness and muscle tone should be

noted during the change in position. Patients who exhibit strong extensor tone and posturing may become flexed and hypotonic once they are upright.

When the patient is sitting on the side of a mat table, the goal is for the patient to achieve a neutral pelvic position with an erect trunk and head. Frequently, it is necessary to use two individuals during sitting activities because of the abnormal tone in the patient's trunk. One person can assist the patient with trunk and head control from behind while the other therapist, facing the patient, works on the position of the patient's pelvis, the position of the upper and lower extremities, and general awareness. Supporting the upper extremities on a large ball in the patient's

Intervention 6-5 ▌ SUPINE-TO-SIT TRANSFER

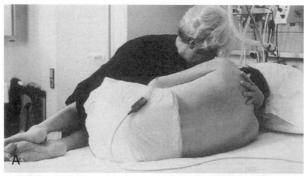

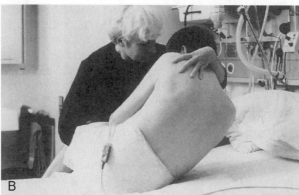

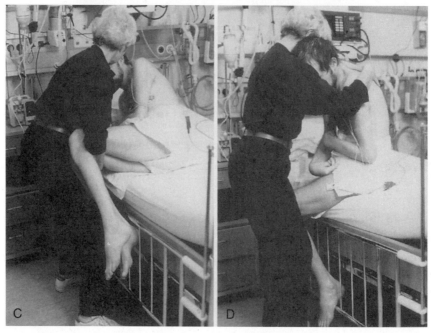

A. The therapist's arm around the patient's flexed knees, her other arm beneath his neck.

B. His legs are brought over the side of the bed.

C. Lifting his trunk toward the vertical.

D. Preventing his knees from sliding forward while supporting his head and trunk.

From Davies PM. Starting Again: Early Rehabilitation after Traumatic Brain Injury or Other Severe Brain Lesion. New York, Springer-Verlag, 1994.

lap can be beneficial for the patient with poor trunk control or hypotonia. The ball assists the therapist in maintaining trunk stabilization and may provide a sensation of support for the patient. Gentle anterior and posterior weight shifts can also be performed with the patient in this position. The weight shifts provide a mechanism to assess the patient's postural responses and also serve to increase awareness. Trunk flexion performed in the short-sitting position also maintains range of motion. Intervention 6–6 depicts this activity.

Other sitting activities can also be employed. Weight bearing on the upper extremities decreases ab-

Intervention 6–6 ▌ **TRUNK FLEXION IN SITTING**

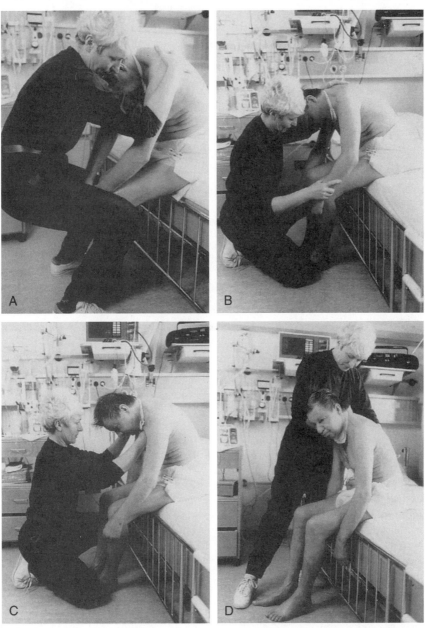

A. Bending the trunk forward with the therapist blocking the patient's knees.

B. Hands reaching toward the feet.

C. Assisting return to an upright position.

D. Assisting extension of the thoracic spine.

From Davies PM. Starting Again: Early Rehabilitation after Traumatic Brain Injury or Other Severe Brain Lesion. New York, Springer-Verlag, 1994.

normal muscle tone and also provides the patient with a greater sense of stability. As the patient progresses, reaching activities, throwing and catching tasks, and the performance of activities of daily living such as donning socks and shoes can be completed when the patient is in a sitting position. Intervention 6–7 shows examples of upper extremity activities performed with the patient in a sitting position.

Care must be taken not to overstimulate the patient with multiple sensory and verbal cues. Only one person should speak to the patient at a time. To maximize the patient's understanding of verbal information, the therapist facing the patient should be designated as the person to interact with him. This approach minimizes the chances that the patient will receive verbal information from multiple sources. In addition, instructions given should be concrete and stated in simple terms.

Transfers

The techniques used to transfer the patient with hemiplegia discussed in Chapter 5 can be used for the patient with TBI. A sit-pivot transfer is recommended for patients who have a low functioning level and who lack trunk control. Intervention 6–8 shows a therapist assisting a patient with a sit-pivot transfer. As the pa-

tient progresses, stand-pivot transfers can be attempted.

Standing Activities

Standing is another excellent position that can provide opportunities for functional tasks while it increases weight bearing and sensory input. If the patient has low functional capabilities, the tilt table may need to be used initially to provide necessary stabilization to maintain a standing posture. Patients can be transferred to a tilt table or a standing table and acclimated to an upright position. Activities aimed at increasing awareness and cognition can be performed while the patient is on the tilt table. Administering different sensory modalities through the use of the CNC or the Multisensory Assessment can be easily accomplished while the patient is on the tilt table. The upright posture may also serve to increase the patient's level of alertness. Performance of simple activities of daily living such as washing one's face or brushing one's teeth is also possible.

As the patient progresses, standing activities at the bedside or mat table can be instituted with appropriate assistance. Readers are advised to review Chapter 5 for specific techniques. Adequate head and trunk control is necessary for standing. Bedside tables, grocery

---

Intervention 6–7 ▌ SITTING ACTIVITIES

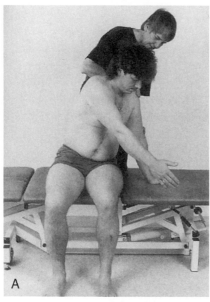 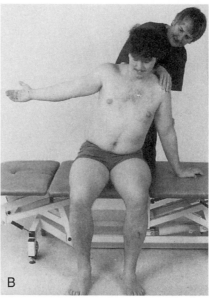

A. Rotating the trunk forward with the arm supported sideways.

B. Trunk rotated back with the contralateral arm abducted.

From Davies PM. Starting Again: Early Rehabilitation after Traumatic Brain Injury or Other Severe Brain Lesion. New York, Springer-Verlag, 1994.

Intervention 6–8 ▌ SIT-PIVOT TRANSFER

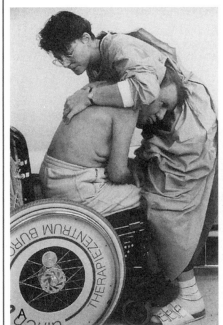
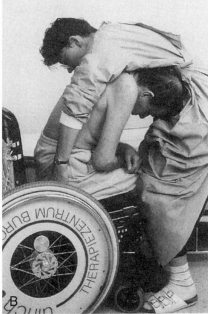
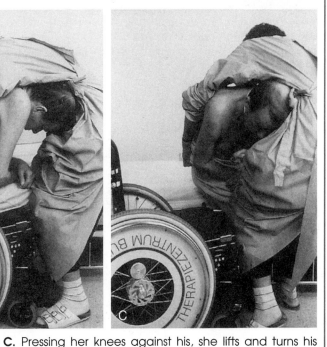

Transferring the patient with his trunk flexed forward.

A. The therapist flexes the patient's trunk and supports his head against her side.

B. She puts one hand under each trochanter.

C. Pressing her knees against his, she lifts and turns his buttocks onto the bed.

From Davies PM. Starting Again: Early Rehabilitation after Traumatic Brain Injury or Other Severe Brain Lesion. New York, Springer-Verlag, 1994.

carts, or high-low mat tables can be used for upper extremity support. As the patient progresses, stepping and gait training activities can be encouraged. Intervention 6–9 demonstrates standing of a patient who is unconscious. Intervention 6–10 demonstrates various examples of assisting the patient with standing.

The Physical Environment

When working with this population, one must consider several things that are different from patients with cerebrovascular accidents. The physical environment must be monitored. Patients who have sustained a TBI often have exaggerated responses to sensory stimuli in the environment. The lighting, noise level, and number of individuals present must be assessed. Think about the amount of activity that takes place in a physical therapy gym. Many people are present, and there is a great deal of auditory stimulation from people talking, background music, and public address systems. Frequently, patients with TBIs cannot filter out extraneous stimuli in the environment. Too much sensory stimuli can overstimulate the patient and can lead to confusion or an adverse behavioral response (Persel

and Persel, 1995). Patients may become more agitated, aggressive, or distracted in this type of environment. In addition, physical performance is often adversely affected when cognitive stress is increased (Wright and Veroff, 1988). Many facilities have smaller private treatment areas for these patients. Structure is also important to the patient with TBI. A daily schedule, a consistent rehabilitation team, and a similar treatment program assist the patient in adjusting to the situation and the rehabilitation environment. In addition, repetition and practice are needed for learning new information and tasks.

INTEGRATING PHYSICAL AND COGNITIVE COMPONENTS OF A TASK INTO TREATMENT INTERVENTIONS

Often, one of the most challenging aspects of treating patients with TBIs is integration of the physical and cognitive components of a task. The cognitive deficits frequently are the more debilitating and difficult to treat. Physical therapists and physical therapist assistants are adept with treatment that addresses the patient's physical limitations; however, they are usually

Intervention 6-9 ▌ STANDING THE UNCONSCIOUS PATIENT

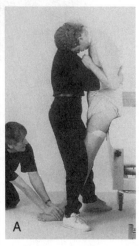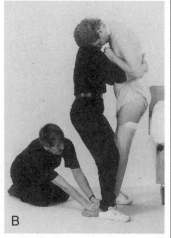

A. Starting position, feet held firmly to prevent forward sliding.

B. Therapist uses key points of control to support the patient.

From Davies P.M. Starting Again: Early Rehabilitation after Traumatic Brain Injury or Other Severe Brain Lesion. New York, Springer-Verlag, 1994.

far less comfortable dealing with cognitive impairments. The following is to be used as a guide in dealing with the various cognitive and behavioral impairments seen in these patients.

Cognitive and Behavioral Impairments

Disorientation

Patients with TBI are often disoriented to place or time. Frequently, you will see caregivers quizzing the patient who is disoriented in the hope that eventually the patient will get the right answers. A better approach to this impairment is to provide the patient with correct information during the treatment session. In essence, the therapist fills in the missing information for the patient. As stated previously, the use of a script or a calendar can be effective in dealing with disorientation. If the patient's orientation level does not improve, the goal will be for the patient to refer to his memory book, where he can obtain information independently. The contents of the memory book vary. Photographs of the patient, family members, and caregivers, therapy schedules, and pertinent information about the patient including name, age, and address may all be components of the memory book.

Intervention 6-10 ▌ SUPPORTING THE PATIENT IN STANDING

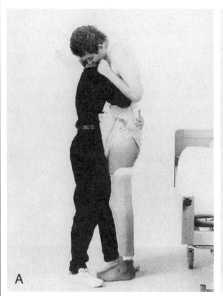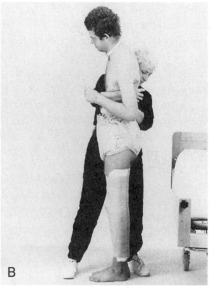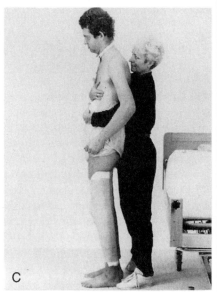

A. Weight is brought forward over his feet.

B. Therapist moves around behind him.

C. Therapist uses tactile cues on the pelvis and trunk to achieve extension.

From Davies P.M. Starting Again: Early Rehabilitation after Traumatic Brain Injury or Other Severe Brain Lesion. New York, Springer-Verlag, 1994.

Attention Deficits

Attention deficits are also a frequent finding in this population. Patients may have difficulty in maintaining attention to a task even for periods as short as 10 to 15 seconds. This deficit becomes a significant challenge during treatment. Early in the recovery process, the therapist will need to keep verbal instructions simple and may wish to have a number of different treatment activities planned and prepared. Treatment will be implemented more efficiently, and the patient may be successfully redirected to an original activity at a later time if the therapist is well prepared. As the patient progresses, the therapist can use a stopwatch or timer to encourage the patient to continue to focus during specific activity performance. For example, the patient can ride a stationary bike for a predetermined amount of time and the therapist can try to increase the time each session. This approach can be used as a means to monitor the patient's progress.

Memory Deficits

Almost all patients who have sustained a TBI have some degree of memory impairments following their injury. As we have already discussed, the use of a day planner or memory book may be recommended. Computerized schedule books, watches, and pillboxes are available. These devices sound alarms to remind patients of important times and events. If the patient has residual memory problems, he must be instructed in the use of compensatory strategies to assist with functioning in the community.

Problem-Solving Deficits

Problem-solving deficits may also be apparent. Patients may have difficulties with abstract thinking. Safety issues are a concern. Patients may not understand the significance of a hot stove or a stranger at the front door. Creation of situations that require attention to safety within the safe confines of the rehabilitation unit can assist the patient in the transition to home. In addition, these types of problem-solving activities help to identify whether constant supervision will be necessary on discharge.

Difficulties with topographic orientation may be apparent in some individuals with TBIs. Patients with these types of deficits are unable to negotiate or find their way around the facility. Route-finding tasks can be employed. Patients are encouraged to use markers or cues such as signs and pictures for guidance as they move through the facility. As the patient progresses, obstacle courses and mazes can be constructed to challenge the patient's problem-solving abilities (Krus, 1988).

Behavioral Deficits

Patients who have sustained a TBI may also exhibit behavioral problems. Some of the more common behavioral impairments include agitation and irritability, decreased control of emotional responses, denial of deficits, impulsiveness, and a lack of inhibition (Krus, 1988). Considering the physiologic cause of these behavioral problems may allow therapists to treat these patients more effectively. Agitation and irritability may be caused or heightened by the patient's level of disorientation. If you can imagine for a moment what it would be like to have little or no memory, not to recognize family and friends, and perhaps to have some significant physical limitations, you may be better able to see why someone with a TBI may be agitated and irritable. Following a consistent schedule, having structure in the environment, and keeping the patient occupied can assist in managing the patient's disorientation. Limited use of television is also recommended. Patients can become easily confused by the events they see within the context of a television program and may have difficulty in distinguishing the television programming from reality.

For patients who are overreacting or exhibiting poor emotional control, the therapist or assistant may elect to ignore the behavior or reinforce positive behaviors. Having the therapist provide appropriate positive alternatives is also advisable because patients often are unable to select appropriate responses on their own. Sometimes offering the patient a choice between two activities assists in redirecting inappropriate responses and allows the patient some control over the situation.

The use of group treatment activities may be of benefit for remediation of some of these behavioral and cognitive issues. Peer support, appropriate modeling of behaviors by others, and pressure to conform can assist patients in the recognition of their deficits.

Aggressive Behaviors

An area of concern for some therapists and assistants working with this patient population is the aggressive and combative behavior that can sometimes be exhibited. Because of this possibility, many rehabilitation facilities require staff members to attend certified programs in crisis intervention. The Rancho Los Amigos Scale of Cognitive Functioning discusses possible patient responses at the confused-agitated level. Although aggressive and combative behaviors can occur, they are not the norm. Our goal is to assist the patient in the development of self-controlling behaviors. Assisting the patient in his ability to deal with stressful and anxiety-producing situations is the first step in managing behavior.

Patients with TBI often have difficulty in dealing with both internal and external environmental stressors. Behavioral changes including physical aggression can occur as patients become afraid or feel threatened. If a patient is unable to manage stress and frustration successfully, a crisis situation can develop. During a crisis, the sympathetic nervous system responds, and certain physical and cognitive changes occur. Heart rate, blood pressure, and respiration rates increase, whereas cognitive skills become depressed. Communication skills, reasoning, and judgment become impaired. Thus, it is important for the physical therapist and physical therapist assistant to recognize how to assist the patient in dealing with stressors and to prevent a crisis from occurring. Several different models of crisis and behavior management have been developed. Many facilities provide crisis training programs for staff involved in the care of patients with TBIs. Individuals who work with this population should attend one of these courses.

Initially, if a patient becomes anxious and overstimulated, it is a good idea to be supportive and attempt to remove the stimulus. Sometimes it is not possible for the physical therapist or assistant to identify the triggering event or source of irritation to the patient. As the patient becomes anxious or distressed, the therapist may notice changes in the patient's tone of voice or other physical changes including pacing, tapping of the feet, or wringing of the hands. If such changes occur, it is advisable to remove the patient from the area, continue to offer emotional support, and redirect the patient to another task. Reorientation may assist in calming the patient because disorientation is an underlying factor in severe behavior disturbances. (Persel and Persel, 1995).

If these techniques do not help the patient to relax, the situation can escalate to a full crisis. During a crisis, a patient can lose control over verbal and physical responses and may exhibit destructive and assaultive behaviors. The patient can be dangerous to himself or to others. Often, when this situation occurs, the health care provider becomes extremely anxious as well. If the physical therapist and physical therapist assistant do not remain calm, they, too, can escalate to a sympathetic state. If you become involved in such an incident and notice yourself becoming excessively stressed, remove yourself from the situation. Once the patient is in a crisis, your role should be to protect the patient from harming himself or others. The episode will need to run its course. As the patient recovers from the situation, the clinician will again need to provide emotional support. Trying to reestablish a rapport with the patient is advisable. The patient will eventually return to his baseline behavioral state. Once the patient has moved through all the stages of crisis, the patient and the health care provider who intervened will develop postcrisis drain or depression. This can last for several hours after the initial episode and manifests itself as exhaustion and withdrawal. It is best to allow the patient to rest following this experience.

Once the patient has returned to a resting state, the clinician will want to reflect with the patient about the incident and what happened. Questioning the patient about the event, object, or individual who triggered the episode is valuable. If the rehabilitation team is able to identify the stressful object or trigger, methods to minimize the patient's response can be developed (Persel and Persel, 1995).

All members of the rehabilitation team should remember that patients who exhibit agitation or aggressive behaviors are demonstrating the need for structure and control over their environments. A health care provider has no reason to take the event personally. Internalizing the event can affect the patient-therapist relationship and may ultimately affect the care the patient receives.

Motor Deficits and Interventions

Much time has been spent discussing the cognitive aspects of treatment for the patient with TBI. Many of the treatments previously discussed for patients following a cerebrovascular accident are appropriate for this patient population as well. The movement transitions presented, as well as the techniques used to facilitate functional movements, can be used. The reader is advised to review the information discussed in Chapter 8 for a thorough discussion of these concepts.

Students and practicing clinicians alike often report that the most challenging patients are those who have good motor skills but significant cognitive deficits. A review of treatment activities for patients who are functioning at a high physical level is now provided. High-level balance activities are challenging for these patients. Patients must maintain postural stability while performing selective movement patterns and attending to a cognitive task. Movable surfaces such as balls, bolsters, or tilt boards can be used. Exercises that can be performed on the ball include the following:

1. Maintaining balance
2. Raising arms overhead
3. Performing proprioceptive neuromuscular facilitation diagonals
4. Rotating or laterally bending the trunk
5. Reciprocally moving the arms
6. Performing anterior and posterior pelvic tilts
7. Marching or knee extension exercises
8. Bouncing in a circle
9. Practicing more difficult exercises, including moving from sitting to supine and from sitting to prone

Bolsters are used for static positioning or to provide the patient with a movable surface. Patients can straddle the bolster and can practice weight shifting and coming to stand. Tilt boards can be used to practice weight shifting and equilibrium responses. Patients can either sit or stand on the tilt board, depending on their motor abilities. Other activities that challenge the patient's static and dynamic balance include one-foot standing, heel-toe walking, walking on a balance beam, braiding (walking sideways, crossing one foot over the other), jumping, and skipping.

The sensory components of an activity can also be modified to make the activity more challenging for the patient. Lighting can be changed, and patients can be asked to work on foam or floor mats to change the proprioceptive input received through the feet. Patients can also progress from working in a quiet environment to working in one that is noisier and busier.

Incorporating Physical and Cognitive Components of a Task

The physical therapist may design a treatment program that is rich in physical and cognitive activities. Throwing and catching, maneuvering through an obstacle course, and following a map allow for the performance of high-level motor and cognitive tasks. Balance activities previously mentioned can also be performed, and an additional cognitive component such as counting the repetitions can be incorporated. Some facilities have access to simulated city environments (Easy Street). A grocery store, bank, fast-food counter, and environmental barriers one would encounter in the community are represented and available for patient practice. Community outings are another therapeutic way to work on physical and cognitive tasks. Many facilities arrange outings for patients at various stages in their rehabilitation. Trips to a restaurant, the zoo, or a bowling alley are common examples of community trips. On these trips, patients are allowed to practice the skills they have been working on in therapy. The benefit of these outings is that therapists are there to assist the patients and can assess areas in which the patients may have difficulty once they are discharged to home.

Cardiovascular and aerobic conditioning activities are good exercises for patients with good motor abilities to perform. Walking on a treadmill, cycling, swimming, and performing an aerobics program are all useful activities to improve cardiovascular responses and to challenge the patient's coordination. As stated previously, many patients who have sustained a TBI are deconditioned, and aerobic exercise is a good way to improve the patient's level of cardiovascular fitness. Exercise can also be used for stress management.

DISCHARGE PLANNING

Discharge planning is an important component of treatment for the patient with TBI. Decisions must be made about the most appropriate discharge destination. It would be nice to assume that all patients will make a full recovery and resume all previous aspects of their lives. We know, however, that this is not the case. Many patients require follow-up care ranging from supervision in the home to placement in an extended care facility. Planning for the patient's discharge should include the patient, the family, and appropriate members of the rehabilitation team. Adaptive equipment, any environmental modifications needed at the patient's home, and necessary home health care services should be arranged prior to the patient's discharge from the facility. Some patients may require additional outpatient services following their discharge from rehabilitation. Outpatient physical therapy may continue to be needed to improve the patient's physical limitations. Other patients may have met their physical therapy goals but need continued intervention to meet their goals for reentry into the community. Programs specifically aimed at assisting patients with this transition back to the community are available. Community reentry programs help patients make the transition back to home, the educational environment, or the workplace by allowing them to practice everyday skills in a group setting. These programs are often staffed by a neuropsychologist, a speech-language pathologist, and an occupational therapist. Examples of tasks that may be practiced include balancing a checkbook, locating resources within the telephone directory, and planning and organizing an event. On a more conceptual basis, activities that stress problem solving, planning, sequencing, and interacting with others are practiced. For individuals with residual deficits, appropriate compensatory strategies are taught. This type of programming is extremely beneficial for patients who continue to have deficits after inpatient rehabilitation but who have the potential for a higher level of motor and cognitive functioning.

CHAPTER SUMMARY

Working with the patient with TBI can be extremely challenging and rewarding. These patients often present in a multitude of ways that vary from coma and no voluntary movement to high motor function with significant cognitive deficits. For many physical therapists and physical therapist assistants, the cognitive component of treatment is most difficult. To provide our patients with the highest quality care possible, we must be able to address motor and cognitive issues together. Creation of interventions that integrate physical and cognitive tasks will provide our patients with the care they need to improve their functional abilities and, one hopes, resume their previous lifestyles.

REVIEW QUESTIONS

1. Describe the clinical manifestations of a subdural hematoma.
2. What are some signs and symptoms of increased ICP?
3. Differentiate between a patient in a coma and a patient in a persistent vegetative state.
4. List four goals of acute physical therapy intervention for the patient with a TBI.
5. Define the eight stages within the Rancho Los Amigos Scale of Cognitive Functioning.
6. Discuss the benefits of hand-over-hand modeling for patients with decreased cognitive functioning.
7. How may the physical environment affect the patient's response to intervention?
8. A patient is exhibiting significant disorientation and attention deficits. How could the physical therapist assistant intervene to assist the patient in therapy?
9. A patient becomes easily agitated and frustrated during therapy. At times, he can escalate into a full crisis. What can the physical therapist assistant do to minimize these episodes? What should the physical therapist assistant do if a crisis should occur?
10. A patient who has had a TBI possesses good motor skills. He is able to walk independently without an assistive device and is able to transfer independently. The patient does exhibit occasional losses of balance. The patient's cognitive abilities are more seriously impaired. He is disoriented and has memory deficits. Identify four treatment activities for this patient that incorporate physical and cognitive components.

REHABILITATION UNIT INITIAL EVALUATION: RICK

Patient: Rick is a 25-year-old divorced male from Indiana. Rick works full-time as a construction worker.

Chart Review: Motor vehicle accident on 3/30/99. At time of admission, Rick presented with ecchymosis about the left ear and lacerations on the scalp. Pupils were small and nonreactive; patient showed increased tone in all extremities, with decerebrate posturing, hyperreflexia, and Babinski present bilaterally. Rick was in a comatose condition with heart rate of 160 to 170, blood pressure, 140/80, and respiration rate, 40. Radiographs of cervical spine were normal, and a CT scan showed no intracranial lesions or midline shift.

Impression: Cerebral brain stem contusion, severe; depressed fracture left midparietal bone with no significant intracranial abnormality noted. A tracheostomy was performed, and Rick was placed on a volume ventilator. Rick was weaned from the ventilator. Seizures are now under control.

Medications: Phenytoin (Dilantin) and diazepam (Valium).

Previous Medical History: Noncontributory.

▌ SUBJECTIVE

Social history could not be obtained because of the condition of the patient and because no family members were present at the initial evaluation; chart review was referred to for information.

▌ OBJECTIVE

Appearance/Equipment: Rick is supine in bed: midline head position; decerebrate posturing with wrist and fingers flexed, ankles plantar flexed, shoulders internally rotated and adducted, lower extremities adducted and extended; tracheostomy plugged; catheter and intravenous line in place.

Vital Signs: Blood pressure, 130/80; heart rate, 85 to 90; respiration rate, 30.

Autonomic Responses: Pupillary response to light is within normal limits bilaterally. No diaphoresis is noted.

Oromotor Function: Rick is able to swallow with facilitated downward stroking to the anterior neck muscles. Rick is producing incomprehensible sounds.

Sensory Awareness: Rick spontaneously opens his eyes in response to light; he presents with an extensor response of all extremities. Rick is able to respond and localize stimuli and follow simple one-step commands inconsistently. He orients toward sound consistently, opens his mouth in response to command inconsistently once in three

REHABILITATION UNIT INITIAL EVALUATION: RICK *Continued*

times, displays partial fixation to light flashes twice in five times; partially fixes on and tracks the physical therapist's face twice in five times, slowly/partially withdraws from a lemon smell with grimacing once in three times, orients his head toward a tap on the shoulder twice in three times, withdraws from pressure across the nail bed twice in three times, and uses nonverbal vocalizations (moans, groaning).

AROM: Right: hip flexion, 0 to 15 degrees; knee flexion, 0 to 10 degrees; ankle lacks 10 degrees from neutral; wrist extension 0 to 5 degrees; all other joints are unable to initiate volitional movement. Left: hip flexion, 0 to 18 degrees; knee flexion, 0 to 10 degrees, ankle lacks 9 degrees from neutral; wrist extension, 0 to 4 degrees; all other joints are unable to initiate volitional movement. Volitional cervical movements of rotation bilaterally were within functional limits.

PROM: Right: hip flexion, 0 to 90 degrees; hip abduction, 0 to 10 degrees, knee flexion, 0 to 89 degrees; ankle, neutral position achieved; elbow extension/flexion, 0 to 110 degrees; all other upper extremity and lower extremity movements are within functional limits. Left: hip flexion, 0 to 95 degrees; hip abduction, 0 to 15 degrees; knee flexion, 0 to 90 degrees; ankle, neutral position achieved; elbow extension/flexion, 0 to 120 degrees; all other upper extremity and lower extremity movements are within functional limits. Cervical passive range of motion is within functional limits. Lack of passive range of motion is due to increased tone and spasticity, particularly in the gastrocnemius, hip adductors, and biceps bilaterally.

Reflexes: Patellar, 4+ bilaterally; Achilles, 4+ bilaterally; biceps, 2+; Babinski reflex was present bilaterally.

Primitive Reflexes: Positive support is present bilaterally with weight bearing in hooklying, palmar and plantar grasp present three out of five times bilaterally. An asymmetric tonic neck reflex is present and consistent on the right; a symmetric tonic neck reflex is present with extension and flexion of the head/neck; a supine tonic labyrinthine reflex is present.

Balance Reactions: No head or trunk righting is noted; protective reactions are not assessed.

Functional Mobility: Rick rolls to the right and left sides nonsegmentally with maximum assistance of one. Rick transfers from supine to sitting and from sitting to standing with maximum assistance of two; he becomes rigid when brought to sit but sits independently with double upper extremity support and maximum assistance of one for head control. No changes in vital signs are noted during movement transitions.

Family Education: The family was not present.

Treatment: Assisted rolling to both sides three times each; trunk elongation performed bilaterally while the patient was in side lying to decrease the rigid trunk and to help promote rotation and trunk/pelvis dissociation: rhythmic rotation to upper extremities and lower extremities to allow for positioning out of the decerebrate posture and into a hooklying position; assisted bridging with facilitation to gluteals bilaterally three times; bottoms-up position with rotation of the trunk and placement of the patient's hands on his face for sensory awareness; from bottoms-up position transitioned to side lying and sitting; weight shifts bilaterally (three times to each side) in sitting using double arm support with forearms on a tabletop to promote weight bearing and sensation; hand-over-hand techniques to promote self-care activities (i.e., brushing teeth and washing face with a cloth); sit-to-stand transfer with maximum assistance of two with weight-shifting exercises for 1.5 minutes.

Reaction to Treatment: No significant changes in vital signs were noted; the patient resumed a rigid decerebrate posture when he was initially placed in sitting, but he was able to relax after rhythmic rotation to the pelvis and shoulder girdles; no other tonal changes were noticed during the rest of the transitions and exercises.

ASSESSMENT

Test Scores

Glasgow Coma Scale: eye opening, 4; motor response, 2; verbal response, 2; 8 total.

Rappaport: 1.25 (near coma) with eight areas assessed.

Continued on following page

REHABILITATION UNIT INITIAL EVALUATION: RICK *Continued*

Assessment *Continued*

***Rancho Los Amigos* (RLA):** Level III (localized response).

Rehabilitation Potential: Rehabilitation potential is fair because of early physical therapy intervention, young age, previous high level of activity, and scores on Glasgow Coma Scale, Rappaport Coma Scale, and Rancho Los Amigos level.

Problem List
1. Dependent in functional mobility skills.
2. Lack of head control in sitting.
3. Decreased active and passive range of motion of upper extremities and lower extremities bilaterally.
4. Decreased level of awareness and response to stimuli.
5. Decreased ability to communicate and focus attention consistently.
6. Lack of patient and family/caregiver education.

Short-Term Goals (2 weeks)
1. Rick will display head control in midline for 10 minutes during weight shifting in sitting with double arm support.
2. Rick will respond consistently to simple commands three out of five times.
3. Rick will transfer from supine to sitting and from sitting to standing with moderate assistance of one.
4. Rick will roll to bilateral sides in bed with standby assistance of one and will display trunk and pelvis dissociation.
5. Rick will demonstrate bilateral volitional movement during self-care activities with moderate verbal cues while sitting independently with one-hand support.
6. Rick will be consistent with communication 75% of the time during therapy sessions with actions such as head nods, eye blinks, and/or hand squeezes.
7. Rick will focus attention during isolated therapy sessions with no external distractions for at least 5 consistent minutes when performing assisted self-care activities.
8. Rick will ambulate with a standard walker on level surfaces with moderate assistance of one to go from his hospital room to the physical therapy gym (approximately 75 to 100 feet).

Long-Term Goals (2 months)
1. Rick will remain focused for 8 to 10 minutes while he practices various vocational activities with environmental distractions.
2. Caregiver will demonstrate an ability to assist the patient with functional mobility skills and activities of daily living.
3. Rick will be independent with bed mobility and transfers for functional return to home setting.
4. Rick will identify safety concerns in the home.
5. Rick will communicate consistently 100% of the time during the treatment session.
6. Rick will be a household ambulator with a straight cane and supervision and will negotiate environmental barriers (e.g., carpet, steps).
7. Rick will be independent in an exercise program.

PLAN

Rick will be seen twice a day for 45-minute treatment sessions. Treatment will include the following:

Positioning: To decrease or eliminate decerebrate rigidity and to prevent contractures, place Rick's upper extremities flexed with arms overhead and hands flat on the mat to facilitate weight bearing through the wrists, and place the lower extremities slightly flexed and abducted with a pillow under the knees in supine. Also position in prone lying on a bolster (longways) under the trunk for upper and lower trunk dissociation. To prevent the influence of asymmetric tonic neck reflex, symmetric tonic reflex, and tonic labyrinthine reflex, place Rick in side lying (to both sides) with the uppermost extremities slightly flexed for dissociation.

Cognitive Retraining: Assist Rick in developing a personalized journal consisting of family pictures, past experiences, and a structured daily schedule of therapy sessions, meals, and sleep.

Establishing a Communication System: Physical actions such as eye blinks and head nods will be used to convey needs and wants.

Functional Activities: These include bed mobility, supine-to-sit and sit-to-stand transfers, weight shifts in standing and sitting to facilitate righting, equilibrium, and protective reactions, and gait activities with a standard walker, progressing to a straight cane.

REHABILITATION UNIT INITIAL EVALUATION: RICK *Continued*

Therapeutic Exercise: This includes assisted proprioceptive neuromuscular facilitation patterns of upper extremities and lower extremities and hand-over-hand techniques for self-care activities to promote strengthening, sensory awareness, and volitional movements. Repetition with all activities will be important to reestablish memory, motor learning, and cardiovascular endurance of the patient.

Discharge Planning: Consult with a speech pathologist and occupational therapist for possible team therapy sessions and discharge planning. Rick will be reevaluated on a weekly basis. Prior to discharge to the home setting, educate the family/caregiver about providing assistance to Rick in activities of daily living and functional mobility skills. At the time of discharge from the rehabilitation unit, Rick will continue with outpatient therapy and will begin vocational training to allow for a gradual return to work environment.

QUESTIONS TO THINK ABOUT

* How will the assistant facilitate the performance of functional activities?
* What other therapeutic interventions could the assistant use to help the patient with motor learning?

* Identify considerations for the patient's discharge to home.

REFERENCES

Bobath B, Bobath K. The neuro-developmental treatment. In Scrutton D (ed). Management of the Motor Disorders in Children with Cerebral Palsy. Clinics in Developmental Medicine. Philadelphia, JB Lippincott, 1984, pp 6–16.

Bontke CF, Boake C. Principles of brain injury rehabilitation. In Braddom RL (ed). Physical Medicine and Rehabilitation. Philadelphia, WB Saunders, 1996, pp 1027–1051.

Bontke CF, Baize CM, Boake C. Coma management and sensory stimulation. Phys Med Rehabil Clin North Am 3:259–272, 1992.

Booth BJ, Doyle M, Montgomery J. Serial casting for the management of spasticity in the head-injured adult. Phys Ther 63:1960–1966, 1983.

Davies PM. Starting Again: Early Rehabilitation after Traumatic Brain Injury or Other Severe Brain Lesion. New York, Springer-Verlag, 1994, pp 23–44, 65–68, 86–88, 316–352, 361–364.

Fitzgerald MJT. Neuroanatomy Basic and Clinical. London, Bailliere Tindall, 1992, p 241.

Gelber DA. The neurologic examination of the traumatically brain-injured patient. In Ashley MJ, Krych DK (eds). Traumatic Brain Injury Rehabilitation. Boca Raton, FL, CRC Press, 1995, pp 23–41.

Gould BE. Pathophysiology for the Health-Related Professions. Philadelphia, WB Saunders, 1997, pp 320–376.

Jennett B, Teasdale G. Management of Head Injuries. Philadelphia, FA Davis, 1981, pp 122–131.

Krus LH. Cognitive and behavioral skills retraining of the brain-injured patient. Clin Manage 8:24–31, 1988.

Leahy P. Traumatic head injury. In O'Sullivan SB, Schmitz TJ (eds). Physical Rehabilitation Assessment and Treatment, 3rd ed. Philadelphia, FA Davis, 1994, pp 491–508.

Lehmkuhl LD, Krawczyk L. Physical therapy management of the minimally-responsive patient following traumatic brain injury: coma stimulation. Neurol Rep 17:10–17, 1993.

Naritoku DK, Hernandez TD. Posttraumatic epilepsy and neurorehabilitation. In Ashley MJ, Krych DK (eds). Traumatic Brain Injury Rehabilitation. Boca Raton, FL, CRC Press, 1995, pp 43–65.

O'Sullivan SB. Strategies to improve motor control and motor learning. In O'Sullivan SB, Schmitz TJ (eds). Physical Rehabilitation Assessment and Treatment, 3rd ed. Philadelphia, FA Davis, 1994, pp 230.

Persel CS, Persel CH. The use of applied behavior analysis in traumatic brain injury rehabilitation. In Ashley MJ, Krych DK (eds). Traumatic Brain Injury Rehabilitation. Boca Raton, FL, CRC Press, 1995, pp 231–273.

Rappaport M, Dougherty AM, Kelting DL. Evaluation of coma and vegetative states. Arch Phys Med Rehabil 73:628–634, 1992.

VanSant AF. Traumatic Head Injury: An Overview of Physical Therapy Care. I. Topics in Neurology. Alexandria, VA, American Physical Therapy Association, 1990a, pp 1–10.

VanSant AF. Traumatic Head Injury: An Overview of Physical Therapy Care. II. Topics in Neurology. Alexandria, VA, American Physical Therapy Association, 1990b, pp 1–7.

Varghese G. Heterotopic ossification. Phys Med Rehabil Clin North Am 3:407–415, 1992.

Winkler PA. Head injury. In Umphred DA (ed). Neurological Rehabilitation, 3rd ed. St. Louis, CV Mosby, 1995, pp 421–453.

Wright KL, Veroff AE. Integration of cognitive and physical hierarchies in head injury rehabilitation. Clin Manage 8:6–9, 1988.

CHAPTER 7

Spinal Cord Injuries

OBJECTIVES

After reading this chapter, the student will be able to

1. Understand the causes, clinical manifestations, and possible complications of spinal cord injury.

2. Differentiate between complete and incomplete types of spinal cord injuries.

3. Understand the various levels of spinal cord injury.

4. Relate segmental level of muscle innervation to level of function in the patient with a spinal cord injury.

5. Teach pulmonary exercises, strengthening exercises, and mat activities to a patient with a spinal cord injury.

6. Teach gait training and wheelchair mobility techniques to the patient, as appropriate.

INTRODUCTION

An estimated 10,000 new cases of spinal cord injury (SCI) occur annually. Within the United States, currently more than 200,000 persons are living with SCIs (National Spinal Cord Injury Statistical Center, 1998; Williams, 1996). SCIs are most likely to occur in young adults between the ages of 16 and 30 years. However, adults 61 years or older comprise approximately 10% of the population with SCIs. Approximately 82% of the individuals with SCIs are male (National Spinal Cord Injury Statistical Center, 1998; Williams, 1996). The etiology of SCIs has changed over the years. Previously, injuries due to motor vehicle accidents and sporting activities were identified as the most likely causes. More recent statistics suggest that motor vehicle accidents (36.6%), followed by acts of violence (27.9%), falls (21.4%), and sports-related injuries (6.5%), are now the most common causes of SCIs in the United States (National Spinal Cord Injury Statistical Center, 1998).

Life expectancies for individuals with SCIs continue to increase but are still somewhat lower than normal. Individuals with SCIs can experience a lifetime of disability and life-threatening medical complications. Po-

tential causes of death that significantly affect life expectancy include pneumonia, pulmonary emboli, and septicemia. The cost of medical care for these individuals is in the billions of dollars. Lifetime medical expenses for persons with high cervical injuries is estimated at $1.3 million, and the estimate is $427,000 for individuals with paraplegia. These figures can exceed the $1 million maximum insurance benefit allowed by many insurance policies. In addition to the direct costs of medical care, there are indirect costs associated with lost wages, employee benefits, and productivity, costs that can average $38,000 a year (National Spinal Cord Injury Statistical Center, 1998).

ETIOLOGY

To understand the etiology of SCIs, it is necessary to review the anatomy of the region. Within the peripheral nervous system are 31 pairs of spinal nerves. The first 7 pairs of spinal nerves, which originate in the cervical area, exit above the first 7 cervical vertebrae. Spinal nerve C8 exits between C7 and T1 because there is no eighth cervical vertebra. The remaining spinal nerve roots exit below the corresponding bony vertebrae. This holds true through T12. At this point, the spinal cord becomes a mass of nerve roots known as the cauda equina. Figure 7–1 illustrates segmental and vertebral levels.

Certain areas of the spinal column are more susceptible to injury than others. In the cervical spine, the spinal segments of C1, C2, and C5 through C7 are often injured, and in the thoracolumbar area, T12 through L2 are most often affected. The biomechanics of the vertebral column predisposes to this situation. Movement (rotation) is greatest at these segments and leads to instability within the regions. In addition, the spinal cord is larger in these areas because of the large number of nerve cell bodies that are located here. Figure 7–2 illustrates this configuration.

NAMING THE LEVEL OF INJURY

To name the level of an individual's injury, the health care professional first identifies the vertebral or bony spine segment involved. For example, cervical injuries are designated with a C, thoracic injuries with a T, and lumbar injuries with an L. This designation is followed by the last spinal nerve root segment in which innervation is present. Therefore, if a patient has an injury in the cervical region and has innervation of the biceps, the lesion would be classified as a C5 injury. Medical personnel have used the following terms to describe the extent of involvement a patient

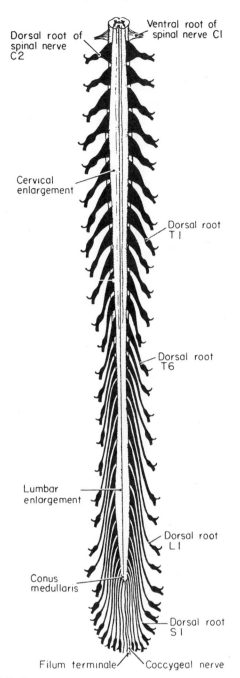

FIGURE 7–2 ■ Posterior view of the spinal cord showing the attached dorsal roots and spinal ganglia. (Modified from Fredericks CM, Saladin CK [eds]. Pathophysiology of the Motor Systems Principles and Clinical Presentations. Philadelphia, FA Davis, 1996.)

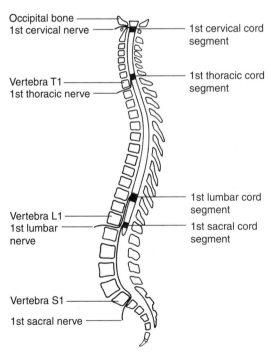

FIGURE 7–1 ■ Segmental and vertebral levels compared. Spinal nerves 1 to 7 emerge above the corresponding vertebrae, and the remaining spinal nerves emerge below them. (From Fitzgerald MJT. Neuroanatomy Basic and Clinical, 3rd ed. London, Bailliere Tindall, 1992.)

may be experiencing. Individuals with injuries to the cervical region of the spine have been classified as having *quadriplegia.* Injuries involving the thoracic spine can produce *paraplegia,* and injuries at L1 or below are called *cauda equina injuries.* The American Spinal Cord Injury Association (ASIA) has adopted the term *tetraplegia,* instead of quadriplegia, to refer to injuries involving the cervical spine.

The ASIA has developed standards to assist health care providers in naming the level of the injury. The *neurologic level* is defined as the caudalmost segment with intact sensory and motor function, as determined by neurologic testing of key *dermatomes* (sensory areas) and *myotomes* (muscles). *Intact muscle function* is further defined as the lowest key muscle with a manual muscle testing grade of fair, provided that the key muscles above this level have at least good or normal strength. The ASIA has defined key muscles as those that provide the patient with the greatest functional improvements because of their innervation (Finkbeiner and Russo, 1990). For example, the triceps comprise a key muscle group. Patients with triceps innervation have the potential to transfer independently without a sliding board because of their ability to extend the elbow and perform a lateral pushup.

The ASIA standards also recognize that muscles are innervated by more than one spinal cord segment. An individual may have poor or trace motor or sensory function in up to three segments below the injury site. This area of innervation is called the *zone of preservation*. If a patient has sparing below the zone of preservation and motor or sensory function in the sacral segments of S4 and S5, then the injury is classified as *incomplete* (Finkbeiner and Russo, 1990).

MECHANISMS OF INJURY

Traumatic impact is a common cause of SCI. Trauma can be precipitated by compression, penetrating injury, and hyperextension or hyperflexion forces. The resultant injury to the spinal cord can be temporary or permanent. Associated injuries to the vertebral bodies may also lead to spinal cord damage. Vertebral subluxation (separation of the vertebral bodies), compression fractures, and fracture-dislocations can further damage the spinal cord by encroachment or addi-

tional compression of the spinal cord. Severe injuries to the vertebral column can also result in partial or complete transection of the spinal cord.

Cervical Flexion and Rotation Injuries

In the cervical region, the most common type of injury is one that involves flexion and rotation. With this type of force, the posterior spinal ligaments rupture, and the uppermost vertebra is displaced over the one below it. Rupture of the intervertebral disc and, in severe cases, the anterior longitudinal ligament can also occur. Transection of the spinal cord is often associated with this type of injury. Rear-end motor vehicle accidents frequently produce flexion and rotation injuries. Figure 7–3*A* provides an example of a flexion and rotation mechanism of injury.

Cervical Hyperflexion Injuries

A pure hyperflexion force causes an anterior compression fracture of the vertebral body with stretching of the posterior longitudinal ligaments. The ligaments remain intact, however. The force sustained by the bony structures leads to a wedge-type fracture of the vertebral bodies. This type of injury frequently severs the anterior spinal artery and results in an incomplete anterior cord syndrome. A head-on collision or a blow to the back of the head is a cause of this type of injury. Figure 7–3*B* depicts an example.

Cervical Hyperextension Injuries

Hyperextension injuries are common in the elderly as a result of a fall. The individual's chin often strikes a stationary object, and this leads to neck hyperexten-

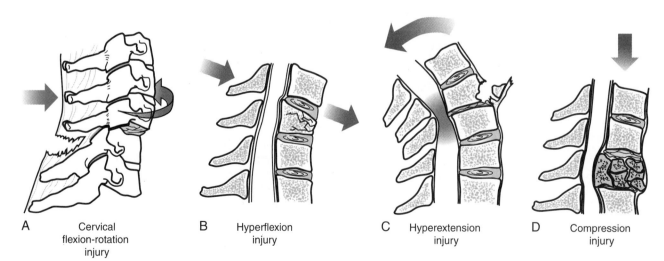

| A | Cervical flexion-rotation injury | B | Hyperflexion injury | C | Hyperextension injury | D | Compression injury |

FIGURE 7–3 ▪ *A* to *D*, Types of spinal cord injuries.

sion. The force ruptures the anterior longitudinal ligament and compresses and ruptures the intervertebral disc. The spinal cord can become compressed between the ligamentum flavum and the vertebral body, with a resulting central cord type of injury. Figure 7–3*C* shows an example.

Compression Injuries

Vertical compressive forces can also injure the cervical or lumbar spine. Diving accidents cause injuries that are a combination of compression and flexion forces. Falls from elevated surfaces can also produce this type of injury. With vertical compression, one sees fracture of the vertebral end plates and movement of the nucleus pulposus into the vertebral body. Bone fragments can be produced and displaced outward. The longitudinal ligaments are stretched but remain intact (Fig. 7–3*D*).

Compression injuries caused by the effects of osteoporosis, osteoarthritis, or rheumatoid arthritis can also produce SCIs in the elderly. A discussion of the pathologic processes that lead to these conditions is beyond the scope of this text.

MEDICAL INTERVENTION

Following an acute SCI, the patient should be immobilized and transferred to a trauma center. Recent advances in the acute medical management include the administration of either methylprednisolone or monosialotetranexxosylyganglioside (GM-1) ganglioside. Methylprednisolone administered within the first 8 hours can limit the extent of initial injury and can decrease the effects of post-traumatic ischemia. GM-1 is thought to enhance function in surviving white matter fiber tracts (Atrice et al, 1995; Yarkony and Chen, 1996).

Once the patient is medically stable, a primary concern of the physician is stabilization of the spine to prevent further spinal cord or nerve root damage. Surgery is indicated in the following situations: (1) to restore the alignment of bony vertebral structures; (2) to decompress neural tissue; (3) to stabilize the spine by fusion or instrumentation; and (4) to allow the individual earlier opportunities for mobilization.

Several different stabilization procedures are available to the surgeon. Skeletal traction may be used on an interim basis while the patient's medical condition is fragile. Traction can reduce the overlapping of fracture fragments and can assist with spinal alignment. Once the patient is medically stable, the physician may schedule the patient for surgery. During surgery, fusion of the fracture fragments is performed. Bone grafting from the iliac crests, combined with placement of internal fixation devices, is often employed during this procedure. In some situations, surgery is not indicated, and external fixation with a halo jacket, a hard cervical collar, or a rigid body jacket may be all that is needed to stabilize the involved spinal segments. Figure 7–4 shows various types of spinal orthoses. Regardless of the method of stabilization employed, recovery for the individual with an SCI will depend on (1) the extent of pathologic changes caused by the trauma, (2) the prevention of further trauma, and (3) the prevention of secondary medical complications (Schmitz, 1994).

PATHOLOGIC CHANGES THAT OCCUR FOLLOWING INJURY

Initially after the injury, hemorrhage into the gray matter of the spinal cord occurs. Necrosis ensues following hemorrhage within the gray matter. Edema develops within the white matter and exerts pressure on the nerve fiber tracts that carry various cutaneous sensations to the cerebral cortex and motor impulses from the cortex to the body. Investigators have hypothesized that norepinephrine is released from the traumatized spinal cord and contributes to the hemorrhagic necrosis. A few hours after the injury, myelin sheathes begin to disintegrate and the axons begin to shrink.

It is extremely important to monitor the patient's level of injury for the first 24 to 48 hours after the injury. The injury may ascend one or two levels because of vascular changes. If loss of function is apparent more than two spinal cord segments above the initial level of the injury, it may mean that the spinal cord was damaged in more than one place. Immediate notification of the patient's primary nurse and physician is necessary.

Immediately after an SCI, the patient exhibits spinal shock. The condition results from interruption of the autonomic nervous system pathways. *Spinal shock* is characterized by a period of flaccidity, areflexia, loss of bowel and bladder function, and autonomic deficits including decreased arterial blood pressure and poor temperature regulation below the level of the injury. Spinal shock normally lasts for approximately 24 to 48 hours; however, certain sources state that it may last up to several weeks. Because of suppressed reflex activity, one cannot accurately assess the patient's level of injury during spinal shock. As spinal shock resolves, reflex activity below the level of the lesion will return, and if motor and sensory tracts have been salvaged, function in these areas will also be evident (Somers, 1992).

TYPES OF LESIONS

SCIs are classified into two primary types: complete and incomplete.

Complete Injuries

If an injury is complete, sensory and motor function will be absent below the level of the injury and in the sacral segments of S4 and S5. *Complete injuries* are most often the result of complete spinal cord transection, spinal cord compression, or vascular impairment.

Incomplete Injuries

Incomplete injuries are described as those injuries in which some motor or sensory function is preserved below the level of the injury and in the lowest sacral segments. Perianal sensation must be present for an injury to be classified as incomplete. Investigators have

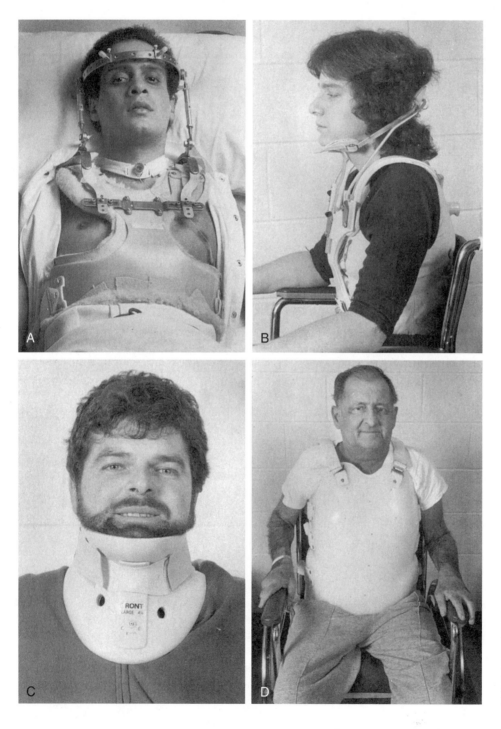

FIGURE 7–4 ■ *A,* Halo vest. *B,* Sternal occipital mandibular immobilization. *C,* Philadelphia collar. *D,* Custom-made body jacket. (From Buchanan LE, Nawoczenski DA. Spinal Cord Injury Concepts and Management Approaches. Baltimore, Williams & Wilkins, 1987.)

estimated that more than 50% of all SCIs are incomplete (Behrman et al, 1993).

The clinical picture of incomplete injuries is highly variable and unpredictable. The area of the spinal cord damaged and the number of spinal cord tracts that remain intact dictate the amount of motor and sensory function preserved. Several clinical findings help to confirm a diagnosis of an incomplete injury. *Sacral sparing* is one such occurrence. Because the sacral tracts run most medially within the spinal cord, they are often salvaged. Patients with sacral sparing present with perianal sensation. They may also be able to flex the great toe and have voluntary control over the rectal sphincter muscle (Finkbeiner and Russo, 1990). These spared motor and sensory functions can be of great functional significance to the patient because they may provide for normal bowel, bladder, and sexual function.

Another clinical finding observed in patients with incomplete injuries is *abnormal tone* or *muscle spasticity*. Patients with incomplete injuries have a tendency to display more abnormal tone than do patients with complete injuries (Maynard et al, 1990). Decreased inhibition from descending supraspinal pathways may be the reason for this finding (Fredericks, 1996).

Brown-Séquard Syndrome

Brown-Séquard syndrome results from an injury involving half of the spinal cord (Fig. 7–5*A*). Penetrating injuries such as those sustained from gunshot or stab wounds are common causes. The patient loses motor function, proprioception, and vibration on the same side as the injury because the fibers within the corticospinal tract and dorsal columns do not cross at the spinal cord level. Pain and temperature sensations are absent on the opposite side of the injury a few segments lower. The reason for the loss of pain and temperature sensations in this distribution is that the lateral spinothalamic tract ascends several spinal segments on the same side of the spinal cord before it crosses to the contralateral side (Fredericks, 1996). Light touch sensation may or may not be preserved in these patients. Prognosis for recovery with this type of injury is good. Many individuals become independent in activities of daily living (ADLs) and are continent of bowel and bladder.

Anterior Cord Syndrome

Anterior cord syndrome results from a flexion injury to the cervical spine in which a fracture-dislocation of the cervical vertebrae occurs. The anterior spinal cord or anterior spinal artery may be damaged (Fig. 7–5*B*). The patient loses motor, pain, and temperature sensation bilaterally below the level of the injury as a result of injury to the corticospinal and spinothalamic tracts.

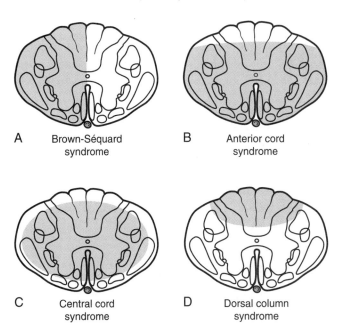

FIGURE 7–5 ■ *A* to *D*, Types of incomplete spinal cord injuries.

The posterior (dorsal) columns remain intact, and therefore the patient retains the ability to perceive position sense and vibration below the injury. The prognosis for functional return is limited because all voluntary motor function is lost.

Central Cord Syndrome

Central cord syndrome is another type of incomplete injury and the most common. This type of SCI can result from progressive stenosis or compression that is a consequence of hyperextension injuries. Bleeding into the central gray matter causes damage to the spinal cord (Fig. 7–5*C*). Characteristically, the upper extremities are more severely involved than the lower extremities. This is because the cervical tracts are located more centrally in the gray matter. Injury to the central spinal cord damages three different motor and sensory tracts including the spinothalamic, corticospinal, and dorsal columns. Sensory deficits tend to be variable. Bowel, bladder, and sexual function are preserved if the sacral portions of the tracts are spared. Ambulation is possible for many patients. Functional independence in ADLs depends on the amount of upper extremity innervation the patient regains.

Dorsal Column Syndrome

Dorsal column syndrome or *posterior cord syndrome* is a rare incomplete injury that results from compression of the posterior spinal artery by a tumor or vascular infarct (Fig. 7–5*D*). A patient with this type of injury loses the ability to perceive proprioception and vibration. The ability to move and to perceive pain remains intact.

Cauda Equina Injuries

A *cauda equina injury* usually occurs after the patient sustains a direct trauma from a fracture-dislocation below L1. This type of injury results in an incomplete or complete lower motor neuron lesion. If the injury occurs at T12 or L1, the patient may present with both upper motor neuron and lower motor neuron symptoms. Flaccidity, areflexia, and a loss of bowel and bladder function are the common clinical manifestations. Regeneration of the involved peripheral nerve root is possible, but it depends on the extent of initial damage. Table 7–1 summarizes the causes and clinical findings seen in patients with incomplete injuries.

Root Escape

Damage to the nerve root within the vertebral foramen can lead to a peripheral nerve injury. *Root escape* is the term used to describe the preservation or return of motor or sensory function in various nerve roots at or near the site of injury. Therefore, a patient may experience some improved function or a return of function in the muscles innervated by the peripheral nerve several months after the initial injury. This increased motor or sensory return should not, however, be mistaken for return of spinal cord function.

CLINICAL MANIFESTATIONS OF SPINAL CORD INJURIES

The clinical picture of a patient who has experienced an SCI can be variable. Much depends on the level of the injury and the muscle and sensory function that remains. In addition, one must consider whether the injury is complete or incomplete. In general, the following signs or symptoms may be present in an individual who has sustained an SCI: (1) motor paralysis or paresis below the level of the injury or lesion; (2) sensory loss (sensory function may remain intact two spinal cord segments below the level of the injury); (3) cardiopulmonary dysfunction; (4) impaired temperature control resulting from sympathetic nervous system damage associated with cervical lesions; (5) spasticity, which can develop as the spinal cord recovers; (6) bladder and bowel dysfunction; and (7) sexual dysfunction.

RESOLUTION OF SPINAL SHOCK

Reflex activity below the injury resumes after spinal shock subsides. The earliest reflexes that return are the sacral level reflexes. As a result, reflexic bowel and bladder function may return. Flexor withdrawal responses may also become apparent. Initially, these reflexes are evoked by a noxious stimulus, and as recovery progresses, they may be evoked by other, less noxious means. As time goes on, upper or lower extremity spasticity can develop in muscle groups that lack innervation. Flexor spasticity in the lower extremities often develops first, secondary to interruption of the vestibulospinal tract. In time, extensor tone usually dominates (Decker and Hall, 1986). Additional muscle tightness and shortening become evident as a result of static positioning and muscle imbalances (Fredericks, 1996). For example, tightness in the hip flexors can develop as the patient spends increased amounts of time sitting upright in a wheelchair.

COMPLICATIONS

Multiple complications can result following an SCI. Careful prevention of possible complications can improve a patient's rehabilitation potential and quality of life.

Table 7–1 ▌ TYPES OF INCOMPLETE SPINAL CORD INJURIES

TYPE	CAUSE	FINDINGS
Brown-Séquard syndrome	Penetrating injury: gunshot or stab wounds	Loss of motor function, proprioception, and vibration on the same side as the injury Pain and temperature lost on the opposite side
Anterior cord syndrome	Flexion injury with fracture-dislocation of the cervical vertebrae	Loss of motor, pain, and temperature sensation bilaterally below the level of the injury Position and vibration sense intact
Central cord syndrome	Progressive stenosis or hyperextension injuries	Damage to all three tracts Upper extremities more involved than lowers Sensory deficits variable
Dorsal column or posterior cord syndrome	Compression of the posterior spinal artery by tumor or vascular infarction	Loss of proprioception and vibration bilaterally
Cauda equina injuries	Direct trauma from a fracture-dislocation below L1	Upper and lower motor neuron signs possible, including flaccidity, areflexia, loss of bowel and bladder function

Pressure Ulcers

One of the most common complications seen after SCI is the development of *pressure ulcers.* Pressure areas develop over bony prominences in response to the patient's inability to perceive the need to shift weight or relieve pressure. The treatment of open wounds that develop as a consequence of excessive pressure is a leading reason for hospitalization of these patients. For health care professionals, prevention of pressure ulcers is of the utmost importance. Patients must be instructed in pressure relief techniques, or family members and caregivers must be taught how to assistance the patient with weight-shifting activities. Patients should be instructed to perform 1 minute of pressure relief for every 15 to 30 minutes of sitting (Yarkony and Chen, 1994). Patients who are able should perform skin inspections independently with the use of a handheld mirror. Patients who require physical assistance with skin inspection should be advised to instruct others in the performance of this activity.

Autonomic Dysreflexia

Autonomic dysreflexia occurs in patients with injuries above T6. This pathologic autonomic reflex is caused by sympathetic nervous system instability. All sympathetic outflow occurs below the T6 level. Consequently, in cervical and upper thoracic injuries, descending excitatory and inhibitory input to sympathetic neurons is lost. Autonomic responses are discharged as a result of a noxious sensory stimulus applied below the level of the lesion. This noxious sensory input causes autonomic stimulation, vasoconstriction, and a rapid and massive rise in the patient's blood pressure. Normally, an increase in an individual's blood pressure would stimulate the receptors in the carotid sinus and aorta and would cause an adjustment in peripheral vascular resistance, thereby lowering the patient's blood pressure. Because of the patient's condition, impulses are unable to travel below the level of the injury to lower the patient's blood pressure. Thus, hypertension persists unless the noxious stimulus is removed or the patient receives medical intervention. This condition can cause life-threatening complications including seizures and subarachnoid hemorrhage if left untreated. Common causes of autonomic dysreflexia can include bladder or bowel distention, disruption of the patient's catheter, noxious cutaneous stimulation, pressure sores, kidney malfunction, environmental temperature changes, and a passive stretch applied to the patient's hip.

Symptoms of autonomic dysreflexia include significant hypertension, severe and pounding headache, profuse sweating, vasoconstriction below the level of the lesion, vasodilation (flushing) above the level of the injury, constricted pupils, goose bumps (piloerection), blurred vision, and a runny nose. Immediate recognition of these signs or symptoms is essential. Patients who are not treated promptly may experience seizures, aphasia, renal failure, or retinal hemorrhage, or they may die (Bloch, 1986; Somers, 1992). Patients experiencing autonomic dysreflexia should be treated as persons in a crisis situation. The first thing one should do is look for the likely source of noxious stimulation. Often, the patient's catheter is kinked or the catheter bag may need emptying. If the source of the problem cannot be identified immediately, one should try to lower the patient's blood pressure by sitting or standing the patient. The patient's primary nurse and physician must be notified as soon as possible. Prevention of recurrent episodes and patient and family education are important. Medications or surgical intervention may be needed to assist the patient in the regulation of this condition.

Postural Hypotension

Another possible complication is *postural hypotension.* Patients who have experienced an SCI often develop low blood pressure. Lack of an efficient skeletal muscle pump, combined with an absent vasoresponse in the lower extremities, leads to venous pooling. Consequently, the amount of blood circulating in the body is decreased, thereby precipitating decreases in stroke volume and cardiac output. Postural hypotension can develop when patients are transferred to sitting, when they are placed in upright standing, or during exercise. Thus, careful monitoring of blood pressure responses must occur during treatment activities. The patient's blood pressure must not drop below 70/40 mm Hg because this may result in cardiac arrest (Morrison, 1994). The use of an abdominal binder during upright activities promotes venous return by minimizing the drops in intra-abdominal pressure that can occur when the patient's position is changed. In addition, elastic stockings can be worn by the patient to prevent venous pooling in the lower extremities.

Pain

Pain may develop as a result of irritation and damage to neural elements such as sensory pathways or as a consequence of mechanical trauma, surgical intervention, or poor handling and positioning. A common pain syndrome seen in patients with SCIs is *dysesthetic pain,* also known as *phantom pain* or *deafferentation pain.* The condition is manifested by poorly localized complaints of numbness, tingling, burning, shooting, and aching pain and visceral discomfort (Atrice et al, 1995; Yarkony and Chen, 1996). The pain can be exaggerated by noxious stimuli, including urinary tract infections, spasticity, bowel impaction, or cigarette smoking. Treatment of dysesthetic pain is challenging for health care practitioners. Medical interventions include patient education about the nature of the pain; administration of acetaminophen or other nonsteroidal anti-inflammatory drugs, tricyclic antidepressants, and anticonvulsants; psychologic pain management techniques; and transcutaneous electrical nerve stimulation. In some situations, neurosurgical intervention is warranted (Yarkony and Chen, 1996). Overuse pain syndromes can also develop in the shoulders as patients rely on upper extremity range of motion and strength for the completion of functional tasks (Atrice et al, 1995; Roth, 1994).

Contractures

Patients tend to develop flexion *contractures* as a result of the flexor reflex activity that develops after the injury and also as a consequence of prolonged sitting. Prevention of contractures is important to maintain maximal function. Patients should be instructed in a good stretching program that they can perform independently or with the assistance of a family member or caregiver. In addition, all patients should be encouraged to perform a regular prone positioning program. Patients should spend at least 20 minutes each day on their stomachs to stretch the hip flexors. The prone position also relieves pressure on the ischial tuberosities and can provide aeration to the buttocks.

Heterotopic Ossification

Heterotopic ossification is another potential secondary complication. Bone can form in the soft tissues below the level of the injury. Usually, heterotopic bone develops adjacent to a large lower extremity joint such as the hip or knee. Researchers have identified several potential causes such as tissue hypoxia, abnormal calcium metabolism, and local trauma. Clinical signs of heterotopic ossification include range-of-motion limitations, swelling, warmth, and pain; fever may or may not be present. The management of this condition is centered around pharmacologic intervention (etidronate disodium), physical therapy range-of-motion exercises, and surgery if the patient has a significant limitation (Yarkony and Chen, 1996).

Deep Vein Thrombosis

The development of *deep vein thrombosis* is a common and life-threatening complication. The risk appears to be greatest during the first 2 weeks after the injury. Because patients are often immobile and are medically fragile during this period, prophylactic anticoagulants such as oral warfarin (Coumadin) or intravenous heparin may be used for the first few months after the injury to prevent blood clotting. Regularly scheduled turning programs and early mobilization, including sitting up in bed and transferring to a wheelchair, are important to prevent venous pooling. Elastic supports and sequential compression devices for the lower extremities may also be prescribed to assist the patient with venous return.

Osteoporosis and Renal Calculi

Osteoporosis and *renal calculi* can be seen after SCIs because of metabolic changes. As a consequence of decreased weight-bearing opportunities, demineralization of bone occurs. Calcium from the bones is absorbed into the blood and is deposited in the kidneys, forming kidney stones. Early mobilization, therapeutic standing, and good dietary management can minimize the development of these potential complications.

Respiratory Compromise

Serious and sometimes life-threatening complications can develop as a result of a patient's decreased respiratory capabilities. These complications develop in response to decreased innervation of the muscles of respiration and immobility. The diaphragm, innervated by cervical nerve roots C3 through C5, is the primary muscle of inspiration. Therefore, patients with high cervical injuries may lose the ability to breathe on their own secondary to paralysis or weakness of the diaphragm muscle. The external intercostal muscles assist with inspiration and are innervated segmentally starting at T1. They act to lift the ribs and increase the dimension of the thoracic cavity. Patients with paraplegia below T12 have innervation of the external intercostals and should be able to exhibit a normal breathing pattern using the chest and diaphragm equally. This is often described as a *two-chest two-diaphragm breathing pattern* (Wetzel, 1985). The abdominals comprise the other important muscle group needed for respiration. The upper abdominal muscles are innervated by T7 through T9, and the lower abdominals are innervated by spinal segments T9 through T11. The abdominals are activated when the patient attempts forceful expiration such as in coughing. Patients who are unable to generate an adequate amount of muscle force to cough will be susceptible to the accumulation of bronchial secretions. This can lead to pneumonia in many individuals. Weakness in the muscles of respiration can also lead to a decreased inspiratory effort and impairment of the patient's ability to tolerate exercise, a factor that ultimately affects endurance for functional activities.

Multiple interventions are used to minimize the effects of impaired respiratory function. These include early acclimation to the upright position, abdominal corsets and binders to assist with positioning of the abdominal contents, assisted cough techniques taught to the patient and caregivers, diaphragmatic strengthening, and incentive spirometry techniques. A more in-depth discussion of these techniques occurs in the treatment section of this chapter.

Bladder and Bowel Dysfunction

Bladder and bowel dysfunction may be considered a clinical finding or a complication of SCI. Patients with SCIs often experience difficulties with this area of function. The bladder is innervated by the lower sacral segments, specifically S2 through S4. During the period of spinal shock, the bladder is flaccid or areflexic. Once spinal shock is over, two possible situations can prevail, depending on the location of the injury. If the patient's injury is above S2, the sacral reflex arc remains intact, and the patient is said to have a *reflex neurogenic bladder*. In this condition, the bladder empties reflexively when the pressure inside it reaches a certain level. Patients can apply specific cutaneous stimulation techniques to the suprapubic region to assist with bladder emptying. If the patient's injury is to the cauda equina or the cona medullaris, the patient is said to have a *nonreflexive bladder*. The sacral reflex arc is not intact, and thus the bladder remains flaccid (Schmitz, 1994).

Bladder training programs are important components of the patient's rehabilitation program. Intermittent catheterization, timed voiding programs, and manual stimulation can be used to empty the bladder and can allow the patient to be catheter free (Schmitz, 1994).

The establishment of a regular bowel program is also part of the patient's comprehensive plan of care. Patients are often placed on a regular schedule of bowel evacuation. High-fiber diets, adequate intake of fluids, the use of stool softeners, and manual stimulation or evacuation may be suggested to assist the patient in the establishment of a bowel program (Schmitz, 1994).

The rehabilitation team needs to be aware of the patient's schedule for bladder and bowel training. Therapies should not be scheduled during times designated for these activities.

Sexual Dysfunction

A common concern expressed by patients following SCI is the impact the injury will have on sexual relationships. As stated previously, physical function depends on the patient's motor level. Males with upper motor neuron injuries have the potential for reflex erections if the sacral reflex arc remains intact. The ability to ejaculate is limited for patients with both upper and lower motor neuron injuries. Therefore, men experience significant problems with fertility. Women with SCIs continue to experience menstruation and thus are able to become pregnant. Women who do become pregnant and are ready to deliver are often hospitalized as a precautionary measure, because they may not be able to feel the uterine contractions that would indicate that they are in labor (Schmitz, 1994).

Physical therapists and physical therapist assistants must feel comfortable discussing this information with their patients. Because of the time we spend working with our patients, questions related to sexual behaviors may be directed to us. We must answer questions honestly and accurately. If you do not feel comfortable fielding these types of questions, you need to refer the patient to someone who can.

Spasticity

Spasticity is a common sequela of SCI. The prevalence of spasticity is higher in patients with cervical and incomplete injuries (Somers, 1992). Research suggests that increased tone is the result of residual influence of supraspinal centers (cortex, red nucleus, reticular system, and vestibular nuclei) on the spinal cord and ineffective modulation of spinal pathways (Craik, 1991). Spasticity may also be greater in those patients who have experienced significant and multiple complications. Investigators have shown that noxious stimuli tend to exacerbate abnormal muscle tone. In most instances, physical therapists and physical therapist assistants focus treatment on ways to decrease or minimize the effects of abnormal muscle tone. However, in some instances, an increase in muscle tone can be advantageous to the patient. Spasticity can help to maintain muscle bulk, prevent atrophy, and assist in the maintenance of circulation. Spasticity can also assist the patient in performing functional activities including transfers, basic bed mobility, and standing when the patient has adequate innervation and sufficient trunk control. In addition, spasticity can provide increased tone to the anal sphincter, tone that may aid the patient in the bowel program.

The management of spasticity can be challenging. At this time, no medical treatment that completely eliminates the effects of abnormal tone is available. Physicians may recommend a multitude of interventions to help the patient. Elimination of the stimuli or factors that contribute to increased sensory input is beneficial. Physical therapy interventions may include positioning, static stretching, weight bearing, cryotherapy, aquatics, and functional electrical stimulation.

These different treatment interventions are discussed in more depth in the treatment section of this chapter. Pharmacologic intervention may be necessary for some patients with significant abnormal tone. The most common oral medications prescribed include baclofen (Lioresal), diazepam (Valium), and dantrolene sodium (Dantrium). All these medications have documented side effects including sedation, decreased attention and memory, and reduced muscle strength and coordination (Katz, 1988; Katz, 1994; Yarkony and Chen, 1996). Patients frequently try these medications and then discontinue their use because of the adverse side effects.

Intrathecal baclofen pumps and *botulism injections* are two newer forms of treatment for spasticity. With the intrathecal pump, a pump and small catheter are implanted subcutaneously into the patient's abdominal wall. Baclofen is then injected directly into the subarachnoid space of the spinal cord, thereby reducing the oral dosage needed and some of the side effects (Katz, 1988). Botulinum toxin A is injected directly into the spastic muscle belly. This neurotoxin inhibits the release of acetylcholine at the neuromuscular junction, thereby causing muscle paralysis (Cromwell and Paquette, 1996).

Surgical intervention is a final type of management of abnormal tone. Neurectomies, rhizotomies, myelotomies, tenotomies, and nerve and motor point blocks may be administered to assist the patient with management of abnormal tone. *Neurectomy* is the surgical excision of a segment of nerve. *Rhizotomy* is a surgical procedure in which the dorsal or sensory root of a spinal nerve is resected. In *myelotomy,* the tracts within the spinal cord are severed. *Tenotomy* is the surgical release of a tendon. Nerve blocks are performed with injectable phenol and reduce spasticity on a temporary basis (3 to 6 months). A more detailed description of these procedures is beyond the scope of this text (Katz, 1988; Katz, 1994; Yarkony and Chen, 1996).

FUNCTIONAL OUTCOMES

A patient's functional outcome following an SCI depends on many factors. Age, the type of injury, the level of the injury, the motor and sensory function preserved, the patient's general health status before the injury, body build, support systems, financial security, motivation, and preexisting personality traits all play a role in the patient's eventual outcome (Lewthwaite et al, 1994).

Key Muscles by Segmental Innervation

Before we can begin to talk about functional capabilities in an individual with an SCI, we must review key muscles and their actions. The innervation of key muscle groups allows patients to achieve a certain level of functional skill and independence. Table 7–2 highlights key muscles at each spinal level.

Functional Potentials

Each successive motor level provides the patient with the potential for greater function. Strength of a muscle must be at least fair plus to perform a functional activity (Alvarez, 1985). Table 7–3 provides a review of functional potentials based on the patient's motor innervation and limitations encountered because of decreased muscle strength or range of motion. A description of each level and the patient's potential for achievement of functional activities is provided.

C1 Through C3

A patient with an injury above C4 has limited muscle innervation. Because the diaphragm is only minimally innervated by C3, most patients with injuries at these levels will likely require mechanical ventilation. The patient will require full-time attendants and will be totally dependent in all ADLs. A power wheelchair with a reclining feature will be needed to allow for pressure relief and rest. The patient should have adequate breath support or neck range of motion to operate a power wheelchair by a sip-and-puff mechanism

Table 7–2 ▍ KEY MUSCLES BY SEGMENTAL INNERVATION

SPINAL LEVEL	MUSCLES
C1–C2	Facial muscles, partial sternocleidomastoid, capital muscles
C3	Sternocleidomastoid, partial diaphragm, upper trapezius
C4	Diaphragm, partial deltoid, sternocleidomastoid, upper trapezius
C5	Deltoid, biceps, rhomboids, brachioradialis, teres minor
C6	Extensor carpi radialis, pectoralis major (clavicular portion), teres major, supinator, weak pronator
C7	Triceps, flexor carpi radialis, latissimus, pronator teres
C8	Flexor carpi ulnaris, extensor carpi ulnaris, patient may have some hand intrinsics
T1–T8	Hand intrinsics, top half of the intercostals, pectoralis major (sternal portion)
T7–T9	Upper abdominals
T9–T12	Lower abdominals
T12	Lower abdominals, weak quadratus lumborum
L1–L2	Quadratus lumborum, weak iliopsoas, weak sartorius, weak rectus femoris
L3–L4	Iliopsoas, sartorius, rectus femoris, anterior tibialis, weak hamstrings
L4–L5	Quadriceps, medial hamstrings, anterior tibialis, posterior tibialis
S1	Plantar flexors, gluteus maximus
S2	Anal sphincter

Table 7–3 ▌ FUNCTIONAL POTENTIAL FOR
PATIENTS WITH SPINAL CORD INJURIES

LEVEL	MUSCLES PRESENT	POTENTIAL	LIMITATIONS
Above C4	C1–C2: Facial muscles C3: Sternocleido- mastoid, upper trape- zius	Vital capacity 20–30% of normal Power wheelchair with breath control or chin control and portable ventilator Full-time attendant required Ability to direct care verbally	Dependent on ventilator Dependent in all ADLs Dependent in pressure relief Dependent in transfers
C4	Diaphragm Upper trapezius	Vital capacity 30–50% of normal Power wheelchair with mouth stick or chin control 30° of cervical motion needed to drive a wheelchair with a chin control Maximum assistance with bed mobility Independent pressure relief with power reclining wheel-chair Full-time attendant required Ability to direct care verbally Use of environmental control units	No upper extremity innervation Dependent in transfers Dependent in all ADLs
C5	Deltoid Biceps Rhomboids Lateral rotators (teres minor and infraspi-natus)	Vital capacity 40–60% of normal Power wheelchair with hand controls Manual wheelchair with rim projections Moderate assistance for bed mobility Maximum assistance with transfers (sliding board or sit pivot) Independent forward raise for pressure relief with loops attached to the back of the wheelchair Possible independence with some self-care activities with adaptive equipment (wrist splints) Attendant needed for activity setup Use of environmental control units	Has only elbow flexors, prone to el-bow flexion contractures Must consider energy and time re-quirements for activity completion
C6	Extensor carpi radialis Pectoralis major (clavic-ular portion) Teres major	Vital capacity 60–80% of normal Independent rolling Independent pressure relief via weight shift Independent sliding board transfers Independent manual wheelchair propulsion with rim pro-jections Independent feeding with adaptive equipment Independent upper extremity dressing; requires assis-tance for lower extremities Ability to drive automobile with hand controls Vocation outside the home possible Prehension with flexor hinge splint Possible a.m. and p.m. care needed Assistance needed for commode transfers	No elbow extension or hand function (patient prone to contractures)
C7	Triceps Latissimus dorsi Pronator teres	Vital capacity 80% of normal Independent living possible Independent pressure relief via lateral pushup Independent self–range of motion of lower extremities Independent transfers, wheelchair propulsion, pressure relief, and upper and lower extremity dressing	No finger muscles Transfers to floor require moderate or maximum assistance Needs assist to right wheelchair
C8	Flexor carpi ulnaris Extensor carpi ulnaris Hand intrinsics	Same potential as individual at C7 Independent living Negotiation of 2- to 4-inch curbs in wheelchair Wheelies in wheelchair	Some intrinsic hand function Writing, fine-motor coordination ac-tivities can be difficult Assistance with floor transfers
T1–T8	Hand intrinsics Top half of intercostals Pectoralis major (ster-nal portion)	Independent in manual wheelchair propulsion on all lev-els and surfaces (6-inch curbs) Therapeutic ambulation with orthoses in parallel bars (T6–T8)	No lower abdominal muscle function Minimal assistance to independent with floor transfers and righting wheelchair
T9–T12	Abdominals	Independent wheelchair mobility Household ambulation with orthoses and assistive devices T10 vital capacity 100%	No hip flexor function
T12–below		Community ambulation	
L1, L2	Quadratus lumborum Weak iliopsoas and sar-torius	Independent in coming to stand and ambulation with orthoses Independent in ambulation on curbs and stairs	No quadriceps function
L3–L5	L3–L4: Iliopsoas, rectus L4–L5: quadriceps, me-dial hamstrings	Same as L1, L2; may only need ankle-foot orthoses and canes for ambulation	No gluteus maximus function
S1–S2	S1: plantar flexors, glu-teus maximus S2: anal sphincter	Ambulation with articulated ankle-foot orthoses	Loss of bowel and bladder function

ADLs, activities of daily living.

or with a chin cup. With a sip-and-puff unit, the patient either sips or blows into a straw mounted in front of her face to provide the stimulus for the wheelchair to move. A few patients may be able to use a chin cup. This device requires that the patient have at least 30 degrees of active cervical motion. Patients with injuries at C1 through C3 may or may not have sufficient active range of motion in the cervical spine. Advances in technology have improved the capabilities of all patients with SCIs, especially those with injuries at higher levels. Environmental control units that can be operated from the wheelchair allow some patients increased control over their home and work environments. These control units can be networked with one's personal computer and can operate appliances, lights, and so forth.

C4

A patient with a C4 level injury likely has some innervation of the diaphragm. This has significant functional implications because it means that a patient may not have to depend on a ventilator. The vital capacity of patients with diaphragmatic innervation is still markedly decreased. Individuals at this level should be able to operate a power wheelchair using a chin cup, chin control, or mouth stick. Patients still must have sufficient range of motion to drive the wheelchair with a chin control. Environmental control units may also be prescribed for these patients. Individuals with C4 innervation continue to require full-time attendants because they are completely dependent in all transfers and ADLs.

C5

Patients with C5 innervation have some functional abilities. A patient with C5 innervation has deltoid, biceps, and rhomboid function. However, even though these muscles are innervated at this level, they may not have normal strength. Each patient presents with different motor capabilities, and the physical therapist must thoroughly evaluate muscle function. Because of innervation of these key muscles, a patient with innervation at C5 should be able to flex and abduct the shoulders, flex the elbows, and adduct the scapulae. The ability to flex and abduct the shoulders means that the patient will be able to raise his arms to assist with rolling and can also bring his hand to his mouth. He cannot, however, extend the elbow because the triceps are not innervated. The patient will be able to operate a power wheelchair with a hand control. A few patients are able to propel a manual wheelchair with rim projections. Although manual wheelchair propulsion may be possible, one must consider the high energy costs associated with this activity. For this reason, power wheelchairs are often prescribed for patients

with innervation at this level. The individual with C5 innervation may be able to be independent with some self-care activities, but the patient will require setup of the activity by an attendant or family member. Patients also need to use adaptive equipment including splints and built-up ADL devices to perform self-care activities. Our experience has shown that even though patients may be able to perform a self-care activity independently after setup, the time and energy required to complete the task are often too great to continue performance on a regular basis. Individuals with innervation at the C5 level can provide minimal assistance with sliding board transfers from their wheelchairs. They can perform independent pressure relief by leaning forward in the wheelchair or by looping one of their upper extremities over the push handles on the back of the wheelchair and performing a weight shift. The rhomboids provide limited scapular stabilization for upper extremity self-care activities and for assuming functional positions such as prone on elbows and long sitting with extended arm support.

C6

Patients with C6 innervation have some greater functional abilities. Because of innervation of the wrist extensors, the pectoralis major, and the teres major, patients at this level are able to be independent with rolling, feeding, and upper extremity dressing. The patient should be able to propel a manual wheelchair independently with rim projections, and the potential exists for the person to be independent with sliding board transfers. Patients may need assistance in the morning and at night with self-care activities, and some patients need assistance for transfers, especially to the commode. Assistance is also required for lower extremity dressing. Gainful employment outside the home is possible for individuals with innervation at this level.

C7

An individual with a C7 injury has the potential for living independently because patients at this level have innervation of the triceps. With triceps strength, the patient can use her upper extremities to lift herself up during transfers. In addition, the person will be able to perform a wheelchair pushup for pressure relief. Independence in self-care activities is possible, including upper and lower extremity dressing. Persons should become independent in wheelchair-to-bed or mat transfers, first with a sliding board and eventually without the use of a board. Additional functional capabilities include independence with pressure relief, self–range of motion to the lower extremities, and operation of a standard motor vehicle with adapted hand controls.

C8

With innervation at C8, a patient can live independently. An individual is able to perform everything that a patient with innervation at a C7 level is able to complete. With the addition of some increased finger control, the patient may also be able to perform wheelies and negotiate 2- to 4-inch curbs in the wheelchair.

T1 Through T8

We look at capabilities of individuals with T1 through T8 innervation as a group. With increased motor return in the thoracic region, the patient demonstrates improved trunk control and breathing capabilities because of increasing innervation of the intercostals. Individuals are able to operate a manual wheelchair on all levels and surfaces and should be able to transfer into and out of the wheelchair to the floor. Patients with innervation at the T1 through T8 level may also be candidates for physiologic standing and limited therapeutic ambulation in the parallel bars with physical assistance and orthoses. *Therapeutic ambulation* is defined as walking for the physiologic benefits that standing and weight bearing provide. The section of this chapter on ambulation discusses this concept in greater detail.

T9 Through T12

Persons with innervation at the T9 through T12 level have abilities similar to those mentioned for individuals with T1 through T8 function. Innervation of the lower abdominal muscles assists the patient with respiratory function because the patient is able to initiate a cough. Therapeutic ambulation and ambulation in the home with orthoses and assistive devices may be possible.

L1 Through L3

The lower trunk musculature is innervated at the L1 level, the hip flexors are innervated at L2, and the quadriceps are partially innervated by L3. The presence of lower extremity innervation improves the patient's capacity for ambulation activities. Patients with innervation at this level should be independent in household ambulation and may become independent in community ambulation. Knee-ankle-foot orthoses or ankle-foot orthoses are necessary.

L4 and L5

Patients with injuries at the L4 and L5 level should be independent with all functional activities including gait. These individuals can ambulate in the community with some type of orthoses and assistive device.

PHYSICAL THERAPY INTERVENTION: ACUTE CARE

The acute care management of the patient with an SCI centers around three primary goals:

1. Prevention of joint contractures and deformities.
2. Improvement of muscle and respiratory function.
3. Acclimation of the patient to an upright position.

The patient's initial physical therapy evaluation includes information on the patient's respiratory function, muscle strength, muscle tone, reflex activity, skin status, cardiac function, and functional mobility skills. The physical therapist develops a treatment plan to address the patient's primary problems. In these early stages, treatment focuses on breathing exercises, selective strengthening exercises, range of motion, functional mobility training, activities to improve the patient's tolerance to the upright position, and patient and family education.

A patient with a cervical or thoracic injury may not immediately undergo surgical stabilization; therefore, the physical therapist may be involved in the care of the patient in the intensive care unit. Any patient with an unstable spine must be carefully assessed by the physician for the appropriateness of physical therapy innervation. Because of the acuteness of the patient's condition and the potential for unpredictable patient responses, it is best for the patient to be treated by the physical therapist at this stage. Co-treatments with the physical therapist assistant or other members of the trauma team may be appropriate.

Breathing Exercises

Exercises performed at the acute stage should emphasize maximizing respiratory function. Much depends on the patient's current level of muscle innervation. For those patients with innervation between C4 and T1, emphasis is on increasing the diaphragm's strength and efficiency. These patients possess diaphragm function and often demonstrate a diaphragmatic breathing pattern. If the diaphragm is weak, use of accessory muscles such as the sternocleidomastoid and scalenes may be evident. A good way to assess respiratory function is to look at the epigastric area and to watch for *epigastric rise*. An exaggerated movement of the abdominal area indicates that the diaphragm is working. The physical therapist assistant can place a hand over this area to determine how much movement is actually taking place, as depicted in Figure 7–6. If the patient is having difficulty, a quick stretch applied before the diaphragm activates can help to facilitate a response. If the patient is able to move the epigastric area at least 2 inches, the strength

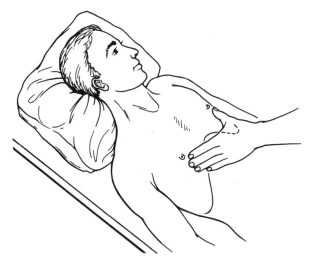

FIGURE 7-6 ■ Placement of the hand for diaphragmatic breathing. (From Myers RS. Saunders Manual of Physical Therapy Practice. Philadelphia, WB Saunders, 1995.)

of the diaphragm is said to be fair (Wetzel, 1985). To strengthen this muscle even more, the assistant can apply manual resistance during the inspiratory phase of respiration. If the patient is able to take resistance to the diaphragm during inspiration, the strength of the muscle is considered good. Care must be taken to gauge the amount of manual resistance used. Early on, patients may experience difficulties in breathing as a consequence of diaphragm weakness. In addition, respiratory muscle fatigue may become evident. Observation of the neck area can provide the clinician with valuable information about accessory muscle use. Patients often use accessory muscles extensively when the diaphragm is weak. Visible contraction of the sternocleidomastoids, scalenes, or platysma indicates accessory muscle use.

Glossopharyngeal Breathing

Patients with injuries at the C1 through C3 level and some patients with injuries at C4 require mechanical ventilation. These patients need to be taught a technique to assist their ability to tolerate short periods of breathing while they are off the ventilator. *Glossopharyngeal breathing* is a technique that can be taught to patients with high-level tetraplegia. The patient takes a breath of air and closes the mouth. The patient raises the palate to trap the air. Saying the words "ah" or "oops" does this. The larynx is then opened. The tongue forces the air through the open larynx. This technique is extremely beneficial if, for some reason, the patient needs to be off the ventilator for a short time because of equipment failure, power outage, or other unforeseeable circumstance. This technique allows the patient to receive adequate breath support until mechanical ventilation can be resumed.

Lateral Expansion

For those patients who have some intercostal innervation (T1 through T12), lateral expansion or basilar breathing should be emphasized. Patients are encouraged to take deep breaths as they try to expand the chest wall laterally. Physical therapist assistants can place their hands on the patient's lateral chest wall and can palpate the amount of movement present. Manual resistance can eventually be applied as the patient gains strength in the intercostal muscles. Progression to a two-diaphragm, two-chest breathing pattern is desirable.

Incentive Spirometry

Another activity that can be used to improve the function of the pulmonary system is *incentive spirometry.* Blow bottles at the patient's bedside can encourage deep breathing. A measurement of a patient's vital capacity can be taken with a handheld spirometer. Vital capacity is the maximum amount of air expelled after maximum inhalation. Measurements of the patient's vital capacity can be taken throughout rehabilitation to document changes in ventilation (Wetzel, 1985). Patients can also be instructed to vary their breathing rate and to hold their breath as a means to promote improved respiratory function.

Chest Wall Stretching

Spasticity and muscle tightness within the chest wall can develop. *Manual chest stretching* may be indicated to increase chest expansion. The assistant can place one hand under the patient's ribs and the other on top of them. The clinician then brings the hands together in a wringing type of motion. The clinician moves segmentally up the chest. This procedure is contraindicated in the presence of rib fractures (Wetzel, 1985). Intervention 7-1 illustrates a clinician performing this technique.

Postural Drainage

Postural drainage with percussion and vibration may be necessary to aid in clearing secretions. Many facilities employ respiratory therapists who are responsible for these activities. However, the physical therapist or physical therapist assistant may be the health care provider responsible for the patient's *bronchial hygiene* (removal of secretions). Postural drainage positions are outlined in Chapter 10.

Physical therapy plays an important role in teaching the patient assisted cough techniques. For patients who lack abdominal innervation, it is imperative to identify ways in which the patient can expel secretions. If the patient is unable to perform these assistive

Intervention 7–1 ▎ CHEST WALL STRETCHING

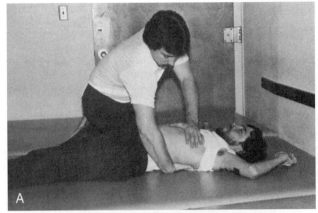

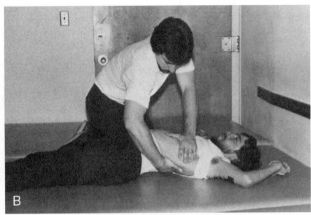

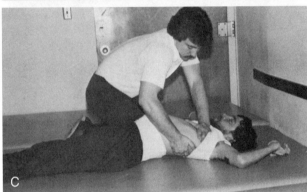

A. Starting position for manual chest stretching with one hand under the patient's ribs and the other on top of the patient's ribs.

B. Ending position of the clinician's hands after applying a wringing-type motion to the patient's chest for manual stretching.

C. The last hand position after the clinician progresses up the patient's chest for manual chest stretching with the clinician's top hand just inferior to the patient's clavicle.

From Adkins HV (ed). Spinal Cord Injury. New York, Churchill Livingstone, 1985.

cough techniques independently, a caregiver or a family member should be taught the technique. These techniques are discussed in the next section. Maintaining good bronchial hygiene assists in the prevention of secondary complications such as pneumonia.

Coughs

Coughs are classified into three different categories, based on the amount of force the individual is able to generate. *Functional coughs* are those that are strong enough to clear secretions. *Weak functional coughs* produce an adequate amount of force to clear the upper airways. *Nonfunctional coughs* are ineffective in clearing the airways of bronchial secretions (Wetzel, 1985).

Assisted Cough Techniques

Several methods are available to assist patients with the ability to cough. Depending on the patient's medical status, these techniques can be initiated in the acute care setting or during the early phases of rehabilitation.

Technique 1. The patient inhales two or three times and, on the second or third inhalation, attempts to cough. Intrathoracic pressure is allowed to build up to allow the patient to generate a greater force to expel secretions.

Technique 2. The patient places her forearms over her abdomen. As the patient tries to cough, the patient pulls downward with her upper extremities to assist with force production. This can be completed in either a supine or a sitting position. This technique can also be modified by having the patient fall toward her knees as she attempts to cough. This is illustrated in Intervention 7–2A.

Technique 3. In a prone on elbows position, the patient raises her shoulders, extends her neck, and inhales. As the patient coughs, the patient flexes her neck downward and leans onto her elbows.

Technique 4. If the patient is unable to master any of the previously mentioned assistive cough techniques, a caregiver can assist the patient with secretion expulsion. A modified Heimlich maneuver can be performed by placing the caregiver's

Intervention 7-2 ▌ ASSISTIVE COUGH TECHNIQUES

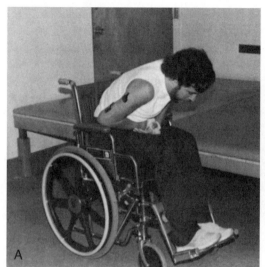

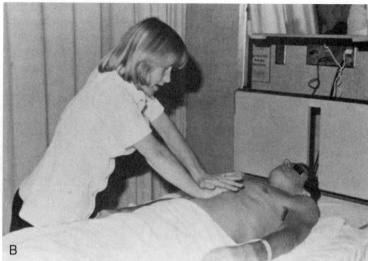

A. Self-manual coughing by the patient.

B. Assistive cough technique administered by the therapist.

From Adkins HV (ed). Spinal Cord Injury. New York, Churchill Livingstone, 1985.

hands on the patient's abdomen just below the rib cage and providing resistance in a downward and upward direction to the cough effort (see Intervention 7–2B).

Range of Motion

Range-of-motion exercises are an important component of the early stage of rehabilitation. For patients with tetraplegia, stretching of the shoulders, elbows, wrists, and fingers is essential. Often, patients with cervical injuries are immobilized in a halo that limits the patient's ability to perform active or passive range of motion of the shoulder. The halo vest sits over the patient's shoulders and thus limits shoulder flexion and abduction to approximately 90 degrees. The following shoulder ranges of motion are necessary to maximize function in the patient with tetraplegia. Approximately 60 degrees of shoulder extension and 90 degrees of shoulder external rotation are desirable. The patient needs shoulder extension to perform transfers from the supine to the long-sitting position. External rotation at the shoulder is needed so the patient can perform an elbow-locking maneuver to assume a sitting position. Full elbow extension must also be maintained to ensure that the patient is able to use elbow locking for the long-sitting position and for transfers. Patients who lack innervation of the triceps (patients with C5 and C6 tetraplegia) use the elbow-

locking mechanism to improve their functional potentials.

Adequate forearm pronation is necessary for feeding. Patients who lack finger function need 90 degrees of wrist extension. When an individual extends the wrist, passive insufficiency causes a subsequent flexing of the finger flexors referred to as *tenodesis*. Tenodesis can be used functionally to allow the patient to grip objects with built-up handles using passive or active wrist extension. As a result of this functional phenomenon, stretching of the extrinsic finger flexors in combination with wrist extension should be avoided. If the finger flexors become overstretched, the patient will lose the ability to achieve a tenodesis grasp. Sitting on the mat with an open hand overstretches the finger flexors. The patient should be encouraged to maintain the proximal interphalangeal joints and the distal interphalangeal joints in flexion. Overstretching of the thumb web space should also be avoided because tightness in the thumb adductors and flexors allows the thumb to oppose the first and second fingers during tenodesis. Patients are then able to use the thumb as a hook for functional activities.

Once the halo is removed, clinicians should also avoid overstretching the cervical extensors. Stretching of the cervical extensors leads to forward head posturing. This head position interferes with the patient's sitting balance and can limit the patient's respiratory capabilities by inhibiting the use of accessory muscles.

Passive Range of Motion

Passive range of motion must be performed to the lower extremities when they are paralyzed. Special attention must be given to the hamstrings. The desired amount of passive hamstring flexibility needed to maintain a long-sitting position and to dress the lower extremities is 110 degrees, although the amount of hamstring range required depends on the length of the patient's upper and lower extremities. When stretching the lower extremities, the assistant should make sure that the patient's pelvis is stabilized so movement is from the hamstrings and not from the low back. Some tightness in the low back musculature is desirable because this assists the patient with rolling, transfers, and maintenance of sitting positions. Tightness in the low back provides the patient with a certain degree of passive trunk stability. In addition, maintenance of a "tight" back prevents the patient from developing a posterior pelvic tilt that can lead to sacral sitting and pressure problems when sitting in the wheelchair. Stretching of the hip extensors, flexors, and rotators is necessary because gravity and increased tone may predispose patients to contractures. Hip flexion range of 100 degrees is needed to perform transfers into and out of the wheelchair. The patient needs 45 degrees of hip external rotation for dressing the lower extremities. Early in rehabilitation, it may not be possible to position the patient in prone to stretch the hip flexors because of respiratory compromise. The prone position can inhibit the diaphragm's ability to work. However, as soon as the patient can safely maintain this position, it should be instituted. Stretching of the ankle plantar flexors is necessary to provide passive stability of the feet during transfers, to allow proper positioning of the feet on the wheelchair footrests, and to allow the use of orthoses if the patient will be ambulatory. Table 7–4 provides a review of passive range-of-motion requirements.

Caution. If the patient's cervical spine is unstable, passive range-of-motion exercises to the shoulders should be limited to 90 degrees of flexion and abduction, to avoid possible movement of the cervical vertebrae. Instability in the lumbar spine requires that passive hip flexion be limited to 90 degrees with knee flexion and 60 degrees with the knees straight (Somers, 1992). Once the spine is stabilized, more aggressive range-of-motion exercises can begin.

Strengthening Exercises

Strengthening exercises are another essential component of the patient's rehabilitation. During the acute phase, certain muscles must be strengthened

Table 7–4 ▮ RANGE-OF-MOTION REQUIREMENTS

MOVEMENT	RANGE NEEDED
Shoulder extension	60°
Shoulder external rotation	90°
Elbow extension	Full elbow extension
Forearm pronation	Full forearm pronation
Forearm supination	Full forearm supination
Wrist extension	90°
Hip flexion	100°
Hip extension	10°
Hip external rotation	45°
Passive straight leg raising	110°
Knee extension	Full knee extension
Ankle dorsiflexion	To neutral

cautiously to avoid stress at the fracture site and possible fatigue. Initially, muscles may need to be exercised in a gravity-neutralized (antigravity) position secondary to weakness. Intervention 7–3A and B illustrates triceps strengthening in a gravity-neutralized position. Application of resistance may be contraindicated in the muscles of the scapulae and shoulders in patients with tetraplegia and in the muscles of the hips and trunk in patients with paraplegia, depending on the stability of the fracture site. When the physical therapist is designing the patient's exercise program, exercises that incorporate bilateral upper extremity movements are beneficial. For example, bilateral upper extremity exercises performed in a straight plane or in proprioceptive neuromuscular facilitation patterns offer the patient many advantages. These types of exercises are often more efficiently performed and reduce the asymmetric forces that can be applied to the spine during upper extremity exercises. Key muscles to be strengthened for patients with tetraplegia include the anterior deltoids, shoulder extensors, and biceps. Key muscles to be emphasized for patients with paraplegia include shoulder depressors, triceps, and latissimus dorsi.

During this early stage of rehabilitation, the assistant may use manual resistance as the primary means of strengthening weakened muscles. In addition, Velcro weights or Theraband may be used (Intervention 7–3C and D). As the patient progresses, these items may be left at the patient's bedside to allow the patient the opportunity to exercise at other times during the day. If you do decide to leave one of these items for the patient, make sure that the patient can apply the device independently. Often, when a patient has decreased hand function, applying one of these devices can be difficult. Fairly rigorous upper extremity exercises can be performed by patients with paraplegia. Barbells, exercise (Nautilus) equipment, free weights, and Theraband can be used for resistive exercise.

Intervention 7–3 I TRICEPS AND UPPER EXTREMITY STRENGTHENING

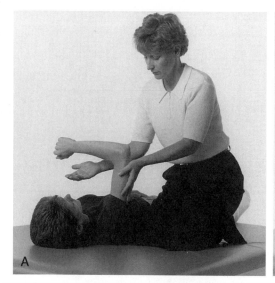

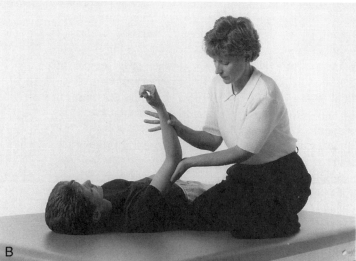

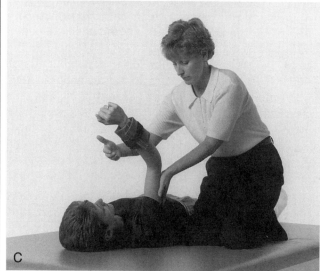

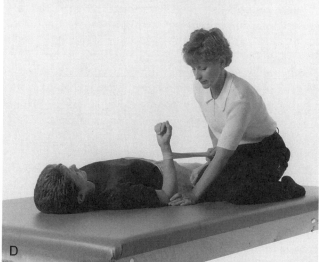

A and B. Triceps strengthening performed in the gravity-neutralized position. The patient's forearm must be carefully guarded. Weakness in the upper extremity may cause the patient's hand to flex toward her face.

C. Using a Velcro weight for additional resistance during triceps strengthening.

D. Using Theraband for biceps strengthening.

Acclimation to Upright

In addition to passive stretching and strengthening exercises, the patient should also begin sitting activities. Because of the injury, the patient may have been in a supine position for several days or weeks. As a consequence, the patient may experience orthostatic hypotension. Initially, nursing and physical therapy can work on raising the head of the patient's bed. One should monitor the patient's vital signs during the performance of sitting activities. Baseline pulse, blood pressure, and respiration rates should be recorded. As stated previously, as long as the patient's blood pressure does not drop below 80/50 mm Hg, kidney perfusion is adequate (Finkbeiner and Russo, 1990). If the patient can tolerate sitting with the head of the bed elevated, the patient can be progressed to sitting in a reclining wheelchair. Often, the patient is transferred to the wheelchair with a draw sheet or buckboard initially. Transfers into and out of hospital beds are often difficult, based on the height of the bed. As the patient is better able to tolerate sitting, the time and degree of elevation can be increased. The tilt table can also be used to acclimate the patient to the upright position (Fig. 7–7).

Weight bearing on the lower extremities has many therapeutic benefits, including reducing the effects of osteoporosis, assisting with bowel and bladder function, and decreasing abnormal muscle tone that may be present. To assist the patient with blood pressure regulation during any of these upright activities, it may be necessary to have the patient wear an abdominal binder, elastic stockings, or elastic wraps. The abdominal binder helps to support the abdominal contents during upright activities to prevent gravity from pulling down on it. Elastic wraps or elastic stockings assist the lower extremities with venous return in the absence of the skeletal muscle action in the lower extremities. The patient should also be carefully monitored for possible autonomic dysreflexia during these early attempts at upright positioning.

PHYSICAL THERAPY INTERVENTIONS DURING INPATIENT REHABILITATION

Once the patient is medically stable, the patient will likely be transferred to a comprehensive rehabilitation

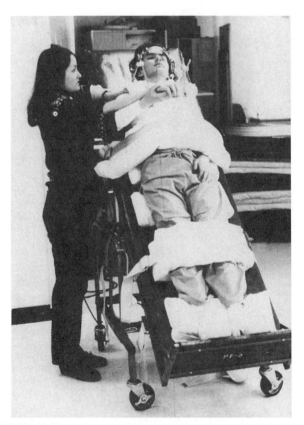

FIGURE 7–7 ■ The tilt table is used to help a patient gradually build up tolerance to the upright position. (From Zejdlik CP. Management of Spinal Cord Injury, 2nd ed. 1991: Jones and Bartlett, Publishers, Sudbury, MA, www.jbpub.com. Reprinted with permission.)

center. During this phase of the patient's recovery, the emphasis is on maximizing functional potential. The average length of inpatient rehabilitation is approximately 44 days (National Spinal Cord Injury Statistical Center, 1998). Activities that were initiated during the acute phase of recovery continue. Treatment focuses on maximizing respiratory function, range of motion, positioning, and strengthening. Additional interventions are addressed to assist the patient in the development of motor control, the performance of functional activities, and improvement in the patient's cardiovascular tolerance to exercise.

Physical Therapy Goals

The goals of treatment at this stage are many and variable. Much depends on the patient's level of innervation and resultant muscle capabilities. Examples of goals for this stage of the patient's recovery include the following:

1. Increased strength of key muscle groups.
2. Independence in skin inspection and pressure relief.
3. Increased passive range of motion of the hamstrings and shoulder extensors.
4. Increased vital capacity.
5. Increased tolerance to upright positioning in bed and the wheelchair.
6. Independence in transfers or independence with directing a caregiver.
7. Independence in bed and mat mobility or independence with directing a caregiver.
8. Independence in wheelchair propulsion on level surfaces.
9. Independence in the operation of a motor vehicle (if appropriate).
10. Return to home, school, and work.
11. Independence in home exercise program performance.
12. Patient and family education.

Goals regarding ambulation may be appropriate, depending on the patient's motivation, motor level, and the philosophy of the clinic and SCI team.

Treatment Planning

The primary physical therapist is responsible for developing the patient's physical therapy treatment plan. In addition to mastery of functional skills, the physical therapist wants to promote certain behaviors in the patient. Patients who have sustained SCIs must become problem solvers. The patient needs to figure out how to move using the remaining innervated muscles. The patient also needs to know what to do in emergency situations. For example, if the patient should fall out of the chair, the patient will need to know how to instruct someone else in a method to assist. In treatment, tasks should be broken down into components, and the assistant should allow the patient to find solutions to movement problems. Patients should practice the whole activity but also work on the steps leading up to the completed activity. An example is practicing getting into a supine on elbows position and then making the transition to long sitting. Patients should also be taught to work in reverse. Once the patient has achieved the desired end position, the patient should practice moving out of that position and back to the start posture.

Patients who have sustained SCIs should experience success during rehabilitation. Activities should be selected that provide the patient with the opportunity to succeed. These tasks should be interspersed with activities that are challenging and difficult. Treatment activi-

ties selected should help the patient to develop a balance of skills between different postures and stages of motor control. The patient does not need to perfect movement in one postural set before moving on to something different. Finally, the patient's treatment plan should be varied. Examples of some of the different components of the patient's treatment plan that are possible include pool therapy, mat programs, group activities, and strengthening exercises.

Early Treatment Interventions

Mat Activities

Early in treatment, the patient should work on rolling. Learning to do this independently can assist with the prevention of pressure ulcers. As the patient prac-

---

Intervention 7–4 ▌ ROLLING FROM SUPINE TO PRONE

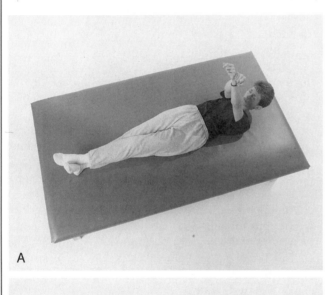

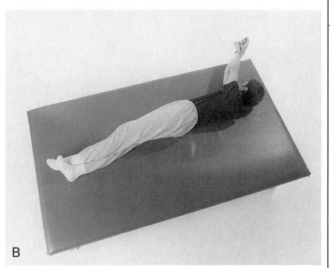

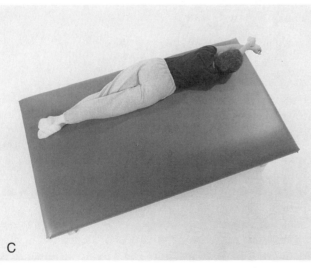

A. Rolling from supine to prone can be facilitated by having the patient flex her head and use upper extremity horizontal adduction for momentum. The patient's lower extremities should be crossed to unweight the hip to assist with rolling.

B and C. With momentum and on the count of three, the patient should flex and turn her head in the direction she wishes to roll while throwing her arms in the same direction.

tices rolling, the assistant can also work on the patient's achievement of the prone position. As stated previously, prone is an excellent position for pressure relief and stretching the hip flexors. If the patient is wearing a halo, it will often be necessary for the assistant to help the patient with rolling. Pre-positioning a wedge under the patient's chest is desirable when the patient is prone. If the patient does not have a halo, rolling can be facilitated in the following way:

Step 1. The patient should flex his head and neck and rotate his head from the right to the left.

Step 2. With both upper extremities extended above the his head (in approximately 90 degrees of shoulder flexion), the patient should move his upper extremities together from side to side.

Step 3. With momentum and on the count of three, the patient should flex and turn his head in the direction he wishes to roll while throwing his arms in the same direction.

Step 4. To make it easier for the patient, the patient's ankles can be crossed at the start of the activity. This pre-positioning allows the patient's lower extremities to move more easily. To roll to the left, you would cross the patient's right ankle over the left. Intervention 7–4 illustrates a patient who is completing the rolling sequence. Cuff weights applied to the patient's wrists can add momentum and can facilitate rolling.

Once the patient has rolled from supine to prone, strengthening exercises for the scapular muscles can also be performed. Shoulder extension, shoulder adduction, and shoulder depression with adduction are three common exercises that can be performed to strengthen the scapular stabilizers. Intervention 7–5 shows a patient who is performing these types of exercises.

Prone

From the prone position, the patient can attempt to assume a prone on elbows position. Prone on elbows is a beneficial position because it facilitates head and neck control, as well as requiring proximal stability of the glenohumeral joint and scapular muscles. For the patient to attain the prone on elbows position, the physical therapist assistant may need to help. The assistant can place his or her hands under the patient's shoulders anteriorly and lift upward (Intervention 7–6A). As the patient's chest is lifted, the assistant should move his or her hands posteriorly to the patient's shoulder or scapular region. If the patient is to attempt achievement of the position independently, the patient should be instructed to place his elbows close to his trunk, hands near his shoulders. The patient is then instructed to push the elbows down into the mat while he lifts his head and upper trunk. To position the elbows under the shoulders, the patient needs to shift his weight from one side to the other to move the elbows into correct alignment. The assistant can facilitate weight shifts in the appropriate direction during these activities (Intervention 7–6B).

Prone on Elbows

Before beginning activities in the prone on elbows position, the patient needs to assume the correct align-

---

Intervention 7–5 ‖ SCAPULAR STRENGTHENING

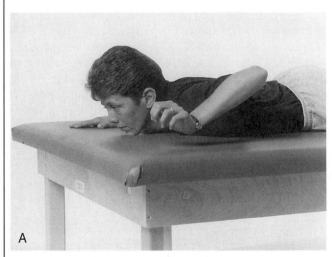 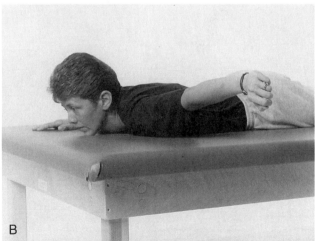

Scapular strengthening exercises can be performed in a prone position.

Intervention 7–6 ▮ PRONE TO PRONE ON ELBOWS

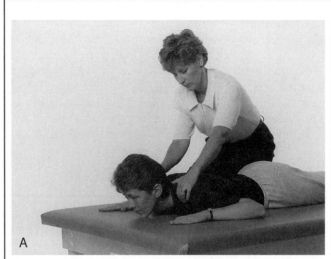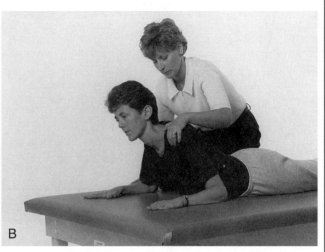

A. The assistant may need to help the patient achieve the prone on elbows position.

B. Weight shifting from one side to the other allows the patient to move her elbows into correct alignment.

ment, as shown in Figure 7–8. The patient should also try to keep the scapulae slightly adducted and downwardly rotated to counteract the natural tendency to hang on the shoulder ligaments. The assistant may need to provide the patient with manual cues on the scapulae to maintain the correct position. Downward approximation applied through the shoulders or tapping to the rhomboids is often necessary to increase scapular stability. Approximation promotes tonic hold-

ing of the muscles. In the prone on elbows position, the patient should practice weight shifting to the right, left, forward, and backward. The patient should be encouraged to maintain good alignment and to avoid shoulder sagging as she exercises in this position.

Once the patient can maintain the position, she can progress to other exercises that will increase proximal control and stability. Alternating isometrics and rhythmic stabilization can be performed. To perform alternating isometrics, the patient should be instructed to hold the desired position as the assistant applies manual resistance to the right or left, forward or backward. Intervention 7–7A illustrates this exercise. With rhythmic stabilization, the patient performs simultaneous isometric contractions of agonist and antagonist patterns as the therapist provides a rotational force. Intervention 7–7B shows an assistant who is performing this activity with a patient. Other activities that can be performed in a prone on elbows position include lifting of one arm, unilateral reaching activities, and serratus strengthening (Intervention 7–8A). To strengthen the serratus, the patient is instructed to push her elbows down into the mat and to tuck the chin while lifting and rounding her shoulders. For patients with paraplegia, the assistant can provide instruction on prone pushups, as depicted in Intervention 7–8B.

Prone to Supine

From a prone on elbows position, the patient can make the transition back to supine. The patient shifts weight onto one elbow and extends and rotates his

FIGURE 7–8 ▮ The elbows should be positioned directly under the shoulders when the patient is in prone on elbows. The assistant is applying a downward force (approximation) through the shoulder to promote tonic holding and stabilization of the shoulder musculature.

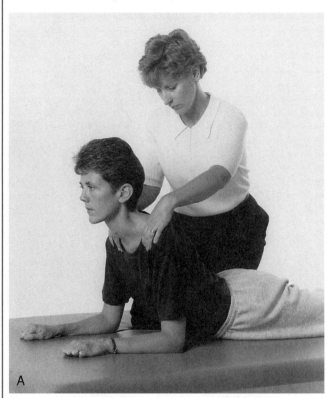

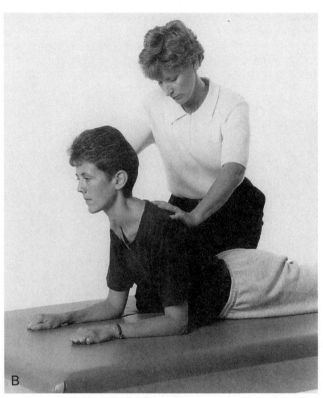

A. The assistant is performing alternating isometrics with the patient in a prone on elbows position. Force is being applied in a posterior direction as the patient is asked to hold the position.

B. Rhythmic stabilization performed in a prone on elbows position. The assistant is applying simultaneous isometric contractions to both agonists and antagonists. As the patient holds the position, a gradual counterrotational force is applied by the assistant.

Intervention 7–8 ▮ OTHER SCAPULAR STRENGTHENING EXERCISES

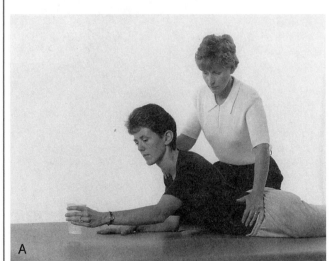

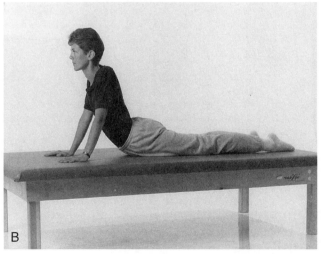

A. The patient reaches for a functional object. The assistant stabilizes the weight-bearing shoulder to prevent collapse.

B. The patient with paraplegia performs a prone pressup.

205

Intervention 7-9 ❚ SUPINE TO SUPINE ON ELBOWS

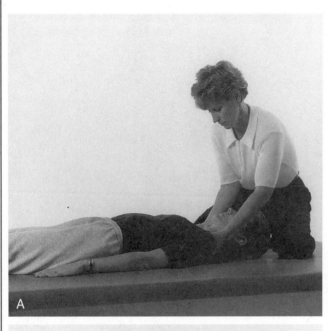

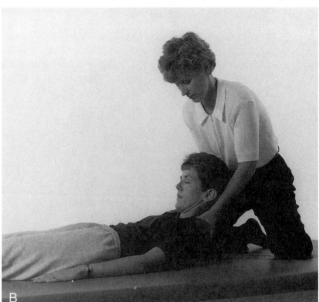

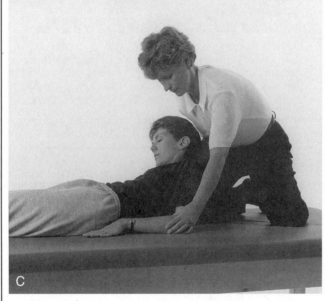

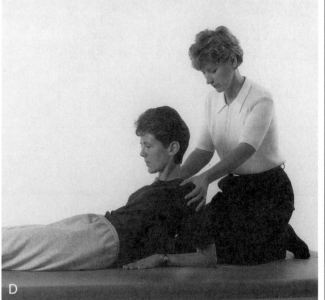

A. The patient flexes her chin to initiate the activity.

B. With her hands on the patient's shoulders, the assistant helps to lift the patient's upper trunk.

C. The head is used to initiate a weight shift to the right so that the left elbow can be brought back.

D. The final position.

head in the same direction. As he does this, the patient "throws" the unweighted upper extremity behind him. The momentum created by this maneuver facilitates the roll back to the patient's back.

Supine on Elbows

The purpose of the supine on elbows position is to assist the patient with bed mobility and to prepare him

to attain long sitting. Patients with innervation at the C5 and C6 levels probably need assistance to achieve the supine on elbows position. Intervention 7–9 depicts a physical therapist assistant who is helping the patient making the transition from the supine position to the supine on elbows position. Several different techniques can be used to assist the patient in learning to achieve this position. A pillow or bolster placed under the patient's upper back can assist the patient

Intervention 7–10 ▌ INDEPENDENT SUPINE TO SUPINE ON ELBOWS

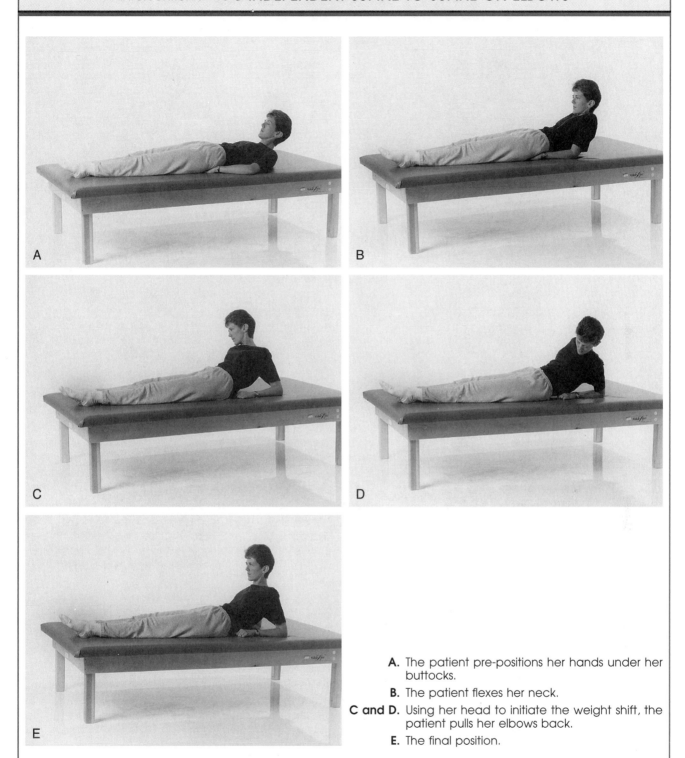

A. The patient pre-positions her hands under her buttocks.

B. The patient flexes her neck.

C and D. Using her head to initiate the weight shift, the patient pulls her elbows back.

E. The final position.

with this activity. This technique helps to acclimate the patient to the position and assists the patient with stretching the anterior shoulder capsule. As the patient is able to assume more independence with the transition from a supine position to supine on elbows, the assistant can have the patient hook his thumbs into his pockets or belt loops or position his hands under his buttocks. Intervention 7–10 illustrates this approach. As the patient does this, he stabilizes himself with one arm as he pulls with the other, using the reverse action of the biceps. The physical therapist or physical therapist assistant may need to position the

Intervention 7–11 ▌ SUPINE ON ELBOWS TO THE LONG-SITTING POSITION

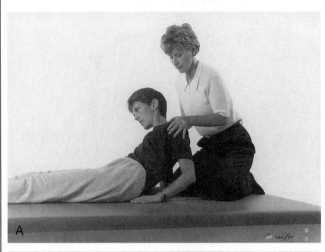

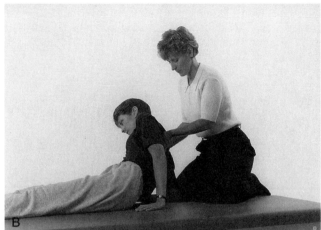

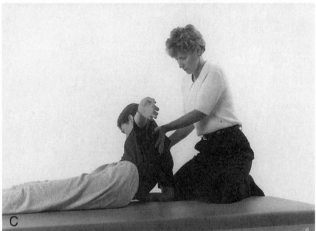

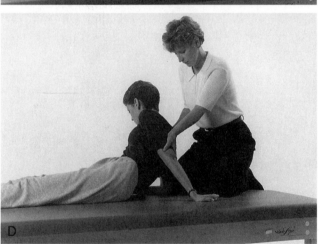

A and B. In supine on elbows, the patient shifts her weight to one side. The patient's head should follow the movement.

C. With her weight on one elbow, the patient throws her other upper extremity behind her buttocks into extension and external rotation.

D. Once the weight is shifted onto the extremity, the elbow is biomechanically locked into extension because of the bony alignment of the joint when it is positioned in shoulder external rotation and then depressed.

patient's arms at the end of the movement. Once the patient is in the supine on elbows position, work can begin on strengthening the shoulder extensors and scapular adductors. Activities to accomplish this include weight shifting in the position, making the transition back to prone, and progressing to long sitting. Supine pullups can also be practiced. While the patient is in a supine position, the assistant holds the patient's supinated forearms in front of the body and has the patient pull up into a modified sit-up position. This exercise helps to strengthen both the shoulder flexors and the biceps. From supine on elbows, the patient can roll to prone by shifting weight onto one

elbow, looking in the same direction, and reaching across the body with the other upper extremity. This maneuver provides the patient with another mechanism to move into prone.

Long Sitting

Long sitting can also be achieved from a supine on elbows position. Long sitting is sitting with both lower extremities extended and is a functional posture for patients with tetraplegia. This position allows patients to perform lower extremity dressing, skin inspection, and self–range of motion. It may be necessary for the assistant to help the patient achieve the position ini-

Intervention 7–11 ▌ SUPINE ON ELBOWS TO THE LONG-SITTING POSITION
Continued

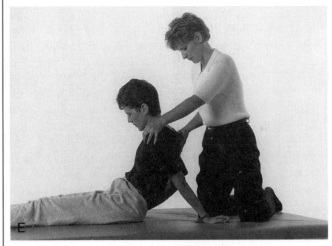

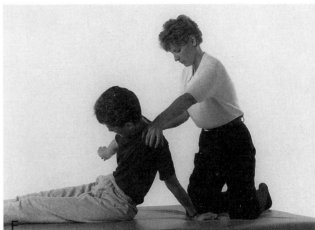

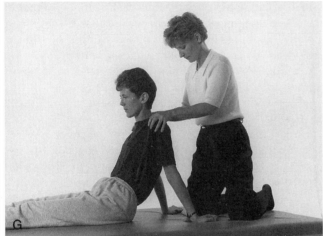

E. The patient shifts her weight back to the midline.

F. Once the patient feels that she has the elbow locked on one side, she repeats the motion with the other upper extremity.

G. The final position.

tially. The technique to assume long sitting is as follows:

Step 1. In the supine on elbows position, the patient shifts her weight to one side. The patient's head should follow the movement (Intervention 7–11A and B).

Step 2. With the weight on one elbow, the patient throws her other upper extremity behind her buttocks into extension and external rotation (Intervention 7–11C). Once weight is shifted onto the extremity, the elbow is biomechanically locked into extension because of the bony nature of the joint when it is aligned in shoulder external rotation and then is depressed (Intervention 7–11D and E).

Step 3. The patient shifts her weight back to the midline (Intervention 7–11E).

Step 4. Once the patient feels that she has the elbow locked on one side, she repeats the motion with the other upper extremity (Intervention 7–11F and G).

Special Note. The fingers should be maintained in flexion (tenodesis) during performance of functional activities to avoid overstretching the finger flexors. This is illustrated in Intervention 7–11F and G.

Initially, the physical therapist assistant may need to help the patient with the movement and placement of the upper extremities. Patients who lack the necessary range of motion in their shoulders have difficulty in performing this maneuver. As mentioned earlier, patients who have developed elbow flexion contractures are not able to achieve and maintain this position because of their inability to extend their elbows passively.

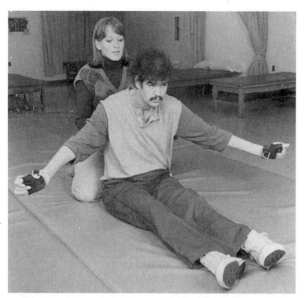

FIGURE 7–9 ■ Balance activities should always be emphasized in the long-sitting position to prepare the patient for numerous functional activities. (From Buchanan LE, Nawoczenski DA. Spinal Cord Injury and Management Approaches. Baltimore, Williams & Wilkins, 1987.)

Patients who do not possess at least 90 to 100 degrees of passive straight leg raising should refrain from performing long-sitting activities. Failure to possess adequate hamstring range of motion causes patients to overstretch the low back and ultimately decrease their functional abilities.

Patients with injuries at C7 and below also use the long-sitting position. However, it is easier for these patients because they possess triceps innervation and may be able to maintain active elbow extension. Once the patient has achieved the long-sitting position with the elbows anatomically locked and is comfortable in the position, additional treatment activities can be practiced. Manual resistance can be applied to the shoulders to foster co-contraction around the shoulder joint and to promote scapular stability. Rhythmic stabilization and alternating isometrics are also useful to improve stability. If the patient has triceps innervation, the assistant will want to work with the patient on the ability, eventually, to sit in a long-sitting position without upper extremity support (Fig. 7–9). The patient moves his hands from behind the hips, to the hips, and finally to forward at the knees. Hamstring range is essential for the patient to be able to perform this transition safely. Once the patient can put his hands in front of his hips and close to his knees, he can try maintaining the position with only one hand for support and eventually with no hands. In this position, the patient learns to perform self–range of motion and self-care activities. The assistant guards the patient carefully during the performance of this activity. In addition, the patient's vital signs should be monitored to minimize the possibility of orthostatic hypotension or autonomic dysreflexia.

A goal for the patient with triceps function is to do a pushup with the upper extremities in a long-sitting position (Intervention 7–12). This activity usually requires that the patient have at least fair-plus strength in the triceps. To complete the movement, the patient straightens her elbows and depresses the shoulders to

---

Intervention 7–12 ▌ **PUSHUP IN THE LONG-SITTING POSITION**

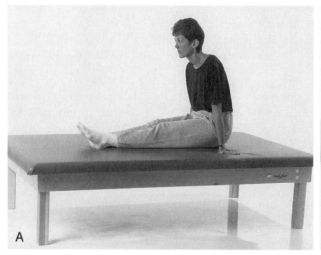
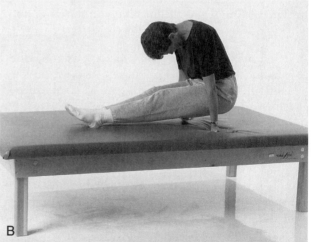

The patient uses the head-hips relationship to assist with lifting the buttocks.

lift the buttocks. The patient should flex her head and upper trunk to facilitate a greater rise of the buttocks. Tightness in the low back also allows this to occur. The patient uses this technique to move herself around on the mat. The same upper extremity movement is used for transfers in and out of the wheelchair and as a means for the patient to perform independent pressure relief.

Transfers

Transfers into and out of the wheelchair are an important skill for the patient with an SCI. Patients with high cervical injuries (C1 through C4 level) are completely dependent in their transfers. A two-person lift, a dependent sit-pivot transfer, or a Hoyer lift must be used.

Preparation Phase

Prior to the transfer, the patient and the wheelchair must be positioned in the correct place. The wheelchair should be positioned parallel to the mat or the bed. The brakes must be locked and the wheelchair

leg rests removed. A gait belt must be applied to the patient before the assistant begins the activity.

Two-Person Lift

A two-person lift may be necessary for the patient with high tetraplegia. This type of transfer is illustrated in Intervention 7–13.

Sit-Pivot Transfer

The technique for a dependent sit-pivot transfer is as follows:

Step 1. The patient must be forward in the wheelchair to perform the transfer safely. The assistant shifts the patient's weight from side to side to move him forward. Often, placing one's hands under the patient's buttocks in the area of the ischial tuberosities is the best way to assist the patient with weight shifting. The assistant must monitor the position of the patient's trunk carefully as he performs this maneuver because the patient does not possess adequate trunk control to maintain trunk stability. Once the patient is forward in the wheelchair, the armrest closest to the mat or bed should be removed.

Intervention 7–13 ▌ TWO-PERSON LIFT

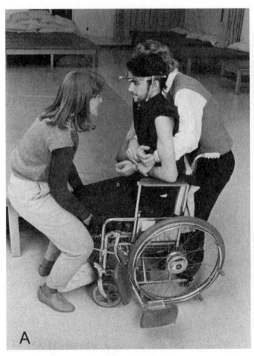 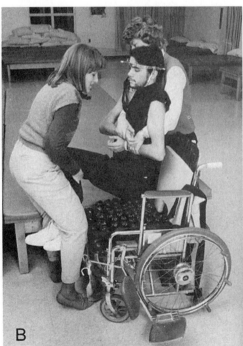

Care must be taken so that the patient's buttocks clear the wheel during the two-person lift. Good body mechanics are equally important for the persons assisting with this type of transfer.

From Buchanan LE, Nawoczenski DA. Spinal Cord Injury and Management Approaches. Baltimore, Williams & Wilkins, 1987.

Intervention 7–14 ▌ SIT-PIVOT TRANSFER

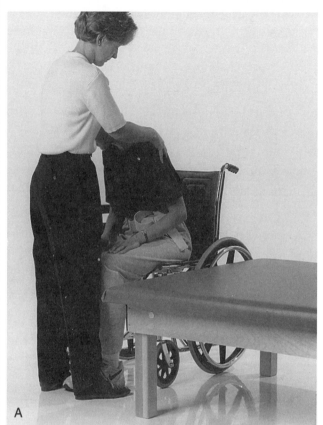

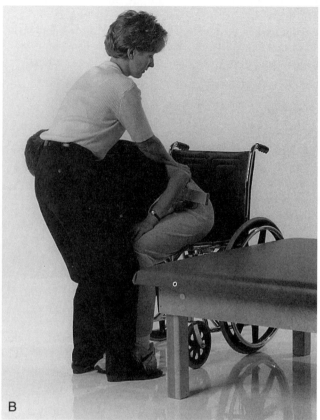

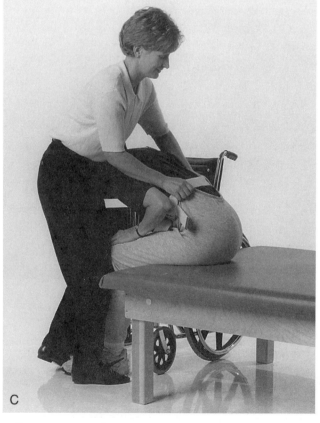

A. The assistant helps the patient to scoot forward in the wheelchair.

B. The patient is flexed forward over the assistant's hip.

C. The patient's hips and buttocks are moved to the transfer surface.

Step 2. The assistant then flexes the patient's trunk over the patient's feet. The assistant brings the patient forward over the assistant's hip that is farther away from the wheelchair. This maneuver allows the assistant to be close to the area where most individuals carry the greatest amount of body weight. The assistant also guards the patient's knees between his or her knees.

Step 3. A second person should be positioned on the mat table or behind the patient to assist with moving the posterior hips and trunk.

Step 4. On a specified count, the assistant in front of the patient shifts the patient's weight forward and moves the patient's hips and buttocks to the transfer surface. The position of the patient's feet must also be monitored to avoid possible injury. Generally, pre-positioning the feet in the direction that the patient will assume at the end of the transfer is beneficial.

Step 5. Once the patient is on the mat, the assistant in front of the patient aligns the patient to an upright position. The assistant does not, however, take his or her hands off the patient because of the patient's lack of trunk control. Without necessary physical assistance, a patient with tetraplegia could lose his balance and fall. Intervention 7–14 shows a physical therapist assistant performing a sit-pivot transfer with a patient.

Modified Stand-Pivot Transfer

A modified stand-pivot transfer can also be used with some patients who present with incomplete injuries and lower extremity innervation. Additionally, patients with lower extremity extensor tone may be able to perform a modified stand-pivot transfer. The steps in completion of this transfer are similar to the ones described earlier and the techniques discussed in Chapter 5. Intervention 7–15 illustrates this type of transfer.

Airlift

The airlift transfer is depicted in Intervention 7–16 and may be the preferred type of transfer for patients with significant lower extremity extensor tone. The patient's legs are flexed and rest on the clinician's thighs. The patient is then rocked out of the wheelchair to the transfer surface. The therapist must maintain proper body mechanics and lift with his or her legs to avoid possible injury to the low back. This type of transfer is often preferred because it prevents shear forces on the buttocks.

Intervention 7–15 ▮ MODIFIED STAND-PIVOT TRANSFER

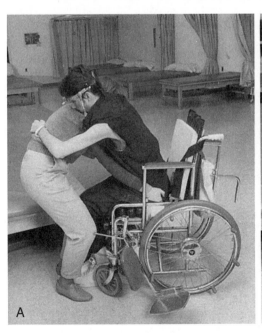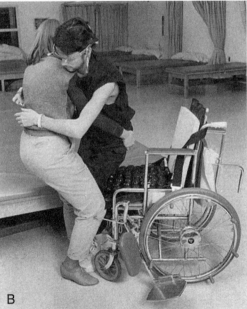

Leverage principles and good body mechanics facilitate this stand-pivot transfer. The patient may assist with this transfer by holding his or her arms around the person who is transferring.

From Buchanan LE, Nawoczenski DA. Spinal Cord Injury and Management Approaches. Baltimore, Williams & Wilkins, 1987.

Intervention 7–16 ▌ AIRLIFT TRANSFER

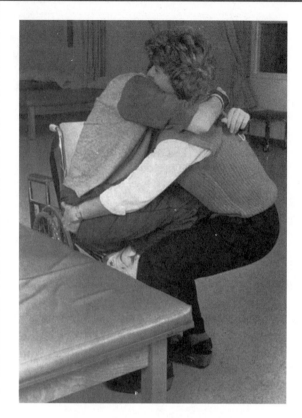

In the airlift transfer, the patient's flexed legs rest on or between the therapist's thighs. The patient can be "rocked" out of the chair and lifted onto the bed or mat. All the patient's weight is carried through the therapist's legs and not the back.

From Buchanan LE, Nawoczenski DA. Spinal Cord Injury and Management Approaches. Baltimore, Williams & Wilkins, 1987.

Sliding Board Transfers

A sliding board can also be used to assist with transfers. The chair should be pre-positioned at a 45-degree angle. As the patient's trunk is flexed forward over his knees, the assistant can place the sliding board under the patient's hip that is closer to the mat table. The assistant may need to lift up the patient's buttocks to assist with board placement. Clinicians must be aware of the patient's active trunk control. Many of these individuals are not able to maintain their trunks in an upright position. Once the board is in the proper position, it helps support the patient's body weight during the transfer. The board also provides the patient's skin some protection during the transfer. The patient's buttocks may be bumped or scraped on various wheelchair parts. This can be dangerous to the patient and can lead to skin breakdown. Intervention 7–17 illustrates a patient who is performing a sliding board transfer with the help of the physical therapist assistant.

Although patients with high cervical injuries are not able to participate in the transfer actively, they must be able to explain the necessary steps to others.

A patient with C6 tetraplegia has the potential to transfer independently using a sliding board. Although the patient has the potential for this type of independence, patients with C6 tetraplegia often use the assistance of a caregiver or family member because of the time and energy involved with transfers. To be independent with sliding board transfers from the wheelchair, the patient must be able to manipulate the wheelchair parts and position the sliding board. Extensions applied to the wheelchair's brakes are common and allow the patient to use wrist movements to maneuver these wheelchair parts. Legrests and armrests may also be equipped with these extensions to provide the patient with a mechanism to negotiate these wheelchair parts independently.

To position the board, the patient can use tightness in the finger flexors to move the board to the proper location. The patient can also place his wrist at the end of the board and use wrist extension to move the board to the right place. Moving the leg that is closer to the mat table by lifting it up under the thigh with the back of the wrist and crossing it over the other leg helps to facilitate board placement under the buttocks and thighs. Loops can be sewn onto the patient's pants to make this easier. Once the board is in position, the patient can reposition his legs by lifting the thigh, as previously described (Intervention 7–18).

Several different transfer techniques can be used for the patient with C6 tetraplegia. When working with this type of patient, one must find the easiest type of transfer for the patient. Trial and error and having the patient engage in active problem solving to complete movement tasks work best. Too often, physical therapists and physical therapist assistants provide patients with all the answers to their movement questions. If a patient is allowed to experiment and to try some things on his own with supervision, the results are often better.

Push-Pull Transfer

Another type of transfer the patient with C6 tetraplegia may perform requires that she rotate her head and trunk to the opposite direction of the transfer while still in the wheelchair. Once the patient is in this position, she flexes both elbows and places them on the wheelchair armrest. The patient then flexes her trunk forward and pushes down on her upper extremities, thus scooting over onto the mat or bed. Some patients may also use the head to assist with the transfer. The patient can place her forehead on the armrest to provide additional trunk stability while she at-

Intervention 7–17 ▌ SLIDING BOARD TRANSFER

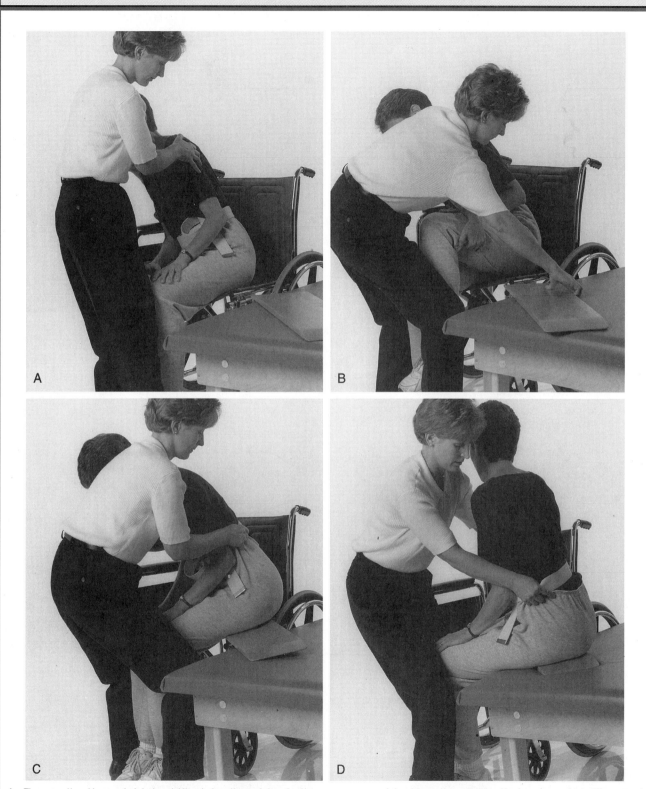

A. The patient's weight is shifted to the side farther from the transfer surface.

B. The patient's thigh is lifted to position the board. The assistant remains in front of the patient, blocking the patient's lower extremities and trunk.

C and D. The patient is transferred over to the support surface.

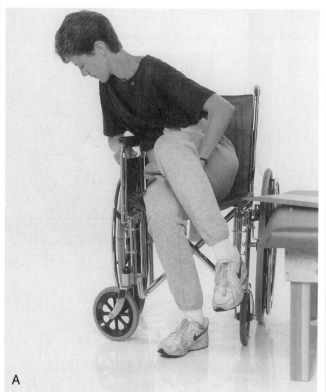

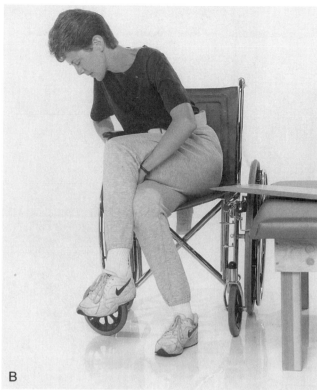

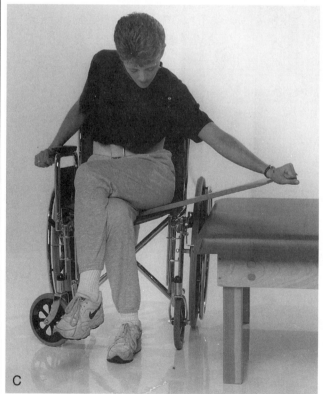

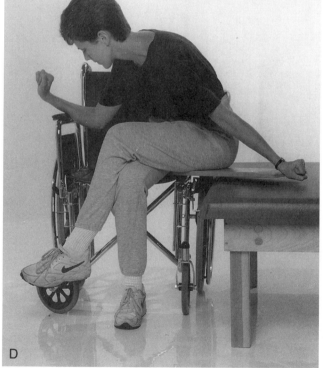

A and B. The patient prepares to position the sliding board by moving the leg closest to the mat table over the other leg.

C. The patient positions the sliding board under the buttock of the leg closest to the mat table.

D. Pushing with the forearm farther from the table against the wheelchair arm and pushing down on the end of the sliding board with the other arm, the patient lifts herself off the wheelchair seat.

Intervention 7-18 ▌ INDEPENDENT SLIDING BOARD TRANSFER *Continued*

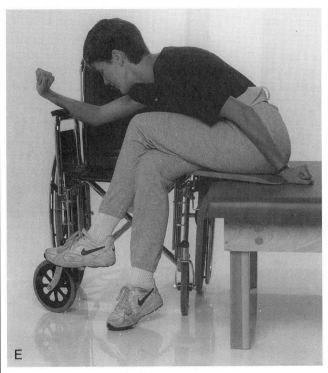

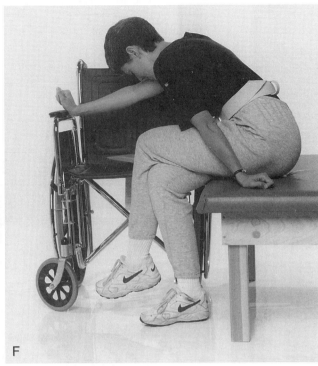

E. The patient then slides her buttocks down the length of the board until she is on the table.

F. Continuing to push off the wheelchair arm and using the other arm on the mat table, the patient scoots off the board and onto the table itself.

tempts to move from the wheelchair. Once the patient is on the mat table, she hooks her arm under her knee and uses the sternal fibers of the pectoralis major to extend the trunk.

Prone on Elbows Transfer

The modified prone on elbows transfer is another method. After removing the wheelchair armrest, the patient rotates his trunk to the mat table. The patient then positions his lower extremities onto the support surface. The patient can use the back of his hand or Velcro loops attached to his pants to lift the lower extremities up onto the support surface. Once the patient's lower extremities are up on the bed, the patient actually rolls out of the wheelchair. The patient can move to a side lying position or can roll all the way over to a prone on elbows position.

Lateral Pushup Transfer

If the patient possesses triceps function, the potential for independent transfers with and without the sliding board is greatly enhanced. As stated earlier, a patient with a C7 injury and good triceps strength should be able to perform a lateral pushup transfer without a sliding board. Initially, when instructing a patient in this type of transfer, the assistant should use a sliding board. The patient positions the board under the posterior thigh. With both upper extremities in a relatively extended position, the patient pushes down with his arms and lifts his buttocks up off the sliding board. The patient's feet and lower extremities should be pre-positioned prior to the start of the transfer. Both feet should be placed on the floor and rotated away from the direction of the transfer. The patient moves slowly, using the board as a place to rest if necessary. As the strength in the patient's upper extremities improves, the patient will be able to complete the transfer faster and will not need to use the sliding board. Patients with high-level paraplegia also perform lateral pushup transfers. Not until a patient possesses fair strength in the lower extremities are stand-pivot transfers possible.

Intermediate Treatment Interventions

Mat Activities

A major component of the patient's treatment plan at this stage of rehabilitation includes mat activities.

Mat activities are chosen to assist the patient in increasing strength and in improving functional mobility skills. The functional mobility activities previously discussed, including rolling, supine to prone, supine to long sitting, and prone to supine, continue to be practiced until the patient masters the tasks. Other, more advanced mat activities are now discussed in more detail.

Independent Self–Range of Motion

A patient with C7 tetraplegia should also be instructed in self–range of motion to the lower extremities. Assuming long sitting without upper extremity support is a prerequisite for becoming independent in self–range of motion. The first exercise that should be addressed is hamstring stretching. Two methods can be employed. The patient can assume a long-sitting position and can lean forward toward his toes. The patient may rest his elbows on his knees to assist in keeping the lower extremities straight. The maintenance of lumbar lordosis is important to prevent overstretching of the low back muscles (Intervention 7–19).

The second method entails having the patient place his hands under his knee and pull the knee back as he leans backward to a supine position. With one

---

Intervention 7–19 ▍ HAMSTRING STRETCHING

A. When stretching the hamstrings in the long-sitting position, the patient may rest her elbows on her knees to assist in keeping the lower extremities straight.

B to E. Stretching the hamstrings in the supine position.

hand at the anterior knee and the other at the ankle, the patient raises the leg while trying to keep the knee as straight as possible. The patient can then try to pull the lower extremity closer to the chest to achieve a better stretch. If the patient does not possess adequate hand function to grasp, he can use the back of his wrist or forearm to complete the activity. Intervention 7–19 shows a patient who is performing hamstring stretching.

The gluteus maximus should also be stretched. In a long-sitting position with one upper extremity used for balance, the patient positions his free hand under the knee on the same side. The patient then pulls the knee up toward his chest and holds the position. Once the lower extremity is in the desired position, the patient can bring the volar surface of the forearm to the anterior shin and can pull the leg toward the patient. This maneuver gives an added stretch to the gluteus maximus (Intervention 7–20).

Patients must also spend some time each day stretching their hip flexors. This is especially important for individuals who spend a majority of their day sitting. The most effective way to stretch the hip flexors is for patients to assume a prone position. Patients should be advised to lie prone for at least 20 to 30 minutes every day. Patients can do this in their beds or on the floor if they are able to transfer into and out of their wheelchairs.

To stretch the hip abductors, adductors, and internal and external rotators, the patient should assume a long-sitting position as described earlier. The knee is brought up into a flexed position. With the nonsupporting hand, the patient should slowly move the lower extremity medially and laterally. The patient can maintain the arm under the knee or can place his hand on the medial or lateral surface of the knee to support the lower extremity (Intervention 7–21).

Stretching of the ankle plantar flexors is also necessary. The patient supports himself with the same upper extremity as the foot he is stretching. With the knee flexed approximately 90 degrees, the patient places either the dorsal or volar surface of the opposite hand on the plantar surface of the foot. Placement of the hand depends on the amount of hand function the patient possesses. Patients with strong wrist extensors can use motion at the wrist to stretch the ankle into dorsiflexion slowly (Intervention 7–22). Patients with paraplegia who possess complete wrist and finger function are able to complete this activity without difficulty. Stretching the ankle plantar flexors with the knee flexed stretches only the soleus muscle. The patient can stretch the gastrocnemius in a long-sitting position with a folded towel placed along the plantar surface of the foot. The ends of the towel are pulled to provide a prolonged stretch.

Advanced Treatment Interventions

Advanced Mat Activities

For the patient with paraplegia, practicing more advanced mat exercises is also appropriate. In a short-sitting or long-sitting position, the patient can practice

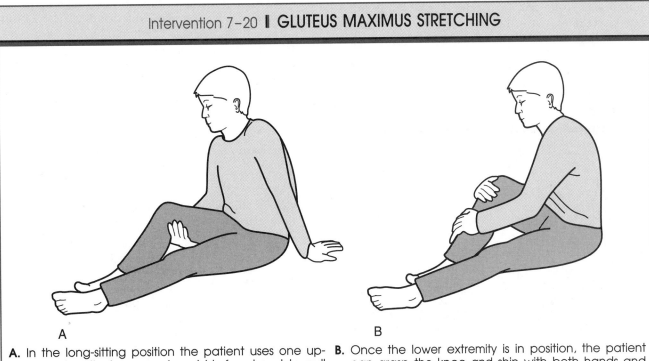

Intervention 7–20 ▌ GLUTEUS MAXIMUS STRETCHING

A. In the long-sitting position the patient uses one upper extremity for support and his free hand to pull the knee on the same side up toward his chest.

B. Once the lower extremity is in position, the patient can grasp the knee and shin with both hands and pull the leg toward his trunk.

Intervention 7–21 ▌ STRETCHING THE HIP ROTATORS

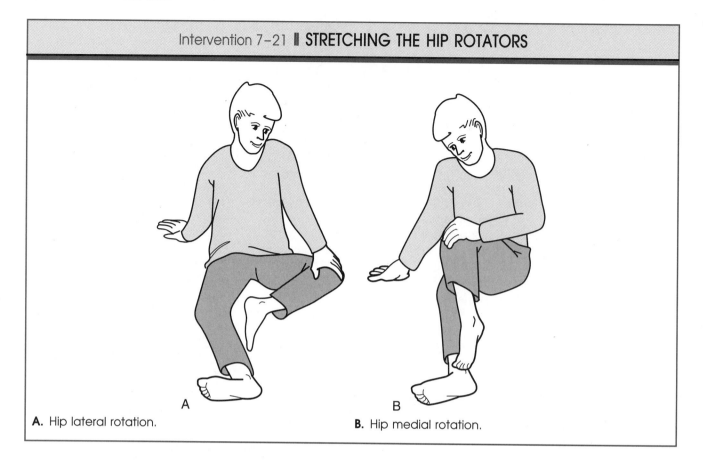

A. Hip lateral rotation.

B. Hip medial rotation.

reaching and other functional upper extremity tasks. Other advanced activities that can be performed include sitting swing-through, hip swayers, trunk twisting and raising, prone pushups, forward reaching in quadruped, creeping, and tall-kneeling. The techniques used to execute each of these activities are as follows.

Intervention 7–22 ▌ ANKLE DORSIFLEXION

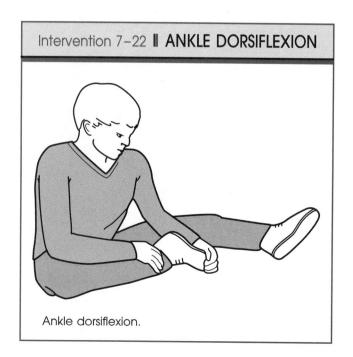

Ankle dorsiflexion.

Sitting Swing-Through

Step 1. The patient assumes a long-sitting position with upper extremity support. The patient's hands should be approximately 6 inches behind the patient's hips.
Step 2. The patient depresses the shoulders and extends the elbows. The buttocks should be lifted off the support surface.
Step 3. The patient swings the hips back between his hands.

Hip Swayer

Step 1. The patient assumes a long-sitting position with upper extremity support.
Step 2. The patient places one hand as close to his hip as possible; the other hand should be placed approximately 6 inches away from the other hip.
Step 3. The patient raises his buttocks and moves his hips toward the hand that is farther away.
Step 4. The patient travels sideways across the mat.
Step 5. The patient should practice moving in both directions.

Trunk Twisting and Raising

Step 1. The patient assumes a side sitting position.
Step 2. The patient places both hands near the hip that is closer to the support surface.

Step 3. The patient straightens his elbows to raise the hips to a semi-quadruped position and then lowers himself to the mat.

Step 4. The activity should also be practiced on the opposite side.

Prone Pushups. In a prone position with the hands positioned next to the shoulders, the patient extends the elbows and lifts the upper body off the support surface.

Forward Reaching

Step 1. The patient assumes a four-point position. Some patients may need assistance into the position. This can be accomplished by having the patient assume the prone position and facilitating a posterior weight shift at the patient's pelvis while the patient extends his elbows. Assistance may be needed. With a gait belt around the patient's low waist or hips, the assistant, in a standing position, straddles the patient and pulls the patient's hips up as the patient pushes.

Step 2. If the patient is having difficulty in maintaining the four-point position, a bolster or other object can be placed under the patient's abdomen to maintain the position. Care must be taken with those patients who have increased lower extremity extensor tone; if the patient is unable to flex the hips and knees, the patient's lower extremities can spasm into extension.

Step 3. Once the patient can maintain the quadruped position, the patient can practice anterior, posterior, medial, and lateral weight shifts, as well as alternating isometrics and rhythmic stabilization.

Step 4. The patient can also practice forward reaching with one upper extremity while maintaining his balance.

Step 5. If the patient possesses innervation of the trunk musculature, the patient can practice arching the back and letting it sag.

Creeping. A patient's ability to creep depends on lower extremity muscle innervation. Strength in the hip flexors is also needed to perform this activity.

Step 1. The patient assumes a quadruped position.

Step 2. The patient alternately advances one upper extremity followed by the opposite lower extremity.

Tall-Kneeling

Step 1. The patient assumes a quadruped position.

Step 2. Using a chair, bench, or bolster, the patient pulls up to a tall-kneeling position. The hips must remain forward while the patient rests on the Y ligaments.

Step 3. Initially, the patient works on maintaining balance in the position.

Step 4. Once the patient can maintain his balance, the patient can work on alternating isometrics, rhythmic stabilization, and reaching activities.

Step 5. The patient can advance to kneeling-height crutches. The patient can balance in the position with the crutches, lift one crutch, advance both crutches forward, or pull both crutches back.

The functional significance of these activities is widespread. The sitting swing-through, hip swayer, and prone pushup exercises work to improve upper extremity strength necessary for transfers and assisted ambulation. The trunk twisting exercise helps to improve the patient's trunk control for transfers, including those from the wheelchair to the floor. Unilateral reaching in the quadruped position assists the patient in developing upper extremity strength and coordination and improves the patient's ability to transfer from the floor into the wheelchair. Creeping on all fours helps to develop the patient's trunk and lower extremity muscle control. It is also a useful position for the patient to be able to assume while on the floor. Tall-kneeling promotes the development of trunk control. It can be used as a position of transition for patients as they transfer from the floor back into their wheelchairs, and it serves as a preambulation activity.

Transfers

Wheelchair-to-Floor Transfers

Patients with paraplegia should be instructed how to fall while in their wheelchairs and how to get back into the chair if for some reason they are displaced. In addition, the floor is a good place to perform hip flexor stretching. In the clinic, the physical therapist or physical therapist assistant will initiate practice of this skill by lowering the patient to the floor as shown in Figure 7–10. The patient should be instructed to tuck his head and to keep his arms in the wheelchair. The patient must be cautioned against trying to soften his fall by using his arms. Extension of the upper

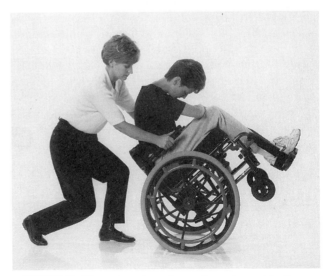

FIGURE 7–10 ■ The assistant lowers the patient to the floor.

extremities can result in wrist fractures. The patient may also want to place one of his upper extremities over his knees to prevent the lower extremities from coming up and hitting the patient in the face.

Once the patient is on the floor, he has several options to get back up. It may be easiest for the patient to right the wheelchair and then to transfer back into it. If the patient can position himself in a supported kneeling position in front of the wheelchair, he can pull himself back into the wheelchair, as depicted in Intervention 7–23. If the patient possesses adequate upper extremity strength and range of motion, he can back up to the wheelchair in a long-sitting position, depress the shoulders, and lift the buttocks back into the wheelchair. The patient's hands are positioned near the buttocks. Flexion of the neck while attempting this maneuver aids in elevating the buttocks through the head-hips relationship. Although this type of transfer is possible, many patients do not have enough strength to complete the transition successfully. In the clinic, one can practice this by using a small step stool or several mats. In a long-sitting position, the patient transfers first to the step stool and then back up into the wheelchair. Intervention 7–24 illustrates a patient who is performing a transfer from the floor back into the wheelchair. Rotating the wheelchair casters forward, the patient places one hand on the caster and the other on the wheelchair seat and pushes upward.

Righting the Wheelchair

Individuals with good upper body strength may be able to right a tipped chair while remaining in it. To be successful with this activity, the individual must be able to push down with the arm in contact with the floor, use the head and upper trunk to shift weight, and remember to push down on the hand in contact with the wheelchair instead of pulling on it. Intervention 7–25 shows an individual who is completing this activity.

Caution. A word of caution must be expressed during the performance of these activities. Patients who lack sensation in the lower extremities and buttocks must monitor the position of their lower extremities during activity performance. Patients can accidentally bump themselves on sharp wheelchair parts, and these injuries can cause skin tears during these activities.

Although patients with tetraplegia cannot complete this activity independently, they should practice the task. These individuals must be able to instruct others in ways to assist them should this situation occur in the community.

Advanced Wheelchair Skills

Patients with innervation and strength in the finger muscles should receive instruction in advanced wheelchair skills. Attaining wheelies and ascending and de-

scending curbs should be taught so that the patient can be as independent in the community as possible.

Wheelies

Before the patient can learn to perform a wheelie independently, the patient must be able to find his balance point in a tipped wheelchair position (Fig. 7–11). The easiest way to do this is to tip the patient gently back onto the rear wheels. The assistant should find the point at which the wheelchair is most perfectly balanced. The patient must keep his back against the wheelchair back. The patient then grasps the hand rims. If the wheelchair begins to tip backward, the patient should be instructed to pull back slightly on the hand rims. If the front casters begin to fall forward, the patient should pull forward. Most patients initially overcompensate while learning to attain a balance point by leaning forward or pulling or pushing too much on the rims.

During these early stages of practice, you must guard the patient carefully. Standing behind the patient with your hands resting near the push handles of the wheelchair and standing near the backrest are the best places to spot the patient. Once the patient is able to maintain a wheelie with your assistance, the patient must learn to achieve the position independently. The patient must master this activity to negotiate curbs independently. To attain the wheelie position, have the patient push forward in his wheelchair. The patient then pulls back on the wheelchair rims and moves his shoulders backward against the back of the wheelchair. The quick forward movement of the chair, combined with the shifting of the patient's weight backward, causes the front casters of the wheelchair to pop up. With practice, the patient learns how

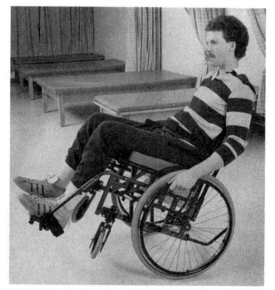

FIGURE 7–11 ■ Finding the balance point is a prerequisite to popping and maintaining a wheelie position. (From Buchanan LE, Nawoczenski DA. Spinal Cord Injury and Management Approaches. Baltimore, Williams & Wilkins, 1987.)

Intervention 7–23 ▌ TRANSFER TO WHEELCHAIR FROM TALL-KNEELING

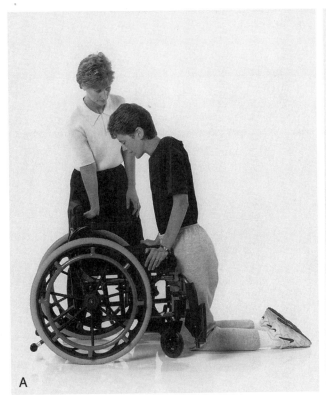

A

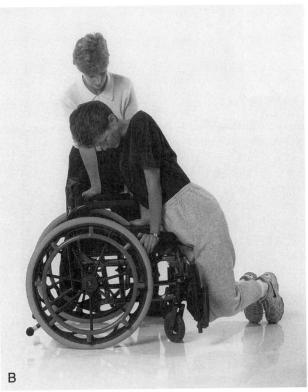

B

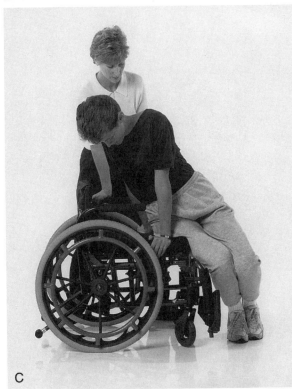

C

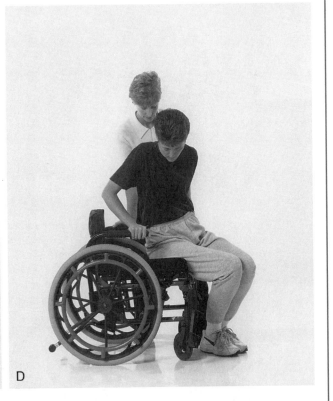

D

The patient pulls herself into the wheelchair from a tall-kneeling position. The patient must rotate over her hips to assume a sitting position. The sequence can be reversed to transfer out of the wheelchair.

much force is needed to attain the position. Eventually, the patient is able to achieve the wheelie position from a stationary or rolling position.

Ascending Ramps

A patient should ascend a ramp while she is in a forward position. The length and inclination must be

considered before the patient attempts to negotiate any ramp. When the patient is going up a ramp, instruct her to lean forward in the wheelchair. If the ramp is long, the patient uses long, strong pushes on the hand rims. If the ramp is relatively short and steep, the patient uses short, quick pushes to acceler-

---

Intervention 7–24 ▌ TRANSFER TO WHEELCHAIR FROM THE LONG-SITTING POSITION

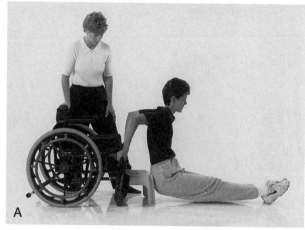

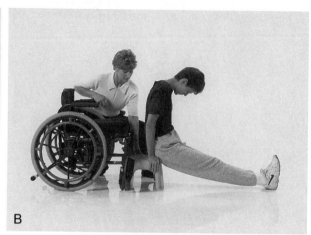

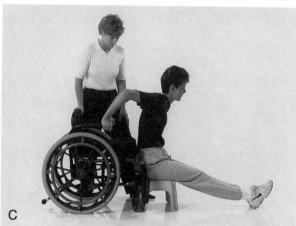

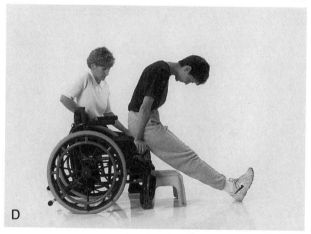

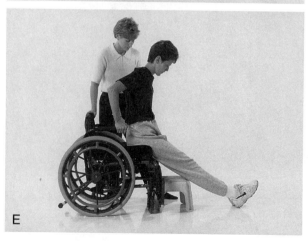

Transfers from the floor to the wheelchair can be practiced in the clinic with a small step stool.

A to C. The patient first transfers from the floor to the stool. The patient uses the head-hips relationship to lift the buttocks.

D and E. From the stool, the patient depresses her shoulders and lifts herself back into the wheelchair.

Intervention 7–25 ▌ RIGHTING THE WHEELCHAIR WHILE SEATED

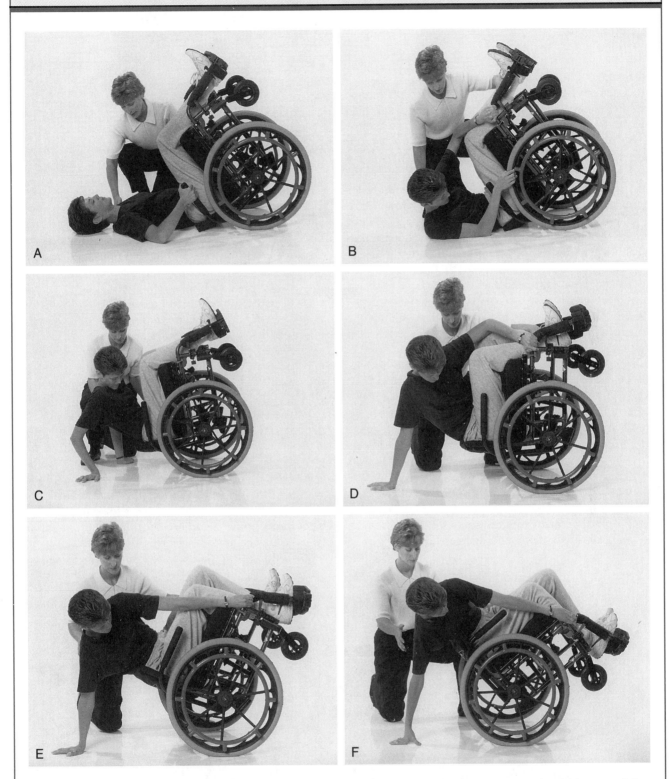

Some patients will be able to right their wheelchairs while they remain seated. Patients should be carefully guarded while they practice this skill.

ate forward. A grade aid on the wheelchair may be needed to prevent the chair from rolling backward between pushes. The grade aid serves as a type of braking mechanism to assist the patient to change hand position for the next push without rolling backward.

Descending Ramps

Patients should be encouraged to descend ramps with their wheelchairs facing forward. The patient is instructed to lean back in the wheelchair. The patient then places both hands on the hand rims or on the rims and wheels themselves. The movement of the wheelchair is controlled by friction applied to the hand rims and wheels by the patient. The patient must let the rims move equally between both hands to guarantee that the wheelchair will move in a straight path. Patients may also elect to apply the wheelchair brakes partially when descending ramps. Although this technique provides added friction to the wheels, it can cause mechanical failure to the braking mechanism of the wheelchair.

Ramps can also be descended with the patient in a backward position if the patient feels safer using this technique. The patient is instructed to line the wheelchair up evenly at the top of the ramp. The patient leans forward and grasps the hand rims near the brakes. The rims are then allowed to slide through the patient's hands during the descent. Patients must be careful at the bottom of the ramp because the casters and footrests can catch on the ramp and can cause the chair to tip backward. Figure 7–12 shows two methods for descending a ramp.

Ramps can also be ascended or descended in a diagonal or zigzag manner. Negotiating the ramp in a diagonal pattern decreases the tendency to roll down the ramp during ascent and decreases speed during descent.

Ascending a Curb

Going up a curb should always be performed with the patient in a forward direction. If the patient is going to be independent with this activity, he must be able to elevate his front casters. As the patient approaches the curb, he pops the front casters up with a wheelie. Once the casters have cleared the curb, the patient leans forward and pushes on the hand rims. Patients require a great deal of practice to master this activity because the timing of the individual components is extremely important and the completion of the task takes considerable muscle strength. Intervention 7–26A and B illustrates this skill.

Descending a Curb

It is often easiest to instruct patients to descend curbs backward; however, most clinicians agree that it does present more danger to the patient because of the risk from unseen traffic. In this technique, the patient backs the wheelchair down the curb. Again, the patient should lean forward and grasp the hand rims near the brakes on the chair. The position of the footplates must also be observed during performance of this activity. The footplates may catch on the curb as the chair goes down. If this occurs, the patient will need to lean back into the chair as the casters clear the curb (see Intervention 7-26C and D).

A second method of descending a curb is for the patient to go down in a forward position. Before the patient attempts this maneuver, he must be able to achieve a wheelie and roll forward while in a tilted position. As the patient approaches the curb, he pops a wheelie. The rear wheels are allowed to roll or bounce off the curb. Once the rear wheels have cleared the curb, the patient leans forward so that the front casters once again are on the ground. Care must be taken when patients learn this task because incorrect shifting of the patient's weight either too far back-

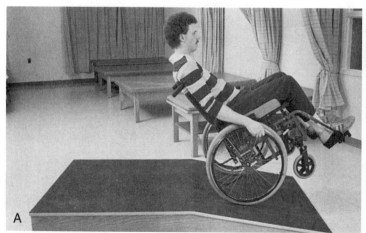 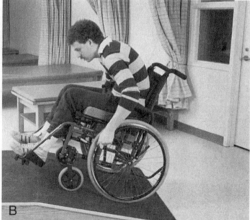

FIGURE 7–12 ▪ *A*, A person with good wheelchair mobility skills may be able to descend a ramp in a wheelie position. *B*, The safest method to descend a ramp is backward. The person must remember to lean forward while controlling the rear wheels. Ascending a ramp is performed in a similar manner. (From Buchanan LE, Nawoczenski DA. Spinal Cord Injury and Management Approaches. Baltimore, Williams & Wilkins, 1987.)

Intervention 7-26 ▎ ASCENDING AND DESCENDING A CURB

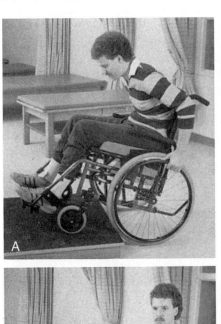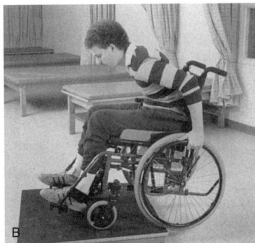
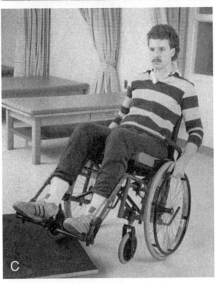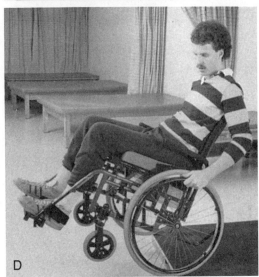

A and B. A person ascends a curb by "popping a wheelie" to place the front casters onto the curb, then pulls the rear wheels upward. Timing and good upper extremity strength are important for this activity.

C. Descending a curb may be performed by lowering the rear wheels evenly off the curb

and completing the activity by spinning the chair to clear the front casters.

D. A person may descend the curb forward in a controlled wheelie position.

From Buchanan LE, Nawoczenski DA. Spinal Cord Injury and Management Approaches. Baltimore, Williams & Wilkins, 1987.

ward or too far forward can cause the patient to fall out of the wheelchair. It is often easiest to begin training the patient to ascend and descend low training curbs. A 1- to 2-inch curb should be used initially with patients as they are trying to perfect these skills.

Powered Mobility

Patients with high-level tetraplegia need to master powered mobility. Often, vendors of wheelchairs pro-

vide power chairs for individuals on a trial basis. A portion of your treatment session should be devoted to assisting the patient with the operation of the power chair. A description of different types of power wheelchairs and of the operation of these units is outside the scope of this text. Clinicians are encouraged to work with facility equipment vendors to become knowledgeable about different wheelchairs and accessories available.

Wheelchair Cushions

Individuals who will be spending a considerable amount of time each day sitting in a wheelchair should also have some type of wheelchair cushion. Specialized cushions are available that reduce some of the pressure applied to the individual's buttocks. No cushion completely eliminates pressure, and individuals must perform some type of pressure relief throughout the day.

Cardiopulmonary Training

Cardiopulmonary training should also be included in the patient's rehabilitation program. Incentive spirometry and diaphragmatic strengthening should be continued to further maximize vital capacity. Endurance activities that can be incorporated into the patient's treatment plan include wheelchair propulsion for extended distances, upper extremity ergometry (arm bikes), swimming, and wheelchair aerobics. Although these activities improve the patient's endurance, the upper extremity muscles are smaller and are able to perform at a higher intensity for a shorter duration of time as compared to the muscles in the lower extremities. Therefore, these muscles fatigue more quickly (Decker and Hall, 1986; Morrison, 1994).

Patients with SCIs lack normal cardiovascular responses to exercise. However, training effects are still possible (Lewthwaite et al, 1994). Blood pressure, heart rate, and sweating responses are altered as a result of autonomic sympathetic dysfunction. Therefore, the use of target heart rate may not be an appropriate indicator of exercise training for patients with cervical and upper thoracic injuries. The Borg Perceived Exertion Scale, which measures how hard a person is exercising, is recommended to assess the patient's response and tolerance to aerobic exercise (Morrison, 1994). Aerobic training effects are possible for these patients. Exercise duration should be 20 to 60 minutes. If the patient is unable to tolerate 20 to 60 minutes of continuous activity, three to four short sessions totaling 20 to 40 minutes can be interspersed throughout the day. Evidence suggests that cardiovascular fitness can be achieved through several shorter bouts of exercise instead of one longer session (Lewthwaite et al, 1994). Frequency of exercise should be at least three times a week and not more than six times a week. A break of 1 to 2 days should be taken to allow for musculoskeletal recovery (Morrison, 1994).

Aquatic Therapy

Pool therapy can be a valuable addition to the patient's overall treatment plan. Water offers an excellent medium for exercising and moving without the effects of gravity and friction. Many facilities have warm water (92 to 96° F) therapeutic pools for their patients. The warm water provides physiologic effects including increased circulation, heart rate, and respiration rate and decreased blood pressure. In addition, general relaxation is usually accomplished with warm water immersion. These effects must be kept in mind as the physical therapist develops a pool program for the patient.

When designing a therapeutic pool program for a patient with an SCI, the physical therapist should consider the following as therapeutic benefits of this type of treatment intervention. Activities performed in the water will help to

1. Decrease abnormal muscle tone
2. Increase muscle strength
3. Increase range of motion
4. Improve pulmonary function
5. Provide opportunities for standing and weight bearing
6. Exercise muscles with fair-minus strength more easily
7. Decrease spasticity

Although most patients can exercise safely in the water, several situations have been identified as contraindications to aquatic programs. A patient with any of the following medical conditions should not be allowed to participate in the program: fever, infectious diseases, a tracheostomy, uncontrolled blood pressure, vital capacities less than 1 liter, urinary or bowel incontinence, and an open wound or sore that cannot be covered by a waterproof dressing. Patients with halo traction devices can be taken into the pool as long as their heads are kept out of the water and components of the device that retain water are replaced. Individuals with catheters may participate in pool programs if the drain tubes are clamped and storage bags are attached to the lower extremity (Giesecke, 1997).

Pool Program

Several logistic factors must be considered prior to taking the patient in the water for a treatment session. As stated previously, warm water is desirable. However, to accommodate the many patients who may need to use a therapeutic pool at a given facility, the temperature of water may be cooler. This factor must be considered when one works with patients with SCIs because their temperature regulation is often impaired. Different facilities have specific requirements regarding safety procedures that must be followed when working with the patient in the water. Previous water safety experience may be necessary. A minimum number of persons may also be needed in the pool area to ensure safety. To prepare the patient for the treatment session, the therapist or assistant must discuss the benefits of the program and describe a typical session. The patient's previous like or dislike of water must also be determined. Many individuals profoundly dislike water and may be apprehensive about the experience. Reassuring the patient should help. The patient should arrive for the treatment session in a swimsuit. Catheters should be clamped to avoid the potential for leakage. The patient should also be instructed to wear socks or elbow or knee pads, depending on the treatment activities to be performed. Because the patient may possess decreased sensation, areas that could become scraped during the session must be protected. Transfers into and out of the pool can occur in a number of different ways and depend on the type of equipment and facilities present. Frequently, a lift transfers the patient into the pool, or the pool may have a ramp, and entrance is in some type of wheelchair or shower chair. Once the patient is in the water, the assistant needs to guard the patient carefully. Patients with tetraplegia and paraplegia have decreased movement, proprioception, and light touch sensation. The patient may have difficulty maintaining his position in the water. At times, the lower extremities may float toward the surface of the water, and the assistant may have a difficult time keeping the patient's feet and lower extremities on the bottom of the pool in a weight-bearing position. Gentle pressure applied to the top of the patient's foot by the assistant's foot can help to alleviate this problem. Flotation vests are helpful and can be reassuring to the patient. Once the patient is more confident in the water, the vest can be removed.

Pool Exercises

Many pools have steps into them or an area where the assistant and the patient can sit down. This feature provides an excellent environment to work on upper extremity strengthening. With the upper extremity supported, the patient moves the arm in the water and uses the buoyancy of the water to complete range-of-motion exercises. The patient can also work on lifting the extremity out of the water, to provide more challenge to the activity. The anterior, middle, and posterior deltoids, as well as the pectoralis major and rhomboids, can be exercised in this position. Triceps strengthening can also occur in a gravity-neutralized or supported position. In addition to working on upper extremity strengthening, use of the sitting position serves to challenge the patient's sitting balance and trunk muscles that remain innervated. Alternating isometrics and rhythmic stabilization can be applied at the shoulder region to work on trunk strengthening.

Exercises to increase pulmonary function can be practiced while the patient is in the water. Having the patient hold his breath or blow bubbles while in the water assists in improving pulmonary capacity.

The patient can practice standing at the side of the pool while he is in the water. The assistant may need to guard the patient at the trunk and to use his or her lower extremities to maintain proper alignment of the patient's legs. Approximation can be applied down through the hips to assist with lower extremity weight bearing. Some therapeutic pools possess parallel bars within the water to assist with standing and ambulation activities. If the patient has an incomplete injury with adequate lower extremity innervation, assisted walking can be performed. As stated previously, this is an excellent way to strengthen weak lower extremity muscles and to improve the patient's endurance. Kickboards can also be used to assist with lower extremity strengthening.

Floating and Swimming

Patients with tetraplegia or paraplegia can be taught to float on their backs. Floating assists with breathing, as well as general body relaxation. Patients can also be instructed in modified or adaptive swimming strokes. Patients with tetraplegia can be taught a modified backstroke and breast stroke. Performance of these swimming strokes assists the patient with upper extremity strengthening and also improves the patient's cardiovascular fitness. Patients with paraplegia can be instructed in the front crawl or butterfly stroke, which also increase upper extremity strength and improve the patient's cardiovascular endurance.

Other Advanced Rehabilitation Interventions

Other treatment activities may be performed as part of the patient's treatment plan. Functional electrical stimulation may be used in patients with muscle weakness to increase strength and to decrease muscle fatigue. Functional electrical stimulation is often suggested when a patient has muscle innervation and weakness associated with an incomplete injury. Electrical stimulation can also be used to decrease range-of-motion limitations, decrease spasticity, minimize muscle imbalances, and provide positioning support for patients who are attempting ambulation.

As stated previously, patients with incomplete injuries often have increased muscle tone that interferes with function. Therefore, a component of the patient's treatment plan is the management of this problem. Stretching, ice, pool therapy, and functional electrical stimulation may be appropriate forms of intervention. Electrical stimulation can be applied either to the antagonist muscle to promote increased strength or to the agonist to induce fatigue. Patients with excessive amounts of abnormal tone may also be receiving pharmacologic interventions, as mentioned previously in this chapter.

Ambulation Training

One of the first questions that your patients with SCIs often ask is whether they will be able to walk again. This question is frequently posed in the acute care center immediately following the injury. Early on, it may be difficult to determine the patient's ambulation potential secondary to spinal shock and the depression of reflex activity. Different philosophies regarding gait training are recognized, and much depends on the rehabilitation team with which you work. Some health care professionals believe that it is best to give patients with the potential to ambulate every opportunity to do so. These individuals believe that most patients, given the opportunity to try walking with orthoses and an assistive device, will not continue to do so after they realize the difficulty encountered. It may be best to allow the patient to come to the decision on his own instead of having the physical therapist or health care team make a decision regarding ambulation for the patient. Other health care professionals believe that a patient should possess strength in the hip flexor musculature before ambulation is even attempted because of the high energy costs, time, and financial resources associated with gait training. Most patients with higher-level injuries choose wheelchair mobility as their preferred method of locomotion after trying ambulation with orthoses and assistive devices (Cerny et al, 1980; Decker and Hall, 1986).

Benefits of Standing and Walking

Although functional ambulation may not be possible for all our patients with SCIs, therapeutic standing has documented benefits. Standing prevents the development of osteoporosis and also helps to decrease the patient's risk for bladder and kidney stones. In addition, standing decreases the risk of heterotopic ossification and decreases abnormal muscle tone (Nixon, 1985).

Guidelines have been established regarding assessment of the patient's likelihood for success with ambulation. Factors to consider include the following: (1) the level of the patient's injury (the lower the injury, the easier it will be for the patient to walk); (2) whether the lesion is incomplete or complete (patients with incomplete injuries usually have a better potential for ambulation); (3) the age of the patient (younger patients have more potential to ambulate); (4) the cardiopulmonary status of the patient (patients with better pulmonary function have an easier time meeting the energy demands of walking); (5) the patient's weight and body build (the heavier the patient is, the more difficult it will be for the patient to walk, and taller patients usually find it more challenging to ambulate with orthoses); (6) the patient's current health status (complicating medical problems or conditions

affect the patient's ability to be successful with orthoses); (7) the amount of spasticity present (lower extremity or trunk spasticity can make wearing orthoses difficult); (8) the amount of proprioception present in lower extremity joints (proprioception in at least the hip joints improves the patient's success with crutch ambulation); (9) the passive range of motion present at the hips, knees, and ankles (hip, knee, or ankle plantar flexion contractures limit the patient's ability to ambulate with orthoses and crutches); in addition, patients need approximately 110 degrees of passive hamstring range of motion to be able to don their orthoses and transfer from the floor if they fall); (10) the financial resources of the patient (long leg orthoses are expensive); depending on the patient's insurance status and other financial resources, the patient may not be able to afford to participate in ambulation training); and (11) the patient's motivation to walk and to continue with ambulation once he is discharged from physical therapy services. Given the opportunity to try assisted ambulation with orthoses and help from the physical therapist or assistant, some patients may decide it is too difficult a task and prefer not to continue with the training. All these factors must be considered by the rehabilitation team when discussing ambulation with the patient.

Depending on the patient's motor level, different types of ambulation potential have been described. The literature varies on the specific motor level and the potential for ambulation. For patients with T2 through T11 injuries, *therapeutic standing* or ambulation may be possible. This means that the patient is able to stand or ambulate in the physical therapy department with assistance. However, functional ambulation is not possible. Therapeutic ambulators require assistance to transfer from sitting to standing and to walk on level surfaces. These patients ambulate for the physiologic and therapeutic benefits it offers. Patients with injuries at the T12 through L2 level have the potential to be household or community ambulators. However, some sources report that patients must have innervation below L2 to achieve functional community ambulation (Atrice et al, 1995).

Individuals who achieve household or community ambulation are able to ambulate in their homes with orthoses and assistive devices. Patients at this level are able to transfer independently, to ambulate on level surfaces of varying textures, and to negotiate doorways and other minor architectural barriers. The energy cost for ambulation in patients with complete injuries above T12 is above the anaerobic threshold and cannot be maintained for an extended period (Atrice et al, 1995). Cerny et al, reported that gait velocities for patients with paraplegia were significantly slower, and gait required a 50% increase in oxygen consumption and a 28% increase in heart rate. Consequently, individuals with paraplegia discontinue ambulation with their orthoses and assistive devices and use their wheelchairs for environmental negotiation (Cerny et al, 1980).

Community ambulation is possible for patients with injuries at L2 or lower. These patients are able to ambulate with or without orthoses and assistive devices. Community ambulators are able to ambulate independently in the community and can negotiate all environmental barriers. (Atrice et al, 1995; Decker and Hall, 1986; Schmitz, 1994).

Orthoses

Patients with paraplegia who decide to pursue ambulation training need some type of orthosis. Figure 7–13 depicts the most common lower extremity orthoses prescribed. Knee-ankle-foot orthoses may be recommended for patients with paraplegia. These orthoses typically have a thigh cuff and an external knee joint with a locking mechanism (drop locks or bail locks are the most common). They have a calf band and an adjustable locked ankle joint. Scott-Craig knee-ankle-foot orthoses are frequently prescribed for patients with paraplegia. These orthoses consist of a single thigh and pretibial band, a bail lock at the knee joint, and modified footplates. The design of this orthosis provides built-in stability for the patient while he is standing.

The reciprocating gait orthosis is another type of orthosis that may be prescribed for patients with SCIs. This device can be used with patients with little trunk control because of the midthoracic and pelvic support. The reciprocating gait orthosis has an external hip joint that is operated by a cable mechanism. When the patient shifts weight onto one lower extremity, the cable system advances the opposite leg. Individuals using reciprocating gait orthoses often use a walker instead of Lofstrand crutches as their preferred assistive device. The reciprocating gait orthosis is frequently prescribed for children with lower extremity weakness secondary to myelomeningocele. Refer to Chapter 9 for a review.

A new type of orthotic system is now available for patients with SCIs. The ARGO system is similar to the reciprocating gait orthosis, but it has a hydraulic lift that allows patients to transfer from sitting to standing more easily. This system appears to have excellent potential for patients with higher level thoracic injuries.

Preparation for Ambulation

The decision to attempt gait training is made by the patient and the rehabilitation team. As stated previously, the patient's motor level and other factors must be considered. In general, the patient should be independent in mat mobility, wheelchair-to-mat transfers, and wheelchair mobility on level surfaces before beginning gait training. Many clinics possess training ortho-

ses that allow the patient to practice standing before permanent orthoses are prescribed and manufactured. An orthotist should work with the patient to assist in identifying and fabricating the best orthosis for the patient.

Depending on the patient's length of stay in the rehabilitation facility, gait training may begin at the end of the patient's inpatient hospitalization, or it may begin in earnest in the outpatient setting.

Once the permanent orthoses have been delivered, it is time to begin the first gait training session. If possible, the orthotist should be present for this session. Having the patient don the orthoses is the first step. It is often easiest for the patient to do this on the mat in a long-sitting position. The patient should be encouraged to do as much for himself as possible on this first attempt. He should start by placing one of his feet into the shoe and then locking the knee joint. During the performance of this activity, one realizes the necessity of possessing 110 degrees of hamstring range. Once the knee is in the orthosis, the patient can tighten the thigh pad. From there, the patient should start to put the other foot in the orthosis. Once both orthoses are on, the therapist and orthotist, if present, will inspect the orthoses and check the fit. The orthoses must not rub the patient's skin. This situation can cause areas of redness and can lead to skin breakdown. If everything looks satisfactory, the patient should then be instructed to transfer back to his wheelchair to begin standing activities in the parallel bars.

Standing in the Parallel Bars

The first thing the patient needs to do is to transfer to standing. The therapist should initially demonstrate this maneuver for the patient. It is easiest to have the patient hold on to the bars and pull forward. In preparation for this transition, the patient needs to move forward in his wheelchair. Having the patient push up and lift the buttocks forward is best, to prevent shearing of the patient's skin. Once the patient is forward in his chair, the therapist will want to make sure the patient's orthoses are locked. If this is the patient's first time to stand up, it will be safest to have two individuals assist. While the patient is wearing the safety belt, one person is positioned in front of the patient, and the other person is at the side or in back of the patient. On a count of three, the patient pulls himself forward on the bars. The individual assisting the patient also provides the patient with the needed strength and momentum to complete the transfer.

Once upright, the patient must work to find his balance point. The patient's lower extremities should be slightly apart, his low back should be in hyperextension, the patient's shoulders are back, and the patient's hands must be forward of his hips and holding on to the parallel bars. Essentially, the patient is rest-

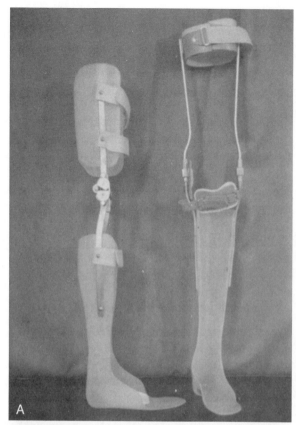

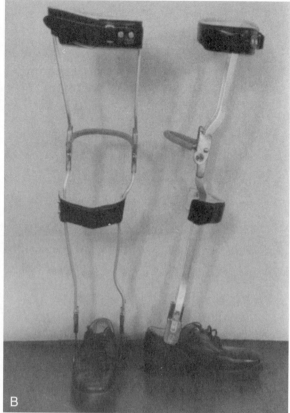

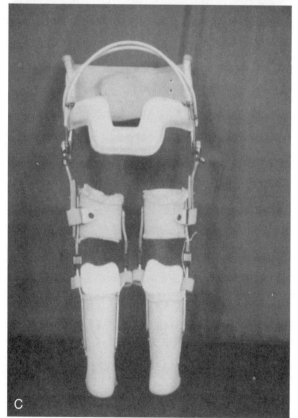

FIGURE 7–13 ■ *A*, Combination plastic and metal knee-ankle-foot orthoses. *B*, The Scott-Craig knee-ankle-foot orthosis is a special design for spinal cord injury. The orthosis consists of double uprights, offset knee joints with locks and bail control, one posterior thigh band, a hinged anterior tibial band, an ankle joint with anterior and posterior adjustable pin stops, a cushion heel, and specially designed foot plates made of steel. *C*, The reciprocating gait orthosis, although generally used with children, is also used with adults. Its main components are a molded pelvic band, thoracic extensions, bilateral hip and knee joints, polypropylene posterior thigh shells, ankle-foot orthosis sections, and cables connecting the two hip joint mechanisms. (From Umphred DA. Neurological Rehabilitation, 3rd ed. St. Louis, CV Mosby, 1995.)

ing on the Y ligaments in the hip and pelvic region. The lower extremity orthoses and positioning allow the patient to move his center of gravity behind his hip joints. Once the patient is able to find his balance point, he will eventually be able to stand and maintain his balance without the use of his upper extremities. To guard the patient during this activity, the therapist will be behind the patient or off to the side. The therapist holds on to the gait belt and should avoid holding on to the patient's upper arms. The therapist may place a supporting hand on the patient's anterior shoulder as long as the therapist does not provide a counterbalancing force.

As the patient is practicing maintaining his balance point, he must keep his hands forward of his hips. If the hands move next to the hips or behind them, the patient will be at risk to jackknife. A *jackknife* can be described as movement of the patient's upper body toward the floor as the patient flexes the hips. The maneuver is similar to the dive of the same name.

During practice of the balance point, the patient should initially practice the activity with both hands on the parallel bars. The patient should be encouraged to hold the bars lightly and to avoid grabbing and pulling on them. Often, just having the patient rest his hands on the bars may be best. Eventually, you will want the patient to balance with one hand and finally with no hands. The patient should ultimately be able to stand in the orthoses without any upper extremity support.

After the patient feels comfortable with his balance point, he can begin to practice pushups in the bars. With his hands in a forward position, the patient pushes down on the bars by depressing the shoulders. Depending on the type of lower extremity orthosis and the presence or absence of a spreader bar, the therapist will want to note what happens to the patient's lower extremities during the pushup. Most often, the legs dangle free. If a spreader bar is attached to the orthoses, the legs will move as one unit. Performing a pushup is a prerequisite activity for the patient to ambulate in a forward direction.

Although jackknifing is an undesirable occurrence, the activity should be practiced in the parallel bars during early gait training sessions. With his hands forward, the patient bends forward at the waist and lowers his trunk down toward the parallel bars. The patient then pushes himself back up to an upright position. Once the patient feels comfortable with this activity, he can practice falling into a jackknife position. The patient can initiate this fall either by moving his hands posterior to his hips or by flexing his head forward. The therapist can also assist the patient with the achievement of the jackknife position by gently pulling the patient's hips and pelvis in a posterior direction.

To review, the jackknife position is the position the patient will likely assume if he loses his balance during ambulation activities. The patient should recognize this position and needs to know what to do if it occurs during gait activities. If this position should occur during gait, the patient will want to straighten his elbows while extending his head and trunk.

Gait Progression

Once the patient can maintain his balance point and can perform a pushup to clear his feet from the floor, he is ready to begin forward ambulation in the parallel bars. You may be wondering how long this typically takes. Normally, you will want to progress the patient to taking a few steps on the first standing and ambulation attempt. However, the clinician has to monitor the patient's responses closely during standing and ambulation. The effects of fatigue, orthostatic hypotension, decreased cardiopulmonary endurance, and the anxiety associated with standing and walking can easily overwhelm the patient. To monitor physiologic responses during the treatment, the clinician should take baseline pulse, respiration, and blood pressure readings before the patient is standing. Careful monitoring of vital signs during the gait training portion of the treatment session is also indicated. In addition, the patient must be instructed to report any feelings of lightheadedness or dizziness immediately.

The assistant should instruct the patient to find his balance point prior to advancing forward in the parallel bars. The patient's head should be held upright, looking forward. The patient then flexes his head, pushes down on his hands, depresses his shoulders, and lifts his lower extremities off the ground. As the patient depresses his shoulders and straightens his elbows, he must extend his head and neck and return it to a neutral position. To maintain his balance, the patient needs to move his hands forward of his hips immediately. If the patient were to maintain his hands in the same place after completing the lift, he would jackknife. After the patient's feet make contact with the floor, he must throw his hips forward to rest on the Y ligaments. This type of gait pattern is known as a *swing-to pattern* because the patient is moving his feet the same distance as his hands. The patient should repeat the steps just described until he progresses to the end of the parallel bars. At this point, someone can pull the wheelchair up behind the patient, or the patient can be instructed in performing a quarter-turn. If the patient is not too tired, he should continue and should learn the turning technique at this time. Intervention 7–27 illustrates the correct head and trunk positions for gait training activities.

Quarter-Turns

To complete a quarter-turn, the patient depresses her shoulders and lifts her legs while she changes her

Intervention 7–27 ▌ GAIT PROGRESSION

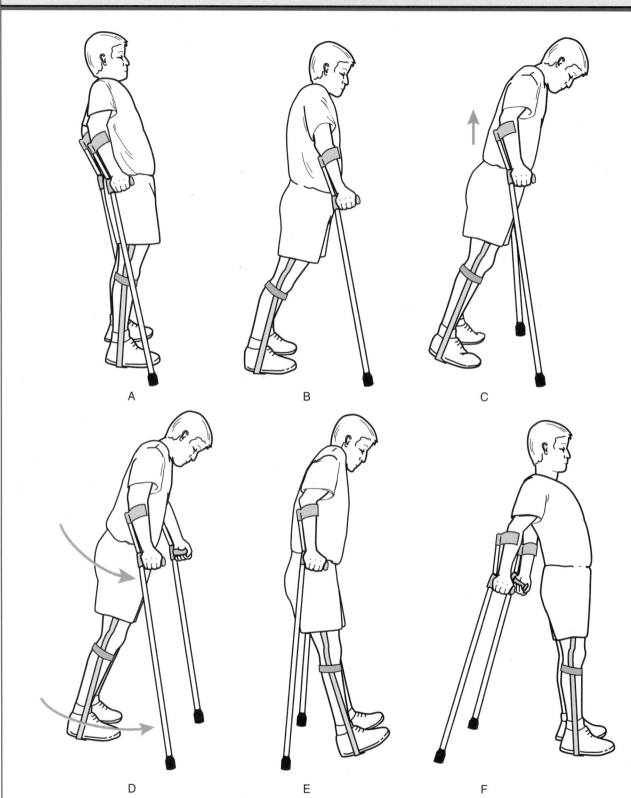

A.

B.

C.

D.

E.

F.

A. The patient finds his balance point.

B. He advances the crutches forward.

C. The patient tucks his head and pushes down on the crutches.

D. His pelvis and lower extremities swing forward.

E. His feet strike the floor.

F. The patient lifts his head and resumes a lordotic posture.

hand position on the parallel bars. In essence, she is completing two quarter-turns to turn around. The patient must practice turning in both directions.

Sitting

Prior to sitting, the patient should have been instructed in the proper technique. You should not pull the wheelchair up to the back of the patient's legs. Remember, the patient transfers from standing to sitting with the lower extremity orthoses locked in extension. For this reason, the chair should at least 12 inches from the patient so he will be able to land in the wheelchair seat. If the chair is too close to the patient, he might tip the chair over backward. The assistant should have the patient keep both his hands on the parallel bars during his descent. In time, the patient will be instructed in other methods to perform transfers from sitting to standing and from standing to sitting without the use of the parallel bars.

Swing-Through Gait Pattern

Once the patient feels comfortable with the swing-to gait pattern, the patient can progress to a swing-through pattern. The technique is the same as the swing-to pattern, except the patient advances his legs a little farther forward, and instead of stopping between steps, the patient moves his hands forward again and takes another step. This gait pattern allows the patient to move forward a little faster and is more energy efficient.

Other Gait Patterns

If the patient possesses lower extremity innervation, specifically hip flexion, the patient may have the potential to use a four-point or two-point gait pattern. Both patterns more closely resemble normal reciprocal gait patterns with upper and lower extremity movement. These patterns are described in standard texts and are not discussed here.

Backing Up

Patients should also be instructed in backing up. This is important when the patient begins to use his crutches on level surfaces within the physical therapy department. Initially, backing up can be practiced in the parallel bars. The patient tucks his head, depresses his shoulders, and extends his elbows. This position causes the patient to perform a mini-jackknife and allows the patient's legs to move backward. The patient repeats this sequence several times to move the desired distance backward.

Progressing the Patient

After the patient has practiced in the parallel bars several times, it is time to progress to ambulation outside them. It is advisable to progress out of the bars without delay because patients can become used to them and may find it difficult to make the transition to ambulation in a less protected environment. To assist with this transition, the clinician may elect to introduce Lofstrand (Canadian or forearm) crutches while the patient is still ambulating in the parallel bars.

Care must be exercised when practicing transitions into and out of the wheelchair. These techniques are best practiced with the back of the wheelchair positioned next to a wall for greater safety. In addition, the patient should check to make sure the wheelchair brakes are locked.

Standing from the Wheelchair

If the patient is to become independent in ambulation activities, he must learn to transfer from sitting to standing independently. Several methods are available to the patient. The first way described is probably the easiest.

Step 1. The patient places the wheelchair against the wall and locks the brakes.

Step 2. The patient places his crutches behind the wheelchair, to rest on the push handles.

Step 3. The patient moves to the edge of his wheelchair. The patient needs to complete mini-push-ups as he does this. Scooting forward can cause unnecessary shearing to the patient's skin.

Step 4. With his orthoses locked, the patient crosses one leg over the other.

Step 5. The patient then pivots over the fixed foot and pushes up to standing.

Step 6. Holding on to the wheelchair armrest, the patient secures one crutch, positions it, and then secures the second crutch.

Step 7. Once the crutches are in place, the patient backs up from the wheelchair, taking two or three steps backward. Intervention 7–28 shows the steps needed to transfer from sitting to standing with lower extremity orthoses and Lofstrand crutches.

An alternative way of completing this transfer is to unlock one of the orthoses and pivot over the unlocked lower extremity. This technique can be less stressful to the hip joint than the one previously described. The patient completes the transition to upright in the same way as noted earlier, except that the patient needs to lock the knee joint of the bent knee once an upright position has been achieved.

The patient can also assume standing from the wheelchair by transferring forward.

Step 1. The patient moves forward to the edge of the chair.

Step 2. With his arms in the crutches, the patient

Intervention 7–28 | SIT-TO-STAND TRANSFER WITH ORTHOSES

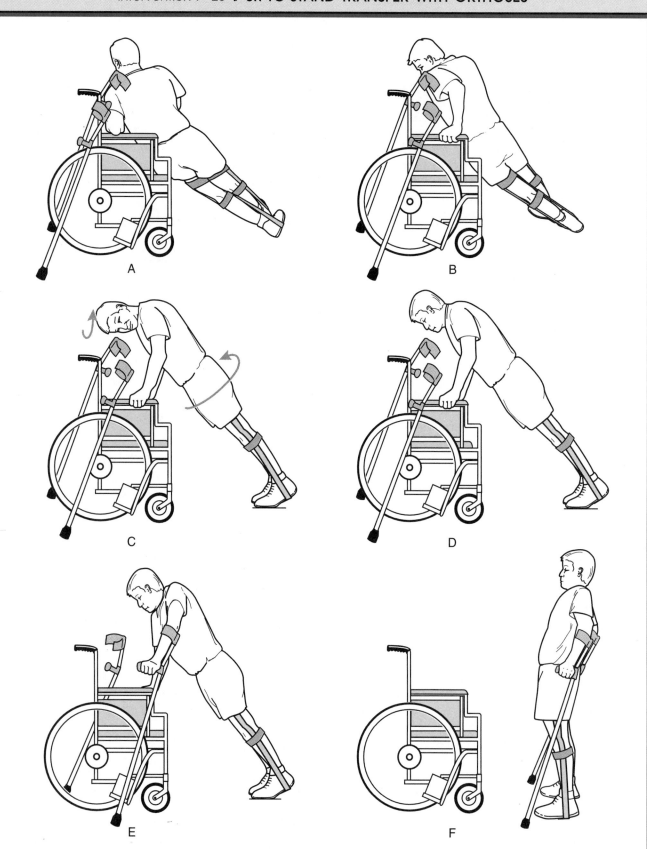

The sequence for transferring from sit to stand with lower extremity orthoses. (See text description, steps 1 through 7.)

places the crutches flat on the floor slightly behind the front wheels.

Step 3. The patient flexes his head and pushes down on the crutches, to propel himself out of the wheelchair.

Step 4. Once standing, the patient must quickly extend his head and trunk, to regain the lumbar lordosis necessary for standing stability.

Step 5. The patient's upper extremities remain behind until the patient feels he has regained his balance. Then he can move his arms and crutches forward. Intervention 7–29 shows a patient completing this activity.

This method is difficult for many patients because it requires a great deal of strength, balance, and coordination.

Once the patient is standing and has regained his balance, he can begin to ambulate using a swing-through gait pattern, as described previously. The clinician guards the patient from behind, with one hand on the gait belt and the other on the patient's posterior shoulder, as depicted in Figure 7–14. The clinician must be careful to avoid the tendency to apply excessive tactile cues to the patient. Pulling on the gait belt or impeding the movement of the patient's upper trunk may, in fact, cause the patient to experience balance disturbances.

To regain a sitting position after walking, the following is recommended:

Step 1. The patient faces the wheelchair initially.

Step 2. The patient places the crutches behind the chair.

Step 3. The patient unlocks one of the knee joints and rotates over that knee to assume a sitting position.

Patients can return to sitting using a straight-back method. This technique is difficult, however, and may be best used when a second person is present to assist with the transition, to stabilize the wheelchair.

Gait Training with Crutches

As the patient begins ambulation training on level surfaces with the crutches, he once again needs to find his balance point. The patient must maintain his hands forward of his hips to prevent jackknifing. Initially, the clinician may elect to perform a swing-to gait pattern with the patient. The clinician should guard the patient from behind by holding on to the gait belt as necessary. Some clinicians may find it easier to guard the patient from the side initially by holding on to the gait belt and placing the other hand on the patient's shoulder (see Fig. 7–14). Verbal and tactile cueing may be necessary to assist the patient with head

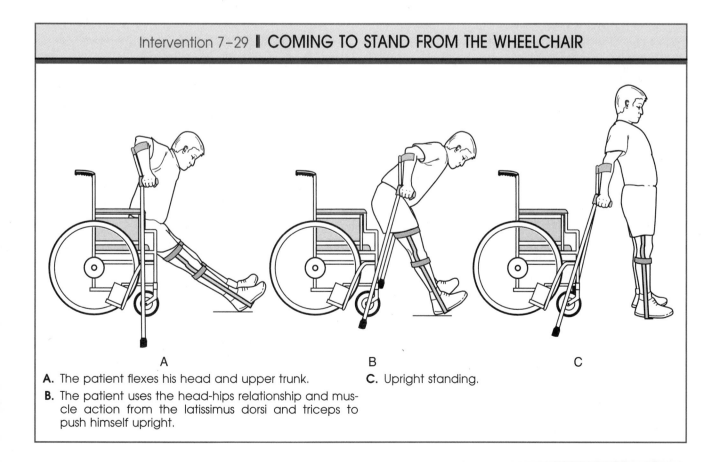

Intervention 7–29 ∎ COMING TO STAND FROM THE WHEELCHAIR

A   B   C

A. The patient flexes his head and upper trunk.

B. The patient uses the head-hips relationship and muscle action from the latissimus dorsi and triceps to push himself upright.

C. Upright standing.

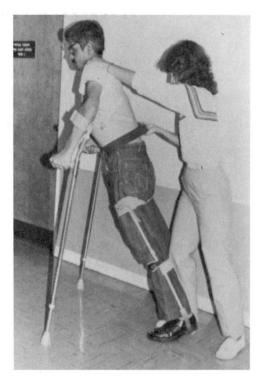

FIGURE 7–14 ▪ Patient with an injury at the T12 level ambulating with crutches and bilateral knee-ankle-foot orthoses for balance and lower extremity advancement. (From Adkins HV [ed]: Spinal Cord Injury. New York, Churchill Livingstone, 1985.)

positioning and the hyperlordotic posture. Should the patient lose his balance and begin to jackknife, the clinician will push the patient's pelvis forward and the shoulders back to resume the hyperextended posture. Because the patient will be moving relatively quickly, the clinician will need to take bigger steps. As the patient becomes more proficient, the patient can begin a swing-through gait pattern.

Falling

All patients who attempt gait training with crutches should also be instructed in proper falling techniques to avoid injury. The first attempts at falling should be completed in a controlled manner. You will want to have the patient fall onto a floor mat. The patient is instructed to let go of his crutches and remove his hands from the hand grips. The patient then reaches toward the ground and flexes his elbows to avoid trauma to the wrist. If the facility has a crash mat (these mats are higher and softer), having the patient fall onto it is an easier starting point for the patient.

Getting Up from the Floor

Once the patient has practiced falling to the floor, the patient must also learn how to get up from the floor. The following steps should be used to assist the patient with this activity. As a note of caution, this transfer should be practiced close to a wall so the patient has something to lean against as he transfers to upright.

Step 1. The patient is instructed to assume a prone position on the floor.

Step 2. The patient positions the crutches with the tips pointing toward his head and the hand grips at the patient's hips.

Step 3. The patient pushes up to a plantigrade position. (The patient ensures that both orthoses are locked prior to attempting this maneuver.)

Step 4. The patient reaches for one of his crutches and puts the crutch tip on the floor to assist in the transition to an upright position. The patient's hand is on the crutch handle, and the crutch rests against his shoulder.

Step 5. The patient uses the crutch on the floor as a point of stability as he reaches for the other crutch and positions it on his forearm.

Step 6. The patient turns the opposite crutch around and places the forearm cuff at his elbow region.

Step 7. The patient regains his balance with the crutches. Intervention 7–30 depicts this sequence.

Negotiating Environmental Barriers

If the patient is to be independent with ambulation in the community, she must be able to negotiate ramps, curbs, and stairs with orthoses and braces.

Ascending a Ramp

Step 1. The patient uses a swing-to gait pattern to move forward up the ramp.

Step 2. To maintain her balance, the patient keeps her crutches several inches in front of her feet.

Step 3. To increase hip stability, the patient's pelvis must be forward in a lordotic posture.

Descending a Ramp

The same technique used for ambulation on level surfaces can be employed. A swing-through gait pattern is recommended.

Ascending a Curb

Step 1. The individual approaches the curb head-on.

Step 2. In a balanced position near the edge of the curb, the patient places his crutch tips on the curb.

Step 3. The patient leans forward, tucks his head, extends his elbows, and depresses his scapulae (jackknifes) to elevate his lower extremities onto the curb. (The patient's toes drag up the elevation of the curb.)

Step 4. The patient can step to or past the crutches.

Step 5. Once the patient's feet land on the curb, he

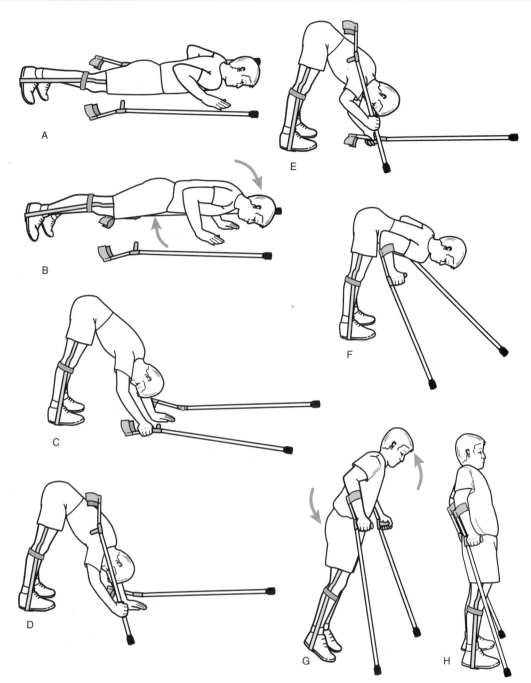

A. Instruct the patient to assume a prone position on the floor. Have the patient position the crutches with the tips pointing toward his head and the hand grips at the patient's hips.

B. The patient pushes up to a plantigrade position. (The patient will want to make sure that both orthoses are locked prior to attempting this.)

C and D. The patient reaches for one of his crutches, using it for balance. The crutch rests against his shoulder.

E and F. The patient uses the crutch on the floor as a point of stability as he reaches for the other crutch and positions it on his forearm.

G and H. The patient regains his balance with the crutches.

will need to regain his balance point.

Descending a Curb

Step 1. The individual approaches the curb head-on.

Step 2. In a balanced position near the edge of the curb, the patient steps off the curb, tucking his head, straightening his elbows, and depressing his scapulae.

Step 3. Once the patient's lower extremities have swung past the edge of the curb, he lowers his legs by eccentrically contracting his elbow and shoulder musculature.

Step 4. When the patient's feet come in contact with the ground, he needs to regain his balance point.

Although the Americans with Disabilities Act increased the accessibility of many public and private buildings, many homes and community buildings are not accessible to certain individuals. For this reason, we review the techniques for instructing the patient in stair negotiation.

Ascending Stairs

Patients can ascend stairs using the same techniques described to go up a single curb. In addition, patients can be instructed in an alternative approach, to ascend the stairs backward.

Step 1. The patient stands with his back to the stairs and in a balanced position.

Step 2. With his crutches on the step above, the patient leans into the crutches, straightens his elbows, and depresses his scapulae. This maneuver causes his lower extremities to be lifted onto the step.

Step 3. Once the patient's feet have landed, he extends his neck and retracts the scapulae to regain a forward pelvis position.

The patient repeats these steps until he has successfully ascended all the required steps.

Descending Stairs

The patient who must descend a series of steps can use the techniques described for going down a curb. However, the patient must be careful because the space in which he can land is limited. The patient must accurately gauge the length of his step so he will not miss a step.

DISCHARGE PLANNING

As stated previously, lengths of stay for inpatient rehabilitation continue to decrease. As a consequence, one must begin discharge planning during the pa-

tient's first visits to physical therapy. All members of the patient's rehabilitation team, including the patient, family members, significant others, and caregivers, must be included in the process. The combined efforts of all these individuals help the patient successfully to make the transition from the hospital to his previous home and work environments.

The discharge planning process ideally includes a number of different activities aimed at improving the patient's functional outcome and providing an easy transition from health care facility to home. Activities that should be a part of the discharge planning process include (1) a discharge planning conference, (2) a trial home pass, (3) an assessment of the home environment to ensure accessibility, (4) development of a vocational plan, (5) procurement of all necessary adaptive equipment and supplies, (6) driver's training, if appropriate, (7) education regarding resource availability, and (8) recommendations regarding additional rehabilitation services.

Discharge Planning Conference

The discharge planning conference should be held approximately 1 to 2 weeks before the patient's anticipated discharge date. At this time, continued medical and rehabilitation follow-up should be addressed, and a review of resources available to both patient and family should be provided. Hopefully, patients will have access to comprehensive follow-up services. Spinal cord clinics that offer routine reassessments at predetermined times are beneficial. At these follow-up appointments, many potential long-term complications are discovered and are successfully managed. Unfortunately, many patients are discharged to areas where medical specialists trained in providing long-term care to this patient population are not available. For this reason, patients must be educated regarding their injuries, possible complications, and potential outcomes for their recovery.

During the discharge planning conference, certain issues must be addressed. Areas of concern include the following:

1. The patient's attitude and discharge plans must be discussed. Is the patient realistic regarding what it will be like at home? Is discharge to home possible?

2. The knowledge base and understanding exhibited by the patient's primary caregivers regarding SCIs and management should be assessed. Do caregivers understand the patient's condition and the level of care required?

3. The availability of a physician who can deal with the medical problems and secondary complications encountered by patients with SCIs should be discussed.

4. The amount and degree of professional and attend-

ant care required by the patient must be addressed. Does the patient possess the financial means (insurance or income) to pay for personal care? Has the patient received all the adaptive and ADL equipment necessary to function at home? Equipment including wheelchairs and seat cushions should be received prior to the patient's discharge, so any necessary training or modifications can be performed in the facility. In addition, a relationship with a durable medical provider is suggested.

5. Transportation issues associated with school, work, leisure activities, and doctors' appointments must be addressed. Patients with power wheelchairs need access to vans with hydraulic chair lift capabilities. Patients who want to resume driving need to have adaptive hand controls installed in their automobiles. The timetable to receive these items can be long. Therefore, one is advised to begin this planning process early.

6. Other issues related to accessibility of community resources and support for the patient and his family members must be discussed. Support groups for patients and their family members are available in many communities. These groups can often provide the patient both emotional support and a social outlet.

Therapeutic passes are often given to patients close to their discharge and are extremely beneficial to the discharge planning process. When a patient is given a pass, the patient is released from the health care facility for several hours or, in some cases, overnight in the care of a family member. The pass is used to determine how the patient will function once he is discharged from the rehabilitation unit. During the pass, the patient and family can practice essential skills that will be needed once the patient is at home full time. These passes also offer opportunities for the patient to solve problems that may be encountered at home such as inaccessibility of various rooms. The passes assist the patient in regaining the confidence needed to function outside the safe confines of the rehabilitation setting. Many patients are often anxious and reluctant about their discharge from rehabilitation. The rehabilitation hospital or unit is considered a safe haven with 24-hour daily care and the comfort of individuals with similar problems and physical deficits.

After the pass, the patient returns to the rehabilitation unit for continued intervention and planning for discharge. The patient and family are expected to share their experiences regarding the pass so that additional training and problem solving can occur. Concomitantly, if additional environmental modifications to the dwelling must be made, the pass provides the information necessary to complete those changes.

As stated previously, during the discharge planning conference, the patient and the rehabilitation team need to discuss vocational planning. A referral to a vocational rehabilitation specialist or, in some instances, a psychologist can foster adjustment toward the patient's disability and can assist the patient in having an optimistic attitude toward the future. Many times, the patient is not ready at this particular point to think about the future, especially his place in the work world. However, beginning a vocational evaluation and discussing the patient's return to school or work is extremely positive and helps to foster the expectation that these activities can be resumed.

Procurement of Equipment

A detailed discussion about securing equipment needed by the patient before discharge from the facility is beyond the scope of this text. Some of the common items that must be considered are presented here. The occupational therapist and the rehabilitation team should be consulted for more specific information.

Items frequently needed by the patient at discharge include the following:

1. Wheelchair: The type and specific requirements are determined by the rehabilitation team. The benefits of power versus manual wheelchairs must be considered. Cost and reimbursement may be concerns for some patients.

2. Wheelchair cushion to assist with pressure relief: Although pressure-relieving devices are beneficial, they do not take the place of regularly performed pressure-relief or weight-shifting activities. Selecting the proper wheelchair cushion depends on the patient's ability to transfer on and off the cushion and the degree of support needed.

3. Hospital or pressure-relieving bed: Patients with high tetraplegia who are to be discharged to home may require hospital beds, other specialized beds, or air mattresses.

4. ADL adaptive equipment: Examples of items that may be needed include dressing sticks to assist with donning clothing, loops attached to pants to assist with putting them on, button and zipper hooks to assist with securing these items, Velcro straps and elastic shoelaces to increase the ease of donning shoes, bath brushes, handheld shower attachments, and tub benches. Built-up utensils, toothbrushes, and handles may be needed for patients with tetraplegia. Dorsal wrist supports or universal cuffs may be necessary to assist the patient with feeding activities.

5. Environmental control units: Environmental control units interfaced with personal computers, the telephone, and appliances within the home may be recommended. These electronic systems allow the patient with tetraplegia some control over the envi-

ronment. By activating the environmental control unit, the patient can turn on the lights, television, or other appliances within the home. Referral to a rehabilitation engineer or other provider with expertise in this area is advisable.

Home Exercise Program

For some patients, discharge from your facility is the end of their rehabilitation. Not all patients receive follow-up services once they are discharged. Therefore, the supervising physical therapist and physical therapist assistant must design a home exercise program for the patient that will meet the patient's immediate and long-term needs. It is not reasonable to expect that once a patient is discharged, he will spend a great deal of time performing a home exercise program. The individual will spend a considerable amount of time each day completing daily care needs. Thus, the physical therapy team should select only a few activities that will provide the patient with the greatest functional benefits.

Things to Consider When Developing a Home Exercise Program

Several factors must be considered when developing a home exercise program for your patient. The following is a list of questions you should ask yourself before you finalize the patient's home program.

1. What activities will the patient be able to perform when he is discharged? Will the patient be able to transfer independently? Is progress likely in other functional skills?
2. What motor and cardiopulmonary capacities will the patient need to continue completion of ADLs? Areas to consider include range of motion, strength, flexibility, balance, and vital capacity.
3. How will the patient maintain his skin integrity and respiratory status and prevent possible complications?
4. What skills and capacities can the patient maintain by completing his daily routine? For example, getting dressed and bathing assist in maintaining upper and lower extremity range of motion.
5. What areas will require extra attention because they are not addressed during routine ADLs? Areas to consider include the maintenance of hip extension and ankle dorsiflexion and cardiopulmonary endurance.

In addition to asking these questions about the patient's motor and cardiopulmonary function, one should also consider the patient and the role of the family or caregivers in designing the home exercise program (Nixon, 1985). As stated earlier, patients who have SCIs must become active problem solvers and must be able to direct and initiate their care. Patients who become reliant on their rehabilitation team for making decisions regarding their care may have difficulty in directing their home exercise program. Failure to understand the possible complications of immobility and contractures may lead to lack of interest in a home exercise program. Stretching activities and active wheelchair propulsion each day will do a great deal to assist the patient in maintaining an optimal level of functional independence.

Family Teaching

As discussed throughout this chapter, family involvement and training are of the utmost importance. Family teaching should be initiated early during the patient's rehabilitation stay and should not wait until a few days before discharge. Family members or caregivers should assist therapists and assistants with patient transfers and range-of-motion exercises. One should be patient with family members as they begin to learn these tasks because they are often anxious and afraid of causing pain or additional injury. Not only is it important to teach families how to assist patients physically, but also families must be educated about the injury, potential complications, precautions, and likely outcome. This instruction is best if given over a period of time, to give the family member or caregiver adequate time to digest and assimilate information. If the patient is to be discharged home, all individuals responsible for assisting with the care of the patient should demonstrate a level of competence with techniques prior to the patient's release from the facility.

Community Reentry

As the patient prepares for discharge, a final area that must be considered is the individual's reentry into the community. The patient should be encouraged to resume previously performed activities as his level of functional independence and interests warrant. Significant advances have been made in the areas of employment, recreational activities, sports, and hobbies for patients with disabilities. Approximately 12 to 13% of persons injured are employed 2 years after injury. This figure increases to 38.3% 12 years later. Factors that positively affect employment following injury include younger age, being a white male, higher educational levels, motivation, and prior employment (DeVivo and Richards, 1992). A thorough review of recreational and sports programs is beyond the scope of this text.

Quality of Life

Research suggests that most individuals who sustain an SCI report that, in time, they achieve a satisfactory quality of life and psychosocial well-being (Lewthwaite et al, 1994). Evidence suggests that the depression and hostility often experienced initially after the injury decrease over time, and the individual gains acceptance of the disability (DeVivo and Richards, 1992). An individual's social support mechanisms can positively affect the individual's adjustment to his injury. Level or extent of the injury does not, however, predict whether an individual is satisfied with his quality of life (DeVivo and Richards, 1992).

Long-Term Health Care Needs

As the population in the United States ages, so do the survivors with SCIs. Investigators have estimated that 40% of persons with SCIs are more than 45 years old. Research studies are just now beginning to address how the normal aging process affects the preexisting musculoskeletal and cardiopulmonary deficits experienced by individuals who have had an SCI and

how cumulative stresses sustained from years of wheelchair propulsion, repetitive upper extremity activities, and assisted ambulation may accelerate problems encountered with aging. As patients age, they can experience declines in function and the need to use greater assistance. Fatigue, weakness, medical complications, shoulder pain, weight gain, and postural changes have been attributed to declines in function. Fortunately, many of these functional limitations are amenable to physical therapy intervention, including the procurement of adaptive equipment, seating systems, and power wheelchairs (Gerhart et al, 1993).

An important point for health care providers working with individuals with SCIs is that many of the problems associated with aging and overuse may be preventable through education, health promotion, and wellness activities. Comprehensive follow-up services are extremely important to these individuals and may decrease the incidence of secondary complications (Gerhart et al, 1993).

CHAPTER SUMMARY

Patients with SCIs benefit from comprehensive rehabilitation services to optimize their functional independence. Physical therapy treatment sessions started shortly after the patient's injury can help to improve the patient's strength, mobility, and cardiopulmonary function. Treatment should continue with admission to a comprehensive rehabilitation center where additional resources can be devoted to the patient's optimal recovery. Multiple therapeutic interventions and modalities are available to assist the patient in achieving the highest level of functional independence. Emphasizing the patient's active participation in the rehabilitation process is essential. In addition, patient and family education must be

included from the very start of rehabilitation to ensure a successful transition from health care facility to home. Early discussions with the patient regarding returning home and to work or school assist the patient with reintegration into the community. Adequate long-term follow-up care remains absolutely essential in order to eliminate or minimize the potential long-term complications that can develop in this patient population. One hopes that as research continues in the areas of spinal cord repair and regeneration, new medical interventions will become available to these patients to improve their functional potentials.

REVIEW QUESTIONS

1. List the four most common causes of SCIs.
2. Differentiate between a complete SCI and an incomplete SCI.
3. What are the characteristics of spinal shock?
4. What is autonomic dysreflexia? Describe the clinical manifestations of a patient experiencing this condition.
5. What is the functional potential of a patient with C7 tetraplegia?
6. List three physical therapy interventions that will improve pulmonary function.
7. List the three primary goals of physical therapy

intervention during the acute care phase of rehabilitation.
8. Discuss a typical mat exercise program for a patient with C6 tetraplegia.
9. What is the most functional type of wheelchair-to-mat transfer for a patient with C7 tetraplegia?
10. List the benefits of a therapeutic pool program.
11. Discuss the gait training sequence for a patient with paraplegia who will be using orthoses.
12. Describe important areas for patient and family teaching for a patient with SCI.

REHABILITATION UNIT INITIAL EVALUATION: BOB

Chart Review: Bob is a 20-year-old male who was admitted to the hospital 1 week ago after diving headfirst into a shallow lake. He sustained a fracture-dislocation of C6 on C7 resulting in a medical diagnosis of complete C7 tetraplegia. He was taken to surgery 4 days ago and underwent posterior fusion and wiring of C5 through C7. Bone graft was taken from the iliac crests. Bob was fitted with a halo body jacket. Pertinent medical history is unremarkable. Nursing states they have been raising the head of the bed to acclimate patient to upright.

SUBJECTIVE

Bob states he is a college sophomore majoring in computer science. Bob enjoys sports and is very active in campus activities. Bob states he is very unhappy about what has happened to him. Will return home to live with parents and two younger siblings. Home is a 2-story with 2 steps to enter (no handrails present) and 10 steps to second floor. Bob's bedroom is upstairs. Bob's goal: To return to prior level of function.

OBJECTIVE

Appearance: Bob is supine in bed. Upper and lower extremities are positioned at the patient's sides. Bob is wearing low-top tennis shoes. Halo with body jacket and catheter is in place.

Cognition: Bob is alert and oriented ×3. Bob is able to follow multistep commands with 100% accuracy.

Pain: Bob denies any pain. Reports some aching in posterior neck.

Cardiopulmonary: HR 70 beats/minute, RR 16 breaths/minute, BP 98/64 in supine. Vital capacity 700 mL taken with spirometer. Bob demonstrates a four-diaphragm breathing pattern. Cough is weak and nonfunctional.

Sensation: Dermatomes intact to sharp/dull and light touch through C7. Sensation absent at C8 and below. No perianal sensation noted.

Reflexes: Biceps 2+ bilaterally, triceps, patellar, and Achilles 1+ bilaterally. Babinski present bilaterally.

PROM: UE PROM limited at bilateral shoulders to 90° flexion and abduction secondary to halo body jacket. Shoulder internal and external rotation WFL. Elbow, wrist, and finger PROM is WFL bilaterally. Bilateral passive hip flexion to 100°. Hip internal/external rotation, abd/adduction, knee flexion/extension are all WFL. Passive straight leg raising to 85° on the right and 90° on the left. Passive ankle dorsiflexion to neutral bilaterally, passive ankle plantar flexion WFL.

AROM: Bob is able to actively flex both shoulders to 60°. Active elbow extension/flexion 20° to 120° on the right and 45–120° on the left. Wrist extension to 40° on the right, 20° on the left. No active movement noted in the lower extremities. Bob's lower extremities are flaccid.

Skin: No redness noted over bony prominences.

Strength: As tested per standard manual muscle testing procedures.

	R	L
Anterior deltoid	3/5	3/5
Middle deltoid	3/5	3/5
Rhomboids	3−/5	3−/5
Pectoralis major	3−/5	3−/5
Serratus anterior	1/5	1/5
Latissimus dorsi	1/5	1/5
Triceps	2/5	2/5
Wrist extensors	2+/5	2+/5
Flexor carpi ulnaris	0/5	0/5
Flexor digitorum profundus	0/5	0/5

Functional Mobility: Bob is dependent in rolling to right and left, requires maximal assist of 1. Supine to long sitting with maximal assist of 1. BP in sitting 90/60. Sliding board transfer with maximal assist of 2. Bob is transferred to a reclining wheelchair. BP remained 90/60.

REHABILITATION UNIT INITIAL EVALUATION: BOB *Continued*

ASSESSMENT

Bob is a 20-year-old male who presents with a diagnosis of C7 complete tetraplegia. Bob's rehabilitation potential is good secondary to patient motivation and family support.

Problem List
1. Decreased respiratory function
2. Decreased tolerance to upright
3. Decreased upper extremity strength
4. Decreased passive range of motion of the hamstrings
5. Dependence in functional mobility and ADLs
6. Dependence is pressure relief and skin inspection
7. Patient lacks knowledge of injury and rehabilitation

Short-Term Goals (2 weeks)
1. Bob will tolerate upright sitting in a wheelchair for 3 hours at a time.
2. Bob will increase strength of innervated muscles of bilateral upper extremities to 4/5.
3. Bob will increase hamstring range to 110°.
4. Bob will roll to the right and the left with minimal assist for halo.
5. Bob will transfer from supine to long sitting with standby assist.
6. Bob will maintain static balance in short and long sitting with upper extremity support for 5 minutes independently.

7. Bob will be independent in skin inspection and pressure relief.
8. Bob will transfer with sliding board and moderate assist of 1.
9. Bob will propel wheelchair approximately 25 feet independently.

Long-Term Goals (6 weeks)
1. Bob will tolerate upright sitting in a wheelchair for 8 hours at a time.
2. Bob will increase strength of innervated muscles of bilateral upper extremities to 5/5.
3. Bob will be independent in bed mobility.
4. Bob will be independent in supine to long-sitting transition.
5. Bob will maintain a long-sitting position independently to complete self-care activities.
6. Bob will perform a lateral transfer without a sliding board independently.
7. Bob will perform a car transfer independently.
8. Bob will be independent in wheelchair negotiation on level surfaces and inclines.
9. Bob will be independent in a home exercise program.
10. Bob will be independent in driving an automobile with adaptive controls.

PLAN

Bob will be seen BID 5×/week and one time on Saturday for the next 6 weeks. Treatment sessions will consist of assisted rolling to the right and left and supine to prone until halo is removed. Bob will use a wedge during prone activities. Bob will be assisted to a prone on elbows position to work on balance and scapular strengthening. Bob will be progressed to reaching activities in the position. Upper extremity strengthening exercises will also be performed using cuff weights, pulleys, and Theraband. Shoulder flexion and abduction will be limited to 90° until halo is removed. Will instruct in supine on elbows to long-sitting position. Initially will instruct patient in elbow locking mechanism until triceps strength improves. Tonic holding progressing to alternating isometrics and rhythmic stabilization will be practiced in a long-sitting position. Bob will receive PROM to both lower extremities and will be instructed in self-ROM in long-sitting and supine. Pressure-relief techniques will also be taught, including wheelchair pushups every 10 to 15 minutes when sitting. Acclimation to upright will continue with increasing time spent in the wheelchair. Standing on the tilt table may also be used to assist patient with acclimation to upright. Resistive diaphragm exercises will be practiced. Patient will also be instructed in assistive cough techniques. Bob will be instructed in wheelchair negotiation on

Continued on following page

REHABILITATION UNIT INITIAL EVALUATION: BOB *Continued*

PLAN *Continued*

level surfaces and negotiation of wheelchair parts. Bob will be instructed in sliding board transfers and eventually progressed to lateral transfers without the board. Will reassess patient weekly. Will begin patient and family education and discharge planning. Will assess school and home environment for any necessary modifications. Will secure necessary equipment including wheelchair, cushion, and adaptive equipment as needed.

QUESTIONS TO THINK ABOUT

- What type of specific upper extremity strengthening exercises should be included in the patient's treatment plan?
- Think of ways to incorporate aerobic conditioning into the patient's treatment program.
- What type of activities would be included in a home exercise program?

REFERENCES

Alvarez SE. Functional assessment and training. In Adkins HV (ed). Spinal Cord Injury. New York, Churchill Livingstone, 1985, pp 131–154.

Atrice MB, Gonter M, Griffin DA, et al. Traumatic spinal cord injury. In Umphred DA (ed). Neurological Rehabilitation, 3rd ed. St. Louis, CV Mosby, 1995, pp 484–534.

Behrman AL, Sawyer KL, Tomlinson SS. I want to walk: an approach to physical therapy management of the individual with an incomplete spinal cord injury. Neurol Rep 17:7–12, 1993.

Bloch RF. Autonomic Dysfunction. In Bloch RF, Basbaum M (eds). Management of Spinal Cord Injuries. Baltimore, Williams & Wilkins, 1986, pp 149–163.

Cerny K, Waters R, Hislop H, et al. Walking and wheelchair energetics in persons with paraplegia. Phys Ther 60:1133–1139, 1980.

Craik RL. Abnormalities of motor behavior. In Contemporary Management of Motor Control Problems. Proceedings of the II Step Conference. Alexandria, VA, Foundation for Physical Therapy, 1991, pp 155–164.

Cromwell SJ, Paquette VL. The effect of botulinum toxin A on the function of a person with poststroke quadriplegia. Phys Ther 76: 395–402, 1996.

Decker M, Hall A. Physical therapy in spinal cord injury. In Bloch RF, Basbaum M (eds). Management of Spinal Cord Injuries. Baltimore, Williams & Wilkins, 1986, pp 320–347.

DeVivo MJ, Richards JS. Community reintegration and quality of life following spinal cord injury. Paraplegia 30:108–112, 1992.

Finkbeiner K, Russo SG (eds). Physical Therapy Management of Spinal Cord Injury: Accent on Independence. Woodrow Wilson Rehabilitation Center, through Project Scientia, a grant from the Paralyzed Veterans of America, Fishersville, VA 1990, pp 51–58.

Fredericks CM. Disorders of the spinal cord. In Fredericks CM, Saladin CK (eds). Pathophysiology of the Motor Systems: Principles and Clinical Presentations. Philadelphia, FA Davis, 1996, pp 394–423.

Giesecke C. Aquatic rehabilitation of clients with spinal cord injury. In Ruoti RG, Morris DM, Cole AJ (eds). Aquatic Rehabilitation. Philadelphia, JB Lippincott, 1997, pp 134–150.

Gerhart KA, Bergstrom E, Charlifue SW, et al. Long-term spinal cord injury: functional changes over time. Arch Phys Med Rehabil 74: 1030–1034, 1993.

Katz RT. Management of spasticity. Am J Phys Med Rehabil 67:108–115, 1988.

Katz RT. Management of spastic hypertonia after spinal cord injury. In Yarkony GM (ed). Spinal Cord Injury Medical Management and Rehabilitation. Gaithersburg, MD, Aspen Publishers, 1994, pp 97–107.

Lewthwaite R, Thompson L, Boyd LA, et al. Reconceptualizing physical therapy for spinal cord injury rehabilitation: physical activity for long term health and function. Infusions: Research into Practice 1:1–9, 1994.

Maynard FM, Karunas RS, Waring WP. Epidemiology of spasticity following traumatic spinal cord injury. Arch Phys Med Rehabil 71:566–569, 1990.

Morrison S. Fitness for the spinal cord population: establishing a program in your facility. Neurol Rep 18:22–27, 1994.

Nixon V. Spinal Cord Injury: A Guide to Functional Outcomes in Physical Therapy Management. Rockville, MD, Aspen Systems, 1985, pp 41–66, 177–188.

Roth EJ. Pain in spinal cord injury. In Yarkony GM (ed). Spinal Cord Injury Medical Management and Rehabilitation. Gaithersburg, MD, Aspen Publishers, 1994, pp 141–158.

Schmitz TJ. Traumatic spinal cord injury. In O'Sullivan SB, Schmitz TJ (eds). Physical Rehabilitation Assessment and Treatment, 3rd ed. Philadelphia, FA Davis, 1994, pp 533–575.

Somers MF. Spinal Cord Injury Functional Rehabilitation. Norwalk, CT, Appleton & Lange, 1992, pp 5–34.

Spinal Cord Injury Facts and Figures at a Glance. Birmingham, AL, National Spinal Cord Injury Statistical Center, 1998.

Wetzel J. Respiratory evaluation and treatment. In Adkins HV (ed). Spinal Cord Injury. New York, Churchill Livingstone, 1985, pp 75–98.

Williams DO. Spinal cord injury under managed care. PT Magazine 4(11):34–42, 1996.

Yarkony GM, Chen D. Rehabilitation of Patients with Spinal Cord Injuries. In Braddom RL (ed). Physical Medicine and Rehabilitation. Philadelphia, WB Saunders, 1996, pp 1149–1179.

SECTION 3

CHILDREN

Positioning and Handling Techniques to Foster Motor Function

INTRODUCTION

The purpose of this chapter is to detail some of the most frequent positioning and handling techniques used in working with children who have neurologic dysfunction. Basic techniques such as positioning are used for many reasons: (1) to meet general patient goals such as improving head or trunk control; (2) to accommodate a lack of muscular support; (3) to provide proper postural alignment; and (4) to decrease high muscle tone. Handling techniques can be used to improve the child's performance of functional tasks such as sitting, walking, and reaching by promoting postural alignment prior to movement. Other specific sensory techniques such as tapping a muscle belly, tactile cuing, or pressure are tailored to specific impairments the child may have. Impairments include such things as difficulty in recruiting a muscle contraction for movement initiation, lack of pelvic control for midline positioning, or inability to control certain body segments during changes of position. The ultimate goal of any type of therapeutic intervention is functional movement.

CHILDREN WITH NEUROLOGIC DYSFUNCTION

Children with neurologic dysfunction may exhibit delays in motor development and impairments in muscle tone, sensation, range of motion, strength, and coordination. These children are at risk for musculoskeletal deformities and contractures and often have or are prone to developing limitations in performing functional activities. Functional limitations in transfers, locomotion, manipulation, and activities of daily living may result from impairments. A list of impairments and functional limitations commonly identified by a physical therapy evaluation is found in Table 8–1. Some or all of these impairments may be evident in

Table 8–1 ▌ COMMON IMPAIRMENTS AND FUNCTIONAL LIMITATIONS IN CHILDREN WITH NEUROLOGIC DYSFUNCTION

IMPAIRMENTS	FUNCTIONAL LIMITATIONS
Impaired strength	Dependent in transfers
Impaired muscle tone	Dependent in mobility
Impaired range of motion	Dependent in activities of
Impaired sensation	daily living
Impaired balance and coordination	
Impaired postural reactions	

any child with neurologic dysfunction. The functional limitations may be related to the impairments documented by the physical therapist during an initial evaluation such as deficits in strength, range of motion, and coordination. A lack of postural reactions, balance, and motor milestone acquisition can be expected, given the specific pathologic features of the neurologic disorder. Specific disorders are presented in more depth in Chapters 9, 10, and 11.

GENERAL PHYSICAL THERAPY GOALS

The guiding goal of therapeutic intervention in working with children with neurologic dysfunction is to improve function. The physical therapist and physical therapist assistant team must strive to provide interventions designed to make the child as independent as possible. Specific movement goals vary, depending on the type of neurologic dysfunction. Children with low tone and joint hypermobility need to be stabilized, whereas children with increased tone and limited joint range need mobility. Joint extensibility may be limited by increased tone. A wider range of motion may enable the child with too much tone to change positions independently. Children must be able to move from one position to another with control. Movement from one position to another is called *transitional movement.* Important movement transitions to be mastered include moving from a supine position to a prone position; moving from a supine or prone position to a sitting position; and moving from a sitting position to a standing position. Additional transitional movements usually acquired during normal development are moving from a prone position to a four-point position, followed by moving to kneeling, half-kneeling, and finally standing.

Children who exhibit excessive and extraneous movement, such as children with athetoid or ataxic cerebral palsy, need practice in maintaining stable postures against gravity because their natural tendency is to be moving all the time. Children with fluctuating muscle tone find it difficult to stabilize or maintain a posture and often cannot perform small weight shifts

from the midline without falling. The ability to shift weight within a posture is the beginning of movement control. With controlled weight shifting comes the ability to change positions safely. Regardless of the type of movement experience needed, all children with neuromuscular difficulties need to be able to function in as many postures as possible. Some postures are more functional than others and may provide therapeutic benefits.

FUNCTION RELATED TO POSTURE

Posture provides a base for movement and function. Impairment of postural control, either in attaining or in maintaining a posture, can produce functional limitations. If an infant cannot maintain postural control in sitting without hand support, then the ability to play with toys is limited. Think of posture as a pyramid, with supine and prone positions at the base, followed by sitting, and erect standing at the apex (Fig. 8–1). As the child gains control, the base of support

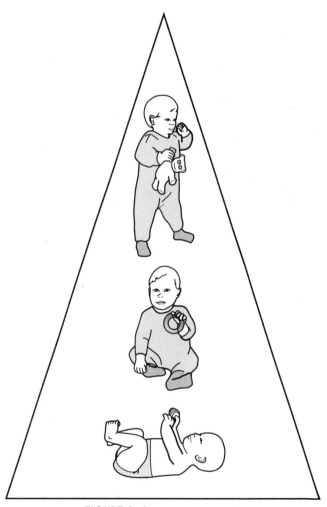

FIGURE 8–1 ▌ Posture pyramid.

becomes smaller. Children with inadequate balance or postural control often widen their base of support to compensate for a lack of stability. A child with decreased postural muscle activity may be able to sit without arm support to play if the legs are straight and widely abducted (abducted long sitting). When the base of support is narrowed by bringing the legs together (long sitting), the child wobbles and may even fall over. The sitting posture, not the child's trunk musculature, was providing the stability.

Supine and Prone

Supine and prone are the lowest postural levels in which a child can function. The supine position is defined as being flat on the back on the support surface. Motor function at this level can involve rolling, reaching with upper extremities, looking, or propelling the body by pushing off flexed lower extremities. The prone position includes lying flat on the tummy with the head turned to one side or lifted, prone on elbows, or prone on extended arms. Mobility in the prone position is possible by means of rolling or crawling on the tummy. Many children push themselves backward when they are prone before they are able to pull themselves forward. Children with weak or uncoordinated lower extremities commonly perform a "commando crawl" using only their arms to pull themselves along the surface. This is also called drag crawling if the lower extremities do not assist in producing the movement but are dragged along by the pull of the arms.

Sitting

Sitting, the next highest posture, affords the child the opportunity to move the extremities while the head and trunk are in a more upright position. In sitting, the child is appropriately oriented to the world, eyes oriented vertically and mouth horizontally. The muscles of the neck and trunk are in the same orientation with gravity, and it is actually easier to maintain head and trunk alignment in this position as compared with prone or supine, in which the force of gravity must be constantly overcome. Sitting upright affords the child the chance to learn to be mobile in a wheelchair or to use the upper extremities for feeding, self-care, and play. Functional use of the upper extremities requires trunk control, whether that comes from postural muscle control or from a seating system. Alternative mobility patterns available to a child who is seated include scooting or hitching along the floor on the buttocks, with or without hand support.

Quadruped

Quadruped, as a developmental posture, allows creeping to emerge sometime between independent sitting and erect standing. In typically developing children, quadruped, or the four-point position, as it may be called, provides quick mobility in a modified prone position before the child has mastered moving in an upright position. Quadruped is considered a dependent and flexed posture; therefore, it has been omitted from the posture pyramid. The child is dependent because the child's head is not always correctly oriented to the world, and with only a few exceptions, the limbs are flexed. It can be difficult for a child to learn to creep reciprocally, so this posture is often omitted as a therapeutic goal. Twelve percent of typically developing children do not creep before walking (Long and Cintas, 1995).

The quadruped position can provide excellent opportunities for the child to bear weight through the shoulders and hips and thereby promote proximal stability at these joints. Such weight-bearing opportunities are essential to preparing for the proximal joint control needed for making the transition from one posture to another. Although the quadruped position does make unique contributions to the development of trunk control because the trunk must work maximally against gravity, other activities can be used to work the trunk muscles without requiring the upper extremities to be fully weight bearing and the hips and knees flexed. Deviating from the developmental sequence may be necessary in therapy because of a child's inability to function in quadruped or because of an increased potential for the child to develop contractures from overutilizing this posture.

Standing

The last and highest level of function is upright standing, in which ambulation may be possible. Most typically developing infants attain an upright standing position by pulling up on furniture at around 9 months of age. By 12 to 18 months, most children are walking independently. Ambulation significantly increases the ability of the toddler to explore the environment. Ask the parent of an infant who has just begun to walk how much more challenging it is to keep up with and safeguard the child's explorations. Attainment of the ability to walk is one of our most frequent therapeutic goals. Being able to move around within our society in an upright standing position is a huge signal that one is "normal." For some parents who are dealing with the realization that their child is not exhibiting typical motor skills, the goal of walking may represent an even bigger achievement, or the final thing the child cannot do. We have worked with parents who have stated that they would rather have their child walk than talk. The most frequently asked questions you will hear when working with very young children are "Will my child walk?" and "When will my child walk?" These are difficult questions. The ambulation potential of children with specific neurologic dysfunction is addressed in Chapters 9, 10, and 11. It is best for the assistant to consult with the supervising therapist before aswering such inquiries.

PHYSICAL THERAPY INTERVENTION

Developmental intervention consists of positioning and handling, including guided movement, and planned environmental experiences that allow the infant and young child to enjoy the feeling of normal movement. These movement experiences must occur within the framework of the infant's or child's role within the family, the home, and, later, the school. An infant's social role is to interact with caregivers and the environment to learn about himself and the world. Piaget called the first 2 years of life the sensorimotor period for that reason. Intelligence (cognition) begins with associations the infant makes between the self and the people and objects within the environment. These associations are formed by and through movement of the body and objects within the environment.

Our intent is to enable the physical therapist assistant to see multiple uses of certain techniques in the context of an understanding of the overall nature of developmental intervention. Initially, when you work with an infant with neuromuscular problems, the child may have a diagnosis of being only "at risk" for developmental delay. The family may not have been given a specific developmental diagnosis. The therapist and physician may have discussed only the child's tight or loose muscles and problems with head control. One of the most important ways to help family members of an "at risk" child is to show them ways to position and handle (hold and move) the child, to make it easier for the child and family to interact. Certain positions may support the infant's head better, thus enabling feeding, eye movement, and looking at the caregiver. Other positions may make diapering easier. Flexing the infant's head, trunk, and limbs while she is being carried is usually indicated because this handling method approximates the typical posture of a young infant and provides a feeling of security for both child and caregiver.

Daily Care

Many handling and positioning techniques can be incorporated into the routine daily care of the child.

Picking a child up and putting her down can be used to provide new movement experiences that the child may not be able to initiate on her own. Optimal positioning for bathing, eating, and playing is in an upright sitting position, provided the child has sufficient head control. As the infant develops head control (4 months) and trunk control, a more upright position can be fostered. If the child is unable to sit with slight support at 6 months, the appropriate developmental time, it may be necessary to use an assistive device such as a feeder seat or a corner chair to provide head or trunk support, to allow the child to experience a more upright orientation to the world.

An upright orientation is also important in developing the child's interest and engaging her socially. Think of how you would automatically position a baby to interact. More than likely, you would pick her up and bring the baby's face toward you. An older child may need only minimal assistance to maintain sitting to perform activities of daily living, as in sitting on a bench to dress or sitting in a chair with arms to feed herself or to color in a book. Some children require only support at the low back to encourage and maintain an upright trunk, as seen in Figure 8–2. Being

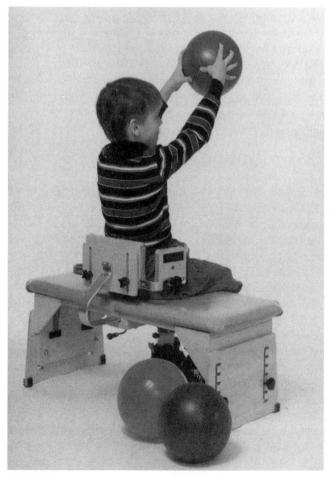

FIGURE 8–2 ❚ Child sitting on a bench with pelvic support. (Courtesy of Kaye Products, Inc., Hillsborough, NC.)

able to sit at the table with the family includes the child in everyday occurrences, such as eating breakfast or reviewing homework. Upright positioning with or without assistive devices provides the appropriate orientation to interact socially while the child plays or performs activities of daily living.

Home Program

Positioning and handling should be part of every home program. When positioning and handling are seen as part of the daily routine, parents are more likely to do these activities with the child. By recognizing all the demands placed on parents' time, you will probably make realistic requests of them. Remember, a parent's time is limited. Stretching can be incorporated into bath time or diaper changes. In addition, by suggesting a variety of therapeutic play positions that can be incorporated into the daily routine of the child, you may make it unnecessary for the caregiver to have to spend as much time stretching specific muscles. Pictures are wonderful reminders. Providing a snapshot of how you want the child to sit can provide a gentle reminder to all family members, especially those who are unable to attend a therapy session. If the child is supposed to use a certain adaptive device such as a corner chair sometime during the day, help the caregiver to determine the best time and place to use the device. Good planning ensures carryover.

POSITIONING AND HANDLING TECHNIQUES

Positioning for Function

One of the fundamental skills a physical therapist assistant learns is how to position a patient. The principles of positioning include alignment, comfort, and support. Additional considerations include prevention of deformity and readiness to move. When positioning the patient's body or body part, the alignment of the body part or the body as a whole must be considered. In the majority of cases, the alignment of a body part is considered along with the reason for the positioning. For example, the position of the upper extremity in relation to the upper trunk is normally at the side; however, when the patient cannot move the arm, it may be better positioned away from the body to prevent tightness of muscles around the shoulder. The patient's comfort is also important to consider because, as we have all experienced, no matter how "good" the position is for us, if it is uncomfortable, we will change to another position. Underlying the rules governing how to position a person in proper body alignment is the need to prevent any potential deformity such as tight heel cords, hip dislocation, or spinal curvature.

Positioning for support may also be thought of as positioning for stability. Children and adults often assume certain positions or postures because they feel safe. For example, the person who has hemiplegic involvement usually orients or shifts weight over the noninvolved side of the body because of better sensory awareness, muscular control, and balance. Although this positioning may be stable, it can lead to potential muscle shortening on the involved side that can impair functional movement. Other examples of postures that provide positional stability include W sitting, wide abducted sitting, and sitting propping on extended arms (Fig. 8–3). All these positions have a wide base of support that provides inherent stability. W sitting is not desirable because the child does not have to use trunk muscles for postural support; the stability of the trunk comes from the position. Asymmetric sitting or sitting with weight shifted more to one side may cause the trunk to develop a muscle imbalance. Common examples of asymmetry are seen in children with hemiplegic cerebral palsy who, even in symmetric sitting postures such as short or long sitting, do so with their weight shifted away from the involved side.

In working with individuals with neurologic dysfunction, the clinician often must determine safe and stable postures that can be used for activities of daily living. The child who uses W sitting because the position leaves the hands free to play needs to be given an alternative sitting position that affords the same opportunities for play. Alternatives to W sitting may include some type of adaptive seating, such as a corner chair or floor sitter (Fig. 8–4). A simple solution may be to have the child sit on a chair at a table to play, rather than sitting on the floor.

The last consideration for positioning is the idea that a position provides a posture from which movement occurs. This concept may be unfamiliar to those who are used to working with adults. Adults have greater motivation to move because of prior experience. Children, on the other hand, may not have experienced movement and may even be afraid to move because they cannot do so with control. Safety is of paramount importance in the application of this concept. A child should be able to be safe in a posture, that is, be able to maintain the posture and demonstrate a protective response if she falls out of the posture. Often, a child can maintain sitting only if she is propped on one or both upper extremities. If the child cannot maintain a posture even when propped, some type of assistance is required to ensure safety while she is in the position. The assistance can be in the form of a device or a person. Proper alignment of the trunk must always be provided to prevent unwanted spinal curvatures, which can hamper independent sitting and respiratory function.

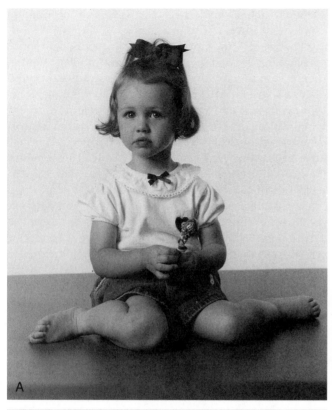

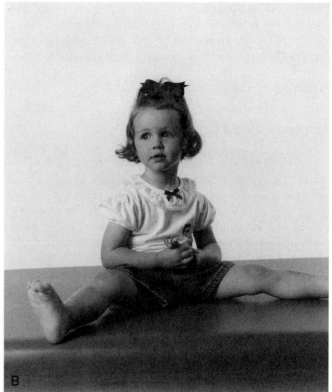

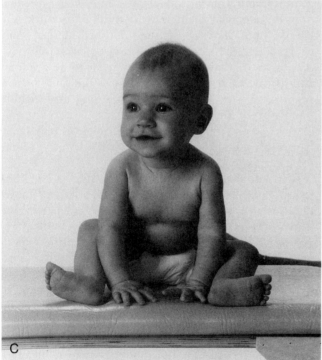

FIGURE 8–3 ■ Sitting postures. *A*, W sitting, which is to be avoided. *B*, Wide abducted long sitting. *C*, Propped sitting with legs abducted.

Any position in which you place a child should allow the child the opportunity to shift weight within the posture for pressure relief. The next movement possibility that should be provided the child is to move from the initial posture to another posture. Many patients, regardless of age and for many reasons, have difficulty in making the transition from one position to another. We often forget this principle of positioning because we are more concerned about the child's safety within a posture than about how the position

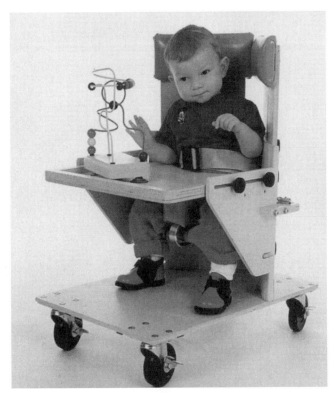

FIGURE 8–4 ■ Corner chair with head support. (Courtesy of Kaye Products, Inc., Hillsborough, NC.)

may affect mobility. When we work with children, we must take into account both mobility and stability to select therapeutic positions that encourage static and dynamic balance. *Dynamic postures* are ones in which controlled mobility can be exhibited, that is, shifting weight so the center of gravity stays within the base of support. In typical development, the child rocks or shifts weight in a hands and knees position for long periods before making the transition to creeping. The ability to shift weight with control within a posture indicates preparation and readiness to move out of that posture into another posture. Dynamic balance is also exhibited when the child moves from the four-point position to a side sitting position. The center of gravity moves diagonally over one hip and down until a new base of support is created by sitting.

The type of activity the child is expected to perform in a particular posture must also be considered when a position is chosen. For example, how an infant or child is positioned for feeding by a caregiver may vary considerably from the position used for self-feeding or for playing on the floor. A child's position must be changed often during the day, so teaching the parent or caregiver only one position rarely suffices. For example, modifications of sitting positions may be required for bathing, dressing, feeding, and toileting, depending on the degree of assistance the child re-

quires with each of these activities. Other positions may be employed to accomplish therapeutic goals related to head control, trunk control, or extremity usage.

The job or occupation of infants and children is merely to play. Although play may appear to be a simple task, it is a constant therapeutic challenge to help parents identify ways to allow their child to participate fully in the world. More broadly, a child's job is interacting with people and objects within the environment and learning how things work. Usually, one of a child's first tasks is to learn the rules of moving, a difficult task when the child has a developmental disability.

Handling at Home

Parents and caregivers should be taught the easiest ways to move the child from one position to another. For example, Intervention 8–1 shows how to assist an infant with head control to move from prone into a sitting position for dressing or feeding. Most children benefit from being picked up while they are in a flexed position and then placed or assisted into sitting. Caregivers are taught how to encourage the infant or child to assist as much as possible during any movement. If the child has head control but decreased trunk control, turning the child to the side and helping her to push up on an elbow or extended arm will result in sitting (Intervention 8–2). Movement transitions are a major part of a home program. The caregiver incorporates into the child's daily routine practicing coming to sit from a supine or prone position and alternates which side of the body the child rolls toward during the maneuver. Trunk rotation from a seated position should also be used when returning the child to a prone or supine position because this requires head control (Intervention 8–3).

If the child does not have head control, it is still appropriate to try to elicit trunk rotation to side lying. Before picking the child up from side lying, the caregiver provides support under the child's shoulders and head with one hand and under the knees with the other hand.

Holding and Carrying Positions

Intervention 8–4 depicts carrying positions with varying amounts of support, depending on whether the child has head or trunk control, hypertonia, or hypotonia. Intervention 8–4A shows an infant cradled for support of the head, trunk, and pelvis. A child with increased lower extremity tone should not be picked up under the arms, as shown in Intervention 8–4B.

Intervention 8-1 ▮ PRONE TO SITTING

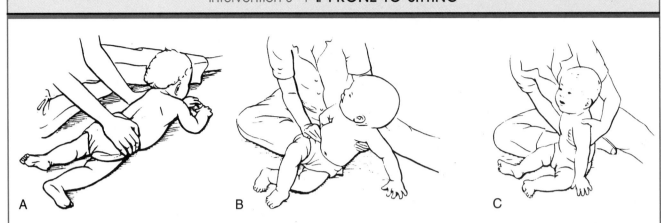

A

B

C

Moving a child with head control from prone into sitting.

A. Place one hand under the arm next to you and the other hand on the child's opposite hip.

B. Initiate rotation of the hip and assist as needed under the shoulder. Allow the child to push up if he is able.

C. Perform the activity slowly to allow the child to help and support the trunk if necessary in sitting.

From Jaeger DL. Home Program Instruction Sheets for Infants and Young Children. Copyright © 1987 by Therapy Skill Builders, A Harcourt Health Sciences Company. Reproduced by permission. All rights reserved.

The legs stiffen into extension and may even cross or "scissor." This way of picking up an infant should also be avoided in the presence of low tone because the child's shoulder girdle stability may not be sufficient for the caregiver to hold the infant safely. Intervention 8-4C and E demonstrates correct ways to hold a child with increased tone. The child's lower extremities are flexed, with the trunk and legs supported. Trunk rotation is encouraged. By having the child straddle the caregiver's hip, as in Intervention 8-4E, the child's hip adductors are stretched, and the upper trunk, which is rotated outward, is dissociated from the lower trunk. The caregiver must remember to carry the child on opposite sides during the day, to avoid promoting asymmetric trunk rotation. The child with low tone needs to be gathered close to you to be given a sense of stability (see Intervention 8-4D). Many infants and children with developmental delay find prone an uncomfortable position but may tolerate being carried in the prone position because of the contact with the caregiver and the movement stimulation (see Intervention 8-4F).

Holding an infant in the prone position over the caregiver's lap can provide vestibular system input to reinforce midline orientation or lifting of the head. Infants with head control and some trunk control can be held on the caregiver's lap while they straddle the caregiver's knee, to abduct their tight lower extremities.

Handling Techniques for Movement Facilitation

Because children with disabilities do have similar problems, grouping possible treatment techniques together is easier based on the position and goal of the technique, such as positioning in prone to encourage head control. The treatment activity should be matched to the child's problem, and one should always keep in mind the overall functional goal. Depending on the severity of neurologic involvement of the child, lower-level developmental milestones may be the highest goal possible. For example, in a child with severe spastic quadriplegic cerebral palsy, therapeutic goals may consist of the development of head control and the prevention of contractures, whereas in a child with quadriplegia and moderate involvement, independent sitting and wheelchair mobility may be the goals of intervention.

Use of Manual Contacts at Key Points of Control

When you are facilitating the child's head or trunk control from the shoulder girdle, placing your hands under the child's axillae while facing him can serve to mobilize the scapulae and lift the extremities away from the body. Your fingers should be spread out in such a way to control both the scapulae and the upper

Intervention 8-2 ▌ SUPINE TO SIDE LYING TO SITTING

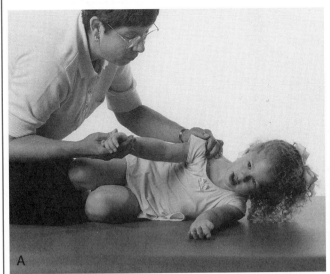

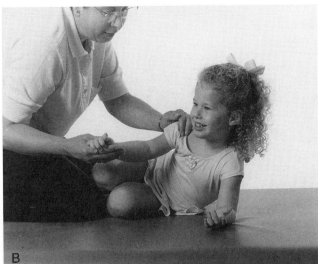

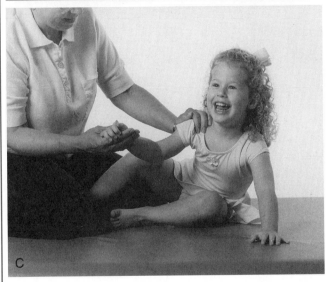

Movement sequence of coming to sit from supine using side lying as a transition.

A. Facilitation of appropriate head lifting in side lying by providing downward pressure on the shoulder.

B. The movement continues as the child pushes up on an extended arm.

C. The child pushes up to an elbow.

arms. By controlling the scapulae in this way, you can facilitate movement of the child's head, trunk, arms, and legs but prevent the arms from pulling down and back, as may be the child's typical movement pattern. If you do not need to control the child's upper extremities, your hands can be placed over the child's shoulders to cover the clavicles, the scapulae, and the heads of the humeri. This second strategy can also promote alignment and therefore can increase stability and can be especially useful in the treatment of a child with too much movement, as in athetoid cerebral palsy. Varying amounts of pressure can be given through the shoulders and can be combined with movement in different directions to provide a stabilizing influence.

Wherever your hands are on the child, the child is not in control, you are, so the child must be given practice controlling the body parts used to guide movement. For example, if you are using the child's shoulders to guide movement, the child needs to learn to control movement at the shoulder. As the child exhibits more proximal control, your points of guidance and handling can be moved more distally to the elbow or hand. Stability can be facilitated by positioning the limbs in a weight-bearing or loaded position. If the child lacks sufficient control, pediatric air splints can be used to control the limb position, thus enabling the child to bear weight on an extended knee or to keep the weight-bearing elbow straight while he reaches with the other arm (Fig. 8–5).

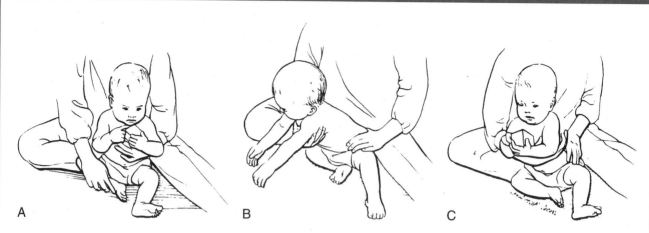

Intervention 8–3 ❙ SITTING TO PRONE

Moving a child with head control from sitting to prone.

A. With the child sitting, bend the knee of the side toward which the child will rotate.

B. Initiate the movement by rotating the child's upper trunk.

C. Complete the rotation by guiding the hip to follow until the child is prone.

From Jaeger DL. Home Program Instruction Sheets for Infants and Young Children. Copyright © 1987 by Therapy Skill Builders, A Harcourt Health Sciences Company. Reproduced by permission. All rights reserved.

Handling Tips

The following should be considered when you physically handle a child with neurologic dysfunction.

1. Allow the child to do as much of the movement as possible. You will need to pace yourself and will probably have to go more slowly than you may think. For example, when bringing a child into a sitting position from supine, roll the child slowly to one side and give the child time to push up onto his hand, even if he can only do this part of the way, such as up to an elbow. In addition, try to entice the child to roll to the side before attempting to have him come to sit. The effects of gravity can be reduced by using an elevated surface such as a wedge.

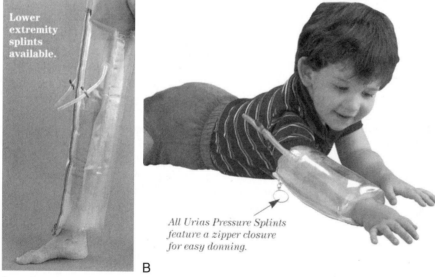

Lower extremity splints available.

All Urias Pressure Splints feature a zipper closure for easy donning.

FIGURE 8–5 ■ *A* and *B*, Use of pediatric air splints for knee control in standing and elbow control in prone reaching. (Courtesy of Sammons Preston, Bowling Brook, IL.)

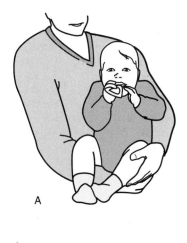

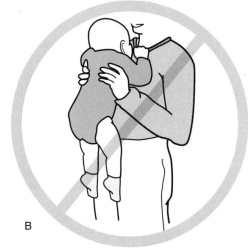

A

B

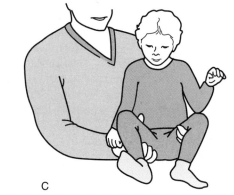

C

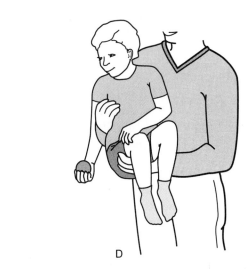

D

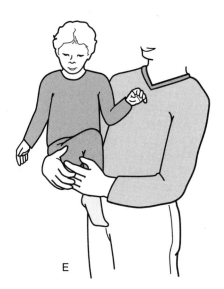

E

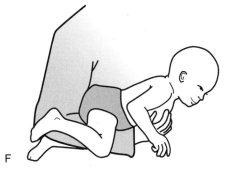

F

A. Place the child in a curled-up position with shoulders forward and hips flexed. Place your arm behind the child's head, *not* behind the neck.

B. INCORRECT: Avoid lifting the child under his arms without supporting the legs. The child with hypertonicity may "scissor" (cross) the legs. The child with hypotonicity may slip through your hands.

C. CORRECT: Bend the child's legs before picking him up. Give sufficient support to the trunk and legs while allowing trunk rotation.

D. Hold the child with low tone close, to provide a feeling of stability.

E. Have the child straddle your hips to separate tight legs. Be sure the child's trunk is rotated forward and both his arms are free.

F. Prone position.

2. When carrying a child, encourage as much head and trunk control as the child can demonstrate. Carry the child in such a way he has to use head and trunk muscles to maintain the head and trunk upright against gravity while you are moving. This allows him to look around and see where you are going.

3. When trying to move the limbs of a child with spasticity, do not pull against the tightness. Do move slowly and rhythmically, starting proximally at the child's shoulders and pelvis. The position of the proximal joints can influence the position of the entire extremity. Changing the position of the proximal joint may also reduce spasticity throughout the extremity.

4. Many children with severe involvement and those with athetosis show an increased sensitivity to touch, sound, and light. These children startle easily and may withdraw from contact to their hands, feet, and mouth. Encourage the child to keep her head in the midline of the body and the hands in sight. Weight bearing on hands and feet is an important activity for these children.

5. Children with low postural tone should be handled more vigorously, but they tire more easily and require more frequent rest periods. Avoid placing these children in the supine position to play because they need to work against gravity in the prone position to develop extensors. Their extensors are so weak that the extremities assume a "frog" position of abduction when these children are supine. Strengthening of abdominal muscles can be done when these children are in a semi-reclined supine position. Encourage arm use and visual learning. By engaging visual tracking, the child may learn to use the eyes to encourage head and trunk movement. Infant seats are appropriate for the young child with low tone, but an adapted corner chair is better for the older child.

6. When encouraging movements from proximal joints, remember that wherever your hands are, the child will not be in control. If you control the shoulders, the child has to control the head and trunk, that is, above and below where you are handling. Keep this in mind anytime you are guiding movement. If you want the child to control a body part or joint, you should not be holding on to that area.

7. Ultimately, the goal is for the child to guide her own movements. Handling should be decreased as the child gains more control. If the child exhibits movement of satisfactory quality only while you are guiding the movement but is not able to assist in making the same movements on her own, you must question whether motor learning is actually taking place. The child must actively participate in move-

ment to learn to move. For movement to have meaning, it must have a goal.

Use of Sensory Input to Facilitate Positioning and Handling

Touch

An infant begins to define the edges of her own body by touch. Touch is also the first way in which an infant finds food and experiences self-calming when upset. Infant massage is a way to help parents feel comfortable about touching their infant. The infant can be guided to touch the body as a prelude to self-calming (Intervention 8–5). Positioning the infant in side lying often makes it easier for him to touch his body and to see his hands and feet, an important factor. Awareness of the body's midline is an essential perceptual ability. If asymmetry in movement or sensation exists, then every effort must be made to equalize the child's awareness of both sides of the body when he is being moved or positioned. Additional tactile input can be given to that side of the body in the form of touch or weight bearing. The presence of asymmetry in sensation and movement can contribute to arm and leg length differences. Shortening of trunk muscles can occur because of lack of equal weight bearing through the pelvis in sitting or as compensation for unilateral muscular paralysis. Trunk muscle imbalance can also lead to scoliosis.

Touch and movement play important roles in developing body and movement awareness and balance. Children with hypersensitivity to touch may need to be desensitized. Usually, gentle but firm pressure is better tolerated than light touch when a child is overly sensitive. Light touch produces withdrawal of an extremity or turning away of the face in children who exhibit tactile defensiveness (Koomar and Bundy, 1991). Most typically developing children like soft textures before rough ones, but children who appear to misperceive tactile input may actually tolerate coarse textures such as terry cloth better than soft textures.

General guidelines for use of tactile stimulation with children with tactile defensiveness have been outlined by Koomar and Bundy (1991). These include the following: (1) having the child administer the stimulation; (2) using firm pressure but realizing that light touch can be used if the child is indeed perceiving light touch as deep pressure; (3) applying touch to the arms and legs before the face; (4) applying the stimulation in the direction of hair growth; and (5) providing a quiet, enclosed area for the stimulation to take place. Textured mitts, paintbrushes, sponges, and vibrators provide different types of tactile stimulation. Theoretically, deep touch or pressure to the extremities has a central inhibitory effect that is more general,

---

Intervention 8–5 ‖ TEACHING SELF-CALMING

A

B

Using touch to self-calm in supported supine and side lying positions.

A. The infant can be guided to touch the body as a prelude to self-calming.

B. Positioning the child in side lying often makes it easier for him to touch his body and to see his hands and feet, important points of reference.

---

even though this touch is applied to a specific body part (Ayres, 1972). The expected outcome is that the child will have an increased tolerance to touch, be able to concentrate better, and exhibit better organized behavior. If handling the child is to be an effective part of intervention, the infant or child must be able to tolerate touch.

A child who is defensive about touch to the face usually also has increased sensitivity to touch inside the mouth. Such children may have difficulty in eating textured foods. Oromotor therapy is a specialized area of practice that requires additional education. A physical, occupational, or speech therapist may be trained to provide this type of care. The physical therapist assistant may be taught specific techniques by the therapist that are applicable to a particular child in a specific setting. However, these techniques are beyond the scope of this book and are only referred to in general terms.

Vestibular System

The three semicircular canals of the vestibular system are fluid filled. Each set of canals responds to movement in different planes. Cartwheels, somersaults, and spinning produce movement in different canals. Linear movement (movement in line with the body orientation) can improve head lifting when the child is in a prone or supine position. This movement is often done with the child prone or supine in a hammock (Fig. 8–6). Movement stimulation often works to

alert a lethargic child or one with low muscle tone because the vestibular system has a strong influence on postural tone and balance. The vestibular system causes a response when the flow of fluid in the semicircular canals changes direction. Constant movement results in the child's habituation or becoming used to the movement and does not produce a response. Rapid, quick movement, as in sitting on a movable

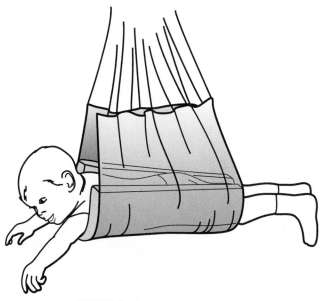

FIGURE 8–6 ■ Child in a hammock.

surface, can alert the child. Fast, jerky movement facilitates low tone. Slow, rhythmic movement inhibits high tone.

Approximation

Application of compression through joints in weight bearing is *approximation.* Rocking on hands and knees and bouncing on a ball in sitting are examples of activities that provide approximation. Additional compression can be given manually through the body parts into the weight-bearing surface. Joints may also be approximated by manually applying constant pressure through the long axis of aligned body parts. Intermittent compression can also be used. Both constant pressure and intermittent pressure provide proprioceptive cues to alert postural muscles to support the body, as in sitting and bouncing on a trampoline. The speed of the compressive force and the give of the support surface provide differing amounts of joint approximation. The direction of movement can be varied while the child is rocking on hands and knees. Compression through the length of the spine is achieved from just sitting, as a result of gravity, but this compression can be increased by bouncing. Axial compression or pressure through the head and neck must be used cautiously in children with Down syndrome because of the 20% incidence of atlantoaxial instability in this population (American Academy of Pediatrics, 1992). External

compression can also be given through the shoulders into the spine while the child is sitting or through the shoulders or hips when the child is in a four-point position (Intervention 8–6). The child's body parts must always be aligned prior to receiving manual compression, with compression graded to the tolerance of the child. Less compression is better in most instances. Use of approximation is illustrated in the following situation involving a young girl with athetoid cerebral palsy. When the clinician placed a hand lightly but firmly on the girl's head as she was attempting to maintain a standing position, the child was more stable within the posture. She was then asked to assume various ballet positions with her feet, to help her learn to adjust to different-sized bases of support and still maintain her balance. During the next treatment session, the girl initiated the stabilization by placing the therapist's hand on her head. Gradually, external stabilization from the therapist's hand was able to be withdrawn.

Intermittent or sustained pressure can also be used to prepare a limb or the trunk to accept weight prior to loading the limb as in gait or laterally shifting weight onto the trunk. Prior to weight bearing on a limb such as in propped sitting, the arm can be prepared to accept the weight by applying pressure from the heel of the hand into the shoulder with the elbow straight, not locked (Intervention 8–7). This is best done with the arm in about 45 degrees of external

---

Intervention 8–6 ❚ COMPRESSION OF PROXIMAL JOINTS

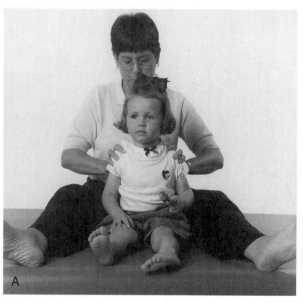 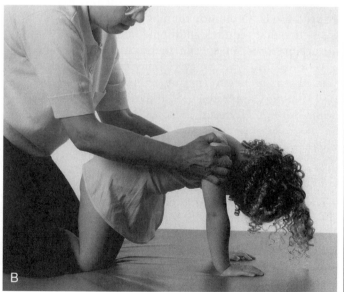

A. Manual approximation through the shoulders in sitting.

B. Manual approximation through the shoulders in the four-point position.

Intervention 8-7 ▌ PREPARATION FOR UPPER EXTREMITY WEIGHT BEARING

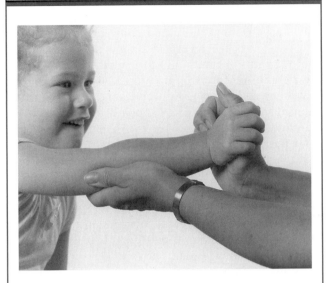

Application of pressure through the heel of the hand to approximate the joints of the upper extremity.

rotation. Think of the typical position of the arm when it is extended as if to catch yourself. The technique of using sustained pressure for the trunk is done by applying firm pressure along the side of the trunk on which the weight will be shifted (Interven-

tion 8–8). The pressure is applied along one side of the trunk from the middle of the trunk out toward the hip and shoulder prior to assisting the child to turn onto that side. This technique can be used as preparation for rolling or coming to sit through side lying. A modification of this technique is used prior to or as you initiate a lateral weight shift to assist trunk elongation.

Vision

Visual images entice a child to explore the environment. Vision also provides important information for the development of head control and balance. Visual fixation is the ability to look with both eyes for a sustained time. To encourage looking, find out whether the child prefers faces or objects. In infants, begin with black and white objects or a stylized picture of a face and then add colors such as red and yellow to try to attract the child's attention. You will have the best success if you approach the infant from the periphery because the child's head will most likely be turned to the side. Next, encourage tracking of objects to the midline and then past the midline. Before infants can maintain the head in the midline, they can track from the periphery toward the midline, then through ever widening arcs. Directional tracking ability then progresses horizontally, vertically, diagonally, and rotationally (clockwise and counterclockwise).

If the child has difficulty using both eyes together or if the eyes cross or turn out, alert the supervising physical therapist, who may suggest that the child see an optometrist or an ophthalmologist. Children who

Intervention 8-8 ▌ PREPARATION FOR WEIGHT ACCEPTANCE

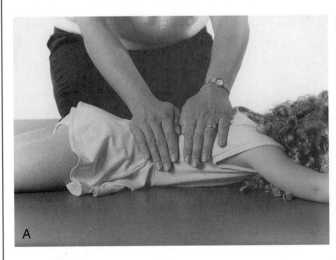
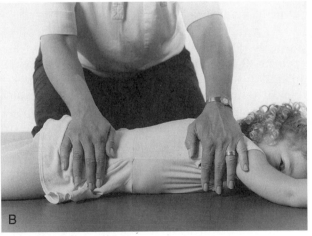

Firm stroking of the trunk in preparation for weight acceptance.
A. Beginning hand position.
B. Ending hand position.

have eye problems corrected early in life may find it easier to develop head control and the ability to reach for objects. Children with permanent visual impairments must rely on auditory signals within the environment to entice them to move. Just as you would use a toy to help a child track visually, use a rattle or other noisemaker to encourage head turning, reaching, and rolling toward the sound. The child has to be able to localize or determine where the sound is coming from before these types of activities are appropriate. Children with visual impairments generally achieve motor milestones later than typically developing children.

Hearing

Although hearing does not specifically play a role in the development of posture and movement, if the acoustic nerve responsible for hearing is damaged, then the vestibular nerve that accompanies it may also be impaired. Impairment of the vestibular nerve or any part of the vestibular system may cause balance deficits because information from head movement is not translated into cues for postural responses. In addition, the close coordination of eye and head movements may be compromised. When working with preschoolers who are hearing impaired, clinicians have often found that these children have balance problems. Studies have shown that both static and dynamic balance can be impaired in this population (Horak et al, 1988; Shumway-Cook and Horak, 1986). Auditory cues can be used to encourage movement and, in the visually impaired, may provide an alternative way to direct or guide movement.

PREPARATION FOR MOVEMENT

Postural Readiness

Postural readiness is the usual preparation for movement. It is defined as the ability of the muscles to exhibit sufficient resting tone to support movement. Sufficient resting tone is evident by the child's ability to sustain appropriate postural alignment of the body before, during, and after performing a movement task. In children with neurologic dysfunction, some positions can be advantageous for movement, whereas others may promote abnormally strong tonic reflexes (Table 8-2). A child in the supine position may be dominated by the effect of the tonic labyrinthine reflex, which causes increased extensor tone and thus decreases the possibility that the child will be able to roll to prone or come to sit easily. If the tone is too high or too low, or if the body is not appropriately aligned, movement will be more difficult, less efficient, and less likely to be successful.

Postural Alignment

Alignment of the trunk is required prior to trying to elicit movement. When you slump in your chair before trying to come to stand, your posture is not prepared to support efficient movement. When the pelvis is either too anteriorly or too posteriorly tilted, the trunk is not positioned to respond with appropriate righting reactions to any weight shift. Recognizing that the patient is lying or sitting asymmetrically should cue repositioning in appropriate alignment. To promote weight bearing on the hands or feet, one must pay attention to how limbs are positioned. Excessive rotation of a limb may provide mechanical locking into a posture, rather than afford the child's muscles an opportunity to maintain the position. Examples of excessive rotation can be seen in the elbows of a child with low tone who attempts to maintain a hands and knees position or whose knees are hyperextended in standing. Advantages and disadvantages of different positions are discussed in Chapter 11 as they relate to the effects of exaggerated tonic reflexes, which are most often evident in children with cerebral palsy.

Key Points of Control

Proximal joints are key points of control from which to guide movement or to reinforce a posture. The shoulders and hips are most commonly used either separately or together to guide movement from one posture to another. Choosing key points is part of movement preparation. The more proximal the manual contacts, the more you control the child's movements. Moving contacts more distally to the elbow or knee or to the hands and feet requires that the child take more control. A description of the use of these key points is given in the section of this chapter on positioning and handling techniques.

Rotation

Slow, rhythmic movement of the trunk and extremities is often helpful in decreasing muscle stiffness (Intervention 8-9). Some children are unable to attempt any change in position without this preparation. When using slow, rhythmic movements, one should begin at proximal joints. For example, if tightness in the upper extremities is evident, then slow, alternating pressure can be applied to the anterior chest wall, followed by manual protraction of the scapula and depression of the shoulder, which is usually elevated. The child's extremity is slowly and rhythmically externally rotated as the arm is abducted away from the body and elevated. The abduction and elevation of the arm allow for some trunk lengthening, which can be helpful prior to rolling or shifting weight in sitting or stand-

Table 8-2 ▍ ADVANTAGES AND DISADVANTAGES OF DIFFERENT POSITIONS

POSITION	ADVANTAGES	DISADVANTAGES
Supine	Can begin early weight bearing through the lower extremities when the knees are bent and feet are flat on the support surface. Positioning of the head and upper trunk in forward flexion can decrease the effect of the STLR. Can facilitate use of the upper extremity in play or object exploration. Lower extremities can be positioned in flexion over a roll, ball, or bolster.	Effect of STLR can be strong and not easily overcome. Supine can be disorienting because it is associated with sleeping. The level of arousal is lowest in this position, so it may be more difficult to engage the child in meaningful activity.
Side lying	Excellent for dampening the effect of most tonic reflexes because of the neutral position of the head; achieving protraction of the shoulder and pelvis; separating the upper and lower trunk; achieving trunk elongation on the down side; separating the right and left sides of the body; and promoting trunk stability by dissociating the upper and lower trunk. Excellent position to promote functional movements such as rolling and coming to sit or as a transition from sitting to supine or prone.	It may be more difficult to maintain the position without external support or a special device such as a sidelyer. Shortening of the upper trunk muscles may occur if the child is always positioned on the same side.
Prone	Promotes weight bearing through the upper extremities (prone on elbows or extended arms); stretches the hip and knee flexors and facilitates the development of active extension of the neck and upper trunk. In young or very developmentally disabled children, it may facilitate development of head control and may promote eye-hand relationships. With the addition of a movable surface, upper extremity protective reactions may be elicited.	Flexor posturing may increase because of the influence of the PTLR breathing may be more difficult for some children secondary to inhibition of the diaphragm, although ventilation may be better. Prone is not recommended for young children as a sleeping posture because of its relationship with an increased incidence of sudden infant death syndrome.
Sitting	Promotes active head and trunk control; can provide weight bearing through the upper and lower extremities; frees the arms for play; and may help normalize visual and vestibular input as well as aid in feeding. The extended trunk is dissociated from flexed lower extremities. Excellent position to facilitate head and trunk righting reactions, trunk equilibrium reactions, and upper extremity protective extension. One or both upper extremities can be dissociated from the trunk. Side sitting promotes trunk elongation and rotation.	Sitting is a flexed posture. A child may be unable to maintain trunk extension because of a lack of strength or too much flexor tone. Optimal seating at 90-90-90 may be difficult to achieve and may require external support. Some floor-sitting postures such as cross-sitting and W sitting promote muscle tightness and may predispose to lower extremity contractures.
Quadruped	Weight bearing through all four extremities with the trunk working against gravity. Provides an excellent opportunity for dissociation and reciprocal movements of the extremities and as a transition to side sitting if trunk rotation is possible.	The flexed posture is difficult to maintain because of the influence of the STNR, which can encourage bunny hopping as a form of locomotion. When trunk rotation is lacking, children often end up W sitting.
Kneeling	Kneeling is a dissociated posture; the trunk and hips are extended while the knees are flexed. Provides a stretch to the hip flexors. Hip and pelvic control can be developed in this position, which can be a transition posture to and from side sitting or to half-kneeling and standing.	Kneeling can be difficult to control, and children often demonstrate an inability to extend at the hips completely because of the influence of the STNR.
Standing	Provides weight bearing through the lower extremities and a stretch to the hip and knee flexors and ankle plantar flexors; can promote active head and trunk control and may normalize visual input.	A significant amount of external support may be required; may not be a long-term option for the child.

PTLR, prone tonic labyrinthine reflex; STLR, supine tonic labyrinthine reflex; STNR, symmetric tonic neck reflex.
Adapted from Lemkuhl LD, Krawczyk L. Physical therapy management of the minimally-responsive patient following traumatic brain injury: coma stimulation. Neurol Rep 17:10–17, 1993.

ing. Always starting at proximal joints provides a better chance for success. Various hand grasps can be used when moving the upper extremity. A handshake grasp is commonly used, as is grasping the thumb and thenar eminence (Fig. 8–7). Extending the carpometacarpal joint of the thumb also decreases tone in the extremity. Be careful to avoid pressure in the palm of the hand if the child still has a palmar grasp reflex. Do not attempt to free a thumb that is trapped in a closed hand without first trying to alter the position of the entire upper extremity.

When a child has increased tone in the lower extremity muscles, begin with alternating pressure on the pelvis (anterior superior iliac spine), first on one side and then the other (Intervention 8–10). As you continue to rock the child's pelvis slowly and gently, externally rotate the hip at the proximal thigh. As the tone decreases, lift the child's legs into flexion; bending the hips and knees can significantly reduce the bias toward extension. With the child's knees bent, continue slow, rhythmic rotation of one or both legs and place the legs into hooklying. Pressure can be given from the knees into the hips and into the feet to reinforce this flexed position. The more the hips and knees are flexed, the less extension is possible, so in cases of extreme increased tone, the knees can be brought to

Intervention 8–9 ▌ TRUNK ROTATION

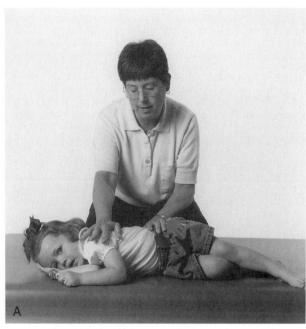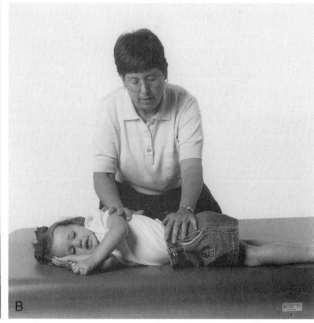

Slow, rhythmic rotation of the trunk in side lying to decrease muscle tone and to improve respiration.

the chest with continued slow rotation of the bent knees across the trunk. By positioning the child's head and upper body into more flexion in supine, you may also flex the child's lower extremities more easily. A wedge, bolster, or pillows can be used to support the child's upper body in the supine position. The caregiver should avoid positioning the child supine without ensuring that the child has a flexed head and upper body because the legs may be too stiff in extension as a result of the supine tonic labyrinthine reflex. Lower trunk rotation initiated with one or both of the child's lower extremities can also be used as a prepara-

Intervention 8–10 ▌ ALTERNATING PELVIC PRESSURE

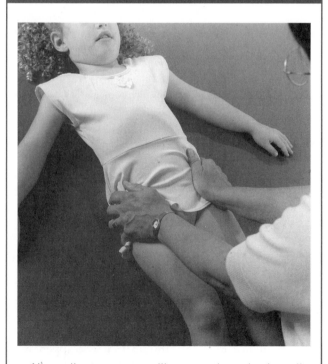

Alternating pressure with manual contact on the pelvis can be used to decrease muscle tone and to facilitate pelvic and lower extremity motion.

FIGURE 8–7 ▪ Handshake grasp.

Intervention 8-11 ▌ LOWER TRUNK ROTATION AND ROLLING FROM SUPINE TO PRONE

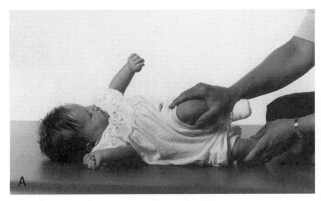 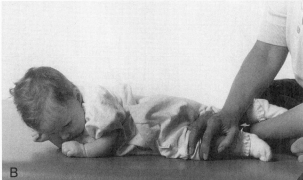

Lower trunk rotation initiated by flexing one leg over the other and facilitating rolling from supine to prone.

tory activity prior to changing position such as rolling from supine to prone (Intervention 8-11). If the child's hips and knees are too severely flexed and adducted, gently rocking the child's pelvis by moving the legs into abduction by means of some outward pressure on the inside of the knees and downward pressure from the knees into the hips may allow you to slowly extend and abduct the child's legs (Intervention 8-12). When generalized increased tone exists, as in a child with quadriplegic cerebral palsy, slow rocking while the child is prone over a ball may sufficiently reduce tone to allow initiation of movement transitions such as rolling to the side or head lifting in prone (Intervention 8-13).

INTERVENTIONS TO FOSTER HEAD AND TRUNK CONTROL

The following positioning and handling techniques can be applied to children with a variety of disorders. They are arranged developmentally, because children need to acquire some degree of head control before they are able to control the trunk in an upright posture. Both head control and trunk control are necessary components for sitting and standing.

Head Control

Several different ways of encouraging head control through positioning in prone, in supine, and while being held upright in supported sitting are presented here. The techniques can be used to facilitate development of head control in children who do not exhibit

appropriate control. Many techniques can be used during therapy or as part of a home program. The decision about which techniques to use should be based on a thorough evaluation by the physical therapist and the therapeutic goals outlined in the child's treatment plan.

Intervention 8-12 ▌ LOWER TRUNK ROTATION AND PELVIC ROCKING

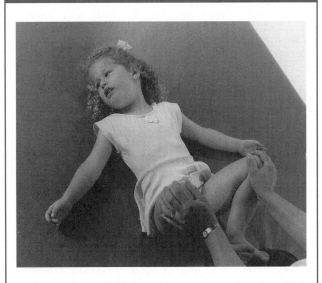

Lower trunk rotation and pelvic rocking to aid in abducting the lower extremities in the presence of increased adductor muscle tone.

Intervention 8-13 ▍ USE OF THE BALL FOR TONE REDUCTION AND HEAD LIFTING

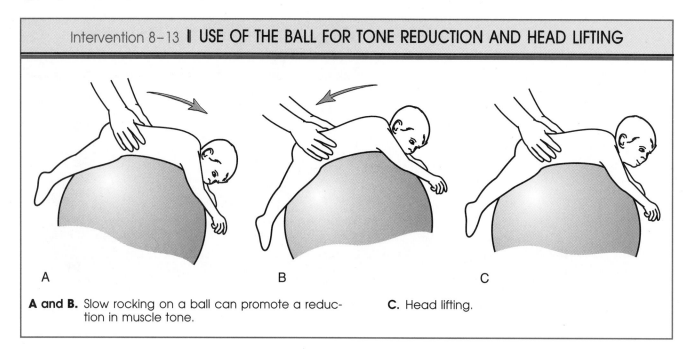

A and B. Slow rocking on a ball can promote a reduction in muscle tone.

C. Head lifting.

Positioning to Encourage Head Control

Prone over a Bolster, Wedge, or Half-Roll. Prone is usually the first position in which the newborn experiences head lifting; therefore, it is one of the first positions used to encourage development of head control. When an infant is placed over a small roll or bolster, the child's chest is lifted off the support surface, and this maneuver takes some weight off the head. In this position, the infant's forearms can be positioned in front of the roll, to add further biomechanical advantage to lifting the head. The child's elbows should be positioned under the shoulders to provide weight-bearing input for a support response from the shoulder girdle muscles. A visual and auditory stimulus such as a mirror, brightly colored toy, or noisemaker can be used to encourage the child to lift the head. Lifting is followed by holding the head up for a few seconds first in any position, then in the midline. A wedge may also be used to support the infant's entire body and to keep the arms forward. The advantage of a half-roll is that because the roll does not move, the child is less likely to "roll" off it. It may be easier to obtain forearm support when the child is positioned over a half-roll or a wedge of the same height as the length of the child's upper arm (Intervention 8–14*A*).

Supine on a Wedge or Half-Roll. Antigravity flexion of the neck is necessary for balanced control of the head. Although most children exhibit this ability at around 5 months of age, children with disabilities may find development of antigravity flexion more of a challenge than head extension, especially children with underlying extensor tone. Preparatory positioning in a supine position on a wedge or half-roll puts the child in a less difficult position against gravity to attempt head lifting (Intervention 8–14*B*). The child should be encouraged to keep the head in the midline while he is positioned in supine. A midline position can be encouraged by using a rolled towel arch or by providing a visual focus. Toys or objects can be attached to a rod or frame, as in a mobile, and placed in front of the child to encourage reaching with the arms. If a child cannot demonstrate any forward head movement, increasing the degree of incline so the child is closer to upright than to supine may be beneficial. This can also be accomplished by using an infant seat or a feeder seat with a Velcro base that allows for different degrees of inclination (Intervention 8–14*C*).

Interventions to Encourage Head Control

Modified Pull-to-Sit Maneuver. The beginning position is supine. The hardest part of the range for the child's head to move through in the pull-to-sit maneuver is the initial part in which the force of gravity is directly perpendicular to the head (Fig. 8–8). The infant or child has to have enough strength to initiate the movement. Children with disabilities have extreme head lag during the pull-to-sit transition. Therefore, the maneuver is modified to make it easier for the child to succeed. The assistant provides support at the child's shoulders and rotates the child toward herself and begins to move the child toward sitting on a diagonal (Intervention 8–15). The assistant may need to wait for the child to bring the head and upper body forward into sitting. The child may be able to help with only the last part of the maneuver as

Intervention 8–14 ▮ POSITIONS TO ENCOURAGE HEAD CONTROL

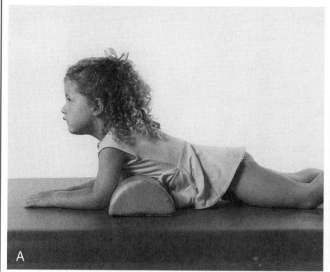

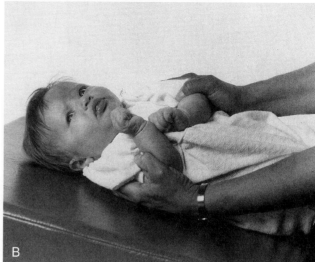

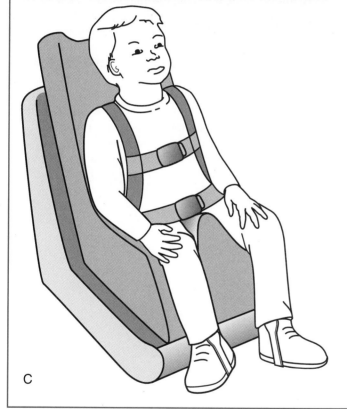

A. Positioning the child prone over a half-roll encourages head lifting and weight bearing on the elbows and forearms.

B. Positioning the child supine on a wedge in preparation for anterior head lifting.

C. A feeder seat/floor sitter that allows for different degrees of inclination.

the vertical position is approached. If the child tries to reinforce the movement with shoulder elevation, the assistant's index fingers can depress the child's shoulders and can thus avoid this substitution. Improvement in head control can be measured by the child's ability to maintain the head in midline in various postures, by exhibiting neck righting reactions, or by assisting in the maneuver earlier during the range. As the child's head control improves, less trunk rotation is used to encourage the neck muscles to work against gravity as much as possible. More distal contacts such as the elbows and finally the hands can be used to initiate

GRAVITY

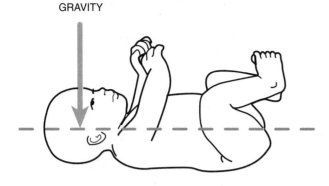

GRAVITY

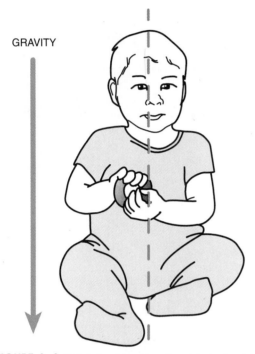

FIGURE 8–8 ■ Relationship of gravity with the head in supported supine and supported sitting positions.

the pull-to-sit maneuver (see Intervention 8–2). These distal points of control are not recommended if the child has too much joint laxity.

Upright in Supported Sitting. In the child's relation to gravity, support in the upright sitting position (Table 8–3) is probably an easier position in which to maintain head control because the orientation of the

Table 8–3 ▎ PROGRESSION OF SUPPORTED SITTING

1. Sitting in the corner of a sofa.
2. Sitting in a corner chair or a beanbag chair.
3. Side sitting with one arm propped over a bolster or half-roll.
4. Sitting with arms forward and supported on an object such as a pillow or a ball.
5. Sitting in a highchair.

head is in line with the force of gravity. The head position and the force of gravity are parallel (see Fig. 8–8), whereas when a child is in the supine or prone position, the force of gravity is perpendicular to the position of the head at the beginning of head lifting. This relationship makes it more difficult to lift the head from either supine or prone than to maintain the head when either held upright in vertical or held upright in supported sitting. This is why a newborn has total head lag as one tries to pull the baby to sit, but once the infant is sitting, the head appears to sit more stably on the shoulders. A child who is supine or prone uses only neck flexors or extensors to lift the head. In the upright position, a balance of flexors and extensors is needed to maintain the head position. The only difference between being held upright in the vertical position and being held upright in supported sitting is that the trunk is supported in the latter position and thus provides some proprioceptive input by approximation of the spine and pelvis. Manual contacts under or around the shoulders are used to support the head (Fig. 8–9). Establishing eye contact with the child also assists head stability because it provides a stable visual input to orient the child to the upright position. To encourage head control further, the child can be placed in supported sitting in an infant seat or a feeder seat as a static position but care should be taken to ensure the infant's safety in such a seat. Never leave a child unattended in an infant seat or other seating device without a seat belt and/or shoulder harness to keep the child from falling forward, and never place such a device on a table unless the child is constantly supervised.

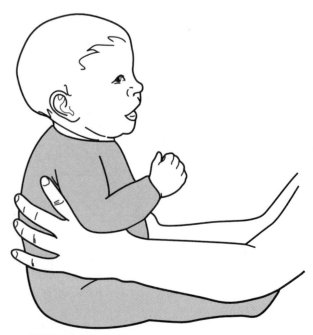

FIGURE 8–9 ■ Early head control in supported sitting.

Intervention 8–15 ‖ MODIFIED PULL-TO-SIT MANEUVER

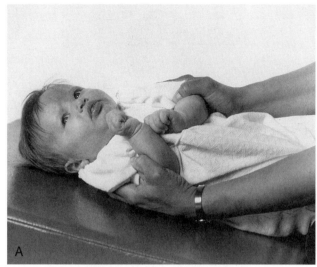 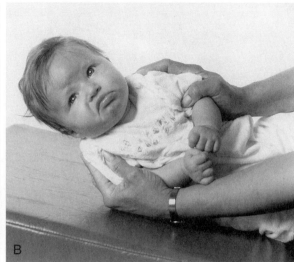

A. Position the child on an inclined surface supine in preparation for anterior head lifting.

B. Provide support at the child's shoulder, rotate the child toward yourself, and begin to move the child toward sitting on a diagonal.

Weight Shifting from Supported Upright Sitting. The beginning position is with the child seated on the assistant's or caregiver's lap and supported under the arms or around the shoulders. Support should be firm, to provide some upper trunk stability without causing any discomfort to the child. Because the child's head is inherently stable in this position, small weight shifts from the midline challenge the infant to maintain the head in the midline. If possible, just visually engaging the child may be enough to assist the child in maintaining head position or righting the head as weight is shifted. As the child becomes able to accept challenges, larger displacements may be given.

Carrying in Prone. The child's beginning position is prone. Because prone is the position from which head lifting is the easiest, when a child is in the prone position with support along the midline of the trunk, this positioning may encourage head lifting, as shown in Intervention 8–4F. The movement produced by the person who is carrying the child may also stimulate head lifting because of the vestibular system's effect on postural muscles. Another prone position for carrying can be used in the case of a child with flexor spasticity (Intervention 8–16A). One of the caregiver's forearms is placed under the child's shoulders to keep the arms forward, while the other forearm is placed between the child's thighs to keep one hip straight. Some lower trunk rotation is achieved as the pelvis is turned from the weight of the dangling leg.

Carrying in Upright. The beginning position is upright. To encourage use of the neck muscles in the development of head control, the child can be carried while in an upright position. The back of the child's head and trunk can be supported against the caregiver's chest (see Intervention 8–16B). The child can be carried, facing forward, in a snuggler or a backpack. For those children with slightly less head control, the caregiver can support around the back of the child's shoulders and head in the crook of an elevated elbow, as shown in Intervention 8–4A. An older child needs to be in a more upright posture than is pictured, with the head supported.

Prone in a Hammock or on a Suspended Platform Swing. The beginning position is prone. Movement stimulation using a hammock or a suspended swing can give vestibular input to facilitate head control when the child is in a prone position. When using a mesh hammock, you should place pillows in the hammock and put the child on top of the pillows. The child's head should be supported when the child is not able to lift it from the midline (see Fig. 8–6). As head control improves, support can gradually be withdrawn from the head. When vestibular stimulation is used, the change in direction of movement is detected, not the continuous rhythm, so be sure to vary the amount and intensity of the stimulation. Always watch for signs of overstimulation, such as flushing of the face, sweating, nausea, or vomiting. Vestibular

Intervention 8-16 ▐ CARRYING POSITIONS TO ENCOURAGE HEAD CONTROL

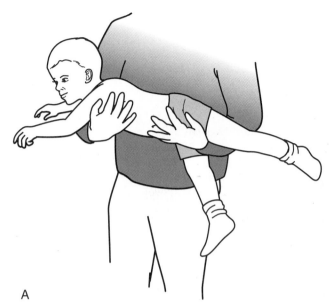

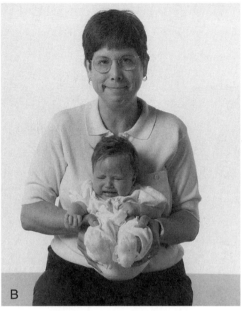

A. In the case of a child with flexor spasticity, the caregiver can place one forearm under the child's shoulders to keep his arms forward and place the other forearm between his thighs, while keeping one hip straight.

B. When the child is carried in the upright position, the back of the child's head is supported against the caregiver's chest.

stimulation may be used with children who are prone to seizures. However, you must be careful to avoid visual stimulation if the child's seizures are brought on by visual input. The child can be blindfolded or wear a baseball cap pulled down over the eyes to avoid visual stimulation.

Trunk Control

Positioning for Independent Sitting

As stated previously, sitting is the position of function for the upper extremities because self-care activities such as feeding, dressing, and bathing require upper extremity use. Positioning for independent sitting may be more crucial to the child's overall level of function than standing, especially if the child's ambulation potential is questionable. Independent sitting can be attained in many ways. Propped sitting can be independent, but it will not be functional unless one or both hands can be freed to perform meaningful activities. Progression of sitting based on degree of difficulty is found in Table 8–4.

Sitting Propped Forward on Both Arms. The beginning position is sitting, with the child bearing weight on extended arms. Various sitting postures can be used, such as abducted long sitting, ring sitting, or tailor sitting. The child must be able to sustain some weight on the arms. Preparatory activities can include forward protective extension or pushing up from prone on elbows. Gentle approximation through the shoulders into the hands can reinforce the posture. Weight bearing encourages a supporting response from the muscles of the shoulder girdle and the upper extremities to maintain the position.

Table 8–4 ▐ PROGRESSION OF SITTING POSTURES BASED ON DEGREE OF DIFFICULTY

1. Sitting propped forward on both arms.
2. Sitting propped forward on one arm.
3. Sitting propped laterally on both arms.
4. Sitting propped laterally on one arm.
5. Sitting without hand support.
6. Side sitting with hand support.
7. Side sitting with no hand support.

Sitting Propped Forward on One Arm. The beginning position is sitting, as described in the previous paragraph. When bilateral propping is possible, weight shifting in the position can encourage unloading one extremity for reaching or pointing and can allow for propping on one arm.

Sitting Propped Laterally on One Arm. If the child cannot support all her weight on one arm laterally, then part of the child's weight can be borne by a bolster placed between the child's side and the supporting arm (Fig. 8–10). Greater weight acceptance can be practiced by having the child reach with the other hand in the direction of the supporting hand. When the location of the object to be reached is varied, weight is shifted and the child may even attempt to change sitting postures.

Sitting Without Hand Support. Progressing from support on one hand to no hand support can be encouraged by having the child shift weight away from the propped hand and then have her attempt to reach with the propped hand. A progression of propping on objects and eventually on the child's body can be used to center the weight over the sitting base. Engaging the child in clapping hands or batting a balloon may also afford opportunities to free the propping hand. Short sitting with feet supported can also be used as a way to progress from sitting with hand support to using one hand to using no hands for support.

Side Sitting Propped on One Arm. Side sitting is a more difficult sitting posture in which to play because trunk rotation is required to maintain the posture to have both hands free for play. Some children are able to attain and maintain the posture only if they prop on one arm, a position that allows only one hand free for play and so negates any bimanual or two-handed activities. Again, the use of a bolster can make it easier to maintain the propped side sitting posture. Asymmetric side sitting can be used to promote weight

bearing on a hip on which the child may avoid bearing weight, as in hemiplegia. The lower extremities are asymmetrically positioned. The lower leg is externally rotated and abducted while the upper leg is internally rotated and adducted.

Side Sitting with No Hand Support. Achievement of independent side sitting can be encouraged in much the same way as described in the previous paragraph.

Movement Transitions That Encourage Trunk Rotation and Trunk Control

Once a child is relatively stable within a posture, the child needs to begin work on developing dynamic control. One of the first things to work on is shifting weight within postures in all directions, especially those directions used in making the transition or moving from one posture to another. The following are general descriptions of movement transitions commonly used in functional activities. These transitions can be used during therapy and can also be an important part of any home program.

Rolling from Supine to Prone Using the Lower Extremity. The beginning position is supine. Intervention 8–17 shows this transition. Using your right hand, grasp the child's right lower leg above the ankle and gently bring the child's knee toward the chest. Continue to move the child's leg over the body to initiate a rolling motion until the child is side lying or prone. Alternate the side toward which you turn the child. Initially, infants roll as a log or as one complete unit. As they mature, they rotate or roll segmentally. If the lower extremity is used as the initiation point of the movement, the pelvis and lower trunk will rotate before the upper trunk and shoulders. As the child does more of the movement, you will need to do less and less until, eventually, the child can be enticed to roll using a sound or visual cue or by reaching with an arm.

Coming to Sit from Supine. The beginning position is supine. Position yourself to one side of the child. Reach across the child's body and grasp the hand farthest away from you. Bring the child's arm across the body so the child has turned to the side and is pushing up with the other arm. Stabilize the child's lower extremities so the rotation occurs in the trunk and is separate from leg rotation.

Coming to Sit from Prone. The beginning position is prone. Elongate the side toward which you are going to roll the child. Facilitate the roll to side lying and proceed as follows in coming to sit from side lying as described in the next paragraph.

Coming to Sit from Side Lying. The beginning position is with the child lying on one side, facing away from you with her head to the right. The child's lower extremities should be flexed. If lower extremity separation is desirable, the child's lower leg should be

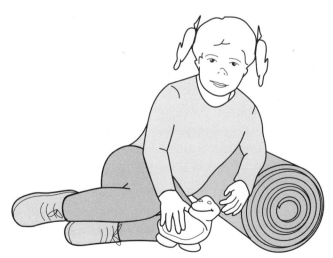

FIGURE 8-10 ■ Sitting propped laterally on one arm over a bolster.

Intervention 8–17 ▎ ROLLING FROM SUPINE TO PRONE

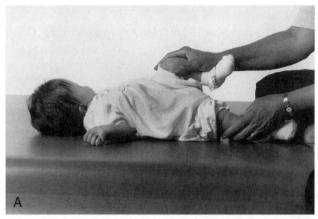

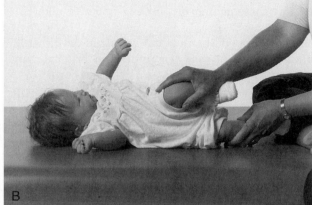

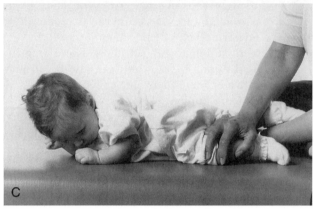

Movement sequence of rolling supine to prone.

A. With the right hand, grasp the child's left lower leg above the ankle and gently bring her knee toward the chest.

B and C. Continue to move the child's leg over the body to initiate a rolling motion until the child is in the side lying or prone position.

flexed and the top leg allowed to remain straight. Apply gentle pressure on the uppermost part of the child's shoulder in a downward and lateral direction. The child's head should right laterally, and the child should prop on the downside elbow. If the child experiences difficulty in moving to propping on one elbow, use one hand to assist the downward arm into the correct position. Your upper hand can now move to the child's top hip to direct the weight shift diagonally back over the flexed hip, while your lower hand assists the child to push up on the downward arm. Part of this movement progression is shown in Intervention 8–2.

The child's movements can be halted anywhere during the progression to improve control within a specific range or to encourage a particular component of the movement. The child ends up sitting with or without hand support, or the support arm can be placed over a bolster or half-roll if more support is needed to maintain the end position. The child's sitting position can range from long abducted sitting, propping forward on one or both extended arms, to half-ring sitting with or without propping. These positions can be maintained without propping if the child is able to maintain them.

Sitting to Prone. This transition is used to return to the floor after playing in sitting. It can be viewed as the reverse of coming to sit from side lying. In other words, the child laterally shifts weight to one side, first onto an extended arm and then to an elbow. Finally, the child turns over the arm and into the prone position. Some children with Down syndrome widely abduct their legs to lower themselves to prone. They lean forward onto outstretched arms as they continue to swing their legs farther out and behind their bodies. Children with hemiplegic involvement tend to move or to make the transition from sitting to prone by moving over the noninvolved side of the body. They need to be encouraged to shift weight toward and move over the involved side and to put as much weight as possible on the involved upper extremity. Children with bilateral involvement need to practice moving to both sides.

Prone to Four-Point. The beginning position is prone. The easiest way to facilitate movement from prone to four-point is to use a combination of cues at the shoulders then the hips, as shown in Intervention 8–18. First, reach over the upper back of the child and lift gently. The child's arms should be flexed be-

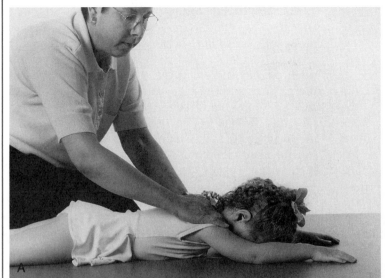

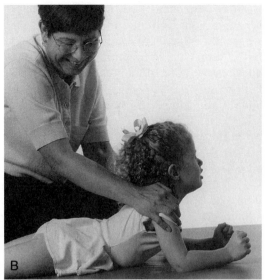

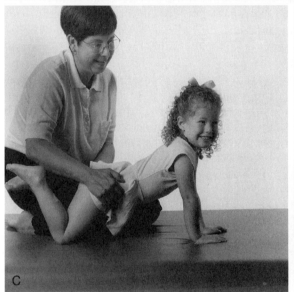

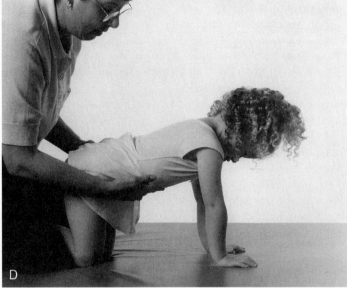

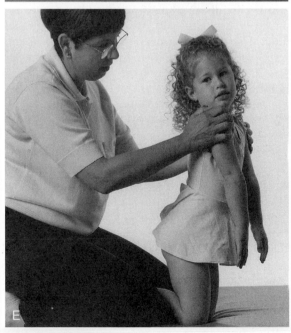

Facilitating the progression of movement from prone to prone on elbows to quadruped position using the shoulders and hips as key points of control.

A. Before beginning, the child's arms should be flexed beside the upper body. Reach over the upper back of the child and lift her shoulders gently.

B. As her shoulders are lifted, the child may bring her forearms under the body in a prone on elbows or puppy position. Continue to lift until the child is able to push up on extended arms.

C and D. Next, lift the child's hips up and bring them back toward her feet, just far enough to achieve a four-point position.

E. Facilitating movement from quadruped to kneeling using the shoulders. The child extends her head before her hips. Use of the hips as a key point may allow for more complete extension of the hips before the head is extended.

side the upper body at the beginning of the movement. By lifting the shoulders, the child may bring the forearms under the body in a prone on elbows or puppy position. Continue to lift until the child is able to push up on extended arms. Weight bearing on extended arms is a prerequisite for assuming a hands and knees position. If the child requires assistance to maintain arms extended, a caregiver can support the child at the elbows, or pediatric air splints can be used. Next, lift the hips up and bring them back toward the feet, just far enough to achieve a four-point position. If the child needs extra support under the abdomen, a bolster, a small stool, or pillows can be used to help sustain the posture. Remember, four-point may just be a transitional position used by the child to go into kneeling or sitting. Not all developmentally normal children learn to creep on hands and knees. Depending on the predominant type of muscle tone, creeping may be too difficult to achieve for some children who demonstrate mostly flexor tone in the prone position. Children with developmental delays and minimal abnormal postural tone can be taught to creep.

Four-Point to Side Sitting. The beginning position is four-point. Once the child can maintain a hands and knees position, start work on moving to side sitting to either side. This transition works on control of trunk lowering while the child is in a rotated position. Dissociation of lower trunk movements from upper trunk movements can also be practiced. A prerequisite is for the child to be able to control or tolerate diagonal weight shifts without falling. So many times, children can shift weight anteriorly and posteriorly, but not diagonally. If diagonal weight shifting is not possible, the child will often end up sitting on the heels or between the feet. The latter position can have a significant effect on the development of lower extremity bones and joints. The degree to which the child performs side sitting can be determined by whether the child is directed to go all the way from four-point to side sitting on the support surface or by whether the movement is shortened to end with the child side sitting on pillows or a low stool. If movement to one side is more difficult, movement toward the other side should be practiced first.

Four-Point to Kneeling. The beginning position is four-point. Kneeling is accomplished from a four-point position by a backward weight shift followed by hip extension with the rest of the child's body extending over the hips (see Intervention 8–18*E*). Some children with cerebral palsy try to initiate this movement by using head extension. The extension should begin at the hips and should progress cephalad (toward the head). A child can be assisted in achieving an upright or tall-kneeling position by placement of extended arms on benches of increasing height, to aid in shifting weight toward the hips. In this way, the child can

practice hip extension in smaller ranges before having to move through the entire range.

Kneeling to Side Sitting. The beginning position is kneeling. Kneeling is an extended position because the child's back must be kept erect with the hips extended. Kneeling is also a dissociated posture because while the hips are extended, the knees are flexed, and the ankles are passively plantar flexed to extend the base of support and to provide a longer lever arm. Lowering from kneeling requires eccentric control of the quadriceps. If this lowering occurs downward in a straight plane, the child will end up sitting on his feet. If the trunk rotates, the lowering can proceed to put the child into side sitting.

Kneeling to Half-Kneeling. The beginning position is kneeling. The transition to half-kneeling is one of the most difficult to accomplish. Typically developing children often use upper limb support to attain this position. To move from kneeling to half-kneeling, the child must unweight one lower extremity. This is usually done by performing a lateral weight shift. The trunk on the side of the weight shift should lengthen or elongate while the opposite side of the trunk shortens in a righting reaction. The trunk must rotate away from the side of the body toward which the weight is shifted to assist the unweighted lower extremity's movement (Intervention 8–19). The unweighted leg is brought forward, and the foot is placed on the support surface. The resulting position is a dissociated one in which the forward leg is flexed at all joints while the loaded limb is flexed at the knee and is extended at the hip and ankle (plantar flexed).

Coming to Stand. The beginning position is sitting. Coming to stand is probably one of *the most functional* movement transitions. Clinicians spend a great deal of time working with people of all ages on this movement transition. Children initially have to roll over to prone, move into a hands and knees position, creep over to a person or object, and pull up to stand through half-kneeling. The next progression in the developmental sequence adds moving into a squat from hands and knees and pulling the rest of the way up on someone or something. Finally, the 18-month-old can usually come to stand from a squat without assistance (Fig. 8–11). As the abdominal muscles become stronger, the child in supine turns partially to the side, pushes with one arm to sitting, then goes to a squat and on up to standing. The most mature standup pattern is to come straight up from supine to sitting with no trunk rotation, assume a squat, and come to stand. From prone, the most mature progression is to push up to four-point, to kneeling and half-kneeling, and then to standing. Independent half-kneeling is a difficult position because of the configuration of the base of support and the number of body parts that are dissociated from each other.

Intervention 8-19 ❙ KNEELING TO HALF-KNEELING

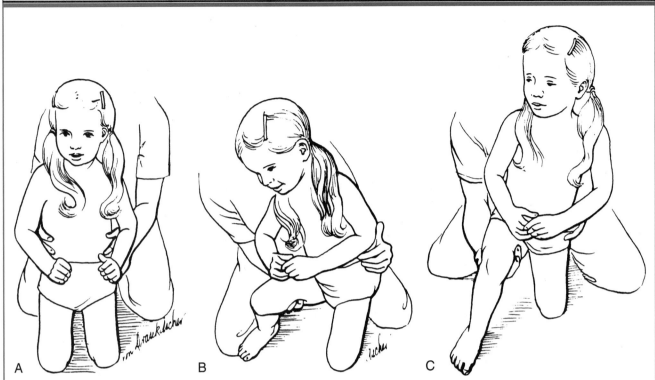

A. Kneel behind the child and place your hands on the child's hips.

B. Shift the child's weight laterally, but do not let the child fall to the opposite side, as is depicted. The child's trunk should elongate on the weight-bearing side, and with some trunk rotation, the child may be able to bring the opposite leg forward.

C. If the child is unable to bring the opposite leg forward, assist as depicted.

From Jaeger DL. Home Program Instruction Sheets for Infants and Young Children. Copyright © 1987 by Therapy Skill Builders, A Harcourt Health Sciences Company. Reproduced by permission. All rights reserved.

ADAPTIVE EQUIPMENT FOR POSITIONING AND MOBILITY

Decisions regarding adaptive equipment for positioning and mobility should be made based on input from the team working with the infant or child. Adaptive equipment can include bolsters, wedges, walkers, and wheeled mobility devices. The decision about what equipment to use is ultimately up to the parents. Barriers to the use of adaptive equipment may include, but are not limited to, architectural, financial, cosmetic, and behavioral constraints. Sometimes, children do not like the equipment the therapist thinks is most therapeutic. Any piece of equipment should be used on a trial basis before being purchased. Regarding wheelchair selection, a team approach is advocated. Members of the assistive technology team may include the physical therapist, the occupational therapist, the speech therapist, the classroom teacher, the re-

habilitation engineer, and the vendor of durable medical equipment. The child and family are also part of the team because they are the ones who will use the equipment. The physical therapist assistant may assist the physical therapist in gathering information regarding the need for a wheel-chair or piece of adaptive equipment, as well as providing feedback on how well the child is able to use the device. For more information on assistive technology, the reader is referred to Carlson and Ramsey (1994).

The 90-90-90 rule for sitting alignment should be observed. In other words, the feet, knees, and hips should be flexed to approximately 90 degrees. This degree of flexion allows weight to be taken on the back of the thighs, as well as the ischial tuberosities of the pelvis. If the person cannot maintain the normal spinal curves while in sitting, thought should be given to providing lumbar support. The depth of the seat should be sufficient to support no more than ⅞ of the

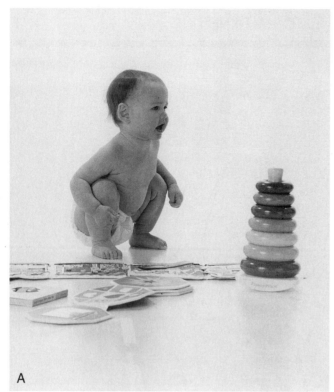

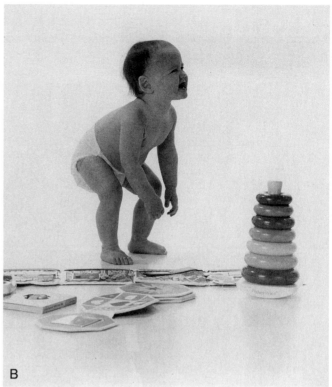

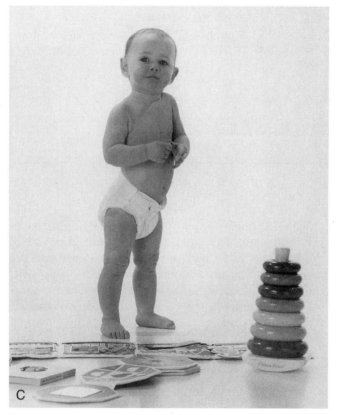

FIGURE 8-11 ▪ *A* to *C*, Coming to stand from a squat requires good lower extremity strength and balance.

thigh (Wilson, 1986). Supporting more than ⅞ of the thigh leads to excessive pressure on the structures behind the knee, whereas less support may require the child to compensate by developing kyphosis. Other po-

tential problems such as neck extension, scapular retraction, and lordosis of the thoracic spine can occur if the child is not able to keep the trunk extended for long periods of time. In such cases, the child may feel as though he is falling forward. Lateral trunk supports are indicated to control asymmetries in the trunk that may lead to scoliosis.

Goals for Adaptive Equipment

Wilson (1993) described eight goals for adaptive equipment that are listed in Table 8–5. Many of these goals reflect what is expected from positioning because adaptive equipment is used to reinforce appropriate positions. For example, positioning should give a child a postural base by providing postural alignment needed for normal movement. Changing the alignment of the trunk can have a positive effect on the child's ability to reach. Supported sitting may counteract the deforming forces of gravity, especially in a child with poor trunk control who cannot maintain an erect trunk posture. Simply supporting the child's feet takes much of the strain off trying to keep weight on the pelvis in a chair that is too high. When at all possible, the child's sitting posture with adaptive equipment should approximate that of a developmentally normal child's by maintaining all spinal curves. The reader is referred to Wilson (1993) for a more in-depth discussion of adaptive equipment. What follows is a general discussion of considerations for positioning in sitting, side lying, and standing.

Supine and Prone Postures

Positioning the child prone over a half-roll, bolster, or wedge is often used to encourage head lifting, as well as weight bearing on forearms, elbows, and even extended arms. These positions are seen in Intervention 8–20. Supine positioning can be used to encourage symmetry of the child's head position and reaching forward in space. Wedges and half-rolls can be used to support the child's head and upper trunk in more flexion. Rolls can be placed under the knees, also to encourage flexion.

Table 8-5 ▌ ANTICIPATED GOALS FOR USE OF ADAPTIVE EQUIPMENT

Gain or reinforce typical movement.
Achieve proper postural alignment.
Prevent contractures and deformities.
Increase opportunities for social and educational interaction.
Provide mobility and encourage exploration.
Increase independence in activities of daily living and self-help skills.
Assist in improving physiologic functions.
Increase comfort.

Wilson, J. Selection and use of adaptive equipment. In Connolly BH, Montgomery PC (eds). Therapeutic Exercise in Developmental Disabilities, 2nd ed. Hixson, TN, Chattanooga Group, 1993, pp 167–182.

Sitting Postures

Many sitting postures are available for the typically developing child who moves and changes positions easily. However, the child with a disability may have fewer positions from which to choose, depending on the amount of joint range, muscle extensibility, and head and trunk control required in each position. Children normally experiment with many different sitting postures, although some of these positions are more difficult to attain and maintain. Sitting on the floor with the legs extended is called long sitting. Long sitting requires adequate hamstring length (Fig. 8–12A) and is often difficult for children with cerebral palsy, who tend to sit on the sacrum with the pelvis posteriorly tilted (Fig. 8–13). During ring sitting on the floor, the soles of the feet are touching, the knees are abducted, and the hips are externally rotated such that the legs form a ring. Ring sitting is a comfortable sitting alternative because it provides a wider base of support; however, the hamstrings can and do shorten if this sitting posture is used exclusively (see Fig. 8–12B). Tailor sitting, or cross-legged floor sitting, also takes some strain off the hamstrings and allows some children to sit on their ischial tuberosities for the first time (see Fig. 8–12C). Again, the hamstrings will shorten if this sitting posture is the only one used by the child. The use of tailor sitting must be carefully evaluated in the presence of increased lower extremity muscle tone, especially in the hamstring and gastrocnemius-soleus muscles. In addition, in many of these sitting positions, the child's feet are passively allowed to plantar flex and invert, thereby encouraging tightening of the heel cords. If independent sitting is not possible, then adaptive seating should be considered.

The most difficult position to move into and out of appears to be side sitting. Side sitting is a rotated posture and requires internal rotation of one lower extremity and external rotation of the other lower extremity (Fig. 8–14A). Because of the flexed lower extremities, the lower trunk is rotated in one direction, a maneuver necessitating that the upper trunk be rotated in the opposite direction. A child may have to prop on one arm to maintain side sitting if trunk rotation is insufficient (see Fig. 8–14B). Some children can side sit to one side but not to the other because of lower extremity range-of-motion limitations. In side sitting, the trunk on the weight-bearing side lengthens to keep the center of gravity within the base of support. Children with hemiplegia may not be able to side sit on the involved side because of an inability to elongate or rotate the trunk. They may be able to side sit only if they are propped on the involved arm, a maneuver that is often impossible. Because weight bearing on the involved side is a general goal with any person with hemiplegia, side sitting is a good position

Intervention 8–20 ▋ ENCOURAGING HEAD LIFTING AND UPPER EXTREMITY WEIGHT BEARING USING PRONE SUPPORTS

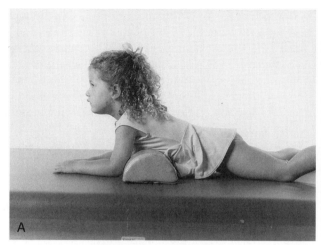

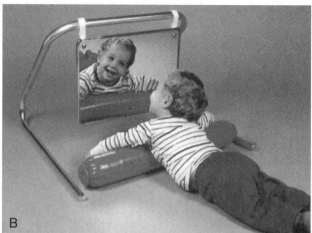

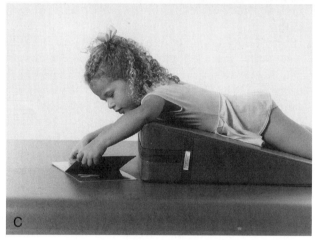

A. Positioning the child prone over a half-roll encourages head lifting and weight bearing on elbows and forearms.

B. Positioning the child prone over a bolster encourages head lifting and shoulder control.

C. Positioning the child prone over a wedge promotes upper extremity weight bearing and function.

B, Courtesy of Kaye Products, Inc., Hillsborough, NC.

to work toward with these children (Intervention 8–21). Actively working into side sitting from a four-point or tall-kneeling position can be therapeutically beneficial because so many movement transitions involve controlled trunk rotation. Advantages of using the four-point position to practice this transition are that some of the weight is taken by the arms and less control is demanded of the lower extremities. As trunk control improves, you can assist the child in moving from tall-kneeling on the knees to heel sitting and finally from tall-kneeling to side sitting to either side. From tall-kneeling, the base of support is still larger than in standing, and the arms can be used for support if needed.

Children with disabilities often have one preferred way to sit, and that sitting position can be detrimental to lower extremity development and the acquisition of trunk control. For example, W sitting puts the hips

into extreme internal rotation and anteriorly tilts the pelvis, thereby causing the spine to be extended (see Fig. 8–3A). In this position, the tibias are subjected to torsional factors that, if sustained, can produce permanent structural changes. Children with low postural tone may accidentally discover this position by pushing themselves back between their knees. Once these children "discover" that they no longer need to use their hands for support, it becomes difficult to prevent them from using this posture. Children with increased tone in the hip adductor group also use this position frequently because they lack sufficient trunk rotation to move into side sitting from prone. Behavior modification has typically been used to attempt to change a child's habit of W sitting. Some children respond to verbal requests of "sit pretty," but often the parent is worn out from constantly trying to have the child correct the posture. As with most habits, if the child can

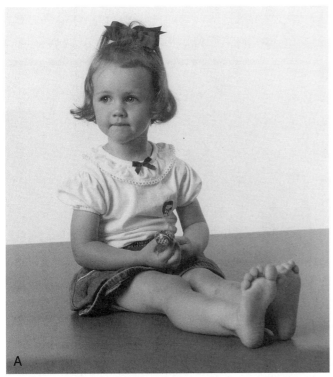

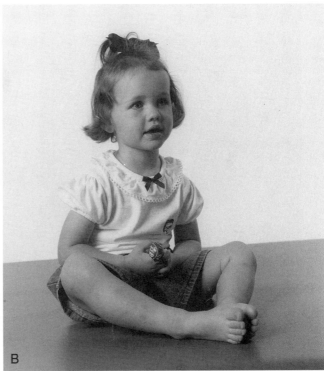

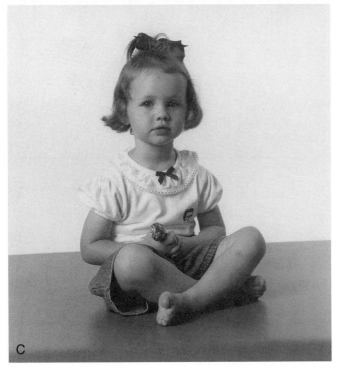

FIGURE 8–12 ■ Sitting postures. *A*, Long sitting. *B*, Ring sitting. *C*, Tailor sitting.

be prevented from ever discovering W sitting, that is optimal. Otherwise, substitute another sitting alternative for the potentially deforming position. For example, if the only way the child can independently sit on the floor is by W sitting, place the child in a corner chair or other positioning device that requires a different lower extremity position.

Adaptive Seating

Many positions can be used to facilitate movement, but the best position for activities of daily living is upright sitting. How that posture is maintained may necessitate caregiver assistance or adaptive equipment for positioning. In sitting, the child can more easily view the world and can become more interested in

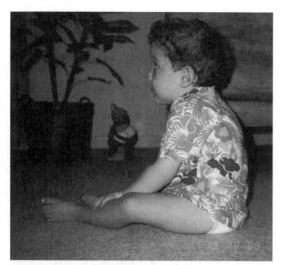

FIGURE 8–13 ▪ Sacral sitting. (From Burns YR, MacDonald J. Physiotherapy and the growing child. London, WB Saunders Company Ltd., 1996.)

interacting with people and objects within the environment. Ideally, the position should allow the child as much independence as possible while maintaining safety. Adaptive seating may be required to meet both these criteria. Some examples of seating devices are shown in Figure 8–15. The easier it is to use a piece of adaptive equipment, the more likely the caregiver will be to use it with the child.

Children without good head control often do not have sufficient trunk control for sitting. Stabilizing the trunk alone may improve the child's ability to main-

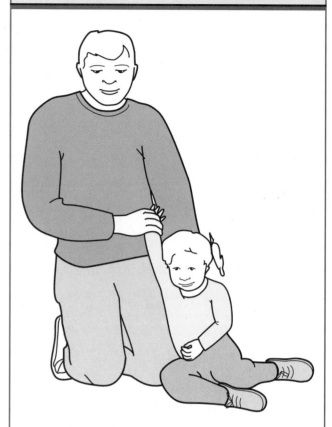

Intervention 8–21 ▮ **ENCOURAGING WEIGHT BEARING ON THE HEMIPLEGIC HIP**

Place the child in side sitting on the hemiplegic side. Elevation of the hemiplegic arm promotes trunk and external rotation elongation.

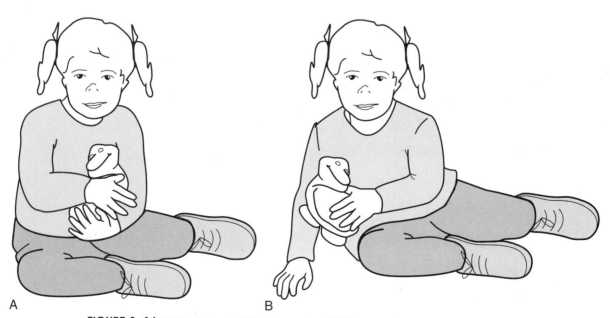

A   B

FIGURE 8–14 ▪ Side sitting. *A*, Without propping. *B*, With propping on one arm for support.

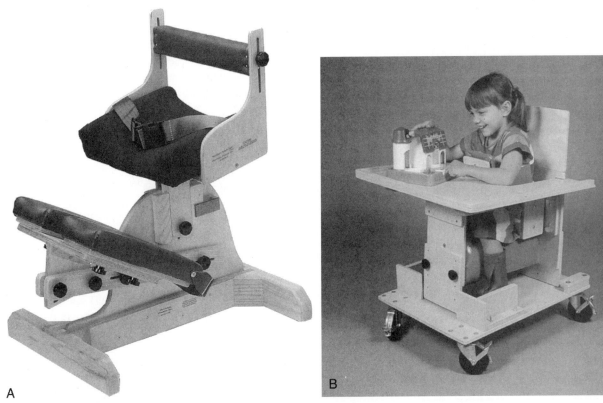

FIGURE 8-15 ∎ Adaptive seating devices. *A*, Posture chair. *B*, Bolster chair. (*A*, Courtesy of TherAdapt Products, Inc., Bensenville, IL; *B*, courtesy of Kaye Products, Inc., Hillsborough, NC.)

tain the head in midline. Additionally, the child's arms can be brought forward and supported on a lap tray. If the child has poor head control, then some means to support the head will have to be incorporated into the seating device (see Fig. 8-4). When sitting a child with poor head and trunk control, the child's back must be protected from the forces of gravity, which accentuate a forward flexed spine. Although children need to be exposed to gravity while they are in an upright sitting position to develop trunk control, postural deviation can quickly occur if muscular control is not sufficient.

Children with low tone often demonstrate flared ribs (Fig. 8-16) as a result of an absence of sufficient trunk muscle development to anchor the rib cage for breath support. Children with trunk muscle paralysis secondary to myelodysplasia may require an orthotic device to support the trunk during sitting. Although the orthosis can assist in preventing the development of scoliosis, it may not totally prevent its development because of the inherent muscle imbalance. The orthosis may or may not be initially attached to lower extremity bracing.

Cristaralla (1975) compared the effect on children with cerebral palsy of sitting on a bolster seat versus a child's chair. She found that sitting on a bolster seat allowed a more vertical position of the child's pelvis than did sitting on the child's chair. The bolster seat

kept the child's hips and knees flexed to 90 degrees. Additionally, sitting astride a bolster puts the child's legs in external rotation and can thus decrease adductor muscle tone. A bolster chair is depicted in Figure

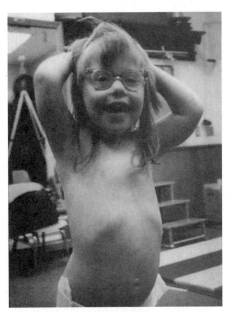

FIGURE 8-16 ∎ Rib flare. (From Moerchen VA: Respiration and motor development: A systems perspective. Neurol Rep 18:9, 1994. Reprinted from the *Neurology Report* with the permission of the Neurology Section, APTA.)

Intervention 8-22 ▐ FACILITATING TRUNK EXTENSION

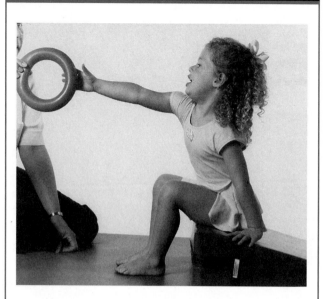

Sitting on a posteriorly inclined wedge may facilitate trunk extension.

8–15B. Sitting on a chair with an anteriorly inclined seat, such as that found in the TherAdapt posture chair (TherAdapt Products, Inc., Bensenville, IL) (see Fig. 8–15A), facilitated trunk extension (Miedaner, 1990). Dilger and Ling (1986) found that sitting a child with cerebral palsy on a posteriorly inclined wedge decreased her kyphosis (Intervention 8–22). Seating requirements must be individually assessed, depending on the therapeutic goals. A child may benefit from several different types of seating, depending on the positioning requirements of the task being performed.

Adjustable-height benches are an excellent therapeutic tool because they can easily grow with the child throughout the preschool years. They can be used in assisting children with making the transition from sitting to standing, as well as in providing a stable sitting base for dressing and playing. The height of the bench is important to consider relative to the amount of trunk control demanded from the child. Depending on the child's need for pelvic support, a bench allows the child to use trunk muscles to maintain an upright trunk posture during play or to practice head and trunk postural responses when weight shifts occur during dressing or playing. Additional pelvic support can be added to some therapeutic benches, as seen in Figure 8–2. The bench can be used to pull up on and to encourage cruising.

Side Lying Position

Side lying is frequently used to orient a child's body around the midline, particularly in cases of severe involvement or when the child's posture is asymmetric when he is placed either prone or supine. In a child with less severe involvement, side lying can be used to assist the child to develop control of flexors and extensors on the same side of the body. Side lying is often a good sleeping posture because the caregiver can alternate the side the child sleeps on every night. For sleeping, a long body pillow can be placed along the child's back to maintain side lying, with one end of the pillow brought between the legs to separate them and the other end under the neck or head to maintain midline orientation. Lower extremities should be flexed if the child tends to be in a more extended posture. For classroom use, a commercial sidelyer or a rolled-up blanket (Intervention 8–23) may be used to promote hand regard, midline play, or orientation.

Positioning in Standing

Positioning in standing is often indicated for its positive physiologic benefits, including growth of the long bones of the lower extremities. Standing can also encourage alerting behavior, peer interaction, and upper extremity usage. The upper extremities can be weight bearing or free to move because they are no longer needed to support the child's posture. The upright orientation can afford the child perceptual opportunities. Many devices can be used to promote an upright standing posture including prone and supine standers, vertical standers, standing frames, and standing boxes.

Intervention 8-23 ▐ USING A SIDELYER

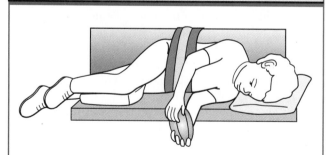

Use of a sidelyer ensures that a child experiences a side lying position and may promote hand regard, midline play, or orientation. Positioning in side lying is excellent for dampening the effects of most tonic reflexes.

Prone standers support the anterior chest, hips, and anterior surface of the lower extremities. The angle of the stander determines how much weight is borne by the lower extremities and feet. When the angle is slightly less than 90 degrees, weight is optimal through the lower extremities and feet (Aubert, 1999). If the child exhibits neck hyperextension or a high guard position of the arms when in the prone stander, its continued use needs to be reevaluated by the supervising physical therapist. Use of a prone stander is indicated if the goal is physiologic weight bearing or hands-free standing.

Supine standers are an alternative to prone standers for some children. A supine stander is similar to a tilt table, so the degree of tilt determines the amount of weight borne by the lower extremities and feet. For children who exhibit too much extension in response to placement in a prone stander, a supine stander may

be a good alternative. However, postural compensations develop in some children with the use of a supine stander. These compensations include kyphosis from trying to overcome the posterior tilt of the body. Asymmetric neck postures or a Moro response may be accentuated because the supine stander perpetuates supine positioning. Use of a supine stander in these situations may be contraindicated.

Vertical standers support the child's lower extremities in hip and knee extension and allow for complete weight bearing. The child's hands are free for upper extremity tasks such as writing at a blackboard (Intervention 8–24). The child controls the trunk. The need to function within different environments must be considered when one chooses adaptive equipment for standing. In a classroom, the use of a stander is often an alternative to sitting, and because the device is adjustable, more than one child may be able to

---

Intervention 8–24 ▌ VERTICAL STANDERS

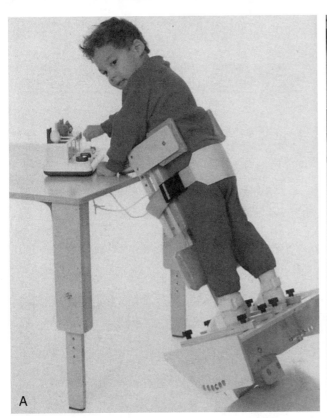 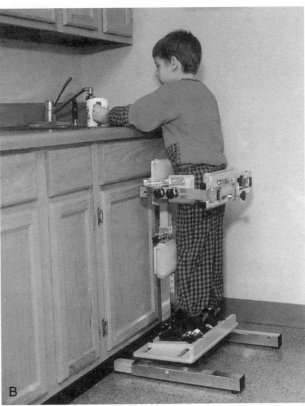

Vertical standers support the child's lower extremities in hip and knee extension and allow for varying amounts of weight bearing depending on the degree of inclination. The child's hands are free for upper extremity tasks, such as writing at a blackboard, playing with toys (A), or working in the kitchen (B).

Courtesy of Kaye Products, Inc., Hillsborough, NC.

benefit from its use. Continual monitoring of a child's response to any type of stander should be part of the physical therapist's periodic reevaluation of the child. The physical therapist assistant should note changes in posture and abilities of any child while using any piece of adaptive equipment.

Positioning in upright standing is important for mobility, specifically ambulation. Orthotic support devices and walkers are routinely used with young children with myelodysplasia. Ambulation aids can also be important to children with cerebral palsy who do not initially have the balance to walk independently. Two different types of walkers are most frequently used in children with motor dysfunction. The standard walker is used in front of the child, and the reverse posture control walker is used behind the child. These walkers can have two wheels in the front. The traditional walker is then called a rollator. Difficulties with the standard walker include a forward trunk lean. The child's line of gravity ends up being anterior to the feet, with the hips in flexion. When the child pushes a reverse walker forward, the bar of the walker contacts the child's gluteal muscles and gives a cue to extend the hips. Because the walker is behind the child, the walker cannot move too far ahead of the child. The reverse walker can have two or four wheels. In studies conducted in children with cerebral palsy, use of the reverse walker (Fig. 8–17) resulted in positive changes

in gait and upright posture (Levangie et al, 1989). Each child needs to be evaluated on an individual basis by the physical therapist to determine the appropriate assistive device for ambulation. The device should provide stability, safety, and an energy-efficient gait pattern.

FUNCTIONAL MOVEMENT IN THE CONTEXT OF THE CHILD'S WORLD

Any movement that is guided by the clinician should have functional meaning. This meaning could be derived as part of a sequence of movement, as a transition from one posture to another, or as part of achieving a task such as touching a toy. Play is a child's occupation and the way in which the child most frequently learns the rules of moving. Physical therapy incorporates play as a means to achieve therapeutic goals. Structuring the environment in which the treatment session occurs and planning which toys you want the child to play with are all part of therapy. Setting up a situation that challenges the child to move in new ways is motivating to older children. Some suggestions from Ratliffe (1998) for toys and strategies to use with children of different ages can be found in Table 8–6.

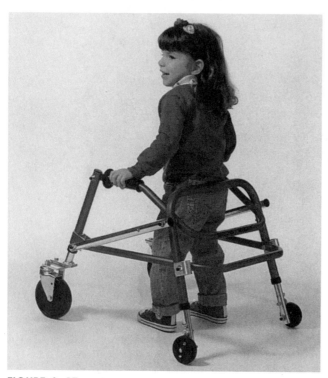

FIGURE 8–17 ■ Reverse posture walker. (Courtesy of Kaye Products, Inc., Hillsborough, NC.)

CHAPTER SUMMARY

Children with neurologic impairments, regardless of the cause of the deficits, need to move. Part of any parent's role is to foster the child's movement exploration of the world. To be a good explorer, the child has to come in contact with the objects and people of the world. By teaching the family how to assist the child to move and by supporting areas of the child's body that the child cannot support, the clinician can encourage functional movement of other body parts such as eyes, hands, and feet. The adage that if the individual cannot get to the world, the world should be brought to the individual, is true. The greatest challenge for physical therapists and physical therapist assistants who work with children with neurologic dysfunction may be to determine how to bring the world to a child who has limited head or trunk control or limited mobility. There is never one answer but rather there are many possibilities to the problems presented by these children. The normal developmental sequence has always been a good source of ideas for positioning and handling. Other sources for ideas are the curiosity of the child and the imagination of the family.

Table 8-6 ▌ APPROPRIATE TOYS AND
MOTIVATIONAL STRATEGIES FOR WORKING WITH
CHILDREN

AGE	TOYS	MOTIVATIONAL STRATEGIES
Infants and toddlers (newborns–3 years)	Rattles, plastic keys Stuffed animals Music boxes Stackable or nesting toys, blocks Mirror Push toys, ride-on toys, tricycles Farm set, toy animals Grocery cart, pretend food Puzzles Computer, age-appropriate software	Smiling, cooing, tickling Present interesting toys Encourage reaching, changing positions by moving toys Use your body as a therapy tool to climb on, under, across Set up enticing environments Include family members Teach caregivers how to do activities with child Read books Demonstrate on doll if child becomes tired
Preschoolers (3–5 years)	Crayons Books Puzzles Playdough Music tapes/tape recorders Building toys such as blocks Dress-up cloths Puppets, dolls Pillows, blankets Art supplies Children's athletic equipment (plastic bats, lightweight balls, portable nets, etc.)	Gross motor play Rough-housing Allow child to explore environment Use peer support through closely planned group activities Use simple, imaginative games Create art projects child can take home; follow child's lead Involve family members or classmates in therapy session
School-age children (5–12 years)	Computer with software Playground equipment Bicycles Athletic equipment (balls, nets, bats, goals, etc.) Dolls and action figures Beads to string Magic sets Trading cards Checkers, dominoes Make-up Water play Board games Music Exercise equipment (stationary bike, rowing machine, kinetic exercise equipment, pulleys, weights, etc.) Model kits Puzzles	Imaginative games (pirates, ballet dancers, gymnastics, baseball, etc.) Draw family members into therapy session Give child sense of accomplishment (help child complete project to take home or learn specific skill that he can demonstrate to family members) Document progress on chart using stars or stickers Find out child's goals and incorporate them into therapy Use small toys/objects as rewards Give child sense of success (make goals small enough that immediate progress can be seen)
Adolescents (12–18 years)	Computer with software Music Exercise equipment Collections Computer with software Athletic equipment	Find out what motivates child (ask child, family members, and peers) Develop system of rewards and consequences for doing home programs or making progress that is attainable and meaningful Use chart to document goals and progress

Ratliffe KT. Clinical Pediatrics Physical Therapy: A Guide for the Physical Therapy Team. St. Louis, CV Mosby, 1998, pp 65–66.

REVIEW QUESTIONS

1. What two activities should always be part of any therapeutic intervention?
2. What are the purposes of positioning?
3. What sensory inputs help to develop body and movement awareness?
4. Identify two of the most important handling tips.
5. Define key points of control.
6. Give three reasons to use adaptive equipment.
7. What are the two most functional postures (positions to move from)?
8. What are the disadvantages of using a quadruped position?
9. Why is side sitting a difficult posture?
10. Why is standing such an important activity?

CASE STUDIES

For each of the case studies listed here, identify appropriate ways to pick up, carry, feed, or dress the child. Additionally, identify any adaptive equipment that could assist in positioning the child for a functional activity.

Case 1

Josh is a 6-month-old with little head control who has been diagnosed as a floppy infant. He does not like the prone position. However, when he is prone, he is able to lift his head and turn it from side to side, but he does not bear weight on his elbows. He eats slowly and well but tires easily.

Case 2

Angie is a 9-month-old who exhibits good head control and fair trunk control. She has low tone in her trunk and increased tone in her lower extremities (hamstrings, adductors, and gastrocnemius-soleus complex). When her mother picks her up under the arms, Angie crosses her legs and points her toes. When Angie is in her walker, she pushes herself backward. Her mother reports that Angie slides out of her highchair, which makes it difficult for her to finger feed.

Case 3

Kelly is a 3-year-old who has difficulty in maintaining any posture against gravity. Head control and trunk control are inconsistent. She can bear weight on her arms if they are placed for her. She can sit on the floor for a short time when she is placed in tailor sitting. When startled, she throws her arms up in the air (Moro reflex) and falls. She wants to help get herself dressed and undressed.

POSSIBLE SUGGESTIONS

Case 1

Picking up/Carrying: Use maximum head and trunk support, facilitate rolling to the side, and gather him in a flexed position before picking him up. You could carry him prone to increase tolerance for the position and for the movement experience.

Feeding: Use an infant seat.

Positioning for Functional Activity: Position him prone over a half-roll with toys at eye level.

Case 2

Picking up/Carrying: From sitting, pick her up, ensuring lower extremity flexion and separation if possible. Carry her astride your hip, with her trunk and arms rotated away from you.

Feeding: Attach a seat belt to the highchair. Support her feet so the knees are higher than the hips. Towel rolls can be used to keep the knees abducted. A small towel roll can be used at the low back to encourage a neutral pelvis.

Mobility: Consult with the supervising therapist about the use of a walker for this child.

Positioning for Functional Activity: Sit her astride a bolster to play at a table. A bolster chair with a tray can also be used.

Case 3

Picking up/Carrying: Assist her to move into sitting using upper extremity weight bearing for stability. Pick her up in a flexed posture and place her in a corner seat on casters to transport or a stroller.

Dressing: Position her in ring sitting on the floor, with the caregiver ring sitting around her for stability. Stabilize one of her upper extremities and guide her free arm to assist with dressing. Another option could include sitting on a low dressing bench with her back against the wall and being manually guided to assist with dressing.

Positioning for Functional Activity: Use a corner floor sitter that would give a maximum base of support. She could sit in a chair with arms, her feet supported, the table at chest height, and one arm holding on to the edge of the table while the other arm manipulates toys or objects.

REFERENCES

American Academy of Pediatrics Task Force on Infant Positioning and SIDS. Positioning and SIDS. Pediatrics 90:264, 1992.

Aubert EK. Adaptive equipment for physically challenged children. In Tecklin JS (ed). Pediatric Physical Therapy, 3rd ed. Philadelphia, JB Lippincott, 1999, pp 314–351.

Ayres AJ. Sensory Integration and Learning Disorders. Los Angeles, Western Psychological Services, 1972.

Carlson SJ, Ramsey C. Assistive technology. In Campell SK (ed). Physical Therapy for Children. Philadelphia, WB Saunders, 1994, pp 621–658.

Cristaralla M. Comparison of straddling and sitting apparatus for the spastic cerebral palsied child. Am J Occup Ther 29:273–276, 1975.

Dilger NJ, Ling W. The influence of inclined wedge sitting on infantile postural kyphosis. Dev Med Child Neurol 28:23, 1986.

Horak F, Shumway-Cook A, Crowe T, et al. Vestibular function and motor proficiency in children with hearing impairments and in learning disabled children with motor impairments. Dev Med Child Neurol 30:64–79, 1988.

Koomar JA, Bundy CA. The art and science of creating direct intervention from theory. In Fisher AG, Murray EA, Bundy AC (eds). Sensory Integration: Theory and Practice. Philadelphia, FA Davis, 1991, pp 251–314.

Levangie P, Chimera M, Johnston M, et al. Effects of posture control walker versus standard rolling walker on gait characteristics of children with spastic cerebral palsy. Phys Occup Ther Pediatr 9: 1–18, 1989.

Long TM, Cintas HL. Handbook of Pediatric Physical Therapy. Baltimore, Williams & Wilkins, 1995.

Miedaner JA. The effects of sitting positions on trunk extension for children with motor impairment. Pediatr Phys Ther 2:11–14, 1990.

Ratliffe KT. Clinical Pediatric Physical Therapy. St. Louis, CV Mosby, 1998.

Shumway-Cook A, Horak F. Assessing the influence of sensory interaction on balance. Phys Ther 66:1548–1550, 1986.

Wilson JM. Achieving postural alignment and functional movement in sitting. Workshop notes, 1986.

Wilson JM. Selection and use of adaptive equipment. In Connolly, BH, Montgomery PC (eds). Therapeutic Exercise in Developmental Disabilities, 2nd ed. Hixson, TN, Chattanooga Group, 1993, pp 167–182.

Myelomeningocele

INTRODUCTION

Myelomeningocele (MMC) is a complex congenital anomaly (Chauvel and Kinsman, 1996). Although it primarily affects the nervous system, it secondarily involves the musculoskeletal and urologic systems. MMC is a specific form of myelodysplasia that is the result of faulty embryologic development of the spinal cord, especially the lower segments. The caudal end of the neural tube or primitive spinal cord fails to close before the 28th day of gestation (Fig. 9–1A). Definitions of basic myelodysplastic defects can be found in Table 9–1. Accompanying the spinal cord dysplasia (abnormal tissue growth) is a bony defect known as spina bifida, which occurs when the posterior vertebral arches fail to close in the midline to form a spinous process (Fig. 9–1C to E). The normal spine at birth is seen in Figure 9–1B. The term *spina bifida* is often used to mean both the bony defect and the various forms of myelodysplasia. When the bifid spine occurs in isolation, with no involvement of the spinal cord or meninges, it is called spina bifida occulta (see Fig. 9–1C). Usually, no neurologic impairment occurs in persons with *spina bifida occulta*. The area of skin over the defect may be marked by a dimple or tuft of hair and can go unnoticed. In *spina bifida cystica*, patients have a visible cyst protruding from the opening caused by the bony defect. The cyst may be covered with skin or meninges. This condition is also called *spina bifida aperta*, meaning open or visible. If the cyst contains only cerebrospinal fluid (CSF) and meninges, it is referred to as a *meningocele* because the "cele" (cyst) is covered by the meninges (see Fig. 9–1D). When the malformed spinal cord is present within the cyst, the lesion is referred to as a *myelomeningocele* (see Fig. 9–1E). In MMC, the cyst may be covered with only meninges or with skin. Motor paralysis and sensory loss are present below the level of the MMC. The most common location for MMC is in the lumbar region.

INCIDENCE

The incidence of MMC varies from source to source, ranging from 1 per 1000 live births (Ratliff, 1998) to 2 per 1000 (Schnieder et al, 1995). The generally accepted range of incidence is 1 to 2 per 1000 live births (Goodman and Miedaner, 1998). If a sibling has already been born with MMC, the risk of recurrence in the family is 2 to 3% (Shurtleff et al, 1986). All types of neural tube defects occur at a rate of 1 in 1000 live births in the United States

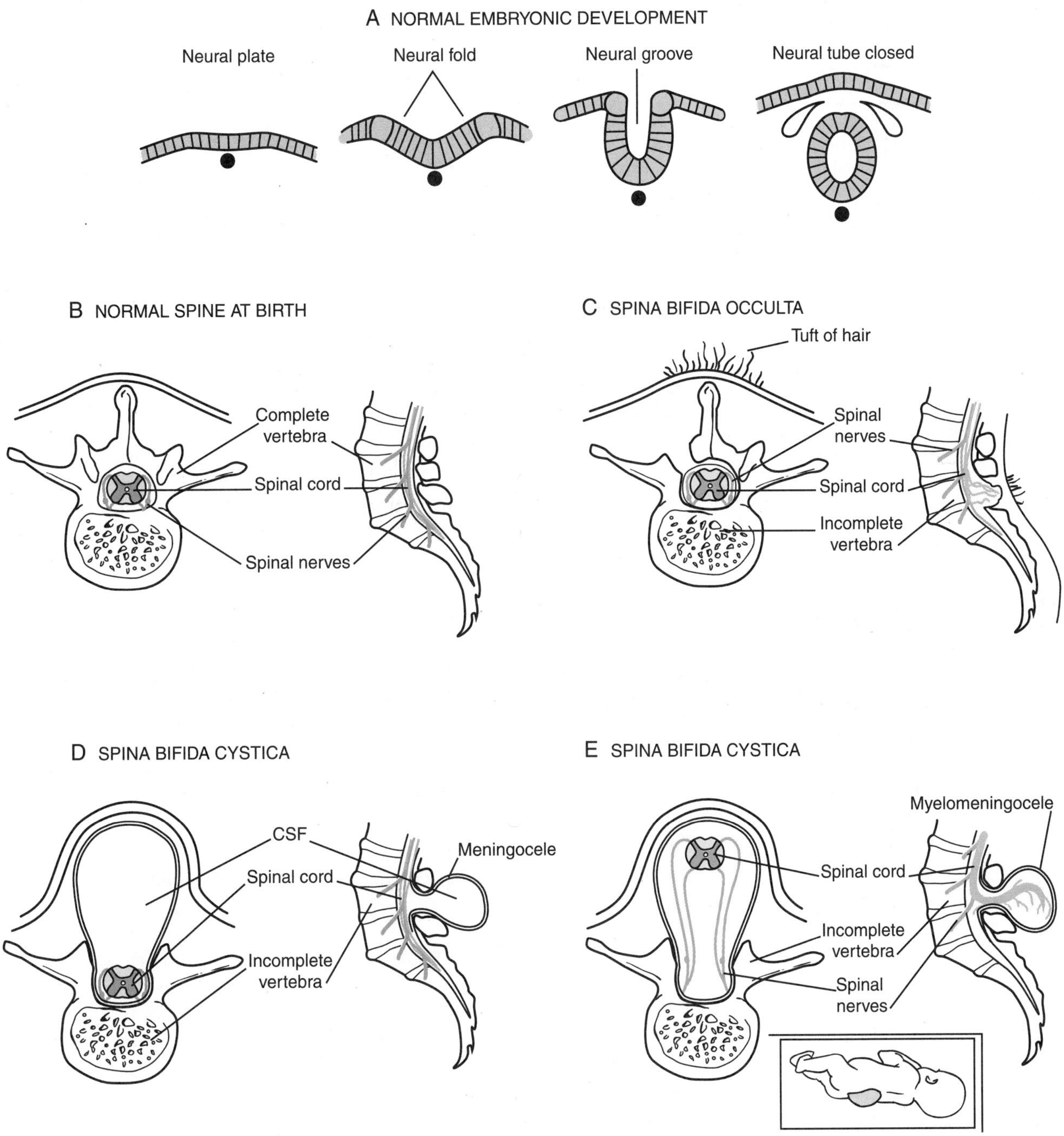

FIGURE 9-1 ■ Types of spina bifida. *A*, Normal formation of the neural tube during the first month of gestation. *B*, Complete closure with normal development in cross-section on the left and in longitudinal section on the right. *C*, Incomplete vertebral closure with no cyst, marked by a tuft of hair. *D*, Incomplete vertebral closure with a cyst of meninges and cerebrospinal fluid (CSF)—meningocele. *E*, Incomplete vertebral closure with a cyst containing a malformed spinal cord—myelomeningocele.

(Hobbins, 1991); China has the highest rate, 10 per 1000 live births (Xiao et al, 1990). These figures include defects of closure of the neural tube at the cephalic end, as well as in the thoracic, lumbar, and sacral regions. The lack of closure cephalically results in *anencephaly,* or failure of the brain to develop beyond the brain stem. These infants rarely survive for any length of time after birth. An *encephalocele* results when the brain tissue protrudes from the skull. It usually occurs occipitally and results in visual impairment.

ETIOLOGY

Many causal factors have been implicated in spina bifida and MMC. Genetic predisposition has been

Table 9–1 ▮ BASIC DEFINITIONS OF MYELODYSPLASTIC DEFECTS

DEFECT	DEFINITION
Spina bifida occulta	Vertebral defect in which posterior elements of the vertebral arch fail to close; no sac; vertebral defect usually not associated with an abnormality of the spinal cord
Spina bifida cystica	Vertebral defect with a protruding cyst of meninges or spinal cord and meninges
Meningocele	Cyst containing cerebrospinal fluid and meninges and usually covered with epithelium; clinical symptoms variable
Myelomeningocele	Cyst containing cerebrospinal fluid, meninges, spinal cord, and possibly nerve roots; cord incompletely formed or malformed; most common in the lumbar area; the higher the lesion, the more deficits present

Adapted from Ryan KD, Ploski C, Emans JB. Myelodysplasia—the musculoskeletal problem: habilitation from infancy to adulthood. Phys Ther 71:935–946, 1991, with permission of the American Physical Therapy Association.

shown to be a factor in some cases. Exposure to alcohol is suggested to cause MMC, in addition to producing fetal alcohol syndrome (Main and Mennuti, 1986). Some ethnic groups, such as the Irish and Americans of Irish descent, demonstrate a higher incidence of MMC (Noetzel, 1989). Lack of folic acid, a B vitamin, has been correlated with neural tube defects. Increasing the amount of folic acid in the diet has been used successfully as a preventive measure in women who have already had an infant with a neural tube defect (MRC, 1991). The use of folic acid prenatally has been shown to decrease the incidence of neural tube defects (CIBA, 1994; Daly et al, 1995).

PRENATAL DIAGNOSIS

A neural tube defect can be diagnosed prenatally by testing for levels of alpha-fetoprotein. If levels of the protein are too high, it may mean that the fetus has an open neural tube defect. This suspicion can be confirmed by high-resolution ultrasonography to visualize the vertebral defect. When an open neural tube defect is detected, the infant should be delivered by cesarean section before labor begins in order to decrease the risk of central nervous system infection and to minimize trauma to the spinal cord during the delivery process (Luthy et al, 1991). Because of this improved medical care, the prevalence of MMC in the population has increased even though the likelihood of having an infant with MMC has declined. (Prevalence is the number of people with a disorder in a population.)

CLINICAL FEATURES

Neurologic Defects and Impairments

The infant with MMC presents with motor and sensory impairments as a result of the spinal cord malformation. The extent of the impairment is directly related to the level of the cyst and the level of the spinal cord defect. Unlike in complete spinal cord injuries, which have a relatively straightforward relationship between the level of bony vertebra involvement and the underlying cord involvement, no clear relationship is present in infants with MMC. Some bony defects may involve more than one vertebral level. The spinal cord may be partially formed or malformed, or part of the spinal cord may be intact at one of the involved levels and may have innervated muscles below the MMC. If the nerve roots are damaged or the cord is dysplastic, the infant will have a flaccid type of motor paralysis with lack of sensation, the classic lower motor neuron presentation. However, if part of the spinal cord below the MMC is intact and has innervated muscles, the potential exists for a spastic type of motor paralysis. In some cases, the child may actually demonstrate an area of flaccidity at the level of the MMC, with spasticity present below the level of flaccidity. Either type of motor paralysis presents inherent difficulty in managing range of motion and in using orthoses for ambulation.

Functional Movement Related to Level

In general, the higher the level of the lesion, the greater the degree of muscular impairment and the less likely the child will be to ambulate functionally. A child with thoracic involvement at T12 has some control of the pelvis because of the innervation of the pelvic elevators and the complete innervation of the abdominal muscles. The gluteus maximus would not be active because it is innervated by L5–S1. A high lumbar level lesion (L1–L2) affects the lower extremities, but hip flexors and hip adductors are able to work. A midlumbar level lesion at L3 means that the child can flex at the hips and can extend the knees but has no ankle or toe movement. In a low lumbar level of paralysis at L4 or L5, the child adds the ability to flex the knees, dorsiflex the ankles, but only weakly extend the hips. Children with sacral level paralysis at S1 have weak plantar flexion for pushoff and good hip abduction. To be classified as having an S2 or S3 level lesion, the child's plantar flexors have to be at least grade 3 and the gluteal muscles a grade 4 on a five-point manual muscle test scale (Hinderer et al, 1994). The lesion is considered "no loss" when the child has normal bowel and bladder function and normal strength in the lower extremity muscles.

Musculoskeletal Impairments

Muscle paralysis results in an impairment of voluntary movement of the trunk and lower extremities. Children with the classic lower motor neuron presentation of flaccid paralysis have no lower extremity motion, and the legs are drawn into a frog-leg position by gravity. Because of the lack of voluntary movement, the lower extremities assume a position of comfort—hip abduction, external rotation, knee flexion, and ankle plantar flexion. Table 9–2 provides a list of typical deformities caused by muscle imbalances seen with a given level of lesion. Rather than memorizing the table, one would be better served to review the appropriate anatomy and kinesiology and see whether one could determine in what direction the limbs would be pulled if only certain muscles were innervated. For example, if there was innervation of only the anterior tibialis (L4 motor level) with no opposing pull from the gastrocnemius or posterior tibialis, in what position would the foot be held? It would be pulled into dorsiflexion and inversion, resulting in a calcaneovarus foot posture. In this situation, what muscle is most likely to become shortened? This may be one of the few instances in which the anterior tibialis needs to be stretched to maintain its resting length.

The child with MMC may also have congenital lower limb deformities, in addition to being at risk of acquiring additional deformities because of muscle imbalances. These deformities may include hip dislocation, hip dysplasia and subluxation, genu varus, and genu valgus. Congenital foot deformities associated with MMC are talipes equinovarus or congenital clubfoot, pes equinus or flatfoot, and convex pes valgus or rocker-bottom foot, with a vertical talus. These are depicted in Figure 9–2. Clubfoot is the most common foot deformity seen in children with MMC who have an L4 or L5 motor level (Tappit-Emas, 1994). The physical therapist may perform taping and gentle manipulation during the early management of this foot problem. The physical therapist assistant may or may not be involved with providing gentle corrective range of motion. Because of pressure problems over the bony prominences, splinting is recommended instead of serial casting. Surgical correction of the foot deformity is probably indicated in all but the mildest cases (Tappit-Emas, 1994).

Most children with MMC begin to ambulate between 1 and 2 years of age. A plantigrade foot, one that can be flat and in contact with the ground, is essential to ensure ambulation. In addition, the foot needs to be able to exhibit 10 degrees of dorsiflexion for toe clearance. This does not have to be active range.

If the child has a spastic type of motor paralysis, limb movements may result from muscle spasms, but such movements are not under the child's voluntary control. Various limb positions may result, depending on which muscles are spastic. The deforming forces will be stronger if spasticity is present. For example, in a child with an L1 or L2 motor level, the hip flexors and adductors may pull strongly because of increased tone that the hip is dislocated. A calcaneal foot is the result of having an innervated anterior tibialis muscle that is not balanced by an innervated gastrocnemius-soleus complex.

Table 9–2 ‖ FUNCTION RELATED TO LEVEL OF LESION

LEVEL OF LESION	MUSCLE FUNCTION	POTENTIAL DEFORMITY
Thoracic	Trunk weakness T7–T9 upper abdominals T9–T12 lower abdominals T12 has weak quadratus lumborum	Positional deformities of hips, knees, and ankles secondary to frog-leg posture
High lumbar (L1–L2)	Unopposed hip flexors and some adductors	Hip flexion, adduction Hip dislocation Lumbar lordosis Knee flexion and plantar flexion
Midlumbar (L3)	Strong hip flexors, adductors Weak hip rotators Antigravity knee extension	Hip dislocation, subluxation Genu recurvatum
Low lumbar (L4)	Strong quadriceps, medial knee flexors against gravity, ankle dorsiflexion and inversion	Equinovarus, calcaneovarus, or calcaneocavus foot
Low lumbar (L5)	Weak hip extension, abduction Good knee flexion against gravity Weak plantar flexion with eversion	Equinovarus, calcaneovalgus, or calcaneocavus foot
Sacral (S1)	Good hip abductors, weak plantar flexors	—
Sacral (S2–S3)	Good hip extensors and ankle plantar flexors	—

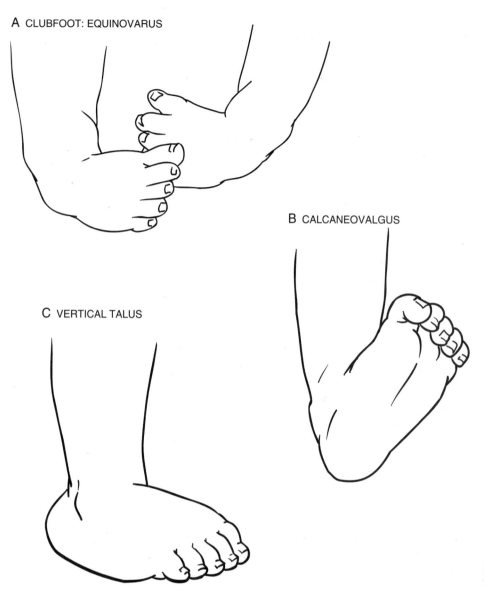

A CLUBFOOT: EQUINOVARUS

B CALCANEOVALGUS

C VERTICAL TALUS

FIGURE 9-2 ■ Common lower extremity deformities.

Osteoporosis

As in adults with spinal cord injury, the loss of the ability to produce a muscle contraction is devastating for voluntary movement, but it also has ramifications for the ongoing development and function of the skeletal system. The skeletal system, including the long bones and axial skeleton, depends on muscle pull and weight bearing to maintain structural integrity and to help balance normal bone loss with new bone production. Children, like adults with spinal cord injury, are at risk of developing *osteoporosis* (Hinderer et al, 1994). Osteoporosis predisposes a bone to fracture; therefore, children with MMC are at greater risk of developing fractures secondary to decreased weight bearing. Researchers have found that children who are household or community ambulators have higher bone mineral density than children who walk only therapeutically (Rosenstein et al, 1987). The reader is referred to Chapter 7 for the definition of the various levels of ambulation.

Neuropathic Fractures

Twenty percent of children with MMC are likely to experience a neuropathic fracture (Lock and Aronson, 1989). *Neuropathic fractures* are those that relate to the underlying neurologic disorder. Paralyzed muscles cannot generate forces through long bones, so that essentially no weight bearing takes place, with resulting osteoporosis. Osteoporosis makes it easier for the bone to fracture. Possible causes of neuropathic fractures in this population include overly aggressive therapeutic exercise and lack of stabilization during transfers (Garber, 1991).

The following clinical example illustrates another possible situation involving a neuropathic fracture.

Once, when placing the lower extremities of a child with MMC into his braces, a clinician felt warmth along the child's tibial crest. The child was biracial, so no redness was apparent, but a definite separation was noted along the tibia. The child was in no pain or distress. His mother later recounted that it had been particularly difficult to put his braces on the day before. A radiograph confirmed the clinician's clinical suspicion that the child had a fracture. The limb was casted until the fracture healed. While the child was in his cast, therapy continued, with an emphasis on upper extremity strengthening and trunk balance. Presence of a cast protecting a fracture is usually not an indication to curtail activity in children with MMC. In fact, it may spark creativity on the part of the rehabilitation team to come up with ways to combat postural insecurity and loss of antigravity muscle strength while the child's limb is immobilized.

Spinal Deformities

Children with MMC can have congenital or acquired *scoliosis. Congenital scoliosis* is usually related to vertebral anomalies, such as a hemivertebra, that are present in addition to the bifid spine. This type of scoliosis is inflexible. *Acquired scoliosis* results from muscle imbalances in the trunk that produce flexible scoliosis. A rapid onset of scoliosis can also occur secondary to a tethered spinal cord or to a condition called hydromyelia. These conditions are explained later in the text. The physical therapist assistant must be observant of any postural changes in treating a child with MMC. Acquired scoliosis should be managed by some type of orthosis until spinal fixation with instrumentation is appropriate. Children with MMC go through puberty at a younger age than typically developing children, and this allows for earlier spinal surgery with little loss of the child's mature trunk height.

Other spinal deformities such as *kyphosis* and *lordosis* may also be seen in these children. The kyphosis may be in the thoracic area or may encompass the entire spine, as seen in a baby. The lordosis in the lumbar area may be exaggerated or reversed. Spinal deformities of all kinds are more likely to be present in children with higher level lesions.

Spinal alignment and potential for deformity must always be considered when one uses developmentally appropriate positions such as sitting and standing. If the child cannot maintain trunk alignment muscularly, then some type of orthosis may be indicated. The child's sitting posture should be documented during therapy, and sitting positions to be used at home should be identified. Spinal deformities may not always be preventable, but attention must be paid to the effect of gravity on a malleable spine when it is in vulnerable developmental postures.

Arnold-Chiari Malformation

In addition to the spinal cord defect in MMC, most children with this neuromuscular problem have an *Arnold-Chiari type II malformation*. The Arnold-Chiari malformation involves the cerebellum, the medulla, and the cervical part of the spinal cord (Fig. 9–3). Because the cerebellum is not fully developed, the hindbrain is downwardly displaced through the foramen magnum. The flow of CSF is obstructed, thus causing fluid to build up within the ventricles of the

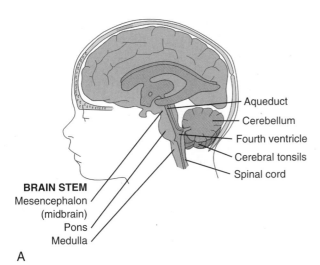
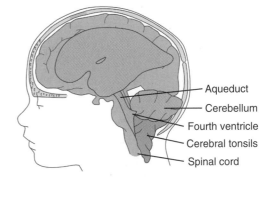

A   B

FIGURE 9–3 ■ *A*, Normal brain with patent cerebrospinal fluid (CSF) circulation. *B*, Arnold-Chiari type II malformation with enlarged ventricles, a condition that predisposes a child with myelomeningocele to hydrocephalus. The brain stem, the fourth ventricle, part of the cerebellum, and the cerebral tonsils are displaced downward through the foramen magnum, and this leads to blockage of CSF flow. Additionally, pressure on the brain stem housing the cranial nerves may result in nerve palsies. (From Goodman CC, Boissonnault WG. Pathology: Implications for the Physical Therapist. Philadelphia, WB Saunders, 1998.)

brain. The abnormal accumulation of CSF results in hydrocephalus, as shown in Figure 9–3. A child with spina bifida and MMC who has an Arnold-Chiari type II malformation has a better than 90% chance of developing hydrocephalus. The Arnold-Chiari type II malformation may also affect cranial nerve and brain stem function because of the pressure exerted on these areas by the accumulation of CSF within the ventricular system. Clinically, this involvement may be manifested by swallowing difficulties.

Hydrocephalus

Hydrocephalus can occur in children with MMC with or without the Arnold-Chiari malformation. Hydrocephalus is treated neurosurgically with the placement of a ventriculoperitoneal shunt, which drains excess CSF into the peritoneal cavity (Fig. 9–4). You will be able to palpate the shunt tubing along the child's neck as it goes under the clavicle and down the chest wall. All shunt systems have a one-way valve that allows fluid to flow out of the ventricles but prevents back-

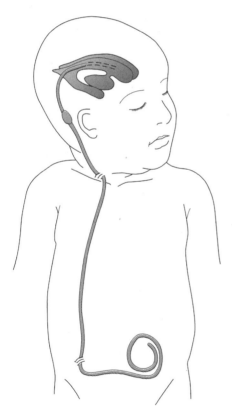

FIGURE 9–4 ▪ A ventriculoperitoneal shunt provides primary drainage of cerebrospinal fluid from the ventricles to an extracranial compartment, usually either the heart or the abdominal or peritoneal cavity, as shown here. Extra tubing is left in the extracranial site to uncoil as the child grows. A unidirectional valve designed to open at a predetermined intraventricular pressure and to close when the pressure falls below that level prevents backflow of fluid. (From Goodman CC, Boissonnault WG. Pathology: Implications for the Physical Therapist. Philadelphia, WB Saunders, 1998.)

Table 9–3 ▌ SIGNS AND SYMPTOMS OF SHUNT MALFUNCTION

SIGN OR SYMPTOM	INFANTS	TODDLERS	SCHOOL-AGE CHILDREN
Bulging fontanelle	X		
Sunset sign of eyes	X		
Excessive rate of growth of head circumference	X		
Thinning of skin over scalp	X		
Irritability	X	X	X
Seizures	X	X	X
Vomiting	X	X	X
Lethargy	X	X	X
Headaches		X	X
Edema, redness along shunt tract	X	X	X
Personality changes			X
Memory changes			X

flow. The child's movements are generally not restricted unless such restriction is specified by the physician. However, the child should avoid spending a prolonged time in a head-down position, such as hanging upside down, because this may disrupt the valve function or may interfere with the flow of the fluid (Williamson, 1987).

Shunts can become blocked or infected, so the clinician must be aware of signs that could indicate shunt malfunction. These signs are listed in Table 9–3. Many of the signs and symptoms, such as irritability, seizures, vomiting, and lethargy, are seen regardless of the age of the child. Other signs are unique to the age of the child. Infants may display bulging of the fontanelles secondary to increased intracranial pressure. The sunset sign of the eyes refers to the finding that the iris is only partially visible because of the infant's downward gaze. Older children may exhibit personality or memory changes.

Central Nervous System Deterioration

In addition to being vigilant about watching for signs of shunt malfunction as the child grows, the clinician must investigate any change in motor and sensory status or functional abilities because it may indicate neurologic deterioration. Common causes of such deterioration are hydromyelia and a tethered spinal cord. All areas of the child's function, such as mobility, activities of daily living (ADLs), and school performance, can be affected by either of these two conditions.

Hydromyelia

Hydromyelia is characterized by an accumulation of CSF in the central canal of the spinal cord. The condition can cause rapidly progressing scoliosis, upper extremity weakness, and increased tone (Long and Cintas, 1995). Other investigators have reported sensory changes (Ryan et al, 1991) and ascending motor loss in the lower extremities (Schneider et al, 1995). The incidence of hydromyelia in children with MMC ranges from 20 to 80% (Byrd et al, 1991). Any time a child presents with rapidly progressing scoliosis, alert your supervising therapist, who will inform the child's physician so that the cause of the symptoms can be investigated and treated quickly.

Tethered Spinal Cord

The relationship of the spinal cord to the vertebral column normally changes with age. At birth, the end of the spinal cord is at the level of L3, rising to L1 in adulthood as a result of skeletal growth. Because of scarring from the surgical repair of the back lesion, adhesions can form and can anchor the spinal cord at the lesion site. The spinal cord is then tethered and is not free to move upward within the vertebral canal as the child grows. Progressive neurologic dysfunction, such as a decline in motor and sensory function, pain, or loss of previous bowel and bladder control, may result. Other signs may include rapidly progressive scoliosis, increased tone in the lower extremities, and changes in gait pattern. Prompt surgical correction can usually prevent any permanent neurologic damage (Banta, 1991; Grief and Stalmasck, 1989). Any deterioration in neuromuscular or urologic performance from the child's baseline or the rapid onset of scoliosis should immediately be reported to the supervising physical therapist.

Sensory Impairment

Sensory impairment from MMC is not as straightforward in children as it is in adults with a spinal cord injury. The sensory losses exhibited by children are less likely to correspond to the motor level of paralysis. Do not presume that because one part of a dermatome is intact, the entire dermatome is intact to sensation. "Skip" areas that have no sensation may be present within an innervated dermatome (Hinderer et al, 1994). Often, the therapist has tested for only light touch or pinprick because the child with MMC is usually unable to differentiate between the two sensations. If the therapist has tested for vibration, intact areas of sensation may be present below those perceived as insensate for either light touch or pinprick (Hinderer and Hinderer, 1990).

The functional implications of loss of sensation are enormous. An increased potential exists for damaging the skin and underlying tissue secondary to extremes of temperature and normal pressure. A child with MMC loses the ability to feel when he has too much pressure on the buttocks from sitting too long. This loss of sensation can lead to the development of pressure ulcers. The consequences of loss of time from school and play and of independent function because of a pressure ulcer can be immeasurable. The plan of care must include teaching skin safety and inspection as well as pressure-relief techniques. These techniques are essential to good primary prevention of complications. The use of seat cushions and other joint protective devices is advised. Insensitive skin needs to be protected as the child learns to move around and explore the environment. The family needs to made aware of the importance of making regular skin inspection part of the daily routine. As the child grows and shoes and braces are introduced, skin integrity must be a high priority when one initiates a wearing schedule for any orthotic devices.

Bowel and Bladder Dysfunction

Most children with MMC have some degree of bowel and bladder dysfunction. The sacral levels of the spinal cord, S2 to S4, innervate the bladder and are responsible for voiding and defecation reflexes. With motor and sensory loss, the child has no sensation of bladder fullness or of wetness. The reflex emptying and the inhibition of voiding can be problematic. If tone in the bladder wall is increased, the bladder cannot store the typical amount of urine and empties reflexively. Special attention must be paid to the treatment of urinary dysfunction because mismanagement can result in kidney damage. By the age of 3 or 4 years, most children begin to work on gaining urinary continence by using clean intermittent catheterization. By 6 years, the child should be independent in self-intermittent catheterization. Functional prerequisites for this skill include sitting balance with no hand support and the ability to do a toilet transfer. These functional activities should be incorporated into early and middle stages of physical therapy management.

Latex Allergy

According to a survey by Pearson and associates (1994), children with MMC are much more likely to have an allergy to latex. These investigators reported that more than 50% of children with MMC surveyed were allergic to latex. Exposure to latex can produce an anaphylactic reaction that can be life-threatening (Dormans et al, 1995). All contact with latex products should be avoided, including catheters, surgical gloves, and Theraband. Any surgery should be performed in a latex-free environment. Toys that contain latex such as rubber balls and balloons should be avoided.

PHYSICAL THERAPY INTERVENTION

Three stages of care are used to describe the continuum of physical therapy management of the child with myelodysplasia. Although similarities exist between adults with spinal cord injuries and children with congenital neurologic spinal deficits, inherent differences are also present. The biggest difference is that the anomaly occurs during development of the body and its systems. Therefore, one of the major foci of a physical therapy plan of care should be to minimize the impact and ongoing development of bony deformation, postural changes, and abnormal tone. Optimizing development encompasses not only motor development but cognitive and social-emotional development as well. Other therapeutic considerations are the same as for an adult who has sustained a spinal cord injury, such as strengthening the upper extremities, developing sitting and standing balance, fostering locomotion, promoting self-care, encouraging safety and personal hygiene, and teaching self-performed range of motion and pressure relief.

First Stage of Physical Therapy Intervention

This stage includes the acute care the infant receives after birth and up to the time of ambulation. Initially, after the birth of a child with MMC, parents are dealing with multiple medical practitioners, each with his or her own contribution to the health of the infant. The neurosurgeon performs the surgery to remove and close the MMC within 24 hours of the infant's birth because of the risk of infection. The placement of a shunt to relieve the hydrocephalus may be done at the same time or may occur within the first week of life. The orthopedist assesses the status of the infant's joints and muscles. The urologist assesses the child's renal status and monitors bowel and bladder function. Depending on the amount of skin coverage available to close the defect, a plastic surgeon may also be involved. Once the back lesion is repaired and a shunt is placed, the infant is medically stabilized in preparation for discharge home. Communication among all members of the team working with the parents and infant is crucial. Information about the infant's present level of function must be shared among all personnel who evaluate and treat the infant.

The physical therapist establishes motor and sensory levels of function; evaluates muscle tone, degree of head and trunk control, and range-of-motion limitations; and checks for the presence of any musculoskeletal deformities. General physical therapy goals during this first stage of care include the following:

1. Prevent secondary complications (contractures, deformities, skin breakdown).
2. Promote age-appropriate sensorimotor development.
3. Prepare the child for ambulation.
4. Educate the family about appropriate strategies to manage the child's condition.

If the physical therapist assistant is involved at this stage of the infant's care, a caring and positive attitude is of utmost importance to foster healthy, appropriate interactions between the parents and the infant. The most important thing to teach the parents is how to interact with their infant. Parents have many things to learn before the infant is discharged from the acute care facility: positioning, sensory precautions, range of motion, and therapeutic handling. Parents need to be comfortable in using handling techniques to promote normal sensorimotor development, especially head and trunk control. Giving parents a sense of competence in their ability to care for their infant is everyone's job and ensures carryover of instructions to the home setting.

Prevention of Deformities: Postoperative Positioning

Positioning after the surgical repair of the back lesion should avoid pressure on the repaired area until it is healed. Therefore, the infant initially is limited to prone and side lying positions. You can show the child's parents how to place the infant prone on their laps and gently rock to soothe and stimulate head lifting. Holding the infant high on the shoulder, with support under the arms, fosters head control and may be the easiest position for the infant with MMC to maintain a stable head. Handling and carrying strategies may be recommended by the physical therapist and practiced by the assistant before being demonstrated to the parents. Parents are naturally anxious when handling an infant with a disability. Use gentle encouragement, and do not hesitate to correct any errors in hand placement. The infant's head should be supported when the infant is picked up and put down. As the child's head control improves, support can gradually be withdrawn. As the back heals, the infant can experience brief periods of supine and supported upright sitting without any interference with wound healing. When the shunt has been inserted, you should always follow any positioning precautions according to the physician's orders.

Prone Positioning

Prone positioning is important to prevent development of potentially deforming hip and knee flexion contractures. Prone is also a position from which the infant can begin to develop head control. Depending on the child's level of motor paralysis and the presence of hypotonia in the neck and trunk, the infant may have more difficulty in learning to lift the head off the support surface in prone than in a supported upright position. Movement in the prone position, as when the infant is placed over the caregiver's lap or when the infant is carried while prone, will also stimulate head control by encouraging lifting the head into extension. Intervention 9–1 demonstrates a way to position an infant prone, lying with lateral supports to maintain proper alignment. Encouraging the infant to use the upper extremities for propping on elbows and for pushing up to extended arms provides a good beginning for upper extremity strengthening.

Effects of Gravity

When the infant is in the supine position, the paralyzed lower extremities will tend to assume positions of

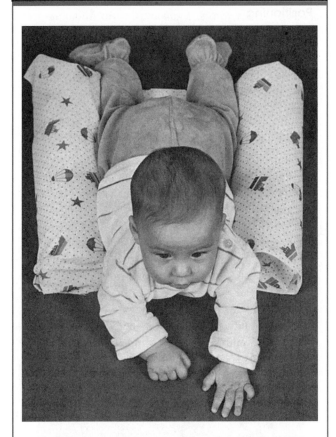

Intervention 9–1 ▌ PRONE LYING WITH SUPPORT

Infant in prone lying position with lateral supports to maintain proper trunk and lower extremity alignment.

From Williamson GG. Children with Spina Bifida: Early Intervention and Preschool Programming. Baltimore, Paul H. Brookes, 1987.

Table 9–4 ▌ **POSITIONS TO BE AVOIDED IN CHILDREN WITH MYELOMENINGOCELE**

Frog-leg position in prone or supine
W sitting
Ring sitting
Heel sitting
Cross-legged sitting

From Hinderer KA, Hinderer SR, Shurtleff DB. Myelodysplasia. In Campbell SK, Palisano RJ, Vander Linden DW (eds). Physical Therapy for Children. Philadelphia, WB Saunders, 1994, pp 571–619.

comfort, such as hip abduction and external rotation, because of the effect of gravity. In children with partial innervation of the lower extremities, hip flexion and adduction can produce hip flexion contractures and can lead to hip dislocation because of the lack of muscle pull from hip extensors or abductors. Certain postures should be avoided, as listed in Table 9–4. *Genu recurvatum* is seen when the quadriceps muscles are not opposed by equally strong hamstring pull to balance the knee extension posture. When only anterior tibialis function is present, a calcaneovarus foot results. Some of these foot deformities are depicted in Figure 9–2.

Orthoses for Lower Extremity Positioning

Orthoses may be needed early to prevent deformities, or the caregiver may simply need to position the child with towel rolls or small pillows to help maintain a neutral hip, knee, and ankle position. An example of a simple lower extremity splint is seen in Figure 9–5. Early on, it is detrimental to adduct the hips completely because the hip joints are incompletely formed and may subluxate or dislocate if they are adducted beyond neutral. Maintaining a neutral alignment of the foot is critical for later plantigrade weight bearing. Children with higher level lesions may benefit initially from a total body splint, to be worn while they are sleeping (Fig. 9–6). Many clinicians recommend night splints for this reason. Any orthosis should be introduced gradually because of lack of skin sensation, and the skin should be monitored closely for breakdown.

Prevention of Skin Breakdown

Lack of awareness of pressure may cause the infant to remain in one position too long, especially once sitting is attained. However, the supine position may pose more danger of skin breakdown over the ischial tuberosities, the sacrum, and the calcaneus. Side lying can be a dangerous position because of the excess pressure on the trochanters. Because of the lack of sensation and decreased awareness of excessive pressure from being in one position too long, the skin of

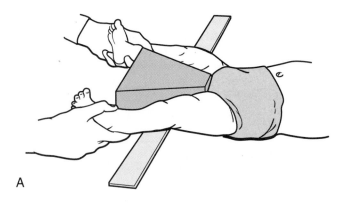

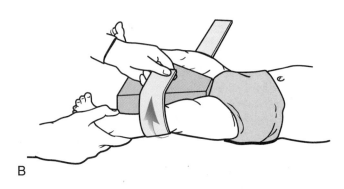

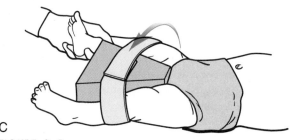

FIGURE 9–5 ■ Simple abduction splint. *A,* A pad is placed between the child's legs with a strap underneath. *B,* The straps are wrapped around the legs and attached with Velcro (*C*), bringing the legs into neutral hip rotation.

children with MMC must be closely monitored for redness. Infants need to have their position changed often. Check for red areas, especially over bony prominences and after the infant wears any orthosis. If redness persists longer than 30 minutes, the orthosis should be adjusted (Tappit-Emas, 1994).

Sensory Precautions

Parents often find it difficult to realize that the infant lacks the ability to feel below the level of the injury. Encouraging parents to play with the infant and to tickle different areas of the child's body will help them to understand where the baby has feeling. It is not appropriate to demonstrate the infant's lack of sensitivity by stroking the skin with a pin, even

though the therapist may use this technique during formal sensory testing. Socks or booties are a good idea for protecting the feet from being nibbled as the infant finds his toes around 6 months. Teach the parents to keep the infant's lower extremities covered to protect the skin when the infant is crawling or creeping. Close inspection for small objects on the floor or carpet that could cause an accidental injury is a necessity. Protecting the skin with clothing also helps with temperature regulation, which is impaired. Skin that is anesthetic does not sweat and cannot conserve heat or give off heat, and therefore it must be protected. Parents must be cautioned always to test bath water before placing the infant into the tub because a burn could easily result. Proper shoe fit is imperative to prevent pressure areas and abrasions. Children with MMC may continue to have a chubby baby foot, so extra room may be needed in shoes.

Prevention of Contractures: Range of Motion

Passive range of motion should be done two to three times a day in an infant with MMC. To decrease the number of exercises in the home program, exercises for certain joints, such as the hip and knee, can be combined. For example, hip and knee flexion on one side can be combined with hip and knee exten-

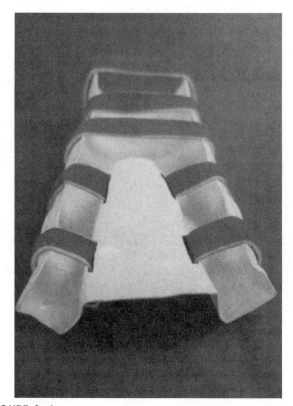

FIGURE 9–6 ■ Total body splint. (From Schneider JW, Krosscheu K, Gabriel KL. Congenital spinal cord injury. In Umphred DA [ed]. Neurological Rehabilitation. St. Louis, CV Mosby, 1995.)

sion on the other side while the infant is supine. Hip abduction can be done bilaterally, as can internal and external rotation. Performing these movements when the infant is prone provides a nice stretch to the hip flexors.

Range of foot and ankle motion should be done individually. Always be sure that the subtalar joint is in a neutral position when doing ankle dorsiflexion range, so that the movement occurs at the correct joint. If the foot is allowed to go into varus or valgus positioning, the motion caused by your stretching will take place in the midfoot, rather than the hindfoot, when stretching a tight heel cord. You may be causing a rocker-bottom foot by allowing the motion to occur at the wrong place. Be sure that your supervising physical therapist demonstrates the correct technique to stretch a heel cord, maintaining subtalar neutral.

Range-of-motion exercises should be done gently, with your hands placed close to the child's joints, to provide a short lever arm. Hold the motion briefly at the end of the available range. Even in the presence of contractures, aggressive stretching is not indicated. Serial casting may be needed as an adjunct to therapy if persistent passive range-of-motion exercise does not improve the range of motion. Always keep your supervising therapist apprised of any problems in this area. Range-of-motion exercises are easy to forget when the infant becomes more active, but these simple exercises are an important part of the infant's program. Once the child is able, she should be responsible for doing her own daily range of motion.

Promotion of Age-Appropriate Sensorimotor Development

Therapeutic Handling: Development of Head Control

Any of the techniques outlined in Chapter 8 to encourage head control can be used in a child with MMC. Some early cautions include being sure that the skin over the back defect is well healed and that care is taken to prevent shearing forces on the lower extremities or trunk when the infant is positioned for head lifting. Additionally, the caregiver should provide extra support if the child's head is larger than normal secondary to hydrocephalus. The infant can be carried at the caregiver's shoulder to encourage head lifting as the body sways, just as you would with any newborn. The caregiver can also support the infant in the prone position during carrying or gentle rocking on the lap to promote head control using vestibular input. Extra support can be given to the infant's head at the jaw or forehead when the child is prone (Intervention 9–2).

Although head control in infants usually develops first in the prone position, it may be more difficult for an infant with myelodysplasia to lift the head from this position because of hydrocephalus and hypotonic neck

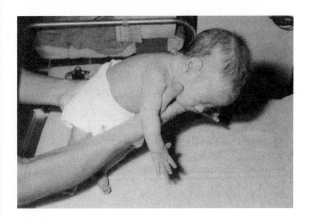

Intervention 9–2 ▮ PRONE CARRYING

Prone carrying with extra support for jaw or forehead.

From Burns YR, MacDonald J. Physiotherapy and the Growing Child. London, WB Saunders Company Ltd., 1996.

and trunk muscles. Extra support from a bolster or a small half-roll under the chest assists in distributing some of the weight farther down the trunk as well as helps to bring the upper extremities under the body to assume a prone on elbows position (Fig. 9–7). Additional support can be provided under the child's forehead, if needed, to give the infant a chance to experience this position. Rolling from supine to side lying with the head supported on a half-roll also gives the child practice in keeping the head in line with the body during rotation around the long axis of the body. Head control in the supine position is needed to balance the development of axial extension with axial flexion. Positioning the child in a supported supine position on a wedge can encourage a chin tuck or forward head lift into flexion. Every time the infant is picked up, the caregiver should encourage active head and trunk movements on the part of the child. Carrying should also be seen as a therapeutic activity to promote postural control, rather than as a passive action performed by the caregiver. The clinician or caregiver should watch for signs that could indicate

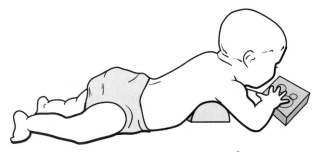

FIGURE 9–7 ▮ Prone position over a half-roll.

medical complications while interacting with and handling a child with MMC and a shunt. Signs of shunt obstruction may include the setting sun sign and increased muscle tone in the upper or lower extremities.

Therapeutic Handling: Developing Righting and Equilibrium Reactions

If the infant uses too much shoulder elevation as a substitute for head control, developing righting reactions of the head and trunk becomes more difficult. Try to modify the position to make it easier for the infant to use neck muscles for stability, rather than the elevated shoulder position. In addition, give more support proximally at the child's trunk to provide a stable base on which the head can work. The infant may carry the elevated position of the shoulders over into propped sitting, with the arms internally rotated and the scapula protracted. Although this posture may be positionally stable, it does not allow the infant to move within or from the posture with any degree of control, thus making it difficult to reach or to shift weight in sitting.

As the infant with MMC develops head control in prone, supine, and side lying positions, righting reactions should be seen in the trunk. Head and trunk righting can be encouraged in prone by slightly shifting the infant's weight onto one side of the body and seeing whether the other side shortens. Righting of the trunk occurs only as far down the body as the muscles are innervated. The clinician should note any asymmetry in the trunk, because this will need to be taken into account for planning upright activities that could predispose the child to scoliosis. As the infant is able to lift the head off the supporting surface, trunk extension develops down the back. The extension of the infant's back and the arms should be encouraged by enticing the child to reach forward from a prone position with one or both arms. As the infant becomes stronger, and depending on how much of the trunk is innervated, less and less anterior trunk support can be given while still encouraging lifting and reaching with the arms and upper trunk. (The goal is to have the child "fly," as in the Landau reflex.) By placing the infant on a small ball or over a small bolster and shifting weight forward, you may elicit head and trunk lifting (Intervention 9–3A), reaching with arms (Intervention 9–3B), or propping on one extended arm and reaching with the other (Intervention 9–3C). If the infant is moved quickly, protective extension of the upper extremities may be elicited. For the infant with a lower level lesion and hip innervation, hip extension should be encouraged when the child is in the prone position.

Trunk rotation must be encouraged to support the child's transition from one posture to another, such as in rolling from supine to prone and back and in coming to sit from side lying. Trunk rotation in sitting encourages the development of equilibrium reactions that bring the center of gravity back within the base of support. Equilibrium reactions are trunk reactions that occur in developmental postures. In prone and supine, trunk incurvation and limb abduction result from a lateral weight shift. Again, the trunk responds only to the degree to which it is innervated, so one should encourage rotation in all directions. Trunk rotation is also used in protective reactions of the upper extremities when balance is lost.

Handling: Developing Trunk Control in Sitting

Acclimation to upright in sitting is begun as close to the developmentally appropriate time (6 to 8 months) as possible. Ideally, the infant should have sufficient head control and the ability to bear weight on extended arms. This propped sitting is a typical beginning to independence in sitting. Always think of the alignment of the back when the child is placed in a sitting position. Floor sitters, a type of adaptive equipment, can be used to support the child's back if kyphosis is present. Some floor sitters have extensions that provide head support if head control is inconsistent. Those floor sitters with head support allow even the child with poor head control to be placed in a sitting position on the floor to play. In children with good head control, sitting balance can be trained by varying the child's base of support and the amount of hand support. Often, a bench or tray placed in front of the child can provide extra support and security as confidence is gained while the child plays in a new position. Certain sitting positions should be avoided because of their potentially deforming forces. These positions are listed in Table 9–4.

Once propped sitting is achieved, hand support is gradually but methodically decreased. Reaching for objects while supporting with one hand can begin in the midline, and then the range can be widened as balance improves. Weight shifting at the pelvis in sitting can be used to elicit head and trunk righting reactions and upper extremity protective reactions. Trunk rotation with extension is needed to foster the ability to protect in a backward direction. Later, the child can work on transferring objects at the midline with no hand support, an ultimate test of balance. Always remember to protect the child's back and skin during weight bearing in sitting. Skin inspection should be done after sitting for short periods of time. If the child cannot maintain an upright trunk muscularly, an orthosis may be indicated for alignment in sitting and for prevention of scoliosis.

Preparation for Ambulation: Acclimation to Upright and Weight Bearing

Acclimation to upright and weight bearing begins with fostering development of head and trunk control and includes sensory input to the lower extremities despite the lack of sensation. Brief periods of weight

Intervention 9–3 **▌ BALL EXERCISES**

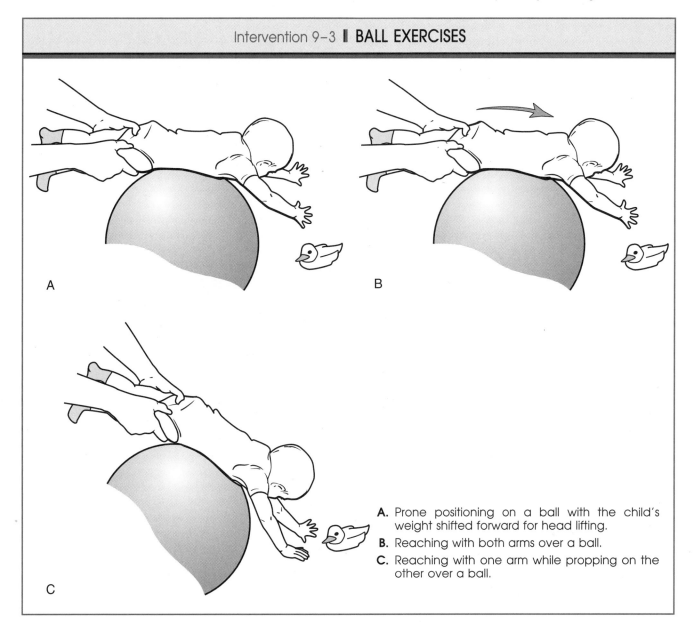

A. Prone positioning on a ball with the child's weight shifted forward for head lifting.

B. Reaching with both arms over a ball.

C. Reaching with one arm while propping on the other over a ball.

bearing on properly aligned lower extremities should be encouraged throughout the day. These periods occur in supported standing and should be done often. Providing a symmetric position for the infant is important for increasing awareness of body position and sensory input. Handling should promote symmetry, equal weight bearing, and equal sensory input. Weight bearing in the upright position provides a perfect opportunity to engage the child in cognitively appropriate play. The physical therapist assistant can serve as a vocal model for speech by making sounds, talking, and describing objects and actions in the child's environment. By interacting with the child, you are also modeling appropriate behavior for the caregiver.

Upper Extremity Strengthening

During early development, pulling and pushing with the upper extremities are excellent ways to foster increasing upper extremity strength. The progression from prone on elbows to prone on extended arms and onto hands and knees can provide many opportunities for the child to use the arms in a weight-bearing form of work. Providing the infant with your hands and requesting her to pull to sit can be done before she turns and pushes up to sit. Pulling on various resistances of latex-free Theraband can be a fun way to incorporate upper extremity strengthening into the child's treatment plan. Other objects can be used for pulling, such as a dowel rod or cane. Pushing on the floor on a scooter board can provide excellent resistance training.

Mat Mobility

Moving around in supine and prone positions is important for exploring the environment and self-care activities, but mat mobility includes movement in upright sitting. Mat mobility needs to be encouraged once trunk balance begins in supported sitting. The child can be encouraged to pull himself up to sitting by using another person, a rope tied to the end of the bed, or an overhead trapeze. Children can and should use pushup blocks or other devices to increase the strength in their upper extremities (Intervention 9–4). They need to have strong triceps, latissimus dorsi, and shoulder depressors to transfer independently. Moving around on the mat or floor is good preparation for moving around in upright standing or doing pushups in a wheelchair. Connecting arm motion with mobility early gives the child a foundation for coordinating other, more advanced transfer and self-care movements.

Standing Frames

Use of a standing frame for weight bearing can begin when the child has sufficient head control and exhibits interest in attaining an upright standing position. Normally, infants begin to pull to stand at around 9 months of age. By 1 year, all children with a motor level of L3 or above should be fitted with a standing frame or parapodium to encourage early weight bearing. The Toronto A-frame is the preambulation orthosis of choice for most children with MMC (Fig. 9–8). A standing frame is usually less expensive than a parapodium and is easier to apply (Ryan et al, 1991). The tubular frame supports the trunk, hips, and knees and leaves the hands free. Some children with L4 or lower lesions may be fitted with some type of hip-knee-ankle-foot orthosis (HKAFO) to begin standing in preparation for walking. The device pictured in Figure 9–9 has a thoracic support. Having the child stand four or five times a day for 20 to 30 minutes seems to be manageable for most parents

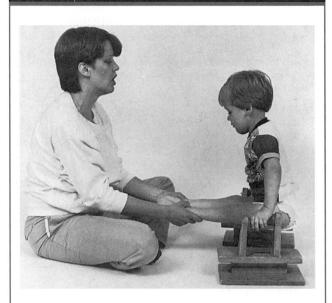

Intervention 9–4 ▌ STRENGTHENING UPPER EXTREMITIES WITH PUSHUP BLOCKS

Pushups on wooden blocks to strengthen scapular muscles. Pushups prepare for transfers and pressure relief.

From Williamson GG. Children with Spina Bifida: Early Invervention and Preschool Programming. Baltimore, Paul H Brookes, 1987.

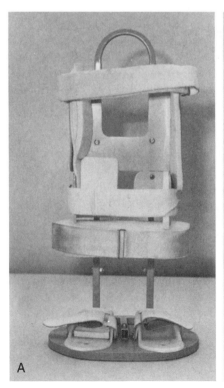

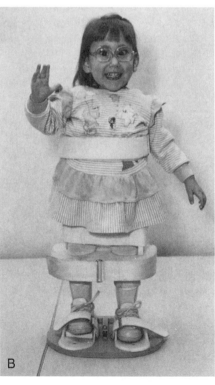

A

B

FIGURE 9–8 ▪ Standing frame. *A*, Anterior view. *B*, The frame is adapted to accommodate the child's leg-length discrepancy and tendency to lean to the right. (From Ryan KD, Ploski C, Emans JB. Myelodysplasia: the musculoskeletal problem: habilitation from infancy to adulthood. Phys Ther 71:935–946, 1991, with permission of the American Physical Therapy Association.)

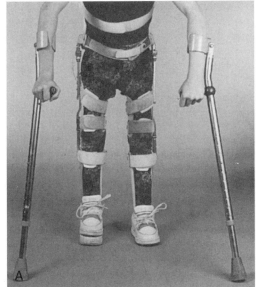
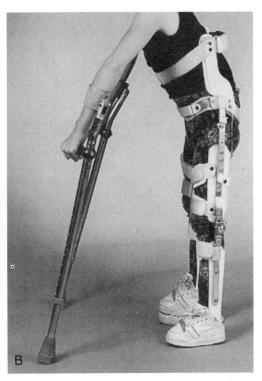
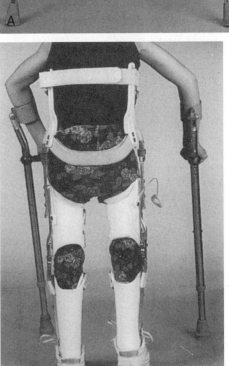

FIGURE 9-9 ■ Hip-knee-ankle-foot orthosis with a thoracic strap. *A*, Front view. *B*, Side view. *C*, Posterior view. (From Nawoczenski DA, Epler ME. Orthotics in Functional Rehabilitation of the Lower Limb. Philadelphia, WB Saunders, 1997.)

(Tappit-Emas, 1994). A more detailed explanation of standing frames is presented later in this chapter.

Family Education

The family must be taught sensory precautions, signs of shunt malfunction, range of motion, handling, and positioning. Most of these activities are not particularly difficult. However, the difficulty comes in trying not to overwhelm the parents with all the things that need to be done. Parents of children with a physical disability need to be empowered to be parents and advocates for their child. Parents are not surrogate therapists and should not be made to think they should be. Literature that may be helpful is available from the Spina Bifida Association of America. As much as possible, many of the precautions, range-of-motion exercises, and developmental activities should become part of the family's everyday routine. Range-of-motion exercises and developmental activities can be shared between the spouses, and a schedule of standing time can be outlined. Siblings are often the best partners in encouraging developmentally appropriate play.

Second Stage of Physical Therapy Intervention

The ambulatory phase begins when the infant becomes a toddler and continues into the school years. The general physical therapy goals for this second stage include the following:

1. Ambulation and independent mobility.
2. Continued improvements in flexibility, strength, and endurance.
3. Independence in pressure relief, self-care, and ADLs.
4. Promotion of ongoing cognitive and social-emotional development.
5. Identification of perceptual problems that may interfere with learning.
6. Collaboration with family, school, and health care providers for total management.

Table 9–5 lists vital components of a physical therapy program.

Orthotic Management

The health care provider's philosophy of orthosis use may determine who receives what type of orthosis and when. Some clinicians do not think that children with high levels of paralysis, such as those with thoracic or high lumbar (L1 or L2) lesions, should be prescribed orthoses because studies show that by adolescence these individuals are mobile in a wheelchair and have discarded walking as a primary means of mobility. Others think that all children, regardless of the level of lesion, have the right to experience upright ambulation even though they may discard this type of mobility later.

Orthotic Selection

The physical therapist, in conjunction with the orthopedist and the orthotist, is involved with the family in making orthotic decisions for the child with MMC. Many factors have to be considered when choosing an orthosis for a child who is beginning to stand and ambulate, including level of lesion, age, central nervous system status, body proportions, contractures, upper limb function, and cognition. Financial considerations also play a role in determining the initial type of orthosis. Any time prior approval is needed, the process must begin in sufficient time so as not to interfere with the child's developmental progress. Even though as a physical therapist assistant you will probably not be directly involved in making orthotic decisions, you do need to be aware of what goes into this decision making.

Level of Lesion. The level of motor function demonstrated by the toddler does not always correspond to the level of the lesion because of individual differences in nerve root innervation. A thorough evaluation needs to be completed by the physical therapist prior to making orthotic recommendations. A chart of possible devices to be considered according to innervation is found in Table 9–6. The age at which such devices may be introduced is found in the same table. Age recommendations vary considerably among different sources and are often linked to the philosophy of orthotic management espoused by a particular facility or clinic. Contractures can prevent a child from being fitted with an orthosis. The child cannot have any significant amount of hip or knee flexion contractures and must have a plantigrade foot—that is, the ankle must be able to achieve a neutral position or 90 degrees—to be able to wear an orthotic device for standing and ambulation.

Age. The type of orthosis used by a child with MMC may vary according to age. A child younger than 1 year of age can be fitted with a night splint to maintain the lower extremities in proper alignment. By 1 year, all children should be fitted with a standing frame or parapodium to encourage early weight bearing. Most children exhibit a desire to pull to stand at around 9 months of age, and the therapist and the assistant should anticipate this desire and should be ready with an orthosis to take advantage of the child's readiness to stand. When a child with MMC exhibits a developmental delay, the child should be placed in a standing device when her developmental age reaches 9 months. If, however, the child does not attain a developmental age of 9 months by 20 to 24 months of chronologic age, standing should be begun for physiologic benefits. A parapodium is the orthosis of choice in this situation (Fig. 9–10).

The level of MMC is correlated with the child's age to determine the appropriate type of orthotic device. A child with a thoracic or high lumbar motor level requires a HKAFO with thoracic support (see Fig. 9–9). Often, the child begins gait training in a parapodium and progresses to a reciprocating gait orthosis (RGO) (Fig. 9–11). A child with a midlumbar (L3 or L4) motor level may begin with a parapodium and may make the transition to standard KAFOs or ankle-foot-orthoses (AFOs) (Figs. 9–12 and 9–13*A*), depending on quadriceps strength. A child with a low

Table 9–5 ▌ VITAL COMPONENTS OF A PHYSICAL THERAPY PROGRAM

Proper positioning in sitting and sleeping
Stretching
Strengthening
Pressure relief and joint protection
Mobility for short and long distances
Transfers and activities of daily living
Self-care

From Hinderer KA, Hinderer SR, Shurtleff DB. Myelodysplasia. In Campbell SK, Palisano RJ, Vander Linden DW (eds). Physical Therapy for Children. Philadelphia, WB Saunders, 1994, pp 571–619.

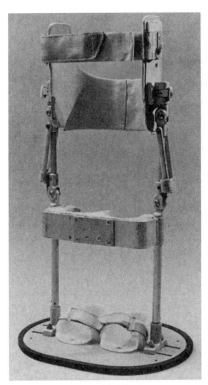

FIGURE 9–10 ■ Front view of the Toronto parapodium. (From Knutson LM, Clark DE. Orthotic devices for ambulation in children with cerebral palsy and myelomeningocele. Phys Ther 71:947–960, 1991, with permission of the American Physical Therapy Association.)

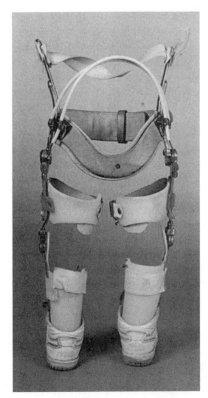

FIGURE 9–11 ■ Reciprocating gait orthosis with a thoracic strap, posterior view. (From Nawoczenski DA, Epler ME. Orthotics in Functional Rehabilitation of the Lower Limb. Philadelphia, WB Saunders, 1997.)

motor level, such as L4 to L5 or S2, may begin standing without any device. When learning to ambulate, children with low lumbar motor levels benefit from AFOs or supramalleolar molded orthoses (Fig. 9–13*A* and *B*). A child with an L5 motor level has hip extension and ankle eversion and may need only lightweight AFOs to ambulate. Although the child with an S2 motor level may begin to walk without any orthosis, she may later be fitted with a foot orthosis (Fig. 9–13*C*).

Types of Orthoses

Parapodiums, RGOs, and swivel walkers are all specially designed HKAFOs. They encompass and control the child's hips, knees, ankles, and feet. A traditional HKAFO consists of a pelvic band, external hip joints, and bilateral long leg braces (KAFOs). Additional trunk components may be attached to an HKAFO if the child has minimal trunk control or needs to control a spinal deformity. The more extensive the orthosis, the less likely the child will be to continue to ambulate as he grows older. The amount of energy expended to ambulate with a cumbersome orthosis is high. Although the child is young, he may be highly motivated to move around in the upright position. As time progresses, it may become more important to keep up with a peer group, and he may prefer an alternative, faster, and less cumbersome means of mobility.

Parapodium. The parapodium (see Fig. 9–10) is a commonly used first orthotic device for standing and ambulating. Its wide base provides support for standing and allows the child to acclimate to upright while

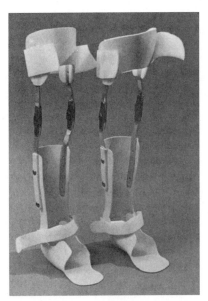

FIGURE 9–12 ■ Oblique view of knee-ankle-foot orthoses with anterior thigh cuffs. (From Knutson LM, Clark DE. Orthotic devices for ambulation in children with cerebral palsy and myelomeningocele. Phys Ther 71:947–960, 1991, with permission of the American Physical Therapy Association.)

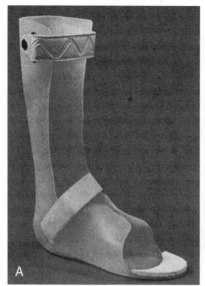

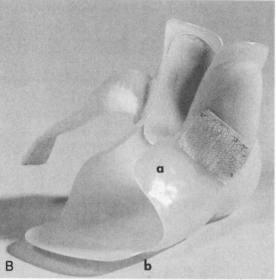

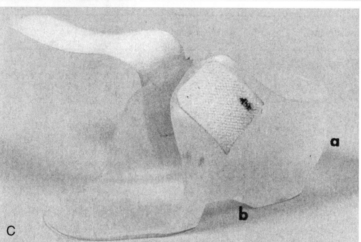

FIGURE 9–13 ▪ *A,* Fixed molded ankle-foot orthosis with an ankle strap to restrain the heel. Extrinsic toe elevation to unload the metatarsal heads is optional. *B,* Supramalleolar orthosis extending proximally to the malleoli. Well-molded medial and lateral walls that wrap over the dorsum of the foot (a) help to control the midtarsal joint and to keep the heel seated. Dorsal flaps also disperse pressure and may reduce sensitivity of the foot. Intrinsic toe elevation (b) can prevent stimulating the plantar grasp reflex. *C,* Foot orthosis designed to oppose pronation by molding the heel cup to grasp the calcaneus firmly (a) and wedging, or posting, the heel medially (b). (From Knutson LM, Clark DE. Orthotic devices for ambulation in children with cerebral palsy and myelomeningocele. Phys Ther 71:947–960, 1991, with permission of the American Physical Therapy Association.)

leaving the arms free for play. The child's knees and hips can be unlocked for sitting at a table or on a bench, a feature that allows the child to participate in typical preschool activities such as snack and circle time. The Toronto parapodium has one lock for the hip and knee, whereas the Rochester parapodium has separate locks for each joint.

Reciprocating Gait Orthosis. An RGO is the orthosis of choice for progressing a child who begins ambulating with a parapodium. The RGO is more energy efficient than a traditional HKAFO because it employs a cable system to cause hip extension reciprocally on the stance side when hip flexion is initiated on the swing side. At least weak hip flexors are needed to operate the cable system (Hinderer et al, 1994). A newer version of the RGO, the isocentric RGO, can be triggered by a lateral and backward weight shift that causes the unweighted leg to swing forward (Schneider et al, 1995; Tappit-Emas, 1994); this feature makes it possible for this type of orthotic device to be used by individuals with a thoracic lesion. This type of gait pattern requires no active movement of the lower extremities.

Swivel Walker. This device is similar to a parapodium, except that the base and footplate assembly allow a swivel motion. An Orthotic Research and Locomotor Assessment Unit (ORLAU) swivel walker is pictured in Figure 9–14. It is prescribed for children with a high level of MMC who require trunk support. By shifting weight from side to side, the child can ambulate without crutches. If arm swing is added, the child can increase the speed of forward progression, and with crutches, the child may be able to learn a swing-to or swing-through gait pattern. Sitting is not possible because this type of orthosis has no locks at the hips and knees.

Donning and Doffing of Orthoses

Ambulating with orthoses and assistive devices requires assistance to don the braces. Teaching donning and doffing of orthoses can be accomplished when the child is supine or sitting. The child may be able to roll into the orthosis by going from prone to supine. Sit-

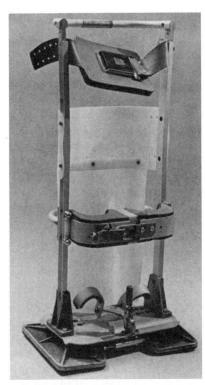

FIGURE 9-14 ■ Front view of the Orthotic Research and Locomotor Assessment Unit (ORLAU) swivel walker. (From Knutson LM, Clark DE. Orthotic devices for ambulation in children with cerebral palsy and myelomeningocele. Phys Ther 71:947–960, 1991, with permission of the American Physical Therapy Association.)

ting is preferable for independent donning of the orthosis if the child can boost into the brace. Next, the child places each foot into the shoe with the knees of the orthosis unlocked, laces or closes the foot piece, locks the knees, and fastens the thigh cuffs or waist belt, if the device has one. Cotton knee-high socks or tights should be worn under the orthosis to absorb perspiration and to decrease any skin irritation. It takes a great deal of practice on the part of the child to become independent in donning the orthosis.

Wearing Time of Orthoses

Caregivers should monitor the wearing time of orthoses, including the gradual increase in time, with periodic checks for any areas of potential skin breakdown. The child can begin wearing the orthosis for 1 or 2 hours for the first few days and can increase wearing time from there. A chart is helpful so that everyone (teacher, aide, family) knows the length of time the child is wearing the orthosis and who is responsible for checking skin integrity. Check for red marks after the child wears the orthosis and note how long it takes for these marks to disappear. If they do not resolve after 20 to 30 minutes, contact the orthotist about making an adjustment. The orthosis should not be worn again until it is checked by the orthotist.

Upper Limb Function

Children with MMC, especially children with hydrocephalus, can often exhibit coordination difficulties with the upper extremities. The difficulties in coordination appear to be related to the timing and smooth control of the movements of the upper extremities. These children do not perform well on tests that are timed and exhibit delayed or mixed hand dominance (Shaffer et al, 1986). A delay could interfere with tasks involving the use of both arms. Difficulties with fine-motor tasks and those related to eye-hand coordination are documented in the literature. Some authors relate the perceptual difficulties to the upper limb dyscoordination rather than to a true perceptual deficit (Hinderer et al, 1994). The low muscle tone often exhibited in the neck and trunk of these children could also add to their coordination problems. The child with MMC must have sufficient upper extremity control to be able to use an assistive device such as a walker. Practicing fine-motor activities has been found to help with the problem and carries over to functional tasks (Fay et al, 1986). Occupational therapists are also involved in the treatment of these children.

Cognition

The child must also be able to understand the task to be performed to master upright ambulation with an orthosis and assistive device. Cognitive function in a child with MMC can vary with the degree of nervous system involvement and hydrocephalus. Results from intelligence testing place them in the normal range but below the population mean (Tappit-Emas, 1994). Problem areas include performance subtests, arithmetic tasks, and visuomotor integration (Willis et al, 1990). Some of the poor performance by children with MMC may be related to their attentional difficulties, slow speed of motor response, and memory deficits.

Cocktail Party Speech

You may encounter a child who seems verbally much more intelligent than she really is when formally tested. "Cocktail party speech" can be indicative of "cocktail party personality," a behavioral manifestation associated with cognitive dysfunction. The assistant must be cautious not to mistake flowery speech for more advanced cognitive ability in a child with MMC. These children are often more severely impaired than one would first think based on their verbal conversation. When they are closely questioned about a topic such as performing daily tasks within their environment, they are unable to furnish details, to solve problems, or to generalize the task to new situations.

Principles of Gait Training

Regardless of the timing and type of orthosis that is used, general principles of treatment can be discussed for this second or middle stage of care. Gait training begins with learning to perform and control weight shifts in standing. If the toddler has had only limited experience in upright standing, a standing program may be initiated simultaneously with practicing weight shifting. If the toddler is already acclimated to standing and has a standing frame, one can challenge the child's balance while she is in the frame. The assistant moves the child in the frame and causes the child to respond with head and trunk reactions (Intervention 9–5). This maneuver can be a good beginning for any standing session. Parents should be taught how to challenge the child's balance similarly at home. The child should not be left unattended in the frame because she may topple over from too much self-initiated body movement. By being placed at a surface of appropriate height, the child can engage in fine-motor

activities such as building block towers, sorting objects, lacing cards, or practicing puzzles.

Children with moderate to severe central nervous system deficits and delayed head and upper extremity development may continue to use the standing frames until age 3 or 4 or until they no longer fit into them (Tappit-Emas, 1994). In this case, an ORLAU swivel walker is used as the ambulation orthosis, with progression to an RGO with thoracic support and a rollator walker.

The physical therapist assistant can play an important role during this second stage of physical therapy management by teaching the child with MMC to ambulate with the new orthosis, usually a parapodium. The child is first taught to shift weight laterally onto one side of the base of the parapodium and to allow the unweighted portion of the base to pivot forward. This maneuver is called a swivel gait pattern. Children can be taught this maneuver in appropriately high parallel bars or with a walker. However, use of the parallel bars may encourage the child to pull rather than push and may make it more difficult to progress to using a walker. The assistant may also be seated on a rolling stool in front of the child and may hold the child's hands to encourage the weight-shifting sequence.

Once the child has mastered ambulation with the new orthosis, consideration can be given to changing the type of assistive device. The child's gait pattern in a parapodium is progressed from a swivel pattern to a swing-to pattern, which requires a walker. Tappit-Emas (1994) recommends using a rollator walker as the initial assistive device for gait training a child with MMC. This type of walker provides a wide base of stability and two wheels; therefore, the child can advance the walker without picking it up. "The child with an L4 or L5 motor level is often able to begin ambulation after one or two sessions of gait training with a rollator walker" (Tappit-Emas, 1994). A child should be independent with one type of orthosis and assistive device before moving on to a different orthosis or different device. After success with a swing-to gait pattern using a walker, the child can be progressed to using the same pattern with Lofstrand crutches.

Once the child has mastered the gait progression with a parapodium and a walker, plans can be made for progression to a more energy-efficient orthosis or a less restrictive assistive device, but not at the same time. A swing-through gait pattern is the most efficient, but it requires using forearm or Lofstrand crutches. The earliest a child may be able to understand and succeed in using Lofstrand crutches is 3 years of age. Tappit-Emas (1994) recommends waiting until the child is 4 or 5 years of age because the use of Lofstrand crutches is complicated. She thinks that the additional time allows the child to be confident in and have perfected additional skills in the upright position.

Intervention 9–5 ❚ WEIGHT SHIFTING IN STANDING

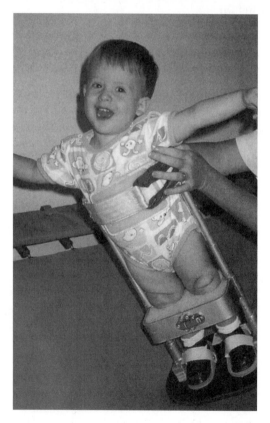

Weight shifting the child while in a standing frame can promote head and trunk righting reactions. These movements prepare the child for later weight shifting during ambulation.

From Burns YR, MacDonald J. Physiotherapy and the Growing Child. London, WB Saunders Company Ltd., 1996.

Lofstrand crutches provide much greater maneuverability than a walker, so whenever possible, the child should be progressed from a walker to forearm crutches.

Orthotic choices following the use of a parapodium include an HKAFO/RGO or a KAFO. The main advantage of the RGO is energy efficiency. A child with only hip flexors can walk faster and has less fatigue using an RGO than using either conventional KAFOs or a parapodium. A walker may still be the assistive device of choice to provide the child with sufficient support during forward locomotion. Transition to an RGO is not recommended before the child is 30 to 36 months of developmental age, according to Knutson and Clark (1991). If the child has some innervated knee musculature, such as a child with an L3 motor level, ambulation with KAFOs protects the knees. A long-term goal may be walking with the knees unlocked, and if quadriceps strength increases sufficiently, the KAFOs could be cut down to AFOs. If the child is able to move each lower extremity separately, a four-point or two-point gait pattern can be taught. Gait instruction progresses from level ground to uneven ground to elevated surfaces such as curbs, ramps, and stairs.

The child's gait pattern should be perfected with one type of orthosis and assistive device before either the orthosis or the assistive device is changed. According to the gait progression principle, when progressing ambulation, change either the orthosis or the assistive device, not both. For example, if a child can ambulate with a parapodium and a walker, she could be progressed to learning to walk with RGOs and a walker, then with RGOs and Lofstrand crutches.

Level of Ambulation

Three levels of ambulation have been identified (Hoffer et al, 1973). These are therapeutic, household, and community. The names of the levels are descriptive of the type and location in which the ambulation takes place and are defined in Chapter 7.

The functional ambulatory level for a child with MMC is linked to the motor level. Table 9–6 relates the level of lesion to the child's ambulation potential over time. A child with thoracic-level involvement can be a therapeutic ambulator. However, children with high thoracic involvement (above T12) rarely ambulate by the time they are teenagers; they prefer to be independently mobile in a wheelchair to be able to keep up with their peers. Children with upper lumbar innervation (L1 or L2) can usually ambulate within the household or classroom. Again, they usually use a wheelchair for quick mobility, and their long-term functional locomotion is independent in a wheelchair. Household or community-aided ambulation is possible for children with either L3 or L4 innervation. The strength of the quadriceps can determine the level of functional ambulation in this group. Children with lower levels of innervation—L5, S1, and below—are community ambulators and should be able to maintain this level of independence throughout adulthood.

Ambulation is a major goal during early childhood, and most children with MMC are successful. Neverthe-

Table 9–6 ▌ AMBULATION POTENTIAL

LEVEL OF LESION	PERAMBULATION ORTHOSIS	AMBULATION ORTHOSIS	AGE	ASSISTIVE DEVICE	AMBULATION POTENTIAL
Thoracic	Standing frame	Parapodium	12–18 months	Walker	Children: therapeutic or household ambulation
		Swivel walker		No device needed	
		RGO	24–36 months	Walker Crutches	Adolescents/adults: wheelchair independent
L1, L2	Standing frame	Parapodium	12–18 months	Walker	Children: household or community
		RGO	24–36 months	Walker Crutches	Adolescents/adults: wheelchair independent
L3, L4	None	RGO/HKAFO	12–18 months	Walker	Children: household or community
		KAFO or AFO	24–36 months	Walker Crutches	Adolescents/adults: variable household or community if quadriceps grade 4 or 5
L5	None	KAFO	12–18 months	None	Children: household or community
		AFO	24–36 months		Adolescents/adults: household or community
S1–S3	None	AFO, FO None	12–18 months	None	Children: community
					Adolescents/adults: community

RGO, reciprocating gait orthosis; HKAFO, hip-knee-ankle-foot-orthosis; KAFO, knee-ankle-foot-orthosis; AFO, ankle-foot orthosis; FO, foot orthosis.
Data from Burns Y, Gilmour J, Kentish M, et al. Physiotherapy management of children with neurological, neuromuscular and neurodevelopmental problems. In Burns YR, MacDonald J (eds). Physiotherapy and the Growing Child. London, WB Saunders, 1996, pp 359–414; Hoffer MM, Feiwell E, Perry R, et al. Functional ambulation in patients with myelomeningocele. Bone Joint Surg Am 55:137–148, 1973; Knutson LM, Clark DE. Orthotic devices for ambulation in children with cerebral palsy and myelomeningocele. Phys Ther 71:947–960, 1991.

Table 9–7 ▋ MOBILITY OPTIONS FOR CHILDREN WITH MYELOMENINGOCELE

Caster cart
Prone scooter
Manual wheelchair
Electric wheelchair
Adapted tricycle
Cyclone

From Hinderer KA, Hinderer SR, Shurtleff DB. Myelodysplasia. In Campbell SK, Palisano RJ, Vander Linden DW (eds). Physical Therapy for Children. Philadelphia, WB Saunders, 1994, pp 571–619.

Table 9–9 ▋ WHEELCHAIR TRAINING FOR TODDLERS AND PRESCHOOLERS

Ability to transfer
Mobility on level surfaces
Exploration of home and classroom
Safety

From Hinderer KA, Hinderer SR, Shurtleff DB. Myelodysplasia. In Campbell SK, Palisano RJ, Vander Linden DW (eds). Physical Therapy for Children. Philadelphia, WB Saunders, 1994, pp 571–619.

less, many children need a wheelchair to explore and have total access to their environment. Studies have shown that early introduction of wheeled mobility does not interfere with the acquisition of upright ambulation. In fact, easy wheelchair use may boost the child's self-confidence. It enables the child to exert control over her environment by independently moving to acquire an object or to seek out attention. Mobility is crucial to the child with MMC, and several options should be made available, depending on the child's developmental status. Table 9–7 is a list of mobility options.

Wheelchair training for the toddler or preschooler should consist of preparatory and actual training activities, as listed in Tables 9–8 and 9–9. The child should have sufficient sitting balance to use her arms to propel the chair or to operate an electric switch. Arm strength is necessary to propel a manual chair and to execute lateral transfers with or without a sliding board. Training begins on level surfaces within the home and classroom. Safety is always a number one priority; therefore, the child should wear a seat belt while she is in the wheelchair.

Strength, Flexibility, and Endurance

All functional activities in which a child participates require strong upper extremities. Traditional strengthening activities can be modified for the shorter stature of the child, and the amount of weight used can be adjusted to decrease the strain on growing bones. Weights, pulleys, latex-free tubing, and pushup blocks

Table 9–8 ▋ PREPARATORY ACTIVITIES FOR WHEELCHAIR MOBILITY

Sitting balance
Arm strength
Ability to transfer
Wheelchair propulsion or operating an electric switch or joystick

From Hinderer KA, Hinderer SR, Shurtleff DB. Myelodysplasia. In Campbell SK, Palisano RJ, Vander Linden DW (eds). Physical Therapy for Children. Philadelphia, WB Saunders, 1994, pp 571–619.

can be incorporated into games of "tug of war" and mat races. Trunk control and strength can be improved by use of righting and equilibrium reactions in developmentally appropriate positions. Refer to the descriptions earlier in this chapter.

Monitoring joint range of motion for possible contractures is exceedingly important at all stages of care. Be careful with repetitive movements because this population is prone to injury from excessive joint stress and overuse. Begin early on to think of joint conservation when the child is performing routine motions for transfers and ADLs. Learning to move the lower extremities by attaching strips of latex-free bands to them can be an early functional activity that fosters learning of self-performed range of motion.

Independence in Pressure Relief

Pressure relief and mobility must also be monitored whether the child is wearing an orthosis or not. When the child has the orthosis on, can she still do a pushup for pressure relief? Does the seating device or wheelchair currently used allow enough room for the child to sit without undue pressure from the additional width of the orthosis, or does it take up too much room in the wheelchair? How many different ways does the child know to relieve pressure? The more ways that are available to the child, the more likely the task is to be accomplished. The obvious way is to do pushups, but if the child is in a regular chair at school, the chair may not have arms. If the child sits in a wheelchair at her desk, the chair must be locked before she attempts a pushup. Forward leans can also be performed from a seated position. Alternative positioning in kneeling, standing, or prone lying can be used during rest and play periods. Be creative!

Independence in Self-Care and Activities of Daily Living

Skin care must be a high priority for the child with MMC, especially as the amount of sitting increases during the school day. Skin inspection should be done twice a day with a handheld mirror. Clothing should be nonrestrictive and sufficiently thick to protect the skin from sharp objects and wheelchair parts and orthoses. An appropriate seat cushion must be used to distribute pressure while the child sits in the wheelchair. Pressure-reducing seat cushions do not, however, decrease the need for performing pressure-relief activities.

Self-care also means dressing and undressing, feeding, and bathing. It also includes bowel and bladder care. Studies done to determine whether children with MMC accomplish self-care activities at the same age as typically developing children have shown delays (Okamoto et al, 1984; Sousa et al, 1983). Interpretation of the data further suggests that the delays may be the result of lower performance expectations. Parents must be encouraged to expect independence from the child with MMC.

By the time the child goes to preschool, she will be aware that her toileting abilities are different from those of her same-age peers (Williamson, 1987). Bowel and bladder care is usually overseen by the school nurse, but everyone working with a child with MMC needs to be aware of the importance of these skills. Consistency of routine, privacy, and safety must always be part of any bowel and bladder program for a young child. Helping the child to maintain a positive self-image while teaching responsible toileting behavior can be especially tricky. The child should be given responsibility for as much of her own care as possible. Even if she is still in diapers, she should wash her hands at the sink after a diaper change. Williamson (1987) suggests these ways to assist the child to begin to participate:

1. Indicate the need for a diaper change.
2. Assist in pulling the pants down and in removing any orthotic devices, if necessary.
3. Unfasten the soiled diaper.
4. Refasten the clean diaper.
5. Assist in donning the orthosis if necessary and in pulling up the pants.
6. Wash hands.

Williamson (1987) provides many excellent suggestions for fostering self-care skills in the preschooler with MMC. The reader is referred to the text by this author for more information.

ADL skills include the ability to transfer. We tend to think of transferring from mat to wheelchair and back as the ultimate transfer goal, but for the child to be as independent as possible, he should also be able to perform all transfers related to ADLs, such as to and from a bed to a dressing bench or a regular chair, to and from a chair to a toilet, to and from a chair to the floor, and to and from the tub or shower.

Promotion of Cognitive and Social-Emotional Growth

Preschoolers are inquisitive individuals who need mobility to explore their environment. They should be encouraged to explore the space around them by physically moving through it, not just visually observing what goes on around them. Scooter boards can be used to help the child to move his body weight with his arms while he receives vestibular input. The use of adapted tricycles that are propelled by arm cranking allows movement through space and could be used on the playground rather than a wheelchair. Difficulty with mobility may interfere with self-initiated exploration and may foster dependence instead of independence. Other barriers to peer interaction or factors that may limit peer interaction are listed in Table 9–10.

Many children with MMC experience healthy emotional development (Williamson, 1987). The task of infancy, according to Erikson, is to develop trust that basic needs will be met. Parents, primary caregivers, and health care providers need to ensure that these emotional needs are met. If the infant perceives the world as hostile, she may develop coping mechanisms such as withdrawal or perseveration. If the child is encouraged to explore the environment and is guided to overcome the physical barriers encountered, she will perceive the world realistically as full of a series of challenges to be mastered, rather than as full of unsurmountable obstacles.

Identification of Perceptual Problems

School-age children with MMC are motivated to learn and to perform academically to the same extent as any other children. During this time, perceptual problems may become apparent. Although some documentation indicates that children with MMC have visual-perceptual difficulties, other researchers have demonstrated that these perceptual problems may be more closely related to upper extremity incoordination. If the child has low muscle tone and delayed upper extremity development, perhaps the motor skills necessary for integrating visual information may be compromised. Visual perception in a child with MMC should be evaluated separately from her visuomotor abilities, to determine whether she truly has a perceptual deficit (Hinderer et al, 1994). For example, a child's difficulty with copying shapes, a motor skill, may be more closely related to her lack of motor control of the upper extremity than to an inaccurate visual perception of the shape to be copied.

Table 9–10 ▌ LIMITATIONS TO PEER INTERACTION

Mobility
Activities of daily living, especially transfers
Additional equipment
Independence in bowel and bladder care
Hygiene
Accessibility

Collaboration for Total Management

The management of the child with MMC in pre-school and subsequently in the primary grades involves everyone who comes in contact with that child. From the bus driver to the teacher to the classroom aide, everyone has to know what the child is capable of doing, in which areas she needs assistance, and what must be done for her. Medical and educational goals should overlap to support the development of the most functionally independent child possible, a child whose psychosocial development is on the same level as that of her able-bodied peers and one who is ready to handle the tasks and issues of adolescence and adulthood.

Third Stage of Physical Therapy Intervention

The third stage of management involves the transition from school age to adolescence and on into adulthood. General physical therapy goals during this last stage are as follows:

1. Reevaluation of ambulation potential
2. Mobility for home, school, and community distances
3. Continued improvements in flexibility, strength, and endurance
4. Independence in ADLs
5. Physical fitness and participation in recreational activities

Reevaluation of Ambulation Potential

The potential for continued ambulation needs to be reevaluated by the physical therapist during the student's school years, and in particular as she approaches adolescence. Children with MMC go through puberty earlier than their able-bodied peers. Surgical procedures that depend on skeletal maturity may be scheduled at this time. The long-term functional level of mobility of these students can be determined as their physical maturity is peaking. The assistant working with the student can provide valuable data regarding length of time upright ambulation is used as the primary means of mobility. Any student in whom ambulation becomes unsafe or whose ambulation skills become limited functionally should discontinue ambulation except with supervision. Physical therapy goals during this time are to maintain the adolescent's present level of function if possible, to prevent secondary complications, to promote independence, to remediate any perceptual-motor problems, to provide any needed adaptive devices, and to promote self-esteem and social-sexual adjustment (Schneider et al, 1995). Developmental changes that may contribute to the loss of mobility in adolescents with MMC are as follows:

1. Changes in length of long bones, such that skeletal growth outstrips muscular growth
2. Changes in body composition that alter the biomechanics of movement
3. Progression of neurologic deficit
4. Immobilization resulting from treatment of secondary problems such as skin breakdown or orthopedic surgery
5. Progression of spinal deformity
6. Joint pain or ligamentous laxity

Physical therapy during this stage focuses on making a smooth transition to primary wheeled mobility if that transition is needed to save energy for more academic, athletic, or social activities. Individuals with thoracic, high lumbar (L1 or L2), and midlumbar (L3 or L4) lesions require a wheelchair for long-term functional mobility. They may have already been using a wheelchair during transport to and from school or for school field trips. School-age children can lose function because of spinal cord tethering, so they should be monitored closely during rapid periods of growth for any signs of change in neurologic status. An adolescent with a midlumbar lesion can ambulate independently within a house or classroom but needs aids to be functional within the community. Long-distance mobility is much more energy efficient if the individual uses a wheelchair. Individuals with lower level lesions (L5 and below) should be able to remain ambulatory for life, unless too great an increase in body weight occurs, thereby making wheelchair use a necessity. Hinderer and colleagues (1988) found a potential decline in mobility resulting from progressive neurologic loss in adolescents even with lower level lesions, so any adolescent with MMC should be monitored for potential progression of neurologic deficit.

Wheelchair Mobility

When an adolescent with MMC makes the transition to continuous use of a wheelchair, you should not dwell on the loss of upright ambulation as something devastating but focus on the positive gains provided by wheeled mobility. Most of the time, if the transition is presented as a natural and normal occurrence, it is more easily accepted by the individual. The wheelchair should be presented as just another type of "assistive" device, thereby decreasing any negative connotation for the adolescent. The mitigating factor is always the energy cost. The student with MMC may be able to ambulate within the classroom but may need a wheelchair to get from class to class and keep up with her friends. "Mobility limitations are magnified once a child begins school because of the increased community mobility distances and skills required" (Hinderer et al, 1994). This requirement becomes a significant problem once a child is in school because the travel distances increase and the skills needed to maneuver within new environments become more complicated. A wheelchair may be a necessity by middle school or whenever the student begins to change classes, has to retrieve books from a locker, and needs to go to the next class in a short time. For the student with all but the lowest motor levels, wheeled mobility is a must to maintain efficient function.

Environmental Accessibility

All environments in which a person with MMC functions should be accessible—home, school, and community. The Americans with Disabilities Act was an effort to make all public buildings, programs, and services accessible to the general public. Under this Act, reasonable accommodations have to be made to allow an individual with a disability access to public education and facilities. Public transportation, libraries, and grocery stores, for example, should be accessible to everyone.

Driver Education

Driver education is as important to a person with MMC as it is to any able-bodied person, and maybe even more so. Some states have programs that evaluate a disabled individual's ability to drive and recommend appropriate devices such as hand controls and types of vehicles. Teaching car transfers should be part of therapy for adolescents along with other activities that prepare them for independent living and a job. The ability to move the wheelchair into and out of the car is also vital to independent function.

Flexibility, Strength, and Endurance

Prevention of contractures must be aggressively pursued during the rapid growth of adolescence because skeletal growth can cause significant shortening of muscles. Stretching should be done at home on a regular basis and at school if the student has problem areas. Areas that should be targeted are the low back extensors, the hip flexors, the hamstrings, and the shoulder girdle (Hinderer et al, 1994). Proper positioning for sitting and sleeping should be reviewed, with the routine use of the prone position crucial to keep hip and knee flexors loose and to relieve pressure on the buttocks. More decubitus ulcers are seen in adolescents with MMC because of increased body weight, less strict adherence to pressure-relief procedures, and development of adult patterns of sweating around the buttocks (Hinderer et al, 1994).

Strengthening exercises and activities can be incorporated into physical education. A workout can be planned for the student that can be carried out both at home and at a local gym. Endurance activities such as wind sprints in the wheelchair, swimming, and wheelchair track, basketball, and tennis are all appropriate ways to work on muscular and cardiovascular endurance while the student is socializing. If wheelchair sports are available, this is an excellent way to combine strengthening and endurance activities for fun and fitness. Check with your local parks and recreation department for information on wheelchair sports available in your area.

Hygiene

Adult patterns of sweating, incontinence of bowel and bladder, and the onset of menses can all contribute to a potential hygiene problem for an adolescent with MMC. A good bowel and bladder program is essential to avoid incontinence, odor, and skin irritation, which could contribute to low self-esteem. Adolescents are extremely body conscious, and the additional stress of dealing with bowel and bladder dysfunction, along with menstruation for girls, may be particularly burdensome. Scheduled toileting and bathing, and meticulous self-care, including being able to wipe properly and to handle pads and tampons, can provide adequate maintenance of personal hygiene.

Socialization

Adolescents are particularly conscious about their body image, so they may be motivated to maintain a normal weight and to provide extra attention to their bowel and bladder programs. Sexuality is also a big concern for adolescents. Functional limitations are discussed in Chapter 7. Abstinence, safe sex, use of birth control to prevent pregnancy, and knowledge of the dangers of sexually transmitted diseases must all be topics of discussion with the teenager with MMC. This is no different than for the teenager without MMC. The clinician must always provide information that is as accurate as possible to a young adult.

Social isolation can have a negative effect on emotional and social development in this population (Baker and Rogosky-Grassi, 1993). Socialization requires access to all social situations at school and in the community. Peer interaction during adolescence can be limited by the same things identified as potential limitations on interaction early in life, as listed in Table 9–10. Additional challenges to the adolescent with MMC can occur if issues of adolescence such as personal identity, sexuality and peer relations, and concern for loss of biped ambulation are not resolved. Adult development is hindered by having to work through these issues during early adulthood (Friedrich and Shaffer, 1986; Shaffer and Friedrich, 1986).

Independent Living

Basic ADLs (BADLs) are those activities required for personal care such as ambulating, feeding, bathing, dressing, grooming, maintaining continence, and toileting (Cech and Martin, 1995). Instrumental ADLs (IADLs) are those skills that require using some equipment such as the stove, washing machine, or vacuum cleaner, and they relate to managing within the home and community. Being able to shop for food or clothes and being able to prepare a meal are examples of IADLs. Mastery of both BADL and IADL skills is needed to be able to live on one's own. Functional limitations that may affect both BADLs and IADLs may become apparent when the person with MMC has difficulty in lifting and carrying objects. Vocational counseling and planning should begin during high school or even possibly in middle school. The student should be encouraged to live on her own if possible after high school as part of a college experience or during vocational training.

"Launching" of a young adult with MMC has been reported in the literature. Launching is the last transition in the family life cycle whereby "the late adolescent is launched into the outside world to begin to develop an autonomous life" (Friedrich and Shaffer, 1986). Challenges during this time include discussion regarding guardianship if ongoing care is needed, placement plans, and a redefinition of the roles of the parents and the young adult with MMC. Employment of only 25% of adults with MMC was reported by Hunt (1990), and few persons described in this report were married or had children. Each period of the life span brings different challenges for the family with a child with MMC. Table 9–11 is a review of the responsibilities and challenges in the care of a child with MMC across the life span.

Table 9–11 ▌ RESPONSIBILITIES AND CHALLENGES IN THE CARE OF A CHILD WITH MYELOMENINGOCELE OVER THE LIFE SPAN

INFANCY (BIRTH TO 2 YEARS)

Initial crisis: grieving; intensive medical services including surgery; hospitalizations that may interfere with bonding process
Subsequent crisis: procurement of therapy services; delay in locomotion and bowel or bladder training

PRESCHOOL (3–5 YEARS)

Ongoing medical monitoring; prolonged dependency of the child requiring additional physical care
Recurrent hospitalizations for CSF shunt revisions and orthopedic procedures

SCHOOL AGE (6–12 YEARS)

School programming; ongoing appraisal of the child's development
Establishment of family roles: dealing with discrepancies in sibling's abilities; parental tasks
Potential for limited peer involvement
Recurrent hospitalizations for CSF shunt revisions and orthopedic procedures

ADOLESCENCE (13–20 YEARS)

Accepting "permanence" of disability
Personal identity
Child's increased size affecting care
More need for adaptive equipment
Issues of sexuality and peer relations
Issues concerning potential loss of biped ambulatory skills
Recurrent hospitalizations for CSF shunt revision and orthopedic procedures

LAUNCHING (21 YEARS AND BEYOND)

Discussion of guardianship issues relating to ongoing care of the young adult
Placement plans for the young adult
Parents redefine roles regarding young adult and themselves

CSF, cerebrospinal fluid.
From Friedrich W, Shaffer J. Family adjustments and contributions. In Shurtleff DB. Myelodysplasias and Exstrophies: Significance, Prevention, and Treatment. Orlando, FL, Grune & Stratton, 1986, pp 399–410.

CHAPTER SUMMARY

The management of the person with MMC is complex and requires multiple levels of intervention and constant monitoring. Early on, intensive periods of intervention are needed to establish the best outcome and to provide the infant and child with MMC the best developmental start possible. Physical therapy intervention focuses primarily on the attainment of motor milestones of head and trunk control within the boundaries of the neurologic insult. Furthermore, the achievement of independent ambulation is expected of most people with MMC during their childhood years. Fostering cognitive and social-emotional maturity should occur simultaneously. The physical therapist monitors the student's motor progress throughout the school years and intervenes during transitions to a new setting. Each new setting may demand increased or different functional skills. Monitoring the student in school also includes looking for any evidence of deterioration of neurologic or musculoskeletal status that may prevent optimum function in school or access to the community. Examples of appropriate intervention times are occasions when the student needs assistance in making the transition to another level of function, such as using a wheelchair for primary mobility, and evaluating a work site for wheelchair access. The physical therapist assistant may provide therapy to the individual with MMC that is aimed at fostering functional motor abilities or teaching functional skills related to use of orthoses or assistive devices, transfers, and ADLs. The physical therapist assistant can provide valuable data to the therapist during annual evaluations as well as ongoing information regarding function to manage the needs of the person with MMC from birth through adulthood most efficiently.

REVIEW QUESTIONS

1. What type of paralysis can be expected in a child with MMC?
2. What complications are seen in a child with MMC that may be related to skeletal growth?
3. What are the signs of shunt malfunction in a child with MMC?
4. What position is important to use in preventing the development of hip and knee flexion contractures in a child with MMC?
5. What precautions should be taken by parents to protect skin integrity in a child with MMC?
6. What determines the type of orthosis used by a child with MMC?
7. What is the relationship of motor level to level of ambulation in a child with MMC?
8. When is the functional level of mobility determined for an individual with MMC?
9. What developmental changes may contribute to a loss of mobility in the adolescent with MMC?
10. When is the most important time to intervene therapeutically with an individual with MMC?

REHABILITATION UNIT INITIAL EVALUATION: PAUL

Chart Review Paul is a talkative, good-natured, 3-year-old boy. He is in the care of his grandmother during the day because both parents work. He is the younger of two children. Paul presents with a low lumbar (L2) MMC with flaccid paralysis. Medical history includes premature birth at 32 weeks' gestation, bilateral hip dislocation, bilateral clubfeet (surgically repaired at 1 year of age), scoliosis, multiple hemivertebrae, and shunted (ventriculoperitoneal) hydrocephalus (at birth).

SUBJECTIVE

Mother reports that Paul's previous physical therapy consisted of passive and active range of motion for the lower extremities and learning to walk with a walker and braces. She expresses concern about his continued mobility now that he is going to preschool.

OBJECTIVE

Physical Therapy Examination
Peabody Developmental Motor Scales (PDMS) Developmental Motor Quotient (DMQ) = 69.
Age equivalent of 12 months. Fine motor development is average for his age (PDMS DMQ = 90).

Muscle Tone: No abnormal tone is noted in the upper extremities; tone is decreased in the trunk, flaccid in the lower extremities.

Deep Tendon Reflexes: Patellar 1+, Achilles 0 bilaterally.

Range of Motion: WFL in the upper and lower extremities. AROM limitations present in the lower extremities secondary to neuromuscular problems.

Strength: As tested per standard manual muscle testing procedures.

	R	L
Hips		
Iliopsoas	3+	3+
Gluteus maximus	0	0
Adductors	3	3
Abductors	0	0
Knee		
Quadriceps	2	2
Hamstrings	0	0
Ankles and feet	0	0

Sensation: Pinprick intact to L2, absent below.

Skin: Intact, no areas of redness.

Continued on following page

REHABILITATION UNIT INITIAL EVALUATION: PAUL *Continued*

OBJECTIVE *Continued*

Posture and Balance: Paul sits independently and stands with a walker and bilateral HKAFOs. He exhibits a mild R thoracic–L lumbar scoliosis. Head and trunk righting present in sitting, upper extremity protective extension present in all directions. Paul exhibits minimal trunk rotation when balance disturbed laterally in sitting.

Mobility: Paul can demonstrate a reciprocal gait pattern for approximately 10 feet when he ambulates with a walker and HKAFOs but prefers a swing-to pattern. Using a swing-to pattern, he can ambulate 25 feet before wanting to rest. He creeps reciprocally but prefers to drag crawl. Paul can creep up stairs with assistance and comes down head first on his stomach.

Movement Transitions: Paul moves into and out of sitting and to and from standing independently. He is unable to transfer into and out of the tub independently.

Self-care: Paul assists with dressing and undressing and is independent in his sitting balance while performing bathing and dressing activities. He feeds himself but is dependent in bowel and bladder care.

ASSESSMENT

Paul is a 3-year-old boy with L2 MMC who is currently ambulatory with a walker and HKAFOs. He is making the transition to a preschool program and has excellent rehabilitation potential to achieve the following goals within the school year.

Problem List
1. Dependent in ambulation with Lofstrand crutches
2. Decreased strength and endurance
3. Dependent in self-care and transfers
4. Lacking knowledge of pressure relief

Short-Term Goals (actions to be accomplished by midyear review)
1. Paul will propel a prone scooter up and down the hall for 5 consecutive minutes.
2. Paul will perform 20 consecutive chinups during recess.
3. Paul will be able to kick a soccer ball 5 to 10 feet 80% of the time.
4. Paul will use a reciprocal gait pattern to ambulate with a walker 100% of the time.
5. Paul will independently brush his teeth twice daily while standing at the sink.

Long-Term Goals (end of the first year in preschool)
1. Paul will ambulate to and from the bus using Lofstrand crutches.
2. Paul will increase strength in the innervated lower extremity muscles to 4+.
3. Paul will dress and undress himself independently within 5 minutes.
4. Paul will transfer to and from a tub bench with standby assist.

PLAN

1. Mat activities that incorporate prone pushups, wheelbarrow walking, movement transitions from prone to long sitting and back to prone, and sitting pushups with pushup blocks.
2. Using a movable surface such as a ball, promote lateral equilibrium reactions to encourage active trunk rotation.
3. Resistive exercises for upper and lower extremities using latex-free Theraband or cuff weights.
4. Resisted creeping to improve lower extremity reciprocation and trunk control.
5. Increased distances walked using a reciprocal gait pattern by 5 feet every 2 weeks first with walker.
6. Increased standing time and ability to shift weight while using Lofstrand crutches.
7. Family instruction and home exercise program.

REHABILITATION UNIT INITIAL EVALUATION: PAUL *Continued*

QUESTIONS TO THINK ABOUT

- What additional interventions could be used to accomplish these goals?
- Which activities should be part of the home exercise program?

- How can fitness be incorporated into Paul's physical therapy program?
- Identify interventions that may be needed as Paul makes the transition to school.

REFERENCES

Baker SB, Rogosky-Grassi MA. Access to the school. In Rowley-Kelly FL, Reigel DH (eds). Teaching the Student with Spina Bifida. Baltimore, Paul H Brookes, 1993, pp 31–70.

Banta J. The tethered cord in myelomeningocele: should it be untethered? Dev Med Child Neurol 133:167–176, 1991.

Byrd SE, Darling CF, McLone DG, et al. Developmental disorders of the pediatric spine. Radiol Clin North Am 29:711–752, 1991.

Cech D, Martin S. Functional Movement Across the Life Span. Philadelphia, WB Saunders, 1995.

Chauvel PJ, Kinsman SL. Spina bifida and hydrocephalus. In Capute AJ, Accardo PJ (eds). Developmental Disabilities in Infancy and Childhood, vol II: The Spectrum of Developmental Disabilities, 2nd ed. Baltimore, Paul H Brookes, 1996, pp 179–187.

CIBA. CIBA Symposium No. 191: Neural Tube Defects. London, CIBA Foundation, 1994.

Daly LE, Kirke PN, Molloy A, et al. Folate levels and neural tube defects: implications for prevention. JAMA 274:1698–1702, 1995.

Dormans JP, Templeton J, Schreiner MS, et al. Intraoperative latex anaphylaxis in children: early detection, treatment, and prevention. Contemp Orthop 30:342–347, 1995.

Fay G, Shurtleff DB, Shurtleff H, Wolf L. Approaches to facilitate independent self-care and academic success. In Shurtleff DB (ed). Myelodysplasias and Exstrophies: Significance, Prevention, and Treatment. Orlando, FL, Grune & Stratton, 1986, pp 373–398.

Friedrich W, Shaffer J. Family adjustments and contributions. In Shurtleff DB (ed). Myelodysplasias and Exstrophies: Significance, Prevention, and Treatment. Orlando, FL, Grune & Stratton, pp 399–410, 1986.

Garber JB. Myelodysplasia. In Campbell SK (ed). Pediatric Neurologic Physical Therapy, 2nd ed. New York, Churchill Livingstone, 1991, pp 169–212.

Goodman CC, Miedaner J. Genetic and developmenal disorders. In Goodman CC, Boissonnault WG (eds). Pathology: Implications for the Physical Therapist. Philadelphia, WB Saunders, 1998, pp 577–616.

Grief L, Stalmasek V. Tethered cord syndrome: a pediatric case study. J Neurosc Nurs 21:86–91, 1989.

Hinderer SR, Hinderer KA. Sensory examination of individuals with myelodysplasia (abstract). Arch Phys Med Rehabil 71:769–770, 1990.

Hinderer KA, Hinderer SR, Shurtleff DB. Myelodysplasia. In Campbell SK, Palisano RJ, Vander Linden DW (eds). Physical Therapy for Children. Philadelphia, WB Saunders, 1994, pp 571–619.

Hinderer SR, Hinderer KA, Dunne K, et al. Medical and functional status of adults with spina bifida (abstract). Dev Med Child Neurol 30 (suppl 57):28, 1988.

Hobbins JC. Diagnosis and management of neural-tube defects today. N Engl J Med 324:690–691, 1991.

Hoffer MM, Feiwell E, Perry R, et al. Functional ambulation in patients with myelomeningocele. J Bone Joint Surg Am 55:137–148, 1973.

Hunt GM. Open spina bifida: outcome for a complete cohort treated unselectively and followed into adulthood. Dev Med Child Neurol 32:108–118, 1990.

Knutson LM, Clark DE. Orthotic devices for ambulation in children with cerebral palsy and myelomeningocele. Phys Ther 71:947–960, 1991.

Lock TR, Aronson DD. Fractures in patients who have myelomeningocele. J Bone Joint Surg Am 71:1153–1157, 1989.

Long T, Cintas H. Handbook of Pediatric Physical Therapy. Baltimore, Williams & Wilkins, 1995.

Luthy DA, Wardinsky T, Shurtleff DB, et al. Cesarean section before the onset of labor and subsequent motor function in infants with myelomeningocele diagnosed antenatally. N Engl J Med 324:662–666, 1991.

Main DM, Mennuti MT. Neural tube defects: issues in prenatal diagnosis and counseling. Obstet Gynecol 67:1–16, 1986.

MRC Vitamin Study Research Group. Prevention of neural tube defects: results of Medical Research Council Vitamin Study. Lancet 338:131–137, 1991.

Noetzel MJ. Myelomeningocele: current concepts of management. Clin Perinatol 16:311–329, 1989.

Okamoto GA, Sousa J, Telzrow RW, et al. Toileting skills in children with myelomeningocele: rates of learning. Arch Phys Med Rehabil 65:182–185, 1984.

Pearson ML, Cole JS, Jarvis WR. How common is latex allergy? A survey of children with myelodysplasia. Dev Med Child Neurol 36: 64–69, 1994.

Ratliffe KT. Clinical Pediatric Physical Therapy. St. Louis, CV Mosby, 1998.

Rosenstein BD, Greene WB, Herrington RT, et al. Bone density in myelomeningocele: the effects of ambulatory status and other factors. Dev Med Child Neurol 29:486–494, 1987.

Ryan KD, Ploski C, Emans JB. Myelodysplasia—the musculoskeletal problem: habilation from infancy to adulthood. Phys Ther 71: 935–946, 1991.

Schneider JW, Krosschell K, Gabriel KL. Congenital spinal cord injury. In Umphred DA (ed). Neurological Rehabilitation, 3rd ed. St Louis, CV Mosby, 1995, pp 454–482.

Shaffer J, Friedrich W. Young adult psychosocial adjustment. In Shurtleff DB (ed). Myelodysplasias and Exstrophies: Significance, Prevention, and Treatment. Orlando, FL, Grune & Stratton, 1986, pp 421–430.

Shaffer J, Wolfe L, Friedrich W, et al. Developmental expectations: intelligence and fine motor skills. In Shurtleff DB (ed). Myelodysplasias and Exstrophies: Significance, Prevention, and Treatment. Orlando, FL, Grune & Stratton, 1986, pp 359–372.

Shurtleff DB, Lemire RJ, Warkany J. Embryology, etiology and epidemiology. In Shurtleff DB (ed). Myelodysplasias and Exstrophies: Significance, Prevention, and Treatment. Orlando, FL, Grune & Stratton, 1986, pp 39–64.

Sousa JC, Telzrow RW, Holm RA, et al. Developmental guidelines for children with myelodysplasia. Phys Ther 63:21–29, 1983.

Stanger M. Use of orthoses in pediatrics. In Nawoczenski DA, Epler ME (eds). Orthotics in Functional Rehabilitaton of the Lower Limb. Philadelphia, WB Saunders, 1997, pp 245–272.

Tappit-Emas E. Spina bifida. In Tecklin JS (ed). Pediatric Physical Therapy, 2nd ed. Philadelphia, JB Lippincott, 1994, pp 135–186.

Williamson GG. Children with Spina Bifida: Early Intervention and Preschool Programming. Baltimore, Paul H Brookes, 1987.

Willis KE, Hombeck GN, Dillon K, et al. Intelligence and achievement in children with myelomeningocele. J Pediatr Psychol 15: 161–176, 1990.

Xiao KZ, Zhang ZY, Su YM, et al. Central nervous system congenital malformations, especially neural tube defects in 29 provinces, metropolitan cities and autonomous regions of China: Chinese Birth Defects Monitoring Program. Int J Epidemiol 19:978–982, 1990.

10

Genetic Disorders

INTRODUCTION

More than 6000 genetic disorders have been identified to date. Some are evident at birth, whereas others present later in life. Most genetic disorders have their onset in childhood. The physical therapist assistant working in a children's hospital, outpatient rehabilitation center, or school system may be involved in providing physical therapy for these children. Some of the genetic disorders discussed in this chapter include Down syndrome (DS), fragile X syndrome, Rett syndrome, cystic fibrosis (CF), Duchenne muscular dystrophy (DMD), and osteogenesis imperfecta (OI). After a general discussion of the types of genetic transmission, the pathophysiology and clinical features of these conditions are outlined, followed by a brief discussion of their physical therapy management. A case study of a child with DS is presented at the end of the chapter to illustrate the physical therapy management of children with low muscle tone.

Genetic disorders in children are often thought to involve primarily only one body system—muscular, skeletal, respiratory, or nervous—and to affect other systems secondarily. However, genetic disorders typi-

cally affect more than one body system, especially when those systems are embryonically linked, such as the nervous and integumentary systems, both of which are derived from the same primitive tissue. For example, individuals with neurofibromatosis have skin defects in the form of café-au-lait spots in addition to nervous system tumors. Genetic disorders that primarily affect one system, such as the muscular dystrophies, eventually have an impact on or stress other body systems, such as the cardiac and pulmonary systems. Because the nervous system is most frequently involved in genetic disorders, similar clinical features are displayed by a large number of affected children.

GENETIC TRANSMISSION

Genes carry the blueprint for how body systems are put together, how the body changes during growth and development, and how the body operates on a daily basis. The color of your eyes and hair is genetically determined. One hair color, such as brown, is more dominant than another color, such as blond. A trait that is passed on as *dominant* is expressed, whereas a *recessive* trait may be expressed only under certain circumstances. All cells of the body carry genetic material in chromosomes. The chromosomes in the body cells are called *autosomes*. Because each of us has 22 pairs of *autosomes,* every cell in the body has 44 chromosomes, and 2 *sex chromosomes.* Reproductive cells contain 23 chromosomes—22 autosomes, and either an X or a Y chromosome. After fertilization of the egg by the sperm, the genetic material is combined during *meiosis,* thus determining the sex of the child by the pairing of the sex chromosomes. Two X chromosomes make a female, whereas one X and one Y make a male. Each gene inherited by a child has a paternal and a maternal contribution. Alleles are alternative forms of a gene, such as H or h. If someone carries identical alleles of a gene, HH or hh, the person is homozygous. If the person carries different alleles of a gene, Hh or hH, the person is heterozygous.

CATEGORIES

The two major categories of genetic disorders are *chromosomal abnormalities* and *specific gene defects.* Chromosome abnormalities occur by one of three mechanisms: nondisjunction, deletion, and translocation. When cells divide unequally, the result is called a *nondisjunction.* Nondisjunction can cause DS. When part or all of a chromosome is lost, it is called a *deletion.* When part of one chromosome becomes detached and reattaches to a completely different chromosome, it is called a *translocation.* Chromosome abnormalities include the following: *trisomies,* in which three of a particular chromosome are present instead of the usual two; *sex chromosome abnormalities,* in which there is an absence or addition of one sex chromosome; and *partial deletions.* The most widely recognized trisomy is DS, or trisomy 21. Turner syndrome and Klinefelter syndrome are examples of sex chromosome errors, but they are not discussed in this chapter. Partial deletion syndromes that are discussed include cri-du-chat syndrome and Prader-Willi syndrome (PWS).

A specific gene defect is inherited in three different ways: (1) as an autosomal dominant trait; (2) as an autosomal recessive trait; or (3) as a sex-linked trait. *Autosomal dominant inheritance* requires that one parent be affected by the gene or that a spontaneous mutation of the gene occur. In the latter case, neither parent has the disorder, but the gene spontaneously mutates or changes in the child. When one parent has an autosomal dominant disorder, each child born has a 1 in 2 chance of having the same disorder. Examples of autosomal dominant disorders include OI, which affects the skeletal system and produces brittle bones, and neurofibromatosis, which affects the skin and nervous system.

Autosomal recessive inheritance occurs when either parent is a carrier for the disorder. A *carrier* is a person

who has the gene but in whom it is not expressed. The condition is not apparent in the person. The carrier may pass the gene on without having the disorder or knowing that he or she is a carrier. In this situation, the carrier parent is said to be *heterozygous* for the abnormal gene, and each child has a 1 in 4 chance of being a carrier. The heterozygous parent is carrying a gene with alleles that are dissimilar for a particular trait. If both parents are carriers, each is heterozygous for the abnormal gene, and each child will have a 1 in 4 chance of having the disorder. If both parents are carriers, there is an increased chance that the child will be homozygous for the disorder. *Homozygous* means that the person is carrying a gene with identical alleles for a given trait. Examples of autosomal recessive disorders that are discussed in this chapter are CF, phenylketonuria, and two types of spinal muscular atrophy (SMA), Werdnig-Hoffmann and Kugelberg-Welander.

Sex-linked inheritance means that the abnormal gene is carried on the X chromosome. Just as autosomes can have dominant and recessive expression, so can sex chromosomes. In X-linked recessive inheritance, females with only one abnormal allele are carriers for the disorder, but they usually do not exhibit any symptoms because they have one normal X chromosome. Each child born to a carrier mother has a 1 in 2 chance of becoming a carrier, and each son has a 1 in 2 chance of having the disorder. The most common examples of X-linked recessive disorders are DMD and hemophilia. Fragile X syndrome is an X-linked disorder that causes mental retardation. It accounts for 8% of all cases of mental retardation in males (Bellenir, 1996). The only X-linked dominant disorder identified to date is Rett syndrome, which presents only in females because the gene is lethal in males. An autosomal dominant type of inheritance for Rett syndrome has not been definitively proven, but theoretically, it is the best explanation for the findings seen in this disorder. A discussion of genetically transmitted disorders follows—first chromosome abnormalities and then specific gene defects.

DOWN SYNDROME

DS is the leading chromosomal cause of mental retardation and the most frequently reported birth defect (Morbidity and Mortality Weekly Report, 1994; Naganuma et al, 1995). Increasing maternal and paternal age is a risk factor. DS occurs in 1 in every 800 live births and is caused by a genetic imbalance resulting in the presence of an extra 21st chromosome in all or most of the body's cells. Trisomy of chromosome 21 is present. Ninety-five percent of DS cases result from a failure of chromosome 21 to split completely during formation of the egg or sperm (nondisjunction). A *gamete* is a mature male or female germ cell (sperm or egg). When the abnormal gamete joins a normal one, the result is three copies of chromosome 21. Fewer than 5% of children have a third chromosome 21 attached to another chromosome. This type of DS is caused by a translocation. The least common type of DS is a mosaic type in which some of the body's cells have three copies of chromosome 21 and others have a normal complement of chromosomes. The severity of the syndrome is related to the proportion of normal to abnormal cells.

Clinical Features

Characteristic features of the child with DS include hypotonicity, joint hypermobility, upwardly slanting epicanthal folds, and a flat nasal bridge and facial profile (Fig. 10–1). The child has a small oral cavity that sometimes causes the tongue to seem to protrude. Developmental findings include delayed development and impaired motor control. Feeding problems may be evident at birth and may require intervention. Forty to 66% of children with DS also have congenital heart disease (Harris and Shea, 1991; Marino and Pueschel, 1996), which can usually be corrected by cardiac surgery (Msall et al, 1991). Musculoskeletal manifestations may include pes planus (flatfoot), thoracolumbar scoliosis, and patellar and possibly atlantoaxial instability.

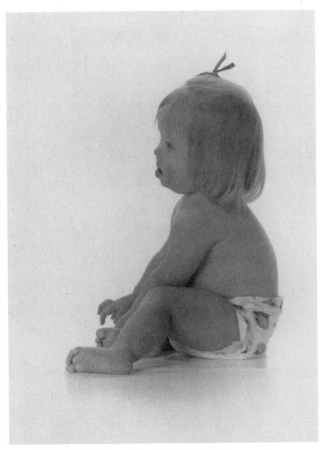

FIGURE 10–1 ▪ Profile of a child with Down syndrome.

The incidence of atlantoaxial instability ranges from 15 to 20% (American Academy of Pediatrics, 1995; Blackston, 1990). Beginning at the age of 2 years, a child's cervical spine can and should be radiographed to determine whether atlantoaxial instability is present. Surgical fusion will be necessary if instability is present. If this condition persists undetected, the child will be at great risk of spinal cord compression, which could result in tetraplegia. Pueschel and associates (1992) reported that only 1% of children with DS become symptomatic, and even those children are unlikely to develop paralysis.

Major sensory systems such as hearing and vision may be impaired in children with DS. Visual impairments may include nearsightedness (myopia), cataracts, crossing of the eyes (esotropia), nystagmus, and astigmatism. Mild to moderate hearing loss is not uncommon. Either a sensorineural loss, in which the eighth cranial nerve is damaged, or a conductive loss, resulting from too much fluid in the middle ear, can result in delayed language development. These problems must be identified early in life and treated aggressively so as to not hinder the child's ability to interact with caregivers and the environment and to develop appropriate language.

Intelligence

As stated earlier, DS is the major cause of mental retardation in children. Intelligence quotients (IQs) within this population range from 25 to 50, with the majority falling in the mildly to moderately retarded range (Ratliffe, 1998). Some intervention programs have appeared to reduce the severity of retardation (Bellenir, 1996).

If effective early intervention programs can be designed and used in the preschool years, the subsequent educational progress of a child with Down syndrome may be altered significantly. An "educable" person is defined as one who is capable of learning such basic skills as reading and arithmetic and is quite capable of self care and independent living (those with mild retardation are generally considered educable). Although trainable (moderately retarded) persons are very limited in educational attainments, they can profit from simple training for self care and vocational tasks (Bellenir, 1996).

Development

Motor development is slow, and without intervention, the rate of acquisition of skills declines. Difficulty in learning motor skills has always been linked to the lack of postural tone and, to some extent, to hypermobile joints. Ligamentous laxity with resulting joint hypermobility is thought to be due to a collagen defect (Shea, 1990). The hypotonia is related not only to structural changes in the cerebellum but also to changes in other central nervous system structures and processes. These changes are indicative of missing or delayed neuromaturation in DS. As a result of the low tone and joint laxity, it is difficult for the child with DS to attain head and trunk control. Weight bearing on the limbs is typically accomplished by locking extremity joints such as the elbows and knees. These children often substitute positional stability for muscular stability, as in W sitting, to provide trunk stability in sitting, rather than dynamically firing trunk muscles in response to weight shifting in a position. Children with DS often avoid activating trunk muscles for rotation and prefer to advance from prone to sitting over widely abducted legs (Fig. 10–2). Table 10–1 compares the age at which motor tasks may be accomplished by children with DS and typically developing children. Infant intervention has been shown to have a positive impact on developing motor skills and overall function in these children (Connolly et al, 1993; Hines and Bennett, 1996).

Whereas in the 1970s, individuals with DS rarely achieved social or economic independence (Scheiner and Abroms, 1980), "today people with Down Syndrome live at home with their families and are active participants in the educational, social, and recreational activities of the community" (Bellenir, 1996). Individuals with DS can live in group communities that foster independence and self-reliance (Blackman, 1983). Some individuals with DS have been employed in small and medium-sized offices as clerical workers or in hotels and restaurants. Batshaw (1997) credits the introduction of supported employment in the 1980s with providing the potential for adults with DS to obtain and to hold a job. In supported employment, the individual has a job coach. Crucial to the individual's job success is the early development and maintenance of a positive self-image and a healthy self-esteem, along with the ability to work apart from the family and to participate in personal recreational activities.

Fitness is decreased in individuals with DS. Dichter and colleagues (1993) found that a group of children with DS had reduced pulmonary function and fitness compared with age-matched controls without disabilities. Other researchers have found children with DS to be less active, and 25% of them become overweight (Pueschel, 1990; Sharav and Bowman, 1992). Lack of cardiorespiratory endurance and weak abdominal muscles have been linked to the reductions in fitness. Because of increased potential longevity, fitness in every person with a disability needs to be explored as another potential area of physical therapy intervention.

Life expectancy for individuals with DS has increased (Carr, 1995); 80% reach the age of 55 years (Bellenir, 1996). The increase has occurred despite the higher incidence of other serious diseases in this population. Of the 40 to 66% of children with DS who are born with congenital heart disease, 76% survive. This percentage drops to 50% by age 30 (Baird and Sadovnick, 1987). Most heart defects can be corrected

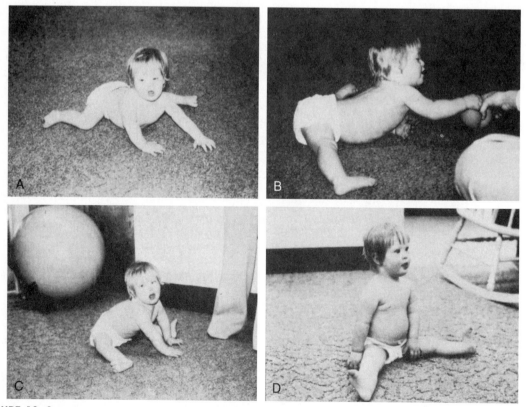

FIGURE 10–2 ■ *A to D,* Common abnormal prone-to-sitting maneuver pattern noted in children with Down syndrome. (Reprinted from Lydic JS, Steele C. Assessment of the quality of sitting and gait patterns in children with Down's syndrome. Phys Ther 59:1489–1494, 1979, with permission of the APTA.)

Table 10-1 ‖ ATTAINMENT OF DEVELOPMENTAL MILESTONES IN DOWN SYNDROME

DEVELOPMENTAL TASK	AGE AT ATTAINMENT IN DOWN SYNDROME	TYPICAL AGE AT ATTAINMENT
Rolls from supine to prone	7 months	6 months
Prone on elbows	7 months	6 months
Sits with back erect	11 months	8 months
Pivots in prone on stomach	12 months	6 months
Creeps on hands and knees	15 months	10 months
Pulls to stand	18 months	9 months
Cruises around furniture	21 months	9 months
Walks with assistance	30 months	12 months
Throws a ball	30 months	24 months
Kicks a ball after demonstration	36 months	24 months
Squats during play	36 months	22 months
Walks down stairs, one hand held	36 months	22 months
Jumps off floor, both feet	48 months	30 months
Walks up stairs, alternating feet	54 months	30 months

Data from Share J, French R. Motor Development of Children with Down Syndrome: Birth to Six Years. Kearney, NE, Educational Systems Association, 1993; Cech D, Martin S. Functional Movement Development Across the Life Span. Philadelphia, WB Saunders, 1995; Long TM, Cintas H. Handbook of Pediatric Physical Therapy. Baltimore, Williams & Wilkins, 1995.

with surgery. Children with DS have a 15 to 20% higher chance of acquiring leukemia during their first 3 years of life. Again, the cure rate is high. The last major health risk faced by these individuals is Alzheimer's disease. Every person with DS who lives past 30 years develops pathologic signs of Alzheimer's disease such as amyloid plaques and tangles, but not all of these persons develop the dementia that is usually part of this condition (Zigman et al, 1996). However, adults with DS who are more than 50 years old are more prone to regression in adaptive behavior than are adults with mental retardation without DS (Zigman et al, 1996).

Child's Impairments and Interventions

The physical therapist's evaluation of the child with DS typically identifies the following impairments to be addressed by physical therapy intervention:

1. Delayed psychomotor development
2. Hypotonia
3. Hyperextensible joints and ligamentous laxity
4. Impaired respiratory function
5. Impaired exercise tolerance

Early physical therapy is important for the child with DS. A case study of a child with DS is presented at the end of the chapter to illustrate general intervention strategies with a child with low muscle tone, because the impairments demonstrated by these children are similar. These interventions could be used with any child who displays low muscle tone or muscle weakness secondary to genetic disorders such as cri-du-chat syndrome, PWS, and SMA.

CRI-DU-CHAT SYNDROME

When part of the short arm of chromosome 5 is deleted, the result is the cat-cry syndrome, or cri-du-chat syndrome. The chromosome abnormality primarily affects the nervous system and results in mental retardation. The incidence is 1 in 50,000 live births according to the latest statistics, an incidence that makes it relatively rare, although 1% of institutionalized individuals with mental retardation may have this disorder (Carlin, 1995; Goodman and Gorlin, 1983). Characteristic clinical features include a catlike cry, microcephaly, widely spaced eyes, and profound mental retardation. The cry is usually present only in infancy and is the result of laryngeal malformation, which is lessened with growth. Although usually born at term, these children exhibit the result of intrauterine growth retardation by being small for their gestational age. *Microcephaly* is diagnosed when the head circumference is less than the third percentile. Together, these features constitute the cri-du-chat syndrome, but any or all of the signs can be noted in many other congenital genetic disorders.

Child's Impairments and Interventions

The physical therapist's evaluation of the child with cri-du-chat syndrome typically identifies the following impairments or potential problems to be addressed by physical therapy intervention:

1. Delayed psychomotor development
2. Hypotonia
3. Delayed development of postural reactions
4. Hyperextensible joints

5. Contractures and skeletal deformities
6. Impaired respiratory function

Musculoskeletal problems that may be associated with cri-du-chat syndrome include clubfeet, hip dislocation, joint hypermobility, and scoliosis. Muscle tone is low, a feature that may predispose the child to problems related to musculoskeletal alignment. In addition, motor delays also result from a lack of the cognitive ability needed to learn motor skills. Postural control is difficult to develop because of the low tone and nervous system immaturity. Physically, the child's movements are laborious and inconsistent. Gravity is a true enemy to the child with low tone. Congenital heart disease is also common, and severe respiratory problems can be present (McEwen, 1994; Naganuma et al, 1995).

PRADER-WILLI SYNDROME

Prader-Willi syndrome is the other example of a syndrome caused by a partial deletion of a chromosome, in this case, chromosome 15. The incidence of this syndrome originally described by Prader, Lablart, and Willi in 1956 is thought to be about 1 in 10,000 to 1 in 20,000 (Seashore and Wappner, 1996). The disorder is more common than cri-du-chat syndrome. Diagnosis is usually made based on the child's behavior and physical features rather than by genetic testing. Features include obesity, underdeveloped gonads, short stature, hypotonia, and mild to moderate mental retardation. These children become obsessed with food at around the age of 2 years, but before this age they have difficulty in feeding secondary to low muscle tone and they gain weight slowly. Obesity can lead to respiratory compromise with impaired breathing and cyanosis.

Child's Impairments and Interventions

The physical therapist's evaluation of the child with PWS typically identifies the following impairments or potential problems to be addressed by physical therapy intervention:

1. Impaired feeding (before age 2)
2. Hypotonia
3. Delayed psychomotor development
4. Obesity (after age 2)
5. Impaired respiratory function

Intervention must match the needs of the child based on age. The infant may need oromotor therapy to improve the ability to feed. Positioning for support and alignment is necessary for feeding and carrying. Techniques for fostering head and trunk control should be taught to the caregivers. As the child's appetite increases, weight control becomes crucial. The physical therapist assistant works to establish and to improve gross-motor abilities in the child with PWS as part of a preschool program. Food control must be understood by everyone working with the child with this condition. Attention in the school years is focused on training good eating habits while improving tolerance for aerobic activity. This is continued throughout adolescence, when behavioral control appears to the most successful means for controlling weight gain.

ARTHROGRYPOSIS MULTIPLEX CONGENITA

One type of arthrogryposis multiplex congenita (AMC) is inherited as an autosomal dominant trait. Only a small percentage of cases have been shown to have a chromosomal etiology. Although AMC is not a primary genetic disorder, it is a nonprogressive neuromuscular syndrome that the physical therapist assistant may encounter in practice. AMC results in multiple joint contractures and usually requires surgical intervention to correct misaligned joints. AMC is also known as multiple congenital contractures (Long and Cintas, 1995). The incidence of the disorder is 1 to 3 per 10,000 live births (Buyse, 1990). Multiple causes have been identified, and its pathogenesis has been related to the muscular, nervous, or joint abnormalities associated with intrauterine movement restriction.

Pathophysiology and Natural History

In 1990, Tachdjian postulated that the basic mechanism for the multiple joint contractures seen in AMC is a lack of fetal movement. Myopathic and neuropathic causes have been linked to multiple nonprogressive joint contractures. If muscles around a fetal joint do not provide enough stimulation (muscle pull), the result is joint stiffness. If the anterior horn cell does not function properly, muscle movement is lessened and contractures and soft tissue fibrosis occur. Muscle imbalances in utero can lead to abnormal joint positions. The first trimester of pregnancy has been identified as the most likely time for the primary insult to occur to produce AMC. Although the contractures themselves are not progressive, the extent of functional disability they produce is significant, as seen in Figure 10–3. Limitation in mobility and in activities of daily living (ADLs) can make the child dependent on family members.

Child's Impairments and Interventions

The physical therapist's evaluation of the child with AMC typically identifies the following impairments to be addressed by physical therapy intervention:

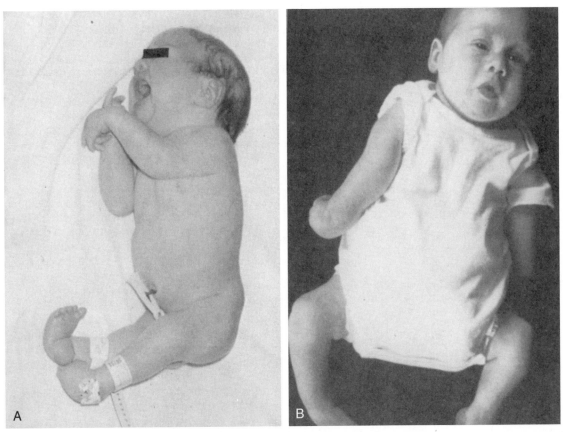

FIGURE 10-3 ■ *A*, An infant with arthrogryposis multiplex congenita (AMC) with flexed and dislocated hips, extended knees, clubfeet (equinovarus), internally rotated shoulders, flexed elbows, and flexed and ulnarly deviated wrists. *B*, An infant with AMC with abducted and externally rotated hips, flexed knees, clubfeet, internally rotated shoulders, extended elbows, and flexed and ulnarly deviated wrists. (From Donohoe M, Bleakney DA. Arthrogryposis multiplex congenita. In Campbell SK [ed]. Physical Therapy for Children, 2nd ed. Philadelphia, WB Saunders, 2000.)

1. Impaired range of motion
2. Impaired functional mobility
3. Limitations in ADLs, including donning and doffing orthoses

Early physical therapy intervention focuses on assisting the infant to attain head and trunk control. Depending on the extent of limb involvement, the child may have difficulty in using the arms for support when initially learning to sit or catch herself if she loses her balance. Most of these children become ambulatory, but they may need some assistance in finding ways to go up and down stairs. An adapted tricycle can provide an alternative means of mobility before walking is mastered (Fig. 10–4). Functional movement and maintenance of range of motion are the two major physical therapy goals for a child with this physical disability. No cognitive deficit is present; therefore, the child with AMC should be able to attend regular preschool and school. Table 10–2 gives an overview of the management of the child with AMC across the life span.

Range of Motion

Range-of-motion exercises and stretching exercises are the cornerstone of physical therapy intervention in children with AMC. Initially, stretching needs to be performed three to five times a day. Each affected joint should be moved three to five times and held for 20 to 30 seconds at the end of the available range.

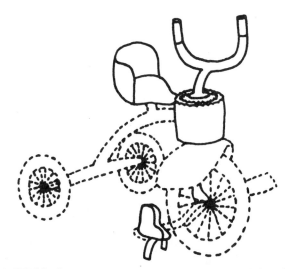

FIGURE 10-4 ■ Adapted tricycle. (Reprinted by permission of the publisher from Connor FP, Williamson GG, Siepp JM [eds]. Program Guide for Infants and Toddlers with Neuromotor and Other Developmental Disabilities [New York, Teachers College Press, © 1978 by Teachers College, Columbia University. All rights reserved.], p. 361.)

Table 10–2 ▌ MANAGEMENT OF
ARTHROGRYPOSIS MULTIPLEX CONGENITA,
OR MULTIPLE CONGENITAL CONTRACTURES

TIME PERIOD	GOALS	STRATEGIES	MEDICAL/SURGICAL	HOME PROGRAM

Infancy	Maximize strength
	Increase ROM
	Enhance sensory and
	  motor development
		Teach rolling
		Floor scooting
		Strengthening
		Stretching
		Positioning
			Clubfoot surgery by
			  age 2 years
			Splints adjusted every
			  4–6 weeks
				Stretching 3–5 times a
				  day
				Standing 2 hours a day
				Positioning

Preschool	Decrease disability
	Enhance ambulation
	Maximize ADLs
	Establish peer relation-
	  ships
		Solve ADL challenges
		Gait training
		Stretching, positioning
		Promote self-esteem
			Stroller for community
			Articulating AFOs
			Splints
				Stretching twice a day
				Positioning
				Playgroups, sleepovers,
				  sports

School age and
  adolescence
	Strengthen peer rela-
	  tionships
	Independent mobility
	Preserve ROM
		Adaptive physical edu-
		  cation
		Environmental adapta-
		  tions, stretching
		Compensatory for
		  ADLs
			Manual wheelchair for
			  community
			Power mobility
			Surgery
				Sports, social activities
				Self-directed stretching
				  and prone posi-
				  tioning
				Personal hygiene

Adulthood	Independent in ADLs
	  with/without assistive
	  devices
	Ambulation/mobility
	Driving
		Joint protection and
		  conservation
		Assess accessibility
		Assistive technology
			Wheelchair	Flexibility
				Positioning
				Endurance

ADLs, activities of daily living; AFOs, ankle-foot orthoses; ROM, range of motion.
From Donohoe M, Bleakney DA. Arthrogryposis multiplex congenita. In Campbell SK (ed). Physical Therapy for Children. Philadelphia, WB Saunders, 1994, pp 261–277.

Because these children have multiple joint involvement, range of motion requires a serious commitment on the part of the family. Incorporating stretching into the daily routine of feeding, bathing, dressing, and diaper changing is warranted. As the child grows older, the frequency of stretching can be decreased. The school-age child should begin to take over responsibility for her own stretching. Although stretching is less important once skeletal growth has ceased, flexibility remains a goal to prevent further deformities from developing. Joint preservation and energy conservation techniques are legitimate strategies for the adult with AMC.

Positioning

Positioning options depend on the type of contractures present. If the joints are more extended in the upper extremity, this will hamper the child's acceptance of the prone position and will require that the chest be supported by a roll or wedge. Too much flexion and abduction in the lower extremities may need to be controlled by lateral towel rolls or a Velcro strap (Fig. 10–5). Quadruped is not a good posture to use because it reinforces flexion in the upper and lower extremities. Prone positioning is an excellent way to stretch hip flexion contractures while encouraging the development of the motor abilities of the prone progression. A prone positioning program should be continued throughout the life span.

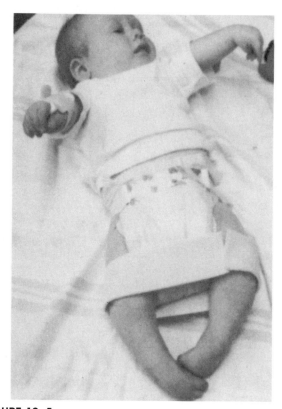

FIGURE 10–5 ■ This child with arthrogryposis multiplex congenita is wearing a wide Velcro band strapped around the thighs to keep the legs in more neutral alignment. (From Donohoe M, Bleakney DA. Arthrogryposis multiplex congenita. In Campbell SK [ed]. Physical Therapy for Children, 2nd ed. Philadelphia, WB Saunders, 2000.)

Functional Activities and Gait

Rolling and scooting on the bottom are used as primary means of floor mobility. Development of independent sitting is often delayed because of the child's inability to attain the position, but most of these children do so by 15 months of age. Placement in sitting and encouragement of static sitting balance with or without hand support should begin early, at around 6 months of age. Focus on dynamic balance and transitions into and out of sitting while using trunk flexion and rotation should follow. Nine months is an appropriate age for the child to begin experiencing weight bearing in standing. For children with plantar flexion contractures, shoes can be wedged to allow total contact of the foot with the support surface. In some cases, a standing frame or parapodium, as is used with children with myelomeningocele, can be beneficial (Fig. 10–6). Other children benefit from use of supine or prone standers. The standing goal for a 1-year-old child is 2 hours a day (Donohoe and Bleakney, 1994). Strengthening of muscles needed for key functional motor skills, such as rolling, sitting, hitching (bottom scooting), standing, and walking, is done in play. Reaching to roll, rotation in sitting and standing, and movement transitions into and out of postures can facilitate carryover into functional tasks. Toys should be adapted with switches to facilitate the child's ability to play, and adaptive equipment should be used to lessen dependence during ADLs.

Ambulation is achieved by most children with AMC by 18 months of age (Donohoe and Bleakney, 1994). Because clubfoot is often a part of the presentation in AMC, its presence must be dealt with in the development of standing and walking. Early surgical correction of the deformity has required later revisions, so investigators have suggested that surgery occur after the child is stronger and wants to walk, at around the end of the first year of life. The operation should be performed by the time the child is 2 years old, to avoid the possibility of having to do more bony surgery, as opposed to soft tissue corrections.

Use of orthoses for ambulation depends on the strength of the lower extremity extensors and the types of contractures found at the hip, knee, and ankle. Less than fair muscle strength at a joint usually indicates the need for an orthosis at that joint. For example, if the quadriceps muscles are scored less than 3/5 on manual muscle testing, then a knee-ankle-foot orthosis (KAFO) is indicated. Children with knee extension contractures tend to require less orthotic control than those with knee flexion contractures (Donohoe and Bleakney, 1994). Children with weak quadriceps or knee flexion contractures may need to walk with the knees of the KAFO locked. Functional ambulation also depends on the child's ability to use an assistive device. Because of upper extremity contractures, this may not be possible, and adaptations to walkers and crutches may be needed. Polyvinyl chloride pipe can often be used to fabricate lightweight walkers or crutches, to give the child maximal independence (Fig. 10–7). Power mobility may provide easy and efficient environmental access for a child with weak lower extremities and poor upper extremity function. Some school-age children or adolescents routinely use a manual wheelchair to keep up with peers in a community setting.

OSTEOGENESIS IMPERFECTA

Osteogenesis imperfecta is an autosomal dominant disorder of collagen synthesis that affects bone metabolism. The four types are listed in Table 10–3. Three of the four types are inherited as an autosomal dominant trait, which occurs in 1 per 20,000 to 1 per 30,000 live births. Each type has a different degree of severity. Depending on the type of OI, the infant may be born with multiple fractures or may not experience any broken bones until reaching preschool age. The more fragile the skeletal system, the less likely it is that

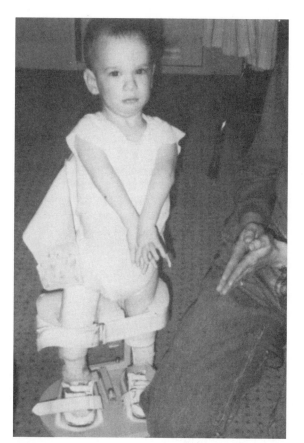

FIGURE 10–6 ∎ A child with arthrogryposis multiplex congenita who is using a standing frame. (From Donohoe M, Bleakney DA. Arthrogryposis multiplex congenita. In Campbell SK [ed]. Physical Therapy for Children, 2nd ed. Philadelphia, WB Saunders, 2000.)

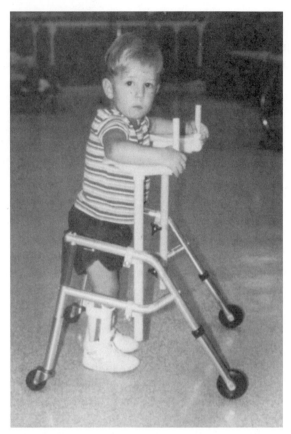

FIGURE 10-7 ■ Thermoplastic forearm supports can be customized to the walker for the child with arthrogryposis multiplex congenita. (From Donohoe M, Bleakney DA. Arthrogryposis multiplex congenita. In Campbell SK [ed]. Physical Therapy for Children, 2nd ed. Philadelphia, WB Saunders, 2000.)

a physical therapist assistant will be involved in the child's therapy. It would be more likely for an assistant to treat children with types I and IV because these are the most common. Individuals with OI have "brittle bones." Many also exhibit short stature, bowing of long bones, ligamentous joint laxity, and kyphoscoliosis. Average or above-average intelligence is typical.

Child's Impairments and Interventions

The physical therapist's evaluation of the child with OI typically identifies the following impairments to be addressed by physical therapy intervention:

1. Impaired range of motion
2. Impaired strength
3. Pathologic fractures
4. Delayed motor development
5. Impaired functional mobility
6. Limitations in ADLs
7. Impaired respiratory function
8. Scoliosis

Children with milder forms of OI are seen for strengthening and endurance training in a preschool

TYPE	CHARACTERISTICS	SEVERITY
I	AD, mild to moderate fragility	Mildest
II	AD, in utero fractures	Most severe, lethal
III	AR, progressive	Intermediate
IV	AD, moderate fragility	More severe than type I

Table 10-3 ▌ CLASSIFICATION OF OSTEOGENESIS IMPERFECTA

AD, autosomal dominant; AR, autosomal recessive.

Data from Naganuma GM, Harris SR, Tada WL. Genetic disorders. In Umphred DA (ed). Neurologic Physical Therapy. St. Louis, CV Mosby, 1995, pp 287–293.

or school setting. Every situation must be viewed as being potentially hazardous for the child with OI. Safety always comes first when dealing with a potential hazard; therefore, orthoses can be used to protect joints, and playground equipment can be padded. No extra force should be used in donning and doffing orthoses. Signs of redness, swelling, or warmth may indicate more than excessive pressure and could indicate a fracture.

Caution. Fracture risk is greatest during bathing, dressing, and carrying. Baby walkers and jumper seats should be avoided. All trunk or extremity rotations should be active, not passive.

Social interaction may need to be structured if the child with OI is unable to participate in many, if any, sports-related activities. Being the manager of the softball or soccer team may be as close as the child with OI can be to participating in sports. Table 10–4 provides an overview of the management of a child with OI across the life span.

Handling and Positioning

Parents of an infant with OI must be taught to protect the child while they carry her on a pillow or in a custom-molded carrier. Handling and positioning are illustrated in Intervention 10–1. All hard surfaces must be padded. Protective positioning must be balanced with permitting the infant's active movement. Sandbags, towel rolls, and other objects may be used. Greatest care is needed when dressing, diapering, and feeding the child. When handling the child, caregivers should avoid grasping her around the ankles, around the ribs, or under the arms because this may increase the risk of fractures. Clothing should be roomy enough to be easily fitted over the child's head. Temperature regulation is often impaired, so light, absorbent clothing is a good idea. A plastic or spongy basin is best for bathing. Despite all precautions, infants may still experience fractures. The physical therapist assistant will most likely not be involved in the initial stages of physical therapy care for the infant with OI because of the patient's fragility but if involved later

Table 10–4 ▌ **THERAPEUTIC MANAGEMENT OF OSTEOGENESIS IMPERFECTA**

TIME PERIOD	GOALS	THERAPEUTIC INTERVENTIONS
Infancy	Safe handling and positioning Development of age-appropriate skills	Even distribution of body weight Padded carrier Prone, side lying, supine, sitting positions Pull-to-sit transfer contraindicated
Preschool	Protected weight bearing Safe independent self-mobility	Use of contour-molded orthoses for compression and support in standing Adaptive devices Light weights, pool therapy
School age and adolescence	Maximizing independence Maximizing endurance Maximizing strength Peer relationships	Mobility cart, HKAFOs, clamshell braces, air splints Ambulation without orthoses as fracture rate declines Wheelchair for community ambulation Adaptive physical education Boy Scouts, Girl Scouts, 4-H
Adulthood	Appropriate career placement	Career counseling Job site evaluation

HKAFOs, hip-knee-ankle-foot orthoses.
From Bleakney DA, Donohoe M. Osteogenesis imperfecta. In Campbell SK (ed). Physical Therapy for Children. Philadelphia, WB Saunders, 1994, pp 279–294.

Intervention 10–1 ▌ **HANDLING A CHILD WITH OSTEOGENESIS IMPERFECTA**

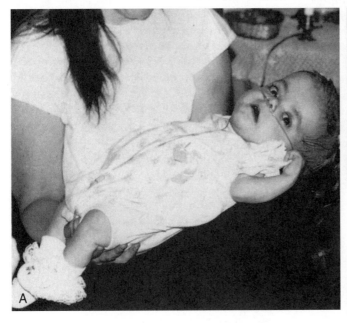

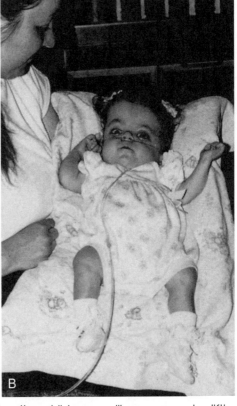

A. In handling a young child with osteogenesis imperfecta, support the neck and shoulders and the pelvis with your hands; do not lift the child from under the arms.

B. Placing the child on a pillow may make lifting and holding easier.

From Myers RS. Saunders Manual of Physical Therapy Practice. Philadelphia, WB Saunders, 1995.

on does need to be knowledgeable about what has been taught to the family.

Positioning should be used to minimize joint deformities. Using symmetry with the infant in supine and side lying positions is good. A wedge can be placed under the chest when the infant is prone to encourage head and trunk movement while providing support (Fig. 10–8). The child's feet should not be allowed to dangle while she is sitting but should always be supported. Water beds are not recommended for this population because the pressure may cause joint deformities.

Range of Motion and Strengthening

By the time the child is of preschool age, not only are the bones still fragile, the joints lax, and the muscles weak but also the child probably has some disuse atrophy and osteoporosis from immobilization secondary to fractures in infancy or childhood. OI has a variable time of onset depending on the type. Range of motion and strengthening are essential. Active movement promotes bone mineralization, and early protected weight bearing seems to have a positive effect on the condition. Range of motion in a straight plane is preferable to diagonal exercises, with emphasis placed on the shoulder and pelvic girdles initially. Light weights can be used to increase strength, but they need to be placed close to the joint to limit excessive torque.

Pool exercise is good because the water can support the child's limbs, and flotation devices can be used to increase buoyancy. Water is an excellent medium for active movement progressing to some resistance as tolerated. The child's respiratory function can be strengthened in the water by having the child blow bubbles and hold his breath. Deep breathing is good

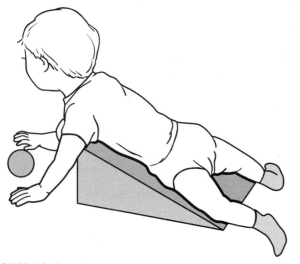

FIGURE 10–8 ▪ Prone positioning of a child on a wedge encourages head and trunk movement and upper extremity weight bearing.

for chest expansion, which may be limited secondary to chest wall deformities. The water temperature needs to be kept low because of these children's increased metabolism (Bleakney and Donohoe, 1994). Increased endurance, protected weight bearing, chest expansion, muscle strengthening, and improved coordination are all potential benefits of aquatic intervention.

Functional Activities and Gait

Developmental activities should be encouraged within safe limits (Intervention 10–2). Use proximal points from which to handle the child and incorporate safe, lightweight toys for motivation. Reaching in supine, side lying, and supported sitting can be used for upper extremity strengthening, as well as for encouraging weight shifting. Rolling is important as a primary means of floor mobility. Pre-positioning one upper extremity beside the child's head as the child is encouraged to roll can be beneficial. All rotations should be active, not passive (Brenneman et al, 1995). Performing a traditional pull-to-sit maneuver is contraindicated. The assistant or caregiver should provide manual assistance at the child's shoulders to encourage head lifting and trunk activation when the assistant is helping the child into an upright position.

Sitting needs to be in erect alignment, as compared with the typical progression of children from prop sitting to no hands, because propping may lead to a more kyphotic trunk posture. External support may be necessary to promote tolerance to the upright position, such as with a corner seat or a seat insert. Sling seats in strollers and other seating devices should be avoided because they do not promote proper alignment. Once head control is present, short sitting or sitting straddling the caregiver's leg or a bolster can be used to encourage active trunk righting, equilibrium, and protective reactions. These sitting positions can also be used to begin protected weight bearing for the lower extremities. Scooting on the bolster or a bench can be the start of learning sitting transfers. Sitting and hitching are primary means of floor mobility for the child with OI after rolling and are used until the child masters creeping.

Transition to Standing

The child with OI should have sufficient upright control to begin standing during the preschool period. Prior to that time, standing and walking with insufficient support will put too much weight on the lower extremities and will produce further bending and bowing of the long bones. A child with OI should be fitted with a standing or ambulatory device by the age of 2 or 3 years (Pauls and Reed, 1996). Hip-knee-ankle-foot orthoses (HKAFOs) are used in conjunction with some type of standing frame such as a prone stander. Ambu-

---

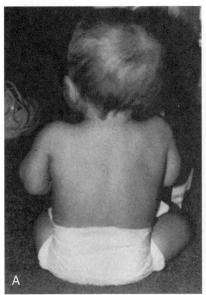 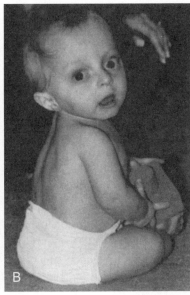 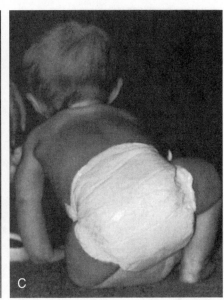

A. The emphasis is on sitting with an erect trunk.
B. All rotations should be active, not passive.

C. Weight bearing is indicated as tolerated on the arms and legs.

From Myers RS. Saunders Manual of Physical Therapy Practice. Philadelphia, WB Saunders, 1995.

---

lation is often begun in the pool because of the protection afforded by the water. The child is then progressed to shallow water. Water can also be used to teach ambulation for the first time or to reteach walking after a fracture, but lightweight plastic splints should also be used. Duffield (1983) suggested the following progression in water: (1) in parallel bars or a standing frame, with a weight shift from side to side, forward, and backward; and (2) forward walking.

Orthotic and Surgical Management

Orthoses are made of lightweight polypropylene and are created to conform to the contours of the child's lower extremity. Initially, the orthosis may have a pelvic band and no knee joints for maximum stability. As strength and control increase, the pelvic band may be removed, and knee joints may be used. Some orthoses have a clamshell design that includes an ischial weight-bearing component, a feature borrowed from lower extremity prostheses. The ambulation potential of a child with OI is highly variable, so orthotic choices are, too. From using a standing frame and orthosis, the child progresses to some type of KAFO with the knees locked in full extension Figure 10-9. The child first ambulates in the safety of the parallel

bars, then moves to a walker, and finally progresses to crutches as limb strength and coordination improve.

Healing time for fractures in children with OI is normally 4 to 6 weeks, the same as in children without the condition. What is not normal is the number of fractures these children can experience. Intramedullary rod fixation is the best way to stabilize fractures that occur in the long, weight-bearing bones. Special telescoping rods developed by Bailey and Dubow (1965) allow the child's bones to grow with the rod in place. This type of surgical procedure is usually done after the child is 4 or 5 years of age to allow for sufficient growth of the femur. However, one study suggests that the operation be performed when the child is between the ages of 2 and 3½ years, potentially to improve the child's neuromotor development (Engelbert et al, 1995). Fortunately, the frequency of fractures tends to decrease after puberty, possibly because of hormonal influences (Bleakney and Donohoe, 1994).

Scoliosis or kyphosis occurs in 50% of children with OI (Tachdjian, 1990). Often, the child cannot use an orthosis to manage a spinal curve because the forces from the orthosis produce rib deformities rather than controlling the spine. Curvatures can progress rapidly after the age of 5 years, with maximum deformity

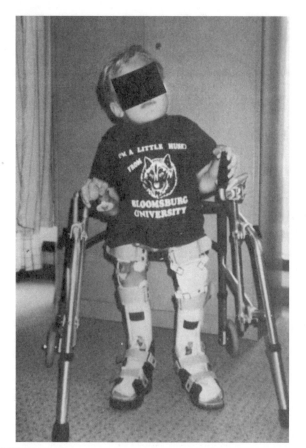

FIGURE 10–9 ■ A child with osteogenesis imperfecta who is using long leg braces and a rollator posture walker. (From Bleakney DA, Donohoe M. Osteogenesis imperfecta. In Campbell SK [ed]. Physical Therapy for Children. Philadelphia, WB Saunders, 1994.)

present by age 12 (Gitelis et al, 1983). Surgical fixation with or without instrumentation is recommended, but few long-term results have been reported (Hanscom et al, 1992). In addition to compounding the short stature in the child with OI, spinal deformities can significantly impair chest wall movement and respiratory function.

School Age and Adolescence

The goals during this period are to maximize all abilities from ambulation to ADLs. One circumstance that may make this more difficult is overprotection of the school-age child by anyone involved with managing the student's care. Strengthening exercise and endurance exercise are continued during this time to improve ambulation. At puberty, the rate of fractures decreases, thus making ambulation without orthoses a possibility for the first time. Despite this change, a wheelchair becomes the primary means of mobility for most individuals for general community mobility. This allows the child with OI to have the energy to keep up and socialize with the peer group. The school-age child with OI has to avoid contact sports, for obvious

reasons, but still needs to have some means of exercising to maintain cardiovascular fitness.

Adulthood

The major challenge to individuals with OI as they move into adulthood is dealing with the secondary problems of the disorder. Spinal deformity may be severe and may continue to progress. Career planning must take into account the physical limitations imposed by the musculoskeletal problems.

CYSTIC FIBROSIS

Cystic fibrosis is an autosomal recessive disorder of the exocrine glands that is caused by a defect on chromosome 7. The pancreas does not secrete enzymes to break down fat and protein in 85% of these individuals. CF produces respiratory compromise because abnormally thick mucus builds up in the lungs. This buildup creates a chronic obstructive lung disorder. A parent can be a carrier of this gene and may not express any symptoms. When one parent is a carrier or has the gene, the child has a 1 in 4 chance of having the disorder. The incidence is 1 in 2000 live births (Boyd et al, 1994).

Diagnosis

CF is the most lethal genetic disease in whites. Diagnosis can be made on the basis of a positive sweat chloride test. Children with CF excrete too much salt in their sweat, and this salt can be measured and compared with normal values. Values greater than 70 mmol/L indicate CF (Harris and Super, 1995). Some mothers have even stated that the child tastes salty when kissed. Because of the difficulty with digesting fat, the child may have foul-smelling stools and may not be able to gain weight. Before being diagnosed with CF, the child may have been labeled as failing to thrive because of a lack of weight gain. Prenatal diagnosis is available, and couples can be screened to detect whether either is a carrier of the gene.

Pathophysiology and Natural History

Even though the genetic defect has been localized, the mechanism that causes the disease is still unidentified. The ability of salt and water to cross the cell membrane is altered, and this change explains the high salt content present when these children perspire. Thick secretions obstruct the mucus-secreting exocrine glands. The disease involves multiple systems: gastrointestinal, reproductive, sweat glands, and respiratory. The two most severely impaired organs are the lungs and the pancreas. Diet and pancreatic enzymes are used to manage the pancreatic involvement.

The structure and function of the lungs are normal at birth. Only after thick secretions begin to obstruct or block airways, which are smaller in infants than in adults, is pulmonary function adversely affected. The secretions also provide a place for bacteria to grow. Inflammation of the airways brings in infiltrates that eventually destroy the airway walls. The combination of increased thick secretions and chronic bacterial infections produces chronic airway obstruction. Initially, this condition may be reversed with aggressive bronchial hygiene and medications. Eventually, repeated infections and bronchitis progress to bronchiectasis, which is irreversible. Bronchiectasis stretches the breathing tubes and leads to abnormal breathing patterns. Pulmonary function becomes more and more severely compromised over the life span, and the person dies of respiratory failure.

Life expectancy for an individual with CF has increased over the last several decades. The median survival is 25 years of age (Garritan, 1994). One source states that approximately 40% of individuals live to an age of 30 years and beyond (Leman et al, 1992). The increase in longevity can be related to improved medical care, pharmacologic intervention, and heart and lung transplantation. The pulmonary manifestations of the disease are those that result in the greatest mortality.

Child's Impairments and Interventions

The physical therapist's evaluation of the child with CF typically identifies the following impairments to be addressed by physical therapy intervention:

1. Retained secretions
2. Impaired ability to clear airways
3. Impaired exercise tolerance
4. Chest wall deformities
5. Nutritional deficits

Chest Physical Therapy

Central to the care of the child with CF is chest physical therapy. It consists of bronchial drainage in specific positions with percussion, rib shaking, vibration, and breathing exercises and retraining. Treatment is focused on reducing symptoms. Respiratory infections are to be avoided or treated aggressively. Signs of pulmonary infection include increased cough and sputum production, fever, and increased respiration rate. Additional findings could include increased white blood cell count, new findings on auscultation or radiographs, and decreased pulmonary function test

values. Unfortunately, bacteria can become resistant to certain medications over time. Parents are taught to perform postural drainage three to five times a day. Adequate fluid intake is important to keep the mucus hydrated and therefore easier to move and expectorate. The child with CF receives medications to provide hydration and to break up the mucus, as well as to keep the bronchial tubes as open as possible and to prevent bronchial spasms. These drugs are usually administered before postural drainage is performed. Antibiotics are a key to the increased survival rate in patients with CF and must be matched to the organism causing the infection.

Exercise

Most individuals with CF can participate in an exercise program (Cerny and Orenstein, 1993; Darbee and Cerny, 1995). Exercise for cardiovascular and muscular endurance plays a major role in keeping these individuals fit and may slow the deterioration of lung function. Bike riding, swimming, tumbling, and walking are all excellent means of providing low-impact endurance training. With decreases in endurance resulting from disease progression, other activities such as table tennis can be suggested. Exercise programs should be based on the results of an exercise test performed by the physical therapist. Children with CF may desaturate with exercise, a condition that indicates the need for an ear or finger pulse oximeter to measure oxygen saturation while the child exercises. Oxygen saturation should remain at 90% during exercise.

Strengthening specific muscles can assist respiration. Target the upper body, with emphasis on the shoulder girdle and chest wall muscles such as the pectoralis major and minor, intercostals, serratus, erector spinae, rhomboids, latissimus dorsi, and abdominals. Stretches to maintain tension relationships of chest wall musculature of optimal length are helpful. Respiratory efficiency can be lost when too much of the work of breathing is done by the accessory neck muscles.

Part of pulmonary rehabilitation is to teach breathlessness positions, use of the diaphragm, and lateral basal expansion. *Breathlessness positions* allow the upper body to rest, to allow the major muscle of inspiration, the diaphragm, to work most easily. Typical postures are seen in Intervention 10–3. *Diaphragmatic breathing* can initially be taught by having the child in a supported back-lying position and using manual cues on the epigastric area (Intervention 10–4A). The child should be progressed from this position to upright sitting, to standing, and then to walking (Intervention 10–4B and C). The diaphragm works maximally when the child breathes deeply. Manual contacts on the lateral borders of the ribs can be used to encourage full expansion of the bases of the lungs (Intervention 10–5).

Intervention 10–3 ▌ BREATHLESSNESS POSTURES

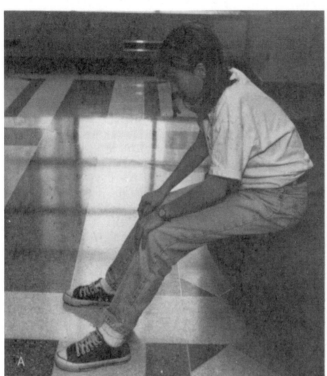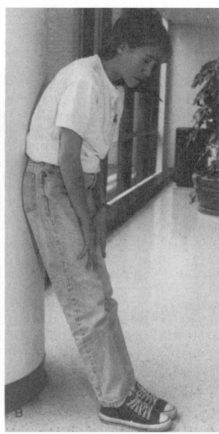

A and B. Breathlessness postures for conserving energy, promoting relaxation, and ease of breathing.

From Campbell SK (ed). Physical Therapy for Children. Philadelphia, WB Saunders, 1994.

Postural Drainage

Postural drainage is the physical act of using gravity or body position to aid in draining mucus from the lungs. The breathing tubes that branch off from the two main stem bronchi are like branches of an upside-down tree, each branch becoming smaller and smaller the farther away it is from the main trunk. The position of the body for postural drainage depends on the direction the branch points. Each segment of the lobes of the lungs has an optimal position for gravity to drain the secretions and allow them to travel back up the bronchial tree to be expelled by coughing. Postural drainage or positioning for drainage is almost always accompanied by percussion and vibration. Manual vibration is shown in Intervention 10–6. *Percussion* is manually applied with a cupped hand while the person is in the drainage positions for 3 to 5 minutes. Proper configuration of the hand for percussion is shown in Figure 10–10. Percussion dislodges secretions within that segment of the lung, and gravity usu-

ally does the rest. The classic 12 positions are shown in Figure 10–11. Percussion and vibration should be applied only to those areas that have retained secretions. Treatment usually lasts no more than 30 minutes total, with the time divided among the lung segments that need to be drained.

Coughing as a form of forced expiration is necessary to clear secretions. Laughing or crying can stimulate coughing. Although most children with CF cough on their own, some may need to be encouraged to do so through laughter. If this technique is unsuccessful, the tracheal "tickle" can be used by placing a finger on the trachea above the sternal notch and gently applying pressure. If you attempt this maneuver on yourself, you will feel the urge to clear your throat. To make coughing more functional and productive, the physical therapist assistant can teach the child a *forced expiration technique.* When the child is in a gravity-aided position, she is asked to "huff" several times after taking a medium-sized breath. This is followed by several relaxed

Intervention 10-4 ▌ DIAPHRAGMATIC BREATHING

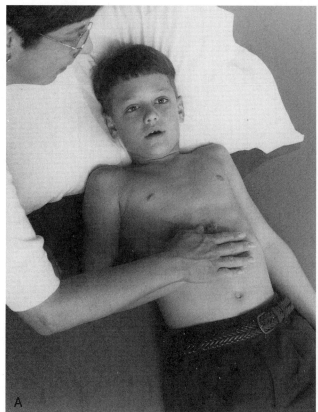

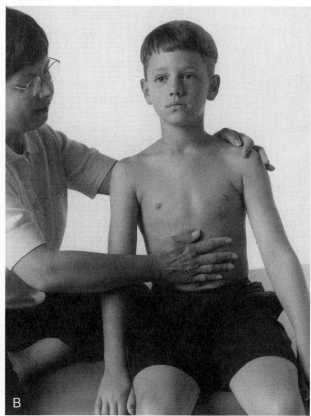

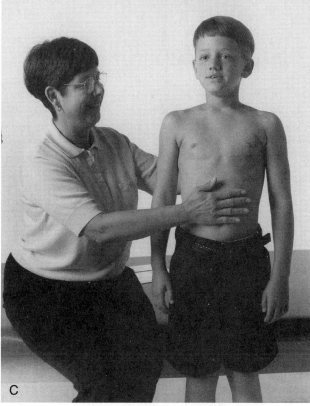

A. Initially, the child can be taught diaphragmatic breathing in a supported back-lying position, with manual cues on the epigastric area.

B and C. Then the child should be progressed to upright sitting, standing, and eventually walking while continuing to use the diaphragm for breathing.

Intervention 10-5 ■ LATERAL BASAL CHEST EXPANSION

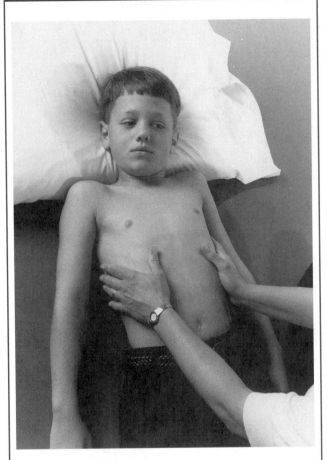

Manual contacts on the lateral borders of the ribs can be used to encourage full expansion of the bases of the lungs.

Intervention 10-6 ■ MANUAL VIBRATION

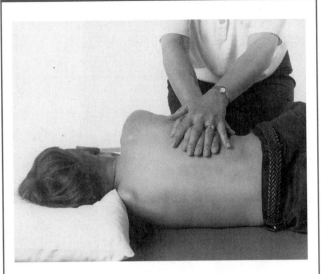

Vibration is used in conjunction with positioning to drain secretions out of the lungs. The chest wall should be vibrated as the child exhales to encourage coughing.

breaths using the diaphragm. The sequence of huffing and diaphragmatic breathing is repeated as long as secretions are being expectorated. The force of the expirations (huffs) can be magnified by manual resistance over the epigastric area or by having the child actively adduct the arms and compress the chest wall laterally. Pauls and Reed (1996) suggested that this technique can be taught to children who are 4 to 5 years of age.

When monitoring exercise tolerance with an individual with CF, use the perceived exertion rating scale and level of dyspnea scale to assess how hard the child is working. These ratings are found in Tables 10–5 and 10–6. If the child is known to desaturate with exercise, monitoring with an oximeter is indicated. If the oxygen saturation level drops below 90%, exercise should be terminated, and the supervising therapist should be notified before additional forms of exercise are attempted. Use of bronchodilating medication 20 minutes prior to exercise may also be beneficial, but again, guidelines for use of any medication should be sought from the supervising therapist in consultation with the child's physician.

SPINAL MUSCULAR ATROPHY

Spinal muscular atrophy is a progressive disease of the nervous system inherited as an autosomal recessive trait. Although most of the genetic disorders discussed so far have involved the central nervous system, in

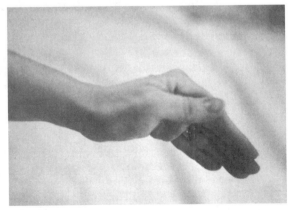

FIGURE 10–10 ■ Proper configuration of the hand for percussion. (From Hillegass EA, Sadowsky HS. Essentials of Cardiopulmonary Physical Therapy. Philadelphia, WB Saunders, 1994.)

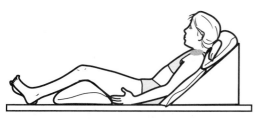

Position 1: Upper lobes, apical segments

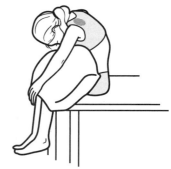

Position 2: Upper lobes, posterior segments

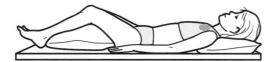

Position 3: Upper lobes, anterior segments

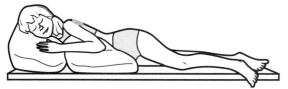

Position 4: Left upper lobe, posterior segments

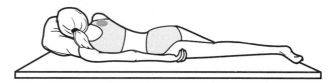

Position 5: Right upper lobe, posterior segments

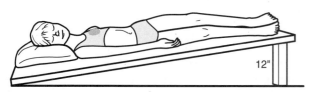

Position 6: Left upper lobe, lingula segment

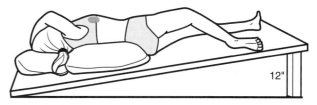

Position 7: Right middle lobe

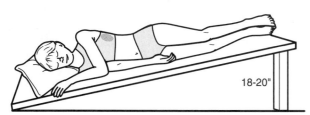

Position 8: Lower lobes, anterior basal segment

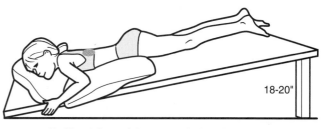

Position 9: Lower lobes, posterior basal segments

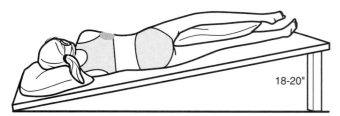

Positions 10 and 11: Lower lobes, lateral basal segments

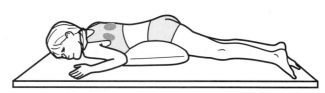

Position 12: Lower lobes, superior segments

FIGURE 10–11 ■ Postural drainage positions.

Table 10-5 ▌ **RATING OF PERCEIVED EXERTION SCALE**

6	
7	Very, very light
8	
9	Very light
10	
11	Fairly light
12	
13	Somewhat hard
14	
15	Hard
16	
17	Very hard
18	
19	Very, very hard
20	

From Borg G. Borg's Perceived Exertion and Pain Scales, Human Kinetics, 1998.

SMA, the anterior horn cell undergoes progressive degeneration. Children with SMA exhibit hypotonia of peripheral, rather than of central, origin. Damage to lower motor neurons produces low muscle tone or flaccidity, depending on whether some or all of the anterior horn cells degenerate. Muscle fibers have little or no innervation from the spinal nerve if the anterior horn cell is damaged, and the result is weakness.

Many types of SMA are recognized. The following discussion is limited to acute infantile SMA and to three forms of chronic childhood SMA. Three of the earliest-occurring types of SMA are also known as Werdnig-Hoffman disease. These are variations of the same disorder involving a gene mutation on chromosome 5. The gene location for a fourth type of SMA, or Kugelberg-Welander SMA, is unknown. All types of SMA differ in age at onset and severity of symptoms. This variability accounts for the wide range of ages at onset reported and some confusion about the number of types of SMA.

As a group of disorders, SMA occurs in 1 of 14,300 live births and is the second most common fatal recessive genetic disorder seen in children, after CF (Seashore and Wappner, 1996).

Acute Infantile SMA. The earliest-occurring, and therefore the most physically devastating, form is type 1, acute infantile SMA. Its onset is between birth and 2

Table 10-6 ▌ **DYSPNEA SCALE**

+1	Mild, noticeable to patient but not observer
+2	Mild, some difficulty, noticeable to observer
+3	Moderate difficulty, but can continue
+4	Severe difficulty, patient cannot continue

From American College of Sports Medicine. Guidelines for Exercise Testing and Prescription, 4th ed. Philadelphia, Lea & Febiger, 1991. Reprinted with permission.

months. The child's limp, "frog-legged" lower extremity posture is evident at birth, along with a weak cry. A third of these children have a history of decreased fetal movements (Seashore and Wappner, 1996). Deep tendon reflexes are absent, and the tongue may fasciculate (quiver) because of weakness. Most infants are sociable and interact appropriately because they have normal intelligence. Motor weakness progresses rapidly, and death results from respiratory compromise at around 7 to 9 months of age.

In the infant with SMA, positioning and family support are the most important interventions. Physical therapy focuses on fostering normal developmental activities and providing the infant with access to the environment. Positioning for feeding, playing with toys, and interacting with caregivers are paramount. The prone position may be difficult for the child to tolerate because it may inhibit diaphragm movement. These infants rely on the diaphragm to breathe because their intercostal and neck accessory muscles are weak. Creative solutions to adaptive equipment needs can often be the result of brainstorming sessions with the entire team and the family. Equipment should be borrowed rather than purchased because the length of time that it will be used is limited. Because of the poor prognosis of children with this type of SMA, listening to the family's concerns is an integral part of the role of physical therapy clinicians.

Chronic Childhood SMA. A chronic childhood type of SMA has a later onset, which is reported to occur between 2 and 18 months. This type is characterized by the onset of proximal weakness, similar to the infantile type. It may be difficult if not impossible for these children to develop the ability to sit or walk without orthotic support. Because of trunk muscle weakness, scoliosis is a pervasive problem and may require surgical intervention. Furthermore, with a reported 12 to 15% fracture rate, weight bearing is also recommended as part of any therapeutic intervention (Ballestrazzi et al, 1989). Stuberg (1994) recommended a supine stander for children who lack adequate head control. Respiratory compromise remains the major cause of death, which usually occurs before 7 years of age.

When the clinician is working with a toddler or preschooler with SMA, physical therapy goals are directed toward mobility, including walking. As stated earlier, an orthosis may be required for the child to attain sitting. Appropriate orthoses for ambulation could include KAFOs, parapodiums, and reciprocating gait orthoses. The reader is referred to Chapter 9 for a discussion of these devices. The physical therapist assistant may be involved in training the child to use and to apply these devices. Wheelchair mobility with either a manual or a power wheelchair may be indicated in this age group. The physical therapist assistant can play a vital role in promoting the child's independence by teaching the child wheeled mobility both in and out of the classroom. Appropriate trunk support when seated must be ensured to decrease the progression of spinal deformities. Although scoliosis cannot always be prevented, every effort should be made to minimize any progression of deformities and therefore to maintain adequate respiratory function. Postural drainage positioning can be incorporated into the preschool and home routine. Deep breathing can be part of the exercise program. Any changes or decreases in strength should be reported by the physical therapist assistant to the supervising therapist (Ratliffe, 1998).

The second type of chronic childhood SMA is the mildest form, *Werdnig-Hoffman*, with an onset at from 1 to 2 years. Again, the pattern of muscle weakness is similar to that in the other types of SMA, but the progression of the disease is more variable. These children usually ambulate, but they require a wheelchair as the disease progresses. Orthotic devices assist ambulation, as does the use of a walker. Safety can be a significant issue as the child becomes weaker, so appropriate precautions such as close monitoring must be taken. Use of a supported walking program has been reported to lessen the incidence of hip dislocation and contractures in these children (Granata et al, 1989). When a wheelchair is needed, a power wheelchair is often recommended. Because of the tendency of the child to lean in the wheelchair even with lateral supports, one should consider alternating placement of the joystick from one side to the other (Stuberg, 1994). The child's ability to participate in school is often hampered by inadequate positioning and lack of ability to access academic materials. Prognosis in this type of SMA depends on the degree and frequency of pulmonary complications. Scoliosis can compound pulmonary problems, with surgical correction indicated only if the child has a good prognosis for survival. Life expectancy is reported to be 19 years (Seashore and Wappner, 1996).

The third type of SMA discussed here is *Kugelberg-Welander* SMA, which occurs later in childhood, with age at onset ranging from 2 to 17 years of age (Seashore and Wappner, 1996). Characteristics include proximal weakness, which is greatest in the hips, knees, and trunk. Developmental progress is slow, with independent sitting achieved by 1 year and independent walking by 3 years. The gait is slow and waddling, often with bilateral Trendelenburg signs (Goodman and Miedenar, 1998). These children have good upper extremity strength, a finding that can differentiate this type of SMA from DMD. Despite the differences in presentation, a child with this type of SMA, more so than all the other types, can be managed in a fashion similar to a child with DMD. However, ambulation is possible until adulthood, at which time the individual will usually need a wheelchair. Life expectancy does

extend into adulthood (Seashore and Wappner, 1996). Because of the variability of the presentation of these disorders, the physical therapy needs are determined by the specific type of SMA, the functional limitations present, and the age of the child.

PHENYLKETONURIA

One genetic cause of mental retardation that is preventable is the inborn error of metabolism called *phenylketonuria* (PKU). PKU is caused by an autosomal recessive trait that can be detected at birth by a simple blood test. The infant's metabolism is missing an enzyme that converts phenylalanine to tyrosine. Too much phenylalanine causes mental and growth retardation along with seizures and behavioral problems. Once the error is identified, infants are placed on a phenylalanine-restricted diet. If dietary management is begun, the child will not develop mental retardation or any of the other neurologic signs of the disorder. If the error is undetected, the infant's mental and physical development will be delayed, and physical therapy intervention is warranted.

DUCHENNE MUSCULAR DYSTROPHY

DMD is transmitted as an X-linked recessive trait, which means that it is manifested only in boys. Females can be carriers of the gene, but they do not express it, although some sources state that a small percentage of female carriers do exhibit muscle weakness. DMD affects 1 in 3700 male births (Seashore and Wappner, 1996). Two thirds of cases of DMD are inherited, whereas one third of cases result from a spontaneous mutation. Boys with DMD develop motor skills normally. However, between the ages of 3 and 5 years, they may begin to fall more often or to experience difficulty in going up and down stairs, or they may use a characteristic Gower maneuver to move into a standing position from the floor (Fig. 10–12). The *Gower maneuver* is characterized by the child's using his arms to push on the thighs to achieve a standing position. This maneuver indicates presenting muscle weakness. The diagnosis is usually made during this time. Elevated levels of creatine kinase are often found in the blood as a result of the breakdown of muscle. This enzyme is a measure of the amount of muscle fiber loss. The definitive diagnosis is usually made by muscle biopsy.

Pathophysiology and Natural History

Children with DMD lack the gene that produces the muscle protein *dystrophin*. Absence of this protein

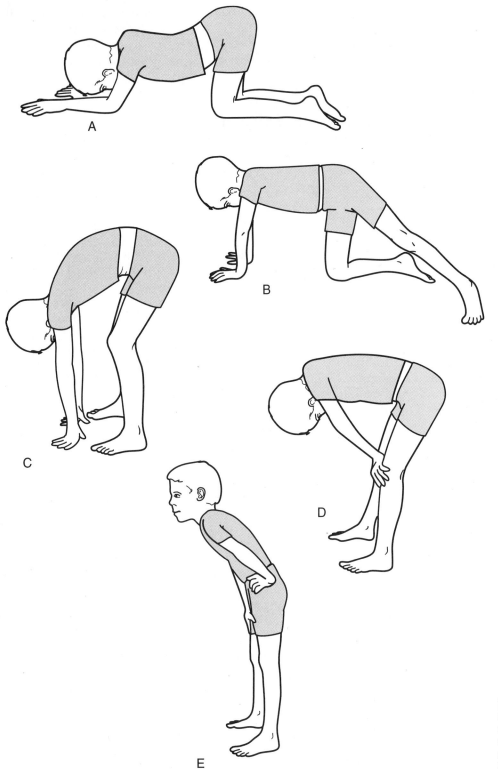

FIGURE 10-12 ■ *A* to *E*, The Gower maneuver. The child needs to push on his legs to achieve an upright position because of pelvic girdle and lower extremity weakness.

weakens the cell membrane and eventually leads to the destruction of muscle fibers. The lack of another protein, *nebulin,* prevents proper alignment of the contractile filaments during muscle contraction. As muscle fibers break down, they are replaced by fat and connective tissue. Fiber necrosis, degeneration, and regeneration are characteristically seen on muscle biopsy.

The replacement of muscle fiber with fat and connective tissue results in a *pseudohypertrophy,* or false hypertrophy of muscles that is most readily apparent in the calves (Fig. 10–13). With progressive loss of muscle, weakness ensues, followed by loss of active and passive range of motion. Limitations in range and ADLs begin at around 5 years of age (Florence, 1994; Stuberg,

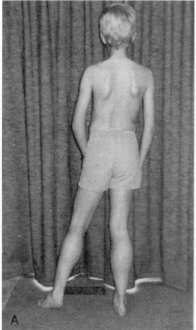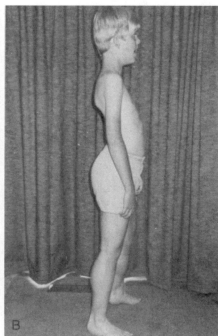

FIGURE 10-13 ■ *A* and *B*, Pseudohypertrophy of the calves. (From Stuberg W. Muscular dystrophy and spinal muscular atrophy. In Campbell SK [ed]. Physical Therapy for Children, 2nd ed. Philadelphia, WB Saunders, 2000.)

1994); an inability to climb stairs is seen between 7 and 13 years of age (Seashore and Wappner, 1996). The ability to ambulate is usually lost between the ages of 9 and 16 years (Seashore and Wappner, 1996). Intellectual function can be less than normal in these children, with 25 to 30% exhibiting some degree of mental retardation (Seashore and Wappner, 1996).

Smooth muscle is also affected by the lack of dystrophin; 84% of boys with DMD exhibit cardiomyopathy, or weakness of the heart muscle. Cardiac failure results either from this weakness or from respiratory insufficiency. As the muscles of respiration become involved, pulmonary function is compromised, with death from respiratory or cardiac failure usually occurring before age 25. Life can be prolonged by use of mechanical ventilation, but this decision is based on the individual's and the family's needs. Bach and colleagues (1991) reported that satisfaction with life was positive in a majority of individuals with DMD who used long-term ventilatory support.

Child's Impairments and Interventions

The physical therapist's evaluation of the child with DMD typically identifies the following impairments or problems to be addressed by physical therapy intervention (Florence, 1994):

1. Impaired strength
2. Impaired active and passive range of motion
3. Impaired gait
4. Impaired functional abilities
5. Impaired respiratory function
6. Spinal deformities—apparent or potential
7. Potential need for adaptive equipment, orthoses, and wheelchair
8. Emotional trauma of the individual and family

The family's understanding of the disease and its progressive nature must be taken into consideration when the physical therapist plans an intervention program. The ultimate goal of the program is to provide education and support for the family while managing the child's impairments. Each problem or impairment is discussed, along with possible interventions.

The physical therapy goals are to prevent deformity, to prolong function by maintaining capacity for ADLs, to facilitate movement, to assist in supporting the family, and to control discomfort. Management is a total approach requiring blending of medical, educational, and family goals. Treatment has both preventive and supportive aspects.

Weakness

Proximal muscle weakness is one of the major clinical features of DMD and is most clearly apparent in the shoulder and pelvic girdles (see Fig. 10-13). The loss of strength eventually progresses distally to encompass all the musculature. Whether exercise can be used to counteract the pathologic weakness seen in muscular dystrophies is unclear. Strengthening exercises have been found to be beneficial by some researchers and not by others. More important, however, exercise has not been found to hasten the progression of the disease (McCartney, 1994). Some therapists do not encourage active resistive exercises (Florence,

1994) and choose instead to focus on preserving functional levels of strength by having the child do all ADLs. Other therapists recommend that submaximal forms of exercise are beneficial but advocate these activities only if they are not burdensome to the family. Movement in some form must be an integral part of a physical therapy plan of care for the child with DMD.

Theoretically, exercise should be able to assist intact muscle fibers to increase in strength to make up for lost fibers. Key muscles to target, if exercise is going to be used to treat weakness, include the abdominals, hip extensors and abductors, and knee extensors. In addition, the triceps and scapular stabilizers should be targeted in the upper extremities. Recreational activities such as bike riding and swimming are excellent choices and provide aerobic conditioning. Walking should be done for a minimum of 2 to 3 hours a day, according to many sources (Siegel, 1978; Ziter and Allsop, 1976). The longer a child can remain ambulatory, the better. Even though the exact role of exercise in these children is unclear, clinicians generally agree that overexertion, exercising at maximal levels, and immobility are detrimental to the child with DMD. Exercise capacity is probably best determined by the stage and rate of disease progression (McCartney, 1994). Exercise may be more beneficial early as opposed to later in the disease process.

Range of Motion

The potential for muscle contractures is high, and every effort should be made to maintain range of motion at all joints. Specifically, attention should be paid to the gastrocnemius-soleus complex and the tensor fasciae latae. Tightness in these muscle groups results in gait deviations and a widened base of support. Stretching of the illiopsoas, iliotibial band, and tensor fasciae latae is demonstrated in Intervention 10–7. Although contractures cannot be prevented, their progression can be slowed (Harris and Cherry, 1974; Scott et al, 1981; Ziter and Allsop, 1976). A prone positioning program is crucial for managing the detrimental effect of gravity. Time in prone counteracts the potential formation of hip and knee flexion contractures, which develop from too much sitting. The physical therapist assistant may teach a home program to the child's parents and may monitor position changes within the classroom. Prolonged sitting can all too quickly lead to lower extremity flexion deformities that can hinder ambulation.

Alternatives to a sitting position should be scheduled several times a day. When the child is in preschool, the prone position can be easily incorporated into nap or rest time. A prone stander can be used during class time when the child is standing and working on the blackboard can be incorporated into the

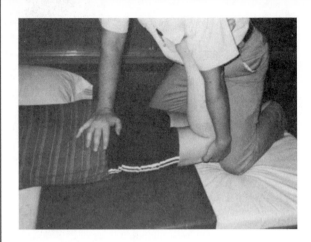

Intervention 10–7 ▌ STRETCHING OF THE ILIOPSOAS, ILIOTIBIAL BAND, AND TENSOR FASCIAE LATAE

Prone stretching of the hip flexors, iliotibial band, and tensor fasciae latae. The hip first is positioned in abduction and then is moved into maximal hip extension and then hip adduction. The knee can be extended to provide greater stretch for the iliotibial and tensor muscles.

From Campbell SK (ed). Physical Therapy for Children. Philadelphia, WB Saunders, 1994.

child's daily classroom routine. Prone positioning over a wedge can also be used. At home, sleeping in the prone position should be encouraged as long as it does not compromise the child's respiratory function.

Skin Care

Skin integrity must always be monitored. Pressure relief and use of a cushion must be part of the daily routine once the child is using a wheelchair for any length of time. If the child is using a splint or orthosis, wearing times must be controlled and the skin must be inspected on a routine basis.

Gait

Children with DMD ambulate with a characteristic waddle as the pelvic girdle musculature weakens. Hip extensor weakness can lead to compensatory lordosis, which keeps the center of mass posterior to the hip joint, as seen in Figure 10–13. Excessive lateral trunk lean during gait may be seen in response to bilateral Trendelenburg signs indicative of hip abductor weakness. Knee hyperextension may be substituted for quadriceps muscle strength, and it can further increase the lumbar lordosis. Failure to keep the body weight in front of the knee joint or behind the hip joint results in a loss of the ability to stand. Plantar flexion contractures can compromise toe clearance, can lead to toe walking, and may make balance even more precarious.

Functional rating scales can be helpful in documenting the progression of disability. Several are available. Table 10–7 depicts simple scales for the upper and lower extremities. The Pediatric Evaluation of Disability Inventory can be used to obtain more specific information about mobility and self-care (Haley et al, 1992). The supervising physical therapist may use this information for treatment planning, and the physical therapist assistant may be responsible for collecting data as part of the ongoing assessment. The physical therapist assistant also provides feedback to the primary therapist for appropriate modifications to be made in the child's treatment plan.

Medical Management

No known treatment can stop the progression of DMD. Steroid therapy has been used to slow the progression of both the Duchenne and Becker forms of muscular dystrophy. Prednisolone has been shown to improve the strength of muscles and to decrease the deterioration of muscle function (Backman and Henriksson, 1995; Hardiman et al, 1993). The immunosup-

Table 10–7 ‖ VIGNOS CLASSIFICATION SCALES FOR CHILDREN WITH DUCHENNE MUSCULAR DYSTROPHY

UPPER EXTREMITY FUNCTIONAL GRADES

1. Can abduct arms in a full circle until they touch above the head.
2. Raises arms above the head only by shortening the lever arm or using accessory muscles.
3. Cannot raise hands above the head, but can raise a 180-mL cup of water to mouth, using both hands, if necessary.
4. Can raise hands to mouth, but cannot raise a 180-mL cup of water to mouth.
5. Cannot raise hands to mouth, but can use hands to hold a pen or pick up a coin.
6. Cannot raise hands to mouth and has no functional use of hands.

LOWER EXTREMITY FUNCTIONAL GRADES

1. Walks and climbs stairs without assistance.
2. Walks and climbs stairs with aid of railing.
3. Walks and climbs stairs slowly with aid of railing (more than 12 seconds for four steps).
4. Walks unassisted and rises from a chair, but cannot climb stairs.
5. Walks unassisted, but cannot rise from a chair or climb stairs.
6. Walks only with assistance or walks independently in long leg braces.
7. Walks in long leg braces, but requires assistance for balance.
8. Stands in long leg braces, but is unable to walk even with assistance.
9. Must use a wheelchair.
10. Bedridden.

From Vignos PJ, Spencer GE, Archibald KC. Management of progressive muscular dystrophy in childhood. JAMA 184:89–96, 1963. Copyright 1963, American Medical Association.

pressant drug cyclosporine has been shown to increase muscle force production (Sharma et al, 1993).

Two additional promising approaches for the treatment of DMD are myoblast transplantation and gene therapy. Both approaches have met with many difficulties, mostly involving immune reactions (Moisset et al, 1998). No reports have been published to date of improved strength in individuals with DMD using the myoblast transfer (Mendell et al, 1995). A report of a pilot study of myoblast transfer in the treatment of subjects with Becker muscular dystrophy stated that myoblast implantation has had limited success (Neumeyer et al, 1998).

Surgical and Orthotic Management

As the quality of the child's functional gait declines, medical management of the child with DMD is broadened. Surgical and orthotic solutions to the loss of range or ambulation abilities are by no means universal. Many variables must be factored into a final decision whether to perform surgery or to use an orthosis. Some clinicians think that it is worse to try to postpone the inevitable, whereas others support the child's and family's right to choose to fight for independence as long as resources are available. Surgical procedures that have been used to combat the progressive effects of DMD are Achilles tendon lengthening procedures, tensor fasciae latae fasciotomy, tendon transfers, tenotomies, and, most recently, myoblast transfers. These procedures must be followed by vigorous physical therapy to make the best gains. Ankle-foot orthoses (AFOs) are often prescribed following heel cord lengthening. Use of KAFOs has also been tried; one source reported that early surgery followed by rehabilitation negated the need for KAFOs (Bach and McKeon, 1991).

Orthoses can be prescribed to maintain heel cord length while the patient is ambulating. A night splint may be fabricated to incorporate the knees, because knee flexion contractures can also be a problem. In the majority of cases, however, as the quadriceps muscles lose strength, the child develops severe lordosis as a compensation. This change keeps the body weight in front of the knee joints and allows gravity to control knee extension. The child's gait becomes lurching, and if the ankles do not have sufficient range to keep the feet plantigrade, dynamic balance becomes impaired. Surgical release of the Achilles tendon followed by use of polypropylene AFOs may prolong the length of time a child can remain ambulatory. However, once ambulation skills are lost, the child will require a wheelchair.

Adaptive Equipment

The physical therapist assistant may participate in the team's decision regarding the type of wheelchair to be prescribed for the child with DMD. The child may not be able to propel a manual wheelchair because of upper extremity weakness, so consideration of a lighter sports wheelchair or a power wheelchair may be appropriate. Energy cost and insurance or reimbursement constraints must be considered. The child may be able to propel a lighter wheelchair during certain times of the day or use it to work on endurance, but in the long term, he may be more mobile in a power wheelchair, as seen in Figure 10–14. If reimbursement limitations are severe and only one wheelchair is possible, power mobility may be a more functional choice. Other adaptive equipment such as mobile arm supports for feeding or voice-activated computer and environmental controls may also be considered to augment the child's level of function.

Respiratory Function

Respiratory function must be targeted for aggressive management. Breathing exercises and range of motion should be part of a home exercise program and incorporated into any therapy session. Flexion of the arms or legs can be paired with inspiration, while extension can be linked to expiration. Diaphragmatic breathing is more efficient than use of accessory muscles and therefore should be emphasized along with lateral basal chest expansion. Chest wall tightness can be discouraged by active trunk rotation, passive counterrotation, and manual stretching (Intervention 10–8). On occasion, postural drainage with percussion may be needed to clear the lungs of retained secretions. Children often miss school because of respiratory involvement. Parents should be taught appropriate postural drainage techniques, as described in the section on CF.

Activities that promote cardiovascular endurance are as important as stretching and functional activities. Always incorporate deep breathing and chest mobility into the child's upper or lower extremity exercises. Wind sprints can be done when the child is in a wheelchair. These are fast, energetic pushes of the wheelchair for set distances. The child can be timed and work to improve or maintain his best time. An exercise program for a child with DMD needs to include an aerobic component because the respiratory system ultimately causes the child to die from the effects of the disease. Swimming is an excellent aerobic exercise for children with DMD.

At least biannual reevaluations are used to document the inevitable progression of the disease. Docu-

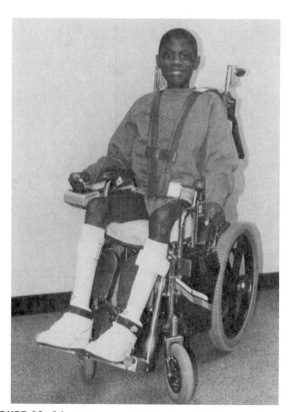

FIGURE 10–14 ▪ A boy with Duchenne muscular dystrophy who is using a power chair. (From Stuberg W. Muscular dystrophy and spinal muscular atrophy. In Campbell SK [ed]. Physical Therapy for Children. Philadelphia, WB Saunders, 1994.)

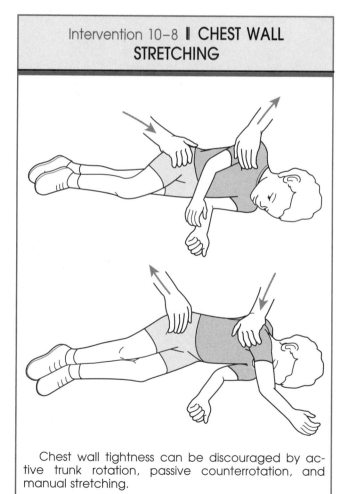

Intervention 10–8 ▌ CHEST WALL STRETCHING

Chest wall tightness can be discouraged by active trunk rotation, passive counterrotation, and manual stretching.

menting progression of the disease is critical for timing of interventions as the child moves from one functional level to another. Whether to have surgical treatment or to use orthotic devices remains controversial. Accurate data must be kept to allow one to intervene aggressively to provide adequate mobility and respiratory support for the individual and his family. Table 10–8 outlines some of the goals, strategies, and interventions that could be implemented over the life span of a patient with DMD.

BECKER MUSCULAR DYSTROPHY

Children with Becker muscular dystrophy have an onset of symptoms between 5 and 10 years of age. This X-linked dystrophy occurs in 3 to 6 per 100,000 males, so it is rarer than DMD. Dystrophin continues to be present but in lesser amounts than normal. Laboratory findings are not as striking as in DMD; one sees less elevation of creatine kinase levels and less destruction of muscle fibers on biopsy. Another significant difference from DMD is the lower incidence of mental retardation with the Becker type of dystrophy. Physical therapy management follows the same general outline as for the child with DMD; however, the progression of the disorder is much slower. Greater potential and expectation exist for the individual to continue to ambulate until his late teens. Prevention of excessive weight gain must be vigorously pursued to avoid use of a wheelchair too early, because life expectancy reaches into the forties. Providing sufficient exercise for weight control may be an even greater challenge in this population because the use of power mobility is more prevalent.

The transition from adolescence to adulthood is more of an issue in Becker muscular dystrophy because of the longer life expectancy. Vocational rehabilitation can be invaluable in assisting with vocational training or college attendance, depending on the patient's degree of disability and disease progression. Regardless of vocational or avocational plans, the adult with Becker muscular dystrophy needs assistance with living arrangements. Evaluation of needs should begin before the completion of high school.

FRAGILE X SYNDROME

Fragile X syndrome, also known as Martin-Bell syndrome, is the leading inherited cause of mental retardation. It occurs in 0.4 to 0.8 per 1000 males and 0.2 to 0.6 per 1000 females (Bellenir, 1996). Detection of a fragile site on the X chromosome at a cellular level makes it possible to confirm this entity as the cause of a child's mental retardation. The disorder is characterized by mental retardation, unusual facies, poor coordination, a generalized decrease in muscle tone, and enlarged testes in male patients after puberty. These children have a long, narrow face with a prominent forehead, jaw, and ears (Fig. 10–15). The clinical manifestations of the disorder vary depending on the completeness of the mutation. Connective tissue involvement can include joint hypermobility, flatfoot, inguinal hernia, pectus excavatum, and mitral valve prolapse (Seashore and Wappner, 1996). The disease appears to worsen in successive generations (Bellenir, 1996). Symptoms in girls are not as severe as in boys. Girls do not usually present with dysmorphic features

Table 10–8 ▌ MANAGEMENT OF DUCHENNE MUSCULAR DYSTROPHY

TIME PERIOD	GOALS	STRATEGIES	MEDICAL/SURGICAL	HOME PROGRAM
School age	Prevent deformity Preserve independent mobility Preserve vital capacity	Stretching Strengthening Breathing exercises	Splints/AFOs Monitor spinal alignment Manual wheelchair as walking becomes difficult Motorized scooter	ROM program Night splints Cycling or swimming Prone positioning Blow bottles
Adolescence	Manage contractures Maintain ambulation Maintain spinal alignment Assist with transfers and ADLs	Stretching Guard during stair climbing or general walking Positioning ADL modifications Strengthening shoulder depressors and triceps	AFOs/KAFOs before ambulation ceases Surgery to prolong ambulatory ability Proper wheelchair fit and support Surgery for scoliosis management	ROM program Night splints Prone positioning Blow bottles Assistance with transfers and ADLs
Adulthood	Monitor respiratory function Manage mobility and transfers	Breathing exercises, postural drainage, assisted coughing Assistive technology	Mechanical ventilation Monitoring oxygen saturation Power mobility	Hospital bed Ball-bearing feeder Hoyer lift

ADLs, activities of daily living; AFOs/KAFOs, ankle-foot orthoses/knee AFOs; ROM, range of motion.
From Stuberg WA. Muscular dystrophy and spinal muscular atrophy. In Campbell SK (ed). Physical Therapy for Children. Philadelphia, WB Saunders, 1994, pp 295–324.

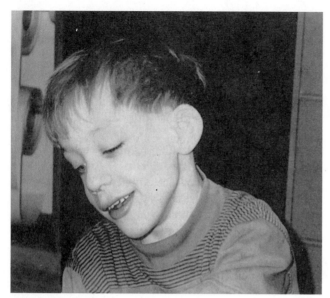

FIGURE 10–15 ▪ A 6-year-old boy with fragile X syndrome. (From *The Fragile X Child,* 1st edition, by Schopmeyer BB, Lowe F [eds]. © 1993. Reprinted with permission of Delmar, a division of Thomson Learning. Fax 800-730-2215.)

(structural differences often seen in the face) or connective tissue abnormalities. Children of female carriers, however, have a greater risk of the disorder than those of male carriers.

Intelligence

Mental retardation in children with fragile X syndrome can range from severe to borderline normal. The average IQ falls between 20 and 60, with a mean of 30 to 45. Additional cognitive deficits may include attention deficit–hyperactivity disorder, learning disability, and autistic-like mannerisms. In fact, girls may be incorrectly diagnosed as having infantile autism or may exhibit only a mild cognitive deficit, such as a learning disability (Seashore and Wappner, 1996).

Motor Development

Gross- and fine-motor development is delayed in the child with fragile X syndrome. The average age of walking is 2 years (Levitas et al, 1983), with 75% of boys exhibiting a flatfooted and waddling gait (Davids et al, 1990). The child's motor skills are at the same developmental age level as the child's mental ability. Even before the diagnosis of fragile X syndrome is made, the physical therapist may be the first to recognize that the child has more problems than just delayed development. Maintaining balance in any developmental posture is a challenge for these children because of their low tone, joint hypermobility, and gravitational insecurity. Mildly affected individuals may present with language delays and behavioral problems, especially hyperactivity (Schopmeyer and Lowe, 1992).

Tactile Defensiveness

Regardless of the severity of the disorder, 90% of these children avoid eye contact, and 80% display tactile defensiveness. The characteristics of tactile defensiveness are listed in Table 10–9. Touch can be perceived as aversive, and light touch may elicit a withdrawal response rather than an orienting response. Treatment involves the use of different-textured surfaces on equipment that the child can touch during play. Vestibular stimulation, firm pressure, and increasing proprioceptive input through weight bearing and movement all are helpful (Schopmeyer and Lowe, 1992).

Sensory Integration

In addition to tactile defensiveness, other sensory integration problems are evident in the decreased ability of these children to tolerate being exposed to multiple sensory inputs at one time. These children become easily overwhelmed because they cannot filter out environmental stimuli. When gaze aversion occurs,

Table 10–9 ▍ TACTILE DEFENSIVENESS

MAJOR SYMPTOM	CHILD'S BEHAVIOR
Avoidance of touch	Avoids scratchy or rough clothing, prefers soft material, long sleeves or pants
	Prefers to stand alone to avoid contact with other children
	Avoids play activities that involve body contact
Aversive responses to nonnoxious touch	Averts or struggles when picked up, hugged, or cuddled
	Averts certain ADL tasks such as baths, cutting fingernails, haircuts, and face washing
	Has an aversion to dental care
	Has an aversion to art materials such as finger-paints, paste, or sand
Atypical affective responses to nonnoxious tactile stimuli	Responds aggressively to light touch to arms, face, or legs
	Increased stress in response to being physically close to people
	Objects to or withdraws from touch contact

ADL, activity of daily living.
From Royeen CB. Domain specifications of the construct of tactile defensiveness. Am J Occup Ther 39:596–599, 1985. Copyright 1985 by the American Occupational Therapy Association, Inc. Reprinted with permission.

it is thought to be related to the child's high degree of anxiety, rather than to autism or social dysfunction. Because low tolerance for frustration often leads to tantrums in these children, always be alert to the child's losing control and institute appropriate behavior modification responses that have been decided on by the team.

Learning

Visual learning is a strength of children with fragile X syndrome, so using a visual cue with a verbal request is a good intervention strategy. Teaching any motor skill or task should be done within the context in which it is expected to be performed, such as teaching hand washing at a sink in the bathroom. Examples of inappropriate contexts are teaching tooth brushing in the cafeteria or teaching ball kicking in the classroom. The physical, social, and emotional surroundings in which learning takes place are significant for the activity to make sense to the child. Teaching a task in its entirety, rather than breaking it down into its component parts, may help to lessen the child's difficulty with sequential learning and tendency to *perseverate*, defined as repeating an action over and over.

RETT SYNDROME

Rett syndrome affects approximately 1 in 12,000 females. The presentation in females suggests an X-linked dominant means of inheritance, with the supposition that the gene is lethal to males during gestation. Early development in affected female infants is normal, with symptoms usually appearing during the first year of life. This neurodegenerative disorder is characterized by mental retardation, ataxia, and growth retardation. These children develop stereotypical hand movements, such as flapping, wringing, and slapping, as well as mouthing. Decline in function during childhood includes a decreased ability to communicate, seizure activity, and later, scoliosis. Expression of the syndrome varies in severity. Girls with Rett syndrome live into adulthood (Seashore and Wappner, 1996).

GENETIC DISORDERS AND MENTAL RETARDATION

Two to 3% of the total U.S. population has psychomotor or mental retardation. *Mental retardation* is "a substantial limitation in present function characterized by subaverage intelligence and related limitations in two or more of the following areas: communication, self-care, home living, social skills, community use,

health and safety, academics, leisure, and work," as defined by the American Association on Mental Retardation (1992). A person must have an IQ of 70 to 75 or less to be diagnosed as having mental retardation. The foregoing definition emphasizes the effect that decreased ability to learn can have on all aspects of a person's life. Educational definitions of mental retardation may vary from state to state because of differences in eligibility criteria for developmental services. An IQ score tells little about the strengths of the individual and may artificially lower the expectations of the child's capabilities. Despite the inclusion of the deficits in adaptive abilities seen in individuals with mental retardation, four classic levels of retardation are reported in the literature. These levels, along with the relative proportion of each type within the population with mental retardation, are listed in Table 10–10.

The two most common genetic disorders that produce mental disability are DS and fragile X syndrome. DS results from a trisomy of one of the chromosomes, chromosome 21, whereas fragile X syndrome is caused by a defect on the X chromosome. This major X-linked disorder explains why the rate of mental retardation is higher in males than females. The defect on the X chromosome is expressed in males when no normal X chromosome is present. Most genetic disorders involving the nervous system produce mental retardation, and children present with low muscle tone as a primary clinical feature.

Child's Impairments and Interventions

The physical therapist's evaluation of the child with low tone secondary to a genetic problem, regardless of whether the child has associated mental retardation, typically identifies similar impairments or potential problems to be addressed by physical therapy intervention:

1. Delayed psychomotor development (only motor delay in SMA)
2. Hypotonia or weakness

Table 10–10 ∎ CLASSIFICATION OF MENTAL RETARDATION

LEVEL OF RETARDATION	INTELLIGENCE QUOTIENT	PERCENTAGE IN MENTALLY RETARDED POPULATION
Mild	55–70	70–89%
Moderate	40–55	20%
Severe	25–40	5%
Profound	<25	1%

Data from Grossman HJ. Classification in Mental Retardation. Washington, DC, American Association on Mental Retardation, 1983; Jones ED, Payne JS. Definition and prevalence. In Patton JR, Payne JS, Beirne-Smith M (eds). Mental Retardation, 2nd ed. Columbus, OH, Charles E. Merrill, 1986, pp 33–75.

3. Delayed development of postural reactions
4. Hyperextensible joints
5. Contractures and skeletal deformities
6. Impaired respiratory function

Intervention to address these impairments is discussed here both generally and within the context of a case study.

Psychomotor Development

Promotion of psychomotor development in children with genetic disorders resulting in delayed motor and cognitive development is a primary focus of physical therapy intervention. Children with mental retardation are capable of learning motor skills and life skills. However, children with mental retardation learn fewer things, and those things take longer to learn. Principles of motor learning can and should be used with this population. Practice and repetition are even more critical in the child with mental retardation than in a child with a motor delay without mental retardation. The clinician must always ensure that the skill or task being taught is part of the child's everyday function. Breaking the task into its component parts improves the potential for learning the original task and for that task to carry over into other skills. The ability to generalize a skill to another task is decreased in children with mental retardation. Each task is new; no matter how similar we may think it is, the process of teaching must start again. Skills that are not practiced on a regular basis will not be maintained, which is another reason for tasks to be made relevant and applicable to everyday life.

Hypotonia and Delayed Postural Reactions

Early in therapy, functional goals are centered around the development of postural control. The child must learn to move through the environment safely and to perform tasks such as manipulating objects within the environment. The mental retardation, hypotonia, joint hypermobility, and delayed development characteristically seen in children with genetic disorders such as DS interact to produce poor postural control. The child with low postural tone cannot easily support a posture against gravity, move or shift weight within a posture, or maintain a posture to use limbs efficiently. Making the transition from one posture to another is accomplished only with a great deal of effort and unusual movement patterns. By improving postural tone in therapy, the therapist provides the child with a foundation for movement. Children with DS benefit from being taught or trained to achieve motor milestones and to improve postural responses (Harris and Shea, 1991). Table 10–1 lists the ages at attainment of developmental milestones in children with DS compared with the typical age at attainment of the same skills.

Ann, as shown in Figure 10–16, is a 17-month-old child with DS. She provides a model for treatment of children with genetic disorders in which hypotonia and delayed motor development are the overriding

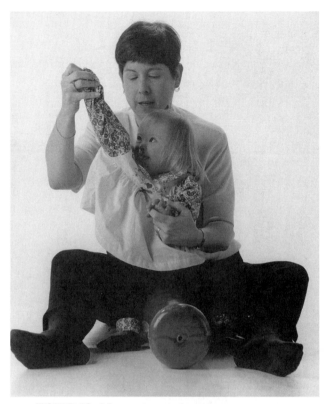

FIGURE 10–16 ■ Trunk weight shift while undressing.

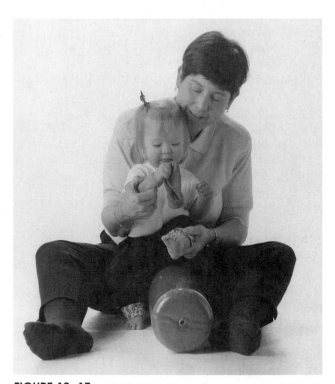

FIGURE 10–17 ■ Child with Down syndrome removing her sock.

impairments. Ann is seen weekly for physical therapy. She creeps and pulls to stand but is not yet walking independently. While Ann undresses, the therapist encourages Ann's ability to balance while her weight is shifted to one side (see Fig. 10–16). In addition, typical help with sock removal is greatly appreciated (Fig. 10–17).

Stability

Preparation for movement in children consists of weight bearing in appropriate joint alignment. Splints of various materials may be used to maintain the required alignment without any mechanical joint locking if the child is unable to do so on her own. Gentle intermittent approximation by manual means helps to prepare a body part to accept weight. Approximation is shown in Intervention 10–9. Approximation through the extremities during weight bearing can reinforce the maintenance of a posture and can provide a stable base on which to superimpose movement, in the form of a weight shift or a movement transition. Intervention 10–10 shows the therapist guiding Ann's movement from sitting to upper extremity weight bearing and Ann reaching with a return to sitting.

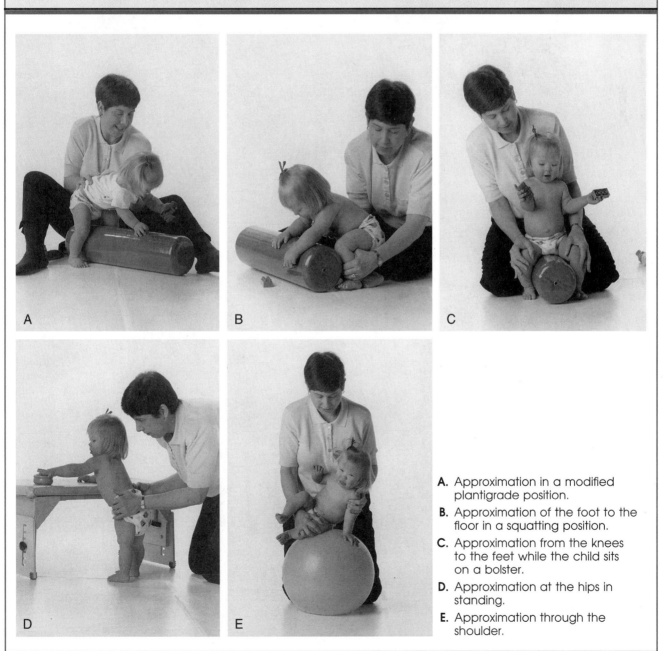

Intervention 10–9 ▌ APPROXIMATION

A. Approximation in a modified plantigrade position.

B. Approximation of the foot to the floor in a squatting position.

C. Approximation from the knees to the feet while the child sits on a bolster.

D. Approximation at the hips in standing.

E. Approximation through the shoulder.

Intervention 10-10 ▌ MOVEMENT TRANSITION

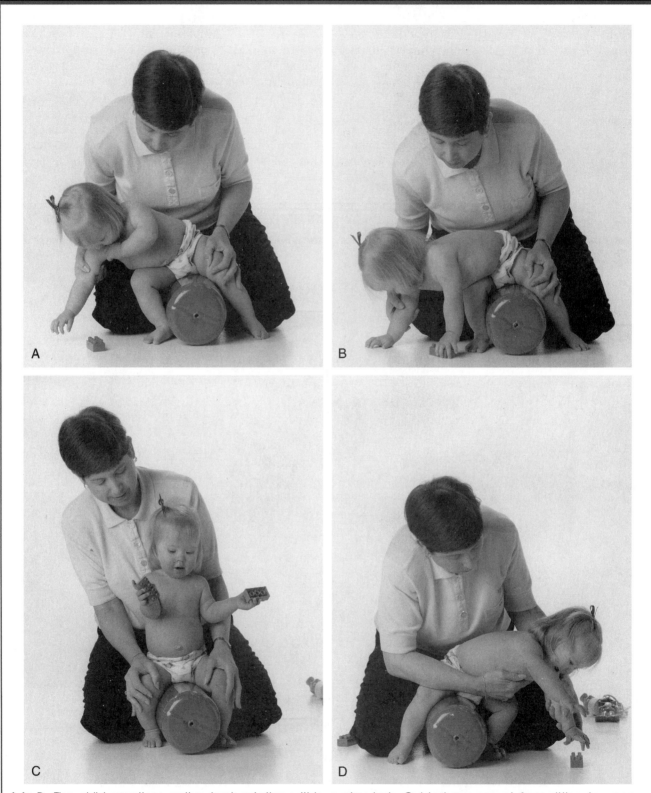

A to D. The child practices active trunk rotation within a play task. Guided movement from sitting to upper extremity weight bearing and reaching with a return to sitting.

Intervention 10–11 ∎ COMING TO STAND

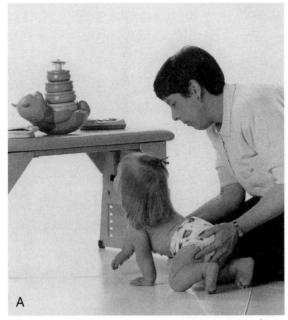
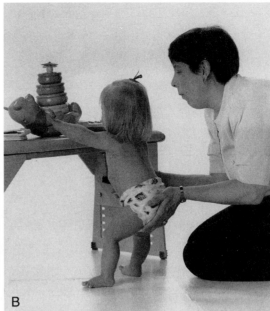
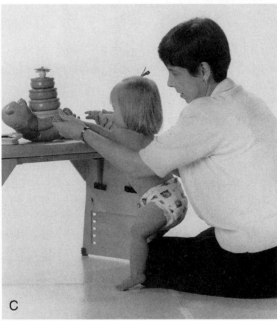

The child is encouraged to stand as follows:

A and B. By pulling up from the floor.

    C. By coming to standing from sitting on the therapist's knee.

Mobility

The child with mental retardation needs to be mobile to explore the environment. Manual manipulation of objects and the ability to explore the surrounding environment are assumed to contribute positively to the development of cognition, communication, and emotion. Even if motor and cognition develop separately, they facilitate one another, so by fostering movement, understanding of an action is made possible. Ann is encouraged to come to stand at a bench to

play both by pulling up and by coming to stand from sitting on the therapist's knee (Intervention 10–11). The use of postural supports such as a toy shopping cart can entice the child into walking (Intervention 10–12). Mobility options facilitate the child's mastery of the environment.

Alternative means of mobility such as a power wheelchair, a cart, an adapted tricycle, or a prone scooter can be used to give the child with moderate to severe mental retardation and impaired motor abilities a way to move independently. McEwen (1994) stated

Intervention 10–12 ▌ WALKING

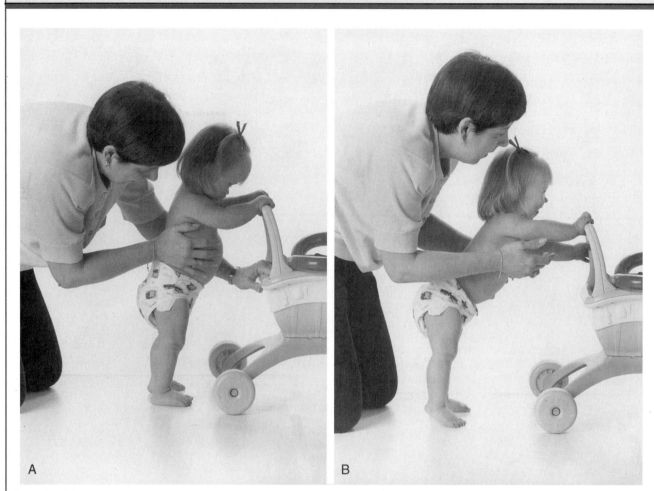

A and B. The use of postural supports such as a toy shopping cart can encourage walking.

that children with mental retardation who have vision and cognition at the level of an 18-month-old are able to learn how to use a powered means of mobility. Orientation in an upright position is important for social interaction with peers and adults. McEwen (1992) also found that teachers interacted more with children who were positioned nearer the normal interaction level of adults, that is, in a wheelchair, than with children who were positioned on the floor.

Postural Control

The child with low tone should be handled firmly, with vestibular input used when appropriate to encourage development of head and trunk control. Joint stability must always be taken into consideration when the clinician uses vestibular sensation or movement to improve a child's balance. The therapist and family should use carrying positions that incorporate trunk support and allow the child's head either to lift against gravity or to be maintained in a midline position. An infant can be carried over the adult's arm, at the adult's shoulder, or with the child's back to the adult's chest (Intervention 10–13). Gathered-together positions in which the limbs are held close to the body and most joints are flexed promote security and reinforce midline orientation and symmetry. Prone on elbows, prone on extended arms, propping on arms in sitting, and four point are all good weight-bearing positions. When the child cannot fully support the body's weight, the use of an appropriate device such as a wedge, a bolster, or a half-roll can still allow the physical therapist assistant to position the child for weight bearing. Upright positioning can enhance the child's arousal and therefore can provide a more optimal condition for learning than being recumbent (Guess et al, 1988).

To develop postural control of the trunk, the clinician must balance trunk extensor strength with trunk

Intervention 10-13 **I CARRYING POSITIONS**

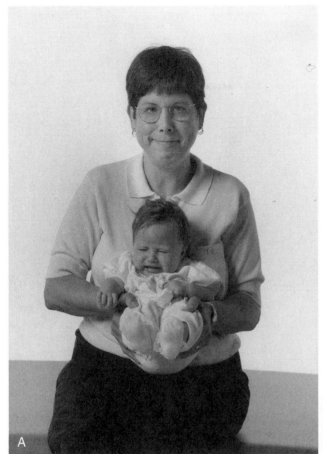

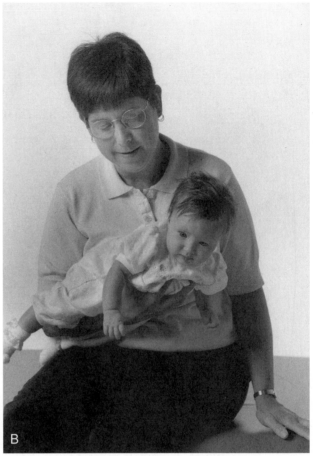

A. Carrying the child with her back to the adult's chest promotes stability.

B. Carrying the child over the arm promotes head lifting and improves tolerance for the prone position.

flexor strength. Trunk extension can be facilitated when the child is in the prone position over a ball by asking the child to reach for an object (Intervention 10-14A). Protective extension of the upper extremities can also be encouraged at the same time, as seen in Activity 10-14B. The ball can also be used to support body weight partially for standing after the hips have been prepared with some gentle approximation (Intervention 10-15). A balanced trunk allows for the possibility of eliciting balance reactions. These reactions can be attempted on a movable surface (Intervention 10-16). The reader is referred to Chapter 8 for descriptions of additional ways to encourage development of motor milestones and ways to facilitate protective, righting, and equilibrium reactions within developmental postures.

When trunk extension is not balanced by abdominal strength, trunk stability may have to be derived from hip adduction and hip extension by using the hamstrings, as seen in Figure 8-16 (Moerchen, 1994).

If a child has such low tone that the legs are widely abducted in the supine position, the hip flexors will quickly tighten. This tightness impairs the ability of the abdominal oblique muscles to elongate the rib cage. The result is inadequate trunk control, a high-riding rib cage, and trunk rotation. Inadequate trunk control in children with low tone not only impairs respiratory function but also impedes the development of dynamic postural control of the trunk, usually manifested in righting and equilibrium reactions.

Contractures and Deformities

Avoiding contractures and deformities may seem to be a relatively easy task because these children exhibit increased mobility. However, muscles can shorten in overly lengthened positions. Because of low tone and excessive joint motion, the child's limbs are at the mercy of gravity. When the child is supine, gravity fosters external rotation of the limbs and the tendency

Intervention 10–14 ▮ TRUNK EXTENSION AND PROTECTIVE EXTENSION

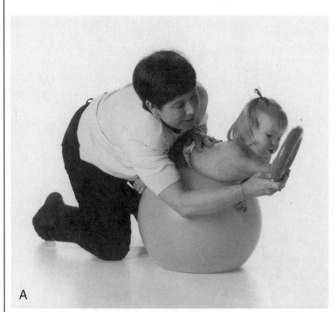

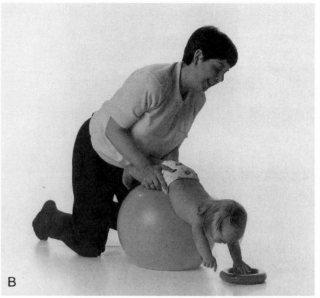

A. Trunk extension can be facilitated with the child in the prone position over a ball by asking the child to reach for an object. The difficulty of the task can be increased by having more of the child's trunk un-supported.

B. Protective extension of the upper extremities can also be encouraged from the same position over a ball if the child is moved quickly forward.

Intervention 10–15 ▮ STANDING WITH SUPPORT FROM THE BALL

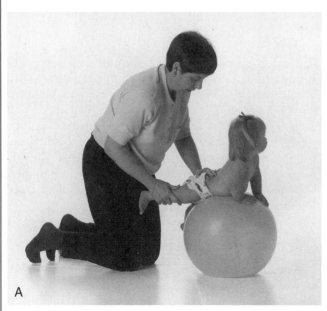

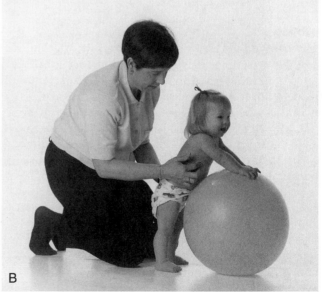

A. Preparing the hips for standing, with some gentle approximation.

B. Use of the ball as a support for standing.

Intervention 10-16 ▌ ELICITING BALANCE REACTIONS

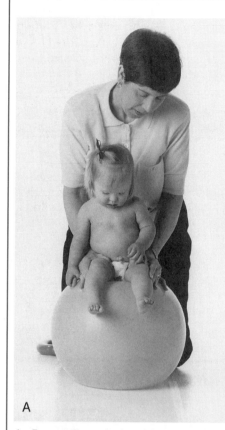 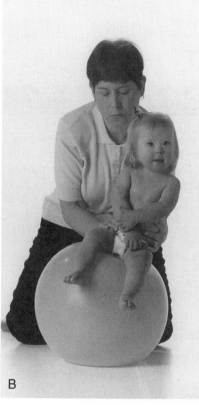 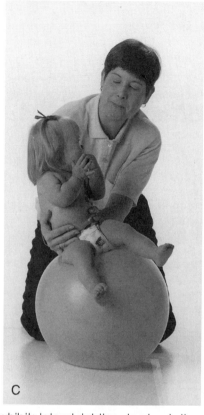

A. Ensure a neutral pelvis, neither anteriorly nor posteriorly tilted.

B. Shift weight to one side, keeping the weight on the down-side hip. This allows the child to respond with lateral head and trunk righting.

C. When the child exhibits lateral righting, trunk rotation can be encouraged as part of an equilibrium reaction.

for the head to fall to one side, thus making it difficult for the child with low tone to maintain the head in midline. Simple positioning devices such as a U-shaped towel roll can be used to promote a midline head position.

Intervention should be aimed at normal alignment and maintenance of appropriate range of motion for typical flexibility and comfort. Positions that provide stability at the cost of continuing excessive range, such as wide abducted sitting, propping on hyperextended arms in sitting, or standing with knee hyperextension, should be avoided. Modify the positions to allow for more typical weight bearing and use of muscles for postural stability rather than maintaining position. Narrow the base of sitting when the child sits with legs too widely abducted. Use air splints or soft splits to prevent elbow or knee hyperextension. Another possibility is to use a vertical stander to support the child so that the knees are in a more neutral position. Good positioning can positively affect muscle use for maintaining posture, for easier feeding, and for breathing.

Respiratory Function

Chest wall tightness may develop in a child who is not able to sit supported at the appropriate time developmentally (6 months). Gravity normally assists in changing the configuration of the chest wall in infants from a triangle to more of a rectangle. If this change does not occur, the diaphragm will remain flat and will not work as efficiently. The child may develop rib flaring as a consequence of the underuse of all the abdominal muscles or the overuse of the centrally located rectus abdominis muscle. If the structural modifications are not made, the diaphragm cannot become an efficient muscle of respiration. The child may continue to belly breathe and may never learn to expand the chest wall fully. Fatigue during physical activity in children with low tone may be related to the inefficient function of the respiratory system (Dichter et al, 1993). Because these children work harder to breathe than other children, they have less oxygen available for the muscular work of performing functional tasks.

Any child with low muscle tone may have difficulty in generating sufficient expiratory force to clear secre-tions. Children who are immobile because of the severity of their neuromuscular deficits, such as those with SMA or late-stage muscular dystrophy, can benefit greatly from chest physical therapy including postural drainage with percussion and vibration. The positions for postural drainage are found in Figure 10–11. Additional expiratory techniques are described in the section of this chapter dealing with CF.

CHAPTER SUMMARY

Working with children with genetic disorders can be challenging and rewarding because of the many variations exhibited within the different disorders. The commonality of clinical features exhibited by children with these disorders, such as low muscle tone, delayed development, and some degree of mental retardation, except for the children with SMA, allows for discussion of some almost universally applicable interventions. Because motor development in children with genetic disorders is generally characterized by immature patterns of movement rather than by abnormal patterns, as seen in children with cerebral palsy, physical therapy management is geared to fostering the normal sequence of sensori-motor development including postural reactions while safeguarding joint alignment. Because of the progressive nature of some of the genetic disorders, physical therapy management must also be focused on preserving motor function or on optimizing function in any body system that is compromised. The physical therapist assistant can play a valuable role in implementing physical therapy treatment for children with any of the genetic disorders discussed in this chapter.

REVIEW QUESTIONS

1. What is the leading cause of inherited mental retardation?
2. When one parent is a carrier for CF, what chance does each child have of being affected?
3. What genetic disorder produces muscle weakness without cognitive impairment?
4. What are the three mechanisms by which chromosome abnormalities occur?
5. What are the two most common clinical features in children with most genetic disorders involving the central nervous system?
6. What principles of motor learning are important to use when working with children with cognitive impairment?
7. What types of interventions are appropriate for a child with low tone?
8. What interventions can be used to prevent secondary complications in children with low tone?
9. What interventions are most often used with a child with OI?
10. What physical therapy goal is most important when working with a child with a progressive genetic disorder?

REHABILITATION UNIT INITIAL EVALUATION: ANN

Chart Review: Ann is a 17-month-old girl with DS. She and her parents have been participants in an infant program since Ann was 3 months old. Ann was born at term with a pneumothorax. During her stay in the neonatal intensive care unit, the DS diagnosis was confirmed by genetic testing. She has had no rehospitalizations. Her health continues to be good. Immunizations are up to date.

REHABILITATION UNIT INITIAL EVALUATION: ANN *Continued*

SUBJECTIVE

The child's mother reports that Ann laughs aloud and sings. She smiles easily and is a good eater. She previously had difficulty with choking on food. Her mother's biggest concern is when Ann is going to walk.

OBJECTIVE

Physical Therapy Examination
Peabody Developmental Motor Scales (PDMS) Gross Motor Developmental Motor Quotient (DMQ) is below average (DMQ = 65). Fine Motor DMQ = 69. Age equivalent of gross- and fine-motor development is 9 months.

Muscle Tone: Low muscle tone is present throughout her extremities and trunk.

Range of Motion: PROM is WFL in all joints, with joint hypermobility present in the hips, knees, and ankles of the lower extremities and in the shoulders and elbows of the upper extremities.
No asymmetry is noted in tone and range.

Deep Tendon Reflexes: Biceps, patellar, and Achilles 1+ bilaterally.

Sensation: Sensation appears to be intact to light touch. Visually, Ann tracks in all directions, although she tends to move her head with her eyes. Quick changes in position such as being picked up or "roughhousing" are tolerated without any crying.

Posture and Balance: Ann sits independently and exhibits head righting reactions in all directions. When she is ring sitting on the floor, her trunk is kyphotic. Trunk righting reactions are present, but equilibrium reactions are delayed and are incomplete in sitting and quadruped positions. Her posture is slightly lordotic in quadruped. Upper extremity protective reactions are present in all directions in sitting but are delayed. Balance in standing requires support of a person or object. She leans forward, flexing her hips and keeping her knees hyperextended.

Mobility: Ann creeps on her hands and knees for up to 30 feet. She pivots in sitting.

Movement Transitions: Ann rolls from supine to prone and pushes herself into sitting over her abducted legs. She pulls to stand by furniture but is unable to come to stand from sitting without pulling with her arms. She is unable to stand from a squat. Ann occasionally exhibits trunk rotation when making the transition from hands and knees to side sitting.

Self-care: Ann finger-feeds. She assists with dressing by removing some clothes.

ASSESSMENT

Ann is a 17-month-old girl with DS who is functioning below her age level in gross- and fine-motor development. She is creeping and pulling to stand but not walking independently. Rehabilitation potential is good for the following goals.

Problem List
1. Delayed gross- and fine-motor development secondary to hypotonia
2. Hypermobile joints
3. Dependent in ambulation
4. Delayed postural reactions

Short-Term Goals (1 month)
1. Ann will walk while pushing an object 20 feet 80% of the time.
2. Ann will demonstrate trunk rotation when moving in and out of side sitting 80% of the time.
3. Ann will rise to standing from sitting on a stool without pulling with her arms 80% of the time.

Continued on following page

REHABILITATION UNIT INITIAL EVALUATION: ANN *Continued*

▌ ASSESSMENT *Continued*

Long-Term Goals (6 months)
1. Ann will ambulate independently without an assistive device for unlimited distances.
2. Ann will go up stairs alternating feet while holding on to a rail.

3. Ann will assist in dressing and undressing as requested.

▌ PLAN

1. Using a movable surface such as a therapeutic ball or roll, encourage Ann to use her trunk muscles to maintain and regain balance.
2. Using appropriate verbal and manual cues, have Ann assist with removing her clothes before therapy and putting them back on after therapy.
3. Work on movement transitions from four point to kneeling, kneeling to half-kneeling, half-kneeling to standing, standing from sitting on a stool, standing to a squat, and returning to standing.
4. Use weight bearing through the upper and lower extremities in developmentally appropriate postures such as four point, kneeling, and standing to increase support responses. Maintain joint alignment to prevent mechanical locking of joints and encourage muscular holding of positions.
5. Use alternating isometrics and rhythmic stability in sitting, quadruped, and standing positions to increase stability.
6. Discuss family instruction and home exercise program.

QUESTIONS TO THINK ABOUT

• What activities could be part of Ann's home exercise program?

• How can fitness be incorporated into Ann's physical therapy program?

REFERENCES

American Academy of Pediatrics Committee on Sports Medicine and Fitness. Atlantoaxial instability in Down syndrome: subject review. Pediatrics 96:151–154, 1995.

American Association on Mental Retardation. Mental Retardation: Definition, Classification, and Systems of Supports, 9th ed. Washington, DC, American Association on Mental Retardation, 1992.

Bach JR, McKeon J. Orthopedic surgery and rehabilitation for the prolongation of brace-free ambulation of patients with Duchenne muscular dystrophy. Am J Phys Med Rehabil 70:323–331, 1991.

Bach JR, Campagnolo DI, Hoeman S. Life satisfaction of individuals with Duchenne muscular dystrophy using long term mechanical ventilatory support. Am J Phys Med Rehabil 70:129–135, 1991.

Backman E, Hendriksson KG. Low-dose prednisolone treatment in Duchenne and Becker muscular dystrophy. Neuromuscul Disord 5:233–241, 1995.

Bailey RW, Dubow HI. Experimental and clinical studies of longitudinal bone growth: utilizing a new method of internal fixation crossing the epiphyseal plate. J Bone Joint Surg Am 47:1669, 1965.

Baird PA, Sadovnick AD. Life expectancy in Down syndrome. J Pediatr 110:849–854, 1987.

Ballestrazzi A, Gnudi A, Magni E, et al. Osteopenia in spinal muscular atrophy. In Merlini L, Granata C, Dubowitz V (eds). Current Concepts in Childhood Spinal Muscular Atrophy. New York, Springer-Verlag, 1989, pp 215–219.

Batshaw ML (ed). Children with Disabilities, 4th ed. Baltimore, PH Brookes, 1997.

Bellenir K (ed). Genetic Disorder Source Book, vol 13: Health Reference Series. Detroit, Omnigraphics, 1996, pp 3–33, 39–40.

Blackman JA (ed). Medical Aspects of Developmental Disabilities in Children Birth to Three Years. Iowa City, University of Iowa, 1983.

Blackston RD. Medical genetics for the orthopaedist. In Morrissy RT (ed). Lovell and Winter's Pediatric Orthopaedics, 3rd ed. Philadelphia, JB Lippincott, 1990, pp 143–174.

Bleakney DA, Donohoe M. Osteogenesis imperfecta. In Campbell SK (ed). Physical Therapy for Children. Philadelphia, WB Saunders, 1994, pp 279–294.

Boyd S, Brooks D, Agnew-Coughlin J, et al. Evaluation of the literature on the effectiveness of physical therapy modalities in the management of children with cystic fibrosis. Pediatr Phys Ther 6: 70–74, 1994.

Brenneman SK, Stanger M, Bertoti DB. Age-related considerations: pediatric. In Myers RS (ed). Saunders Manual of Physical Therapy. Philadelphia, WB Saunders, 1995, pp 1229–1283.

Buyse ML (ed). Birth Defects Encyclopedia, vol 2. Cambridge, MA, Blackwell Scientific Publications, 1990.

Carlin ME. 5p−/Cri-du-Chat Syndrome. Stanton, CA, 5p− Society, 1995.

Carr JH. Down's Syndrome: Children Growing Up. New York, Cambridge University Press, 1995.

Cerny F, Orenstein D. Cystic fibrosis. In Skinner JS (ed). Exercise Testing and Exercise Prescription for Special Cases: Theoretical Basis and Clinical Application, 2nd ed. Philadelphia, Lea & Febiger, 1993, pp 241–250.

Connolly BH, Morgan SB, Russell FF, et al. A longitudinal study of children with Down syndrome who experienced early intervention programming. Phys Ther 73:170–81, 1993.

Darbee J, Cerny F. Exercise testing and exercise conditioning for children with lung dysfunction. In Irwin S, Tecklin JS (eds). Cardiopulmonary Physical Therapy, 3rd ed. St. Louis, CV Mosby, 1995, pp 563–578.

Davids JR, Hagerman RJ, Eilkert RE. Orthopaedic aspects of fragile X syndrome. J Bone Joint Surg Am 72:889–896, 1990.

Dichter CG, Darbee JC, Effgen SK, et al. Assessment of pulmonary function and physical fitness in children with Down syndrome. Pediatr Phys Ther 5:3–8, 1993.

Donohoe M, Bleakney DA. Arthrogryposis multiplex congenita. In Campbell SK (ed). Physical Therapy for Children. Philadelphia, WB Saunders, 1994, pp 261–277.

Duffield MH. Physiological and therapeutic effects of exercise in warm water. In Skinner AT, Thomson AM (eds). Duffield's Exercise in Water, 3rd ed. London, Bailliere Tindall, 1983.

Engelbert RH, Helders PJ, Keessen W, et al. Intramedullary rodding in type III osteogenesis imperfecta: effects on neuromotor development in 10 children. Acta Orthop Scand 66:361–364, 1995.

Florence JM. Neuromuscular disorders in childhood and physical therapy intervention. In Tecklin SJ (ed). Pediatric Physical Therapy, 2nd ed. Philadelphia, JB Lippincott, 1994, pp 390–411.

Garritan SL. Chronic obstructive pulmonary diseases. In Hillegass EA, Sadowsky HS (eds). Essentials of Cardiopulmonary Physical Therapy. Philadelphia, WB Saunders, 1994, pp 262–267.

Gitelis S, Whiffen J, DeWald RL. Treatment of severe scoliosis in osteogenesis imperfecta. Clin Orthop 175:56–59, 1983.

Goodman CC, Miedaner J. Genetic and developmental disorders. In Goodman CC, Boissonnault WG (eds). Pathology: Implications for the Physical Therapist. Philadelphia, WB Saunders, 1998, pp 577–616.

Goodman RM, Gorlin RS. The Malformed Infant and Child. New York, Oxford University Press, 1983, pp 98–99.

Granata C, Marini ML, Capelli T, et al. Natural history of scoliosis in spinal muscular atrophy and results of orthopaedic treatment. In Merlini L, Granata C, Dubowitz V (eds). Current Concepts in Childhood Spinal Muscular Atrophy. New York, Springer-Verlag, 1989, pp 153–164.

Guess D, Mulligan-Ault M, Roberts S, et al. Implications of biobehavioral states for the education and treatment of students with the most profoundly handicapping conditions. J Assoc Persons Severe Handicaps 13:163–174, 1988.

Haley SM, Coster WF, Ludlow LH, et al. The Pediatric Evaluation of Disability Inventory: Development Standardization and Administration Manual. Boston, New England Medical Center Publications, 1992.

Hanscom DA, Winter RB, Lutter L, et al. Osteogenesis imperfecta. J Bone Joint Surg Am 74:598–616, 1992.

Hardiman O, Sklar RM, Brown RH Jr. Methylprednisolone selectively affects dystrophin expression in human muscle cultures. Neurology 43:342–345, 1993.

Harris A, Super M. Cystic Fibrosis: The Facts, 3rd ed. New York, Oxford University Press, 1995.

Harris SE, Cherry DB. Childhood progressive muscular dystrophy and the role of physical therapy. Phys Ther 54:4–12, 1974.

Harris SR, Shea AM. Down syndrome. In Campbell SK (ed). Pediatric Neurologic Physical Therapy, 2nd ed. New York, Churchill Livingstone, 1991, pp 131–168.

Hines S, Bennett, F. Effectiveness of early intervention for children with Down syndrome. Ment Retard Dev Disabil Res Rev 2:96–101, 1996.

Leman RJ, Parce GS, Loughlin G, et al. Pediatric lung diseases. Chest 1992:102(Suppl):232S–242S.

Levitas A, Braden M, Van Norman K, et al. Treatment and intervention. In Hagerman RJ, McBogg P (eds). The Fragile X Syndrome: Diagnosis, Biochemistry, and Intervention. Dillon, CO, Spectra Publishing, 1983, pp 201–226.

Long TM, Cintas H. Handbook of Pediatric Physical Therapy. Baltimore, Williams & Wilkins, 1995, pp 130–131.

Marino B, Pueschel SM (eds). Heart Diseases in Persons with Down Syndrome. Baltimore, PH Brookes, 1996.

McCartney N. Physical activity, fitness, and the physically disabled (neuromuscular disorders). In Bouchard C, Shephard RJ, Stephens T (eds). Physical Activity, Fitness and Health: International Proceedings and Consensus Statement. Champaign, IL, Human Kinetics, 1994, pp 840–850.

McEwen I. Assistive positioning as a control parameter of social-communicative interactions between students with profound multiple disabilities and classroom staff. Phys Ther 72:534–647, 1992.

McEwen I. Mental retardation. In Campbell SK (ed). Physical Therapy for Children. Philadelphia, WB Saunders, 1994, pp 459–488.

Mendell FR, Kissel JT, Amato AA, et al. Myoblast transfer in the treatment of Duchenne's muscular dystrophy. N Engl J Med 333:832–838, 1995.

Moerchen V. Respiration and motor development: a systems perspective. Neurol Rep 18:8–10, 1994.

Moisset PA, Skuk D, Asselin I, et al. Successful transplantation of genetically corrected DMD myoblasts following ex vivo transduction with the dystrophin minigene. Biochem Biophys Res Commun 247:94–99, 1998.

Morbidity and Mortality Weekly Report. Down syndrome prevalence at birth: United States, 1983–1990. MMWR Morb Mortal Weekly Rep 43:617–622, 1994.

Msall ME, Diguadio C, Malone AF. Health, developmental and psychosocial aspects of Down syndrome. Infants Young Child 4:35–45, 1991.

Naganuma G, Harris SR, Tada WL. Genetic disorders. In Umphred DA (ed). Neurologic Rehabilitation, 3rd ed. St. Louis, Mosby-Year Book, 1995, pp 287–311.

Neumeyer AM, Cros D, McKenna-Yasek D, et al. Pilot study of myoblast transfer in the treatment of Becker muscular dystrophy. Neurology 51:589–92, 1998.

Pauls JA, Reed KL. Quick Reference to Physical Therapy. Gaithersburg, MD, Aspen Publishers, 1996, pp 407–409, 440–445, 464–469, 519–524.

Pueschel SM. Clinical aspects of Down syndrome from infancy to adulthood. Am J Med Genet 7(Suppl):52–56, 1990.

Pueschel SM, Scola FH, Peaaullo JC. A longitudinal study of atlanto-dens relationships in asymptomatic individuals with Down syndrome. Pediatrics 89:1194–1198, 1992.

Ratliffe KT. Clinical Pediatric Physical Therapy. St. Louis, CV Mosby, 1998.

Scheiner AP, Abroms IF. The Practical Management of the Developmentally Disabled Child. St. Louis, CV Mosby, 1980, p 225.

Schopmeyer BB, Lowe F (eds). The Fragile X Child. San Diego, Singular Publishing Group, 1992.

Scott OM, Hyde SA, Goddard C, et al. Prevention of deformity in Duchenne muscular dystrophy: a prospective study of passive stretching and splintage. Physiotherapy 67:177–180, 1981.

Seashore MR, Wappner RS. Brain and nervous system. In Seashore MR, Wappner RS (eds). Genetics in Primary Care and Clinical Medicine. Norwalk, CT, Appleton & Lange, 1996, pp 132–152.

Sharav T, Bowman T. Dietary practices, physical activity and body-mass index in a selected population of Down syndrome children and their siblings. Clin Pediatr 31:341–344, 1992.

Sharma KR, Mynhier MA, Miller RG. Cyclosporine increases muscular force generation in Duchenne muscular dystrophy. Neurology 43:527–532, 1993.

Shea AM. Growth and Development in Down Syndrome in Infancy an Early Childhood: Implications for the Physical Therapist. Topic in Pediatrics: Lesson 5. Alexandria, VA, American Physical Therapy Association, 1990.

Siegel IM. The management of muscular dystrophy: a clinical review. Muscle Nerve 1:453–460, 1978.

Stuberg W. Muscular dystrophy and spinal muscular atrophy. In Campbell SK (ed). Physical Therapy for Children. Philadelphia, WB Saunders, 1994, pp 95–324.

Tachdjian M (ed). Pediatric Orthopedics, 2nd ed, vol 2. Philadelphia, WB Saunders, 1990, pp 758–782, 2086–2114.

Zigman W, Silverman W, Wisniewski HM. Aging and Alzheimer's disease in Down syndrome: clinical and pathological changes. Ment Retard Dev Disabil Res Rev 2:73–79, 1996.

Ziter FA, Allsop K. The diagnosis and management of childhood muscular dystrophy. Clin Pediatr 15:540–548, 1976.

11
Cerebral Palsy

OBJECTIVES

After reading this chapter, the student will be able to

1. Understand the incidence, etiology, and classification of cerebral palsy (CP).

2. Describe the clinical manifestations and associated deficits seen in children with CP throughout the life span.

3. Understand the physical therapy management of children with CP throughout the life span.

4. Understand the medical and surgical management of children with CP.

5. Understand the role of the physical therapist assistant in the treatment of children with CP.

6. Recognize the importance of functional training throughout the life span of a child with CP.

INTRODUCTION

Cerebral palsy (CP) is a disorder of posture and movement that occurs secondary to damage to the immature brain before, during, or after birth. This disorder is called a *static encephalopathy* because it represents a problem with brain structure or function. Once an area of the brain is damaged, the damage does not spread to other areas of the brain, as occurs in a progressive neurologic disorder such as a brain tumor. However, because the brain is connected to many different areas of the nervous system, the lack of function of the originally damaged areas may interfere with the ability of these other areas to function properly. Despite the static nature of the brain damage in CP, the clinical manifestations of the disorder may appear to change as the child grows older. Although movement demands increase with age, the child's motor abilities may not be able to change quickly enough to meet these demands.

CP is characterized by decreased functional abilities, delayed motor development, and impaired muscle tone and movement patterns. How the damage to the central nervous system manifests depends on the developmental age of the child at the time of the brain injury and on the severity and extent of that injury. In CP, the brain is damaged early in the developmental process, and this injury results in disruption of voluntary movement. When damage occurs before birth or during the birth process, it is considered *congenital cerebral palsy*. The earlier in prenatal development that a system of the body is damaged, the more likely it is that the damage will be severe. The infant's nervous system is extremely vulnerable during the first trimester of intrauterine development. Brain damage early in gestation is more likely to produce moderate to severe motor involvement of the entire body, or quadriplegia, whereas damage later in gestation may result in primarily lower extremity motor involvement, or diplegia. If the brain is damaged after birth, up to 3 years of age, the CP is considered to be *acquired*. Capute and Accardo (1996) recognized 3 years of age as the time at which the child's brain has achieved three fourths of its adult size.

INCIDENCE

The reported incidence of CP in the general population ranges from 0.6 to 4.2 cases per 1000 live births, depending on the source (Goodman and Miedaner, 1998; Paneth and Kiely, 1984). The prevalence of CP, or the number of individuals within a population who have the disorder, is reported based on the disease's severity. The prevalence of moderately severe to severe CP is 1.5 to 2.5 cases per 1000 people (Kuban and Leviton, 1994). Smaller preterm infants are more likely to demonstrate moderately severe CP because the risk of CP is greater with increasing prematurity and lower birth weights (Sweeney and Swanson, 1995).

ETIOLOGY

CP can have multiple causes, some of which can be linked to a specific time period. Not all causes of CP are well understood. Typical causes of CP and the relationship of these causes with prenatal, perinatal, or postnatal occurrences are listed in Table 11–1.

Prenatal Causes

When the cause of CP is known, it is most often related to problems experienced during intrauterine development. A fetus exposed to maternal infections such as rubella, herpes simplex, cytomegalovirus, or toxoplasmosis early in gestation can incur damage to the brain's motor centers. If the placenta, which provides nutrition and oxygen from the mother, does not remain attached to the uterine wall throughout the pregnancy, the fetus can be deprived of oxygen and other vital nutrients. Inflammation of the placenta occurs in 50 to 80% of premature births (Steer, 1991) and is a risk factor for CP (Nelson and Ellenberg, 1985).

Rh factor is found in the red blood cells of 85% of the population. When blood is typed for transfusion or crossmatching, both ABO classification and Rh status are determined. Rh incompatibility occurs when a mother who is Rh negative delivers a baby who is Rh positive. The mother becomes sensitive to the baby's blood and begins to make antibodies if she is not given the drug RhoGAM (Rh immune globulin). The development of maternal antibodies predisposes subsequent Rh-positive babies to *kernicterus,* a syndrome characterized by CP, high-frequency hearing loss, visual problems, and discoloration of the teeth. When the antibody injection of RhoGAM is given after the mother's first delivery, the development of kernicterus in subsequent infants can be prevented.

Additional maternal problems that can place an infant at risk for neurologic injury include diabetes and toxemia during pregnancy. In diabetes, the mother's metabolic deficits can cause stunted growth of the fetus and delayed tissue maturation. Toxemia of pregnancy causes the mother's blood pressure to become so high that the baby is in danger of not receiving sufficient blood flow and, therefore, oxygen.

Maldevelopment of the brain and other organ systems is commonly seen in children with CP (Nelson and Ellenberg, 1985). Genetic disorders and exposure to teratogens can produce brain malformations. A *teratogen* is any agent or condition that causes a defect in the fetus, including radiation, drugs, infections, and chronic illness. The greater the amount of exposure to the teratogen, the more significant the malformation (Graham and Morgan, 1997).

Perinatal Causes

An infant may experience asphyxiation resulting from *anoxia* (a lack of oxygen) during labor and delivery. Prolonged or difficult labor because of a *breech presentation* (bottom first) or the presence of a prolapsed umbilical cord also contributes to *asphyxia.* The brain may be compressed, or blood vessels in the brain can rupture during the birth process. Although asphyxia has generally been accepted as a significant cause of CP, some reports indicate that most infants who survive major asphyxiation are healthy (Nelson, 1996). The children who do have subsequent neurologic deficits were probably compromised in utero and therefore had an increased susceptibility to experiencing problems during labor and delivery. Even those children with CP who are born at term (40 weeks of gestation) probably experienced some developmental problem before the onset of labor (Kuban and Leviton, 1994).

The two biggest risk factors for CP are prematurity and low birth weight. A baby who is born prematurely and who weighs less than 1500 g (3.3 lb) has a 25 to 31 times greater risk of developing CP than a typically sized newborn who weighs 3500 g (7.7 lb) (Stanley,

Table 11–1 ‖ **RISK FACTORS ASSOCIATED WITH CEREBRAL PALSY**

PRENATAL FACTORS	PERINATAL FACTORS	POSTNATAL FACTORS
Maternal infections	Asphyxia	Cerebrovascular accident
Rubella	Prolonged labor	
Herpes simplex	Breech birth	Intraventricular hemorrhage
Toxoplasmosis	Prolapsed cord	
Cytomegalovirus	Rupture of blood vessels or compression of brain	Brain infections
Placental abnormalities		Meningitis
		Encephalitis
Rh incompatibility	Premature separation of placenta, placenta previa	Seizures
Maternal diabetes		Head trauma
Toxemia		Near-drowning
Brain maldevelopment	Prematurity	
	Low birth weight	

Modified from Goodman C, Miedaner J. Genetic and developmental disorders. In Goodman C, Boissonnault WG (eds). Pathology: Implications for the Physical Therapist. Philadelphia, WB Saunders, 1998, p 579.

1991). One third of infants born early and weighing less than 2500 g (5.5 lb) are found to have CP (Kuban and Leviton, 1994). Decreasing gestational age and small size for gestational age are compounding risk factors for neurologic deficits. A birth weight of less than 1500 g, regardless of gestational age, is a strong risk factor for CP. Thus, any full-term infant weighing less than 1500 g may be at risk for CP. Although CP is more likely to be associated with premature birth, 25 to 40% of cases have no known cause (Bleck, 1987; Russman and Gage, 1989).

Postnatal Causes

An infant or toddler may acquire brain damage secondary to cerebral hemorrhage, trauma, infection, or anoxia. These conditions can be related to motor vehicle accidents, child abuse in the form of shaken baby syndrome, near-drowning, or lead exposure. Meningitis and encephalitis, inflammatory disorders of the brain, account for 60% of cases of acquired CP (Bleck, 1987).

CLASSIFICATION

The designation "cerebral palsy" does not convey much specific information about the type or severity of movement dysfunction a child exhibits. CP can be classified at least three different ways: (1) by distribution of involvement; (2) by type of abnormal muscle tone and movement; and (3) by severity.

Distribution of Involvement

The term *plegia* is used along with a prefix to designate whether four limbs, two limbs, one limb, or half the body is affected by paralysis or weakness. Children with *quadriplegic* CP have involvement of the entire body, with the upper extremities usually more severely affected than the lower extremities (Fig. 11–1*A*). These children have difficulty in developing head and trunk control, and they may or may not be able to ambulate. If they do learn to walk, it may not be until middle childhood. Children with *diplegia* have primarily lower extremity involvement, although the trunk is almost always affected to some degree (Fig. 11–1*B*). Some definitions of *diplegia* state that all four limbs are involved, with the lower extremities more severely involved than the upper ones. *Diplegia* is often related to premature birth, especially if the child is born at around 32 weeks of gestation, or 2 months premature. For this reason, *spastic diplegia* has been labeled the CP of prematurity. Children with *quadriplegia* and *diplegia* have bilateral brain damage.

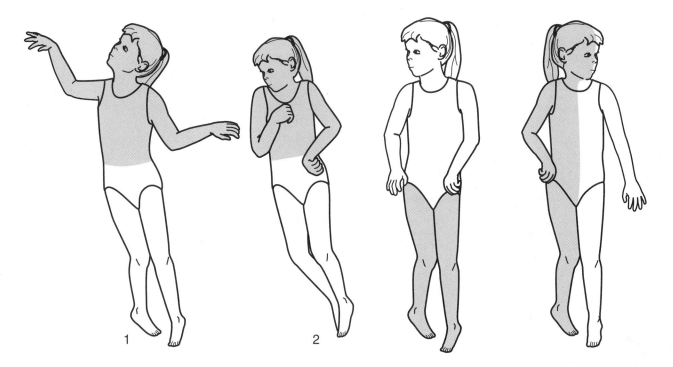

A SPASTIC QUADRIPLEGIA

1 Dominant extension
2 Dominant flexion

B SPASTIC DIPLEGIA   C RIGHT SPASTIC HEMIPLEGIA

FIGURE 11–1 ▪ *A* to *C*, Distribution of involvement in cerebral palsy.

Children with *hemiplegic* CP have one side of the body involved, as is seen in adults after a stroke (Fig. 11–1C). Children with hemiplegia have incurred unilateral brain damage. Although these designations seem to focus on the number of limbs or the side of the body involved, the limbs are connected to the trunk. The trunk is always affected to some degree when a child has CP. The trunk is primarily affected by abnormal tone in hemiplegia and quadriplegia, or it is secondarily affected, as in diplegia, when the trunk compensates for lack of controlled movement in the involved lower limbs.

Abnormal Muscle Tone and Movement

CP is routinely classified by the type and severity of abnormal muscle tone exhibited by the child. Tone abnormalities run the gamut from almost no tone to high tone. Children with the *atonic* type of cerebral palsy present as floppy infants (Fig. 11–2). In reality, the postural tone is hypotonic or below normal. Uncertainty exists regarding the ultimate impairment of tone when an infant presents with hypotonia because tone can change over time as the infant attempts to move against gravity. The tone may remain low, it may increase to normal, it may increase beyond normal to hypertonia, or it may fluctuate from high to low to normal. Continual low tone in an infant impedes the development of head and trunk control, and it inter-

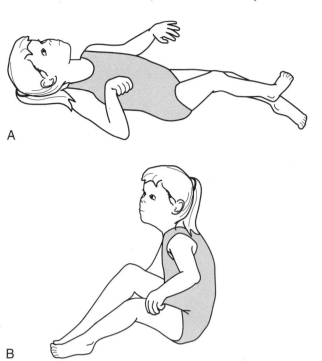

FIGURE 11–3 ■ *A*, Child in extension in the supine position. *B*, The same child demonstrating a flexed sitting posture.

feres with the development of mature breathing patterns. Tonal fluctuations are characteristically seen in the child with a dyskinetic or *athetoid* type of CP. Although abnormal tone is easily recognized, the relationship between abnormal tone and abnormalities in movement is less than clear.

The abnormal tone manifested in children with CP may be the nervous system's response to the initial brain damage, rather than a direct result of the damage. The nervous system may be trying to compensate for a lack of feedback from the involved parts of the body. The distribution of abnormal muscle tone may change when the child's body position changes relative to gravity. A child whose posture is characterized by an extended trunk and limbs when in supine may be totally flexed (head and trunk) when in sitting because the child's relationship with gravity has changed (Fig. 11–3). Tonal differences may be apparent even within different parts of the body. A child with spastic diplegia may exhibit some hypertonic muscles in the lower extremities and may display hypotonic trunk muscles. The pattern of tone may be consistent in all body positions, or it may change with each new relationship with gravity. The degree or amount of abnormal tone is judged relative to the degree of resistance encountered with passive movement. Rudimentary assessments can be made based on the ability of the child to initiate movement against gravity. Usually, the greater the resistance to passive movement, the greater the difficulty seen in the child's attempts to move.

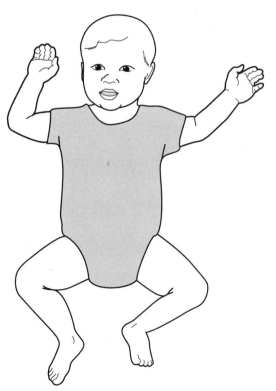

FIGURE 11–2 ■ Hypotonic infant.

Spasticity

By far the most common type of abnormal tone seen in children with CP is *spasticity*. Spasticity is a velocity-dependent increase in muscle tone. *Hypertonus* is increased resistance to passive motion that may not be affected by the speed of movement. Clinically, these two terms are often used interchangeably. Classification and differentiation of the amount of tone above normal are subjective and are represented by a continuum from mild to moderate to severe. The mild and moderate designations usually describe a person who has the ability to move actively through at least part of the available range of motion. Severe hypertonus and spasticity indicate extreme difficulty in moving, with an inability to complete the full range of motion. In the latter instance, the child may have difficulty even initiating movement without use of some type of inhibitory technique. Prolonged increased tone predisposes the individual to contractures and deformities because, in most situations, an antagonist muscle cannot adequately oppose the pull of a spastic muscle.

Hypertonus tends to be found in antigravity muscles, specifically the flexors in the upper extremity and the flexors and extensors in the lower extremity. The most severely involved muscles in the upper extremity tend to be the scapular retractors and the elbow, forearm, wrist, and finger flexors. The same lower extremity muscles that are involved in children with diplegia are seen in quadriplegia and hemiplegia: hip flexors and adductors; knee flexors, especially medial hamstrings; and ankle plantar flexors. The degree of involvement among these muscles may vary, and additional muscles may also be affected. Trunk musculature may exhibit increased tone as well. Increased trunk tone may impair breath control for speech by hampering the normal excursion of the diaphragm and chest wall during inspiration and expiration.

As stated earlier, spasticity may not be present initially at birth, but it can gradually replace low muscle tone as the child attempts to move against gravity. Spasticity in CP is of cerebral origin; that is, it results from damage to the central nervous system by a precipitating event such as an intraventricular hemorrhage. *Spastic paralysis* results from a classic upper motor neuron lesion. Which muscles are affected depends on the type of CP—quadriplegia, diplegia, or hemiplegia. Figure 11–1 depicts typical involvement in these types of spastic CP.

Rigidity

Rigidity is an uncommon type of tone seen in children with CP. It indicates severe damage to deeper areas of the brain, rather than to the cortex. Muscle tone is increased to the point that postures are held rigidly, and movement in any direction is impeded.

Dyskinesia

Dyskinesia means disordered movement. *Athetosis*, the most common dyskinetic syndrome, is characterized by disordered movement of the extremities, especially within their respective midranges. Movements in the midrange are especially difficult because of the lack of postural stability on which to superimpose movement. As the limb goes farther away from the body, motor control diminishes. Involuntary movements result from attempts by the child to control posture and movement. These involuntary movements can be observed in the child's entire extremity, distally in the hands and feet, or proximally in the mouth and face. The child with athetosis must depend on external support to improve movement accuracy and efficiency. Feeding and speech difficulties can be expected if the oral muscles are involved. Speech usually develops, but the child may not be easily understood. *Athetoid* CP is characterized by decreased static and dynamic postural stability. Children with dyskinesia lack the postural stability necessary to allow purposeful movements to be controlled for the completion of functional tasks (Fig. 11–4). Muscle tone often fluctuates from low to high to normal to high such that the child has difficulty in maintaining postural alignment in all but the most

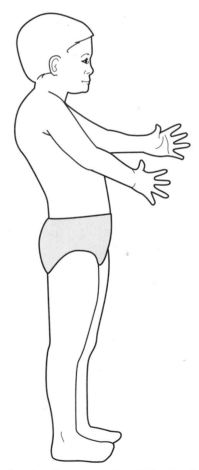

FIGURE 11–4 ■ Standing posture in a child with athetoid cerebral palsy.

firmly supported positions and exhibits slow, repetitive involuntary movements.

Ataxia

Ataxia is classically defined as a loss of coordination resulting from damage to the cerebellum. Children with ataxic CP exhibit loss of coordination and low postural tone. They usually demonstrate a diplegic distribution, with the trunk and lower extremities most severely affected. This pattern of low tone makes it difficult for the child to maintain midline stability of the head and trunk in any posture. Ataxic movements are jerky and irregular. Children with ataxic CP ultimately achieve upright standing, but to maintain this position, they must stand with a wide base of support as a compensation for a lack of static postural control (Fig. 11–5). Postural reactions are slow to develop in all postures, with the most significant balance impairment demonstrated during gait.

Children with ataxia walk with large lateral displacements of the trunk in an effort to maintain balance. Their gait is often described as "staggering" because of these wide displacements, which are a natural consequence of the lack of stability and poor timing of

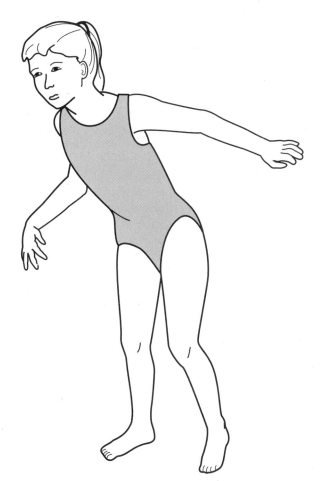

FIGURE 11–5 ■ Ataxic cerebral palsy.

postural corrections. Together, these impairments may seem to spell imminent disaster for balance, but these individuals are able, with practice, to adjust to the wide displacements in their center of gravity and to walk without falling. Wide displacements and slow balance reactions are counteracted by the wide base of support. The biggest challenge for the clinician is to allow the child to ambulate independently using what looks like ·a precarious gait. Proper safety precautions should always be taken, and some children may need to wear a helmet for personal safety. Assistive devices do not appear to be helpful during ambulation unless they can be adequately weighted, and even then, these devices may be more of a deterrent than a help. The use of weighted equipment may prevent excessive upper extremity movements. However, these arm movements are typically used as a compensatory strategy to counteract excessive truncal weight shifts.

DIAGNOSIS

Many children are not formally diagnosed as having CP until after 6 months of age. In children with a severely damaged nervous system, as in the case of quadriplegic involvement, early diagnosis may not be difficult. However, children with hemiplegia or diplegia with mild involvement may not be identified as having a problem until they have difficulty in pulling to stand at around 9 months of age. Lack of early detection may deprive these children of beneficial early intervention. Hypotonic infants who develop athetosis can usually be diagnosed by 10 to 12 months of age, according to Sweeney and Swanson (1995), but other investigators relate that diagnosis cannot occur until the child is 18 months old (Olney and Wright, 1994). Many years of research have been devoted to developing sensitive assessment tools that will allow pediatricians and pediatric physical therapists to identify infants with CP as early as 4 to 6 months of age. Observation of a child's movements in certain antigravity postures may be more revealing than testing reflexes or assessing developmental milestones (Pathways, 1992).

PATHOPHYSIOLOGY (Table 11–2)

Spastic diplegia, quadriplegia, and hemiplegia can be caused by varying degrees of intraventricular hemorrhage. Depending on which fibers of the corticospinal tract are involved and whether the damage is bilateral or unilateral, the resultant neurologic deficit manifests as quadriplegia, diplegia, or hemiplegia. *Spastic quadriplegia* is most often associated with grade III or IV intraventricular hemorrhage in extremely immature infants (Pape and Wigglesworth, 1979) or birth

Table 11–2 ▌ PATHOPHYSIOLOGY OF CEREBRAL PALSY

CAUSE	DEFICIT
Intraventricular hemorrhage	Spastic diplegia
	Spastic quadriplegia
	Spastic hemiplegia
Selective neuronal necrosis of the cerebellum	Ataxia
Status marmoratus (hypermyelination in basal ganglia)	Athetosis

Adapted from Umphred DA (ed). Neurological Rehabilitation, 3rd ed. St. Louis, CV Mosby, 1995.

asphyxia in term infants (Bennett et al, 1981). The higher the grade (number) of hemorrhage, the more severe the damage. Premature infants born at 32 weeks of gestation are especially vulnerable to decreased tissue oxygenation from decreased blood flow to the area around the ventricles where the fibers of the corticospinal tract are most exposed. This ischemia may result in *spastic diplegia*. *Spastic hemiplegia*, the most common type of CP, can result from unilateral brain damage secondary to an intraventricular hemorrhage or other anoxic event. *Athetosis* involves damage to the basal ganglia and has been associated with erythroblastosis fetalis, anoxia, and respiratory distress. *Erythroblastosis*, a destruction of red blood cells, occurs in the newborn when an Rh incompatibility of maternal-fetal blood groups exists. *Ataxia* is related to damage to the cerebellum.

ASSOCIATED DEFICITS (Table 11–3)

The deficits associated with CP are presented in the order in which they may become apparent in the infant with CP. Early signs of motor dysfunction in an infant often present as problems with feeding and breathing.

Feeding and Speech Impairments

Poor suck-swallow reflexes and uncoordinated sucking and breathing may be evidence of central nervous system dysfunction in a newborn. Persistence of infantile oral reflexes such as rooting or suck-swallow or

Table 11–3 ▌ DEFICITS ASSOCIATED WITH CEREBRAL PALSY

Feeding and speech impairments
Breathing inefficiency
Visual impairments
Hearing impairments
Mental retardation
Seizures

exaggerations of normally occurring reflexes such as a tonic bite or tongue thrust can indicate abnormal oromotor development. A hyperactive or hypoactive response to touch around and in the mouth is also possible. Hypersensitivity may be seen in the child with spastic hemiplegia or quadriplegia, whereas hyposensitivity may be evident in the child with low tone or atonic CP.

Feeding is considered a precursor to speech, so the child who has feeding problems may well have difficulty in producing intelligible sounds. Lip closure around the nipple is needed to prevent loss of liquids during sucking. Lip closure is also needed in speech to produce "p," "b," and "m" sounds. If the infant cannot bring the lips together because of tonal problems, feeding and sound production will be hindered. The tongue moves in various ways within the mouth during sucking and swallowing and later in chewing; the patterns change with oromotor development. These changes in tongue movements are crucial not only for taking in food and swallowing but also for the production of various sounds requiring specific tongue placement within the oral cavity.

Breathing Inefficiency

Breathing inefficiency may compound feeding and speech problems. Typically developing infants are belly breathers and only over time develop the ability to use the rib cage effectively to increase the volume of inspired air. Gravity promotes developmental changes in the configuration of the rib cage that place the diaphragm in a more advantageous position for efficient inspiration. This developmental change is hampered in children who are delayed in experiencing upright posture because of lack of attainment of age-appropriate motor abilities such as head and trunk control. Lack of development in the upright posture can result in structural deformities of the ribs, such as rib flaring, and functional limitations, such as poor breath control and shorter breath length that is inadequate for sound production. Abnormally increased tone in the trunk musculature may allow only short bursts of air to be expelled and produce staccato speech. Low muscle tone can predispose children to rib flaring because of lack of abdominal muscle development. Mental retardation, hearing impairment, or central language processing impairment may further impede the ability of the child with CP to develop effective oral communication skills.

Mental Retardation

Children with CP have many other problems associated with damage to the nervous system that also relate to and affect normal development. The most common of these are vision and hearing impairments,

Table 11-4 ▌ RELATIONSHIP OF SEVERITY OF CEREBRAL PALSY AND INTELLIGENCE (IQ)

SEVERITY	MOTOR FUNCTION	IQ	FUNCTIONAL LEVEL
Mild	Independent ambulation	>70	Independent
Moderate	Supported ambulation	50–70	Needs assistance
Severe	Nonambulatory	<50	Dependent

From Russman BS, Gage JR. Cerebral palsy. Curr Probl Pediatr 29:75, 1989.

feeding and speech difficulties, seizures, and mental retardation. The classification of retardation is given in Chapter 10 and is not repeated here. Although no direct correlation exists between the severity of motor involvement and the degree of mental disability, the percentage of children with CP who have mental retardation has been reported to range from 38 to 92%, depending on the type of CP. Intelligence tests require a verbal or motor response, either of which may be impaired in these children. Capute and Accardo (1996) reported that 60% of children with CP have associated mental retardation. They further suggested that children of normal intelligence who have CP may be at risk of having learning disabilities or other cognitive impairments. Russman and Gage (1989) also related intelligence quotient (IQ) to severity of CP (Table 11–4). Generally, children with spastic hemiplegia or diplegia, athetosis, or ataxia are more likely to have normal or higher than normal intelligence. Children with spastic quadriplegia, rigidity, atonia, or mixed types of CF are more likely to exhibit mental retardation (Molnar, 1985; Pellegrino, 1997). However, as with any generalizations, exceptions always exist. It is extremely important to not make judgments about a child's intellectual status based solely on the severity of the motor involvement.

Seizures

The site of brain damage in CP may become the focal point of abnormal electrical activity, which can cause seizures. Approximately 50% of children with CP experience seizures that must be managed by medication (Aksu, 1990; Gersh, 1991). A smaller percentage may have a single seizure episode related to high fever or increased intracranial pressure. Children with CP or mental retardation are more likely to develop seizures than are typically developing children. Seizures are classified as generalized, partial, or unclassified and are listed in Table 11–5. *Generalized seizures* are named for the type of motor activity the person exhibits. *Partial seizures* can be simple or complex, depending on whether the child experiences a loss of consciousness. Partial seizures can have either sensory or motor manifestations or both. *Unclassified seizures* do not fit in any other category.

Children with CP and mild mental retardation tend to exhibit partial seizures, whereas children with more severe involvement display more generalized seizures (Steffenburg et al, 1996). When working with children, the clinician should question parents and caregivers about the children's history of seizure activity. The

Table 11-5 ▌ CLASSIFICATION OF SEIZURES

INTERNATIONAL CLASSIFICATION OF SEIZURES	OLDER TERMS FOR CLASSIFYING SEIZURES	MANIFESTATIONS OF SEIZURES
Generalized seizure	Generalized seizure	Seizures that are generalized to the entire body; always involve a loss of consciousness
Tonic-clonic seizure	Grand mal seizure	Begin with a tonic contraction (stiffening) of the body, then change to clonic movements (jerking) of the body
Tonic seizure		Stiffening of the entire body
Clonic seizure	Minor motor seizure	Myoclonic jerks start and stop abruptly
Atonic seizure	Drop attacks	Sudden lack of muscle tone
Absence seizure	Petit mal seizure	Nonconvulsive seizure with a loss of consciousness; blinking, staring, or minor movements lasting a few seconds
Akinetic seizure		Lack of movement, "freezing" in place
Partial seizure	Focal seizure	Seizures not generalized to the entire body; a variety of sensory or motor symptoms may accompany this type of seizure
Simple partial seizure	Jacksonian seizure	No loss of consciousness or awareness
• With motor symptoms		Jerking may begin in one small part of the body, and spread to other parts; usually limited to one half of the body
• With sensory symptoms		Sensory aura may precede a motor seizure
Complex partial seizure	Psychomotor seizure Temporal lobe seizure	Loss of consciousness occurs during the seizure, at either the beginning or the end of the event; may develop from a simple partial seizure or develop into a generalized seizure; may include automatisms such as lip smacking, staring, or laughing
Unclassified seizure		Seizures that do not fit into the above categories including some neonatal and febrile seizures

From Ratliffe KT. Clinical Pediatric Physical Therapy. St. Louis, CV Mosby, 1998, p 410.

physical therapist assistant should always document any seizure activity observed in a child, including time of occurrence, duration, loss of consciousness, motor and sensory manifestations, and status of the child after the seizure.

Visual Impairments

Vision is extremely important for the development of balance during the first 3 years of life (Shumway-Cook and Woollacott, 1995). Any visual difficulty may exacerbate the inherent neuromotor problems that typically accompany a diagnosis of CP. Eye muscle control can be negatively affected by abnormal tone and can lead to either turning in (*esotropia*) or turning out (*exotropia*) of one or both eyes. *Strabismus* is the general term for an abnormal ocular condition in which the eyes are crossed. In *paralytic strabismus*, the eye muscles are impaired. Strabismus is present in 50% of children with CP (Capute and Accardo, 1996), with the highest incidence in children with quadriplegia and diplegia (Styer-Acevedo, 1994).

Nystagmus is most often seen in children with ataxia. In nystagmus, the eyes move back and forth rapidly in a horizontal, vertical, or rotary direction. Normally, nystagmus is produced in response to vestibular stimulation and indicates the close relationship between head movement and vision. The presence of nystagmus may complicate the task of balancing the head or trunk. Some children compensate for nystagmus by tilting their heads into extension, a move that can be mistaken for neck retraction and abnormal extensor tone. The posteriorly tilted head position gives the child the most stable visual input. Although neck retraction is generally to be avoided, if it is a compensation for nystagmus, the extended neck posture may not be avoidable. Children with hemiplegic CP may exhibit *homonymous hemianopia,* or loss of vision in half the visual field. This condition occurs in 25% of cases (Molnar, 1985).

Children with visual impairments may have more difficulty in developing head and trunk control and in exploring their immediate surroundings. Visual function should be assessed in any infant or child who is exhibiting difficulty in developing head control or in reaching for objects. Clinically, the child may not follow a familiar face or turn to examine a new face. If you suspect that a child has a visual problem, report your suspicions to the supervising physical therapist.

Hearing, Speech, and Language Impairments

Almost one third of children with CP have hearing, speech, and language problems. As already mentioned, some speech problems can be secondary to poor motor control of oral muscles or respiratory impairment.

Language difficulties in the form of expressive or receptive aphasia can result when the initial damage that caused the CP also affects the brain areas responsible for understanding speech or producing language. For most of the right-handed population, speech centers are located in the dominant left hemisphere. Clinically, the child may not turn toward sound or be able to localize a familiar voice. Hearing loss may be present in any type of CP, but it occurs in a higher percentage of children with quadriplegia. These children should be evaluated by an audiologist to ascertain whether amplification is warranted.

PHYSICAL THERAPY EVALUATION

The physical therapist conducts a thorough evaluation and examination of the child with CP that includes a history, observation, and administration of specific standardized tests of development. Test selection is based on the reason for the evaluation: screening, information gathering, treatment planning, eligibility determination, or outcomes measurement. A discussion of developmental assessment is beyond the scope of this text, and the reader is referred to Connolly and Montgomery (1993), Long and Cintas (1995), or Ratliffe (1998) for information on specific developmental assessment tools. The physical therapist assistant needs to have an understanding of the purpose of the evaluation and an awareness of the tools commonly used and of the process used within the particular treatment setting.

The physical therapist assistant should be familiar with the information reported by the physical therapist in the child's evaluation: social and medical history; range of motion; muscle tone, strength, and bulk; reflexes and postural reactions; mobility skills; transfers; activities of daily living (ADLs), recreation, and leisure; and adaptive equipment. The assistant needs to be aware of the basis on which the physical therapist makes decisions about the child's plan of care. The physical therapist's responsibility is to make sure that the goals of therapy and the strategies to be used to implement the treatment plan are thoroughly understood by the physical therapist assistant.

Neuromuscular Impairments and Functional Limitations

The physical therapy evaluation should identify the neuromuscular impairments and the present or anticipated functional limitations of the child with CP. Many physical impairments such as too much or too little range of motion or muscle extensibility can be related to the type of tone exhibited, its distribution, and the severity. Functional limitations such as lack of head control and trunk control or use of the extremities result from these impairments. In the spastic type of CP, the impairments are often related to lack of range and movement resulting from too much muscle tone. Children with athetoid or ataxic CP may have some of the same functional limitations, but their impairments are related to too much mobility and too little stability. Because the impairments and functional limitations of the child with hypotonic CP are similar to those of children with Down syndrome, the reader is referred to Chapter 10 for a discussion of intervention strategies.

Impairments and Functional Limitations in the Child with Spastic Cerebral Palsy

The child with spasticity often moves slowly and with difficulty. When movement is produced, it occurs in predictable, *stereotypical* patterns that happen the same way every time with little variability. The child with spasticity can have functional limitations in head and trunk control, performance of movement transitions, ambulation, use of the extremities for balance and reaching, and ADLs (Table 11–6).

Head Control

The child with spasticity can have difficulty in developing head control because of increased tone, persistent primitive reflexes, exaggerated tonic reflexes, or absent or impaired sensory input. Because the child often has difficulty in generating enough muscle force to maintain a posture or to move, substitutions and compensatory movements are common. For example, an infant who cannot control the head when held upright or supported in sitting may elevate the shoulders to provide some neck stability.

Trunk Control

Lack of trunk rotation and a predominance of extensor or flexor tone can impair the child's ability to roll. Inadequate trunk control prevents independent sitting. In a child with predominantly lower extremity problems, the lack of extensibility at the hips may

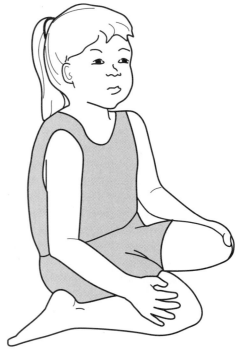

FIGURE 11–6 ■ W sitting.

prevent the attainment of an aligned sitting position. The child compensates by rounding the upper back to allow for sitting (see Fig. 11–3B). Trunk rotation can be absent or impaired secondary to a lack of balanced development of the trunk extensors and flexors. Without this balance, controlled lateral flexion is not possible, nor is rotation. Absent trunk rotation makes transitional movements, that is, moving from one posture to another, extremely difficult. The child with spasticity may discover that it is possible to achieve a sitting position by pushing the body backward over passively flexed and adducted legs, to end up in a W sitting position (Fig. 11–6). This posture should be avoided because its use can impede further development of trunk control and lower extremity dissociation.

Table 11–6 ‖ IMPAIRMENTS, FUNCTIONAL LIMITATIONS, AND FOCUS OF TREATMENT IN CHILDREN WITH SPASTICITY

IMPAIRMENTS	FUNCTIONAL LIMITATIONS	TREATMENT FOCUS
Increased muscle stiffness	Stereotypical movement patterns	Decrease stiffness, increase movement
Slow, labored movement	Poor static and dynamic balance; postural insecurity	Establish head and trunk righting and equilibrium reactions, extremity protective reactions
Decreased trunk rotation	Poor movement transitions	Practice movement transitions involving trunk rotation, i.e., rolling, coming to sit, and walking
Decreased range of motion	Reaching, walking	Increase ease of movement in all ranges; vary speed and excursion of goal-directed movements
Skeletal malalignment	Scoliosis, musculoskeletal deformities	Position properly for function; use orthoses
Muscle weakness	Movements against gravity	Strengthen through movement experiences
Inaccurate muscle recruitment	Inefficient movement; high energy cost	Use novel environments and encourage appropriate sequences of muscle activation

Influence of Tonic Reflexes

Tonic reflexes are often obligatory in children with spastic CP. When a reflex is obligatory, it dominates the child's posture. Obligatory tonic reflexes produce increased tone and postures that can interfere with adaptive movement. When they occur during the course of typical development, they do not interfere with the infant's ability to move. The retention of these reflexes and their exaggerated expression appear to impair the acquisition of postural responses such as head and neck righting reactions and use of the extremities for protective extension. The retention of these tonic reflexes occurs because of the lack of normal development of motor control associated with CP. Tonic reflexes consist of the tonic labyrinthine reflex (TLR), the asymmetric tonic neck reflex (ATNR), and the symmetric tonic neck reflex (STNR), all of which are depicted in Figure 11–7.

The TLR affects tone relative to the head's relationship with gravity. When the child is supine, the TLR causes an increase in extensor tone, whereas when the child is prone, it causes an increase in flexor tone (see Fig. 11–7A and B). Typically, the reflex is present at birth and then is integrated by 6 months. It is thought

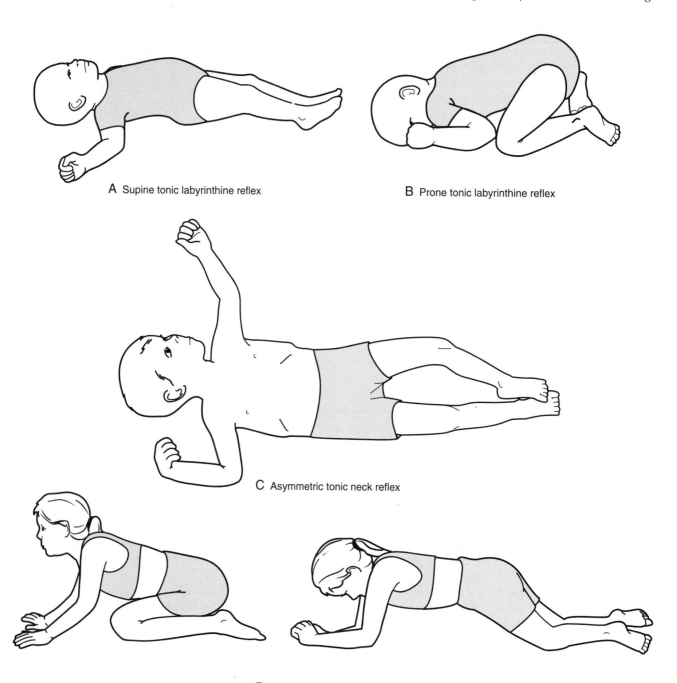

A Supine tonic labyrinthine reflex

B Prone tonic labyrinthine reflex

C Asymmetric tonic neck reflex

D Symmetric tonic neck reflex

FIGURE 11–7 ▪ Tonic reflexes.

to afford some unfolding of the flexed infant to counter the predominance of physiologic flexor tone at birth. If this reflex persists, it can impair the infant's ability to develop antigravity motion (to flex against gravity in supine and to extend against gravity in prone). An exaggerated TLR affects the entire body and can prevent the child from reaching with the arms in the supine position or from pushing with the arms in the prone position to assist in coming to sit. The TLR can affect the child's posture in sitting because the reflex is stimulated by the head's relationship with gravity. If the child loses head control posteriorly during sitting, the labyrinths sense the body as being supine, and the extensor tone produced may cause the child to fall backward and to slide out of the chair. Children who slump into flexion when the head is flexed may be demonstrating the influence of a prone TLR.

The ATNR causes associated upper extremity extension on the face side and flexion of the upper extremity on the skull side (see Fig. 11–7C). For example, turning the head to the right causes the right arm to extend and the left arm to bend. This reflex is usually apparent only in the upper extremities in a typically developing child; however, in the child with CP, the lower extremities may be affected by the reflex. The ATNR is typically present from birth to 4 to 6 months. If this reflex persists and is obligatory, the child will be prevented from rolling or bringing the extended arm to her mouth. The asymmetry can affect the trunk and can predispose the child to scoliosis. In extreme cases, the dominant ATNR can produce hip dislocation on the flexed side.

The STNR causes the arms and legs to flex or extend, depending on the head position (see Fig. 11–7D). If the child's head is flexed, the arms flex and the legs extend, and if the head is extended, vice versa. This reflex has the potential to assist the typically developing infant in attaining a four-point or hands and knees position. However, its persistence prevents reciprocal creeping and allows the child only to "bunny hop" as a means of mobility in the four-point position. When the STNR is obligatory, the arms and legs imitate or contradict the head movement. The child either sits back on the heels or thrusts forward. Maintaining a four-point position is difficult, as are any dissociated movements of the extremities needed for creeping. The exaggeration of tonic reflexes and the way in which they may interfere with functional movement by producing impairments are found in Table 11–7.

Movement Transitions

The child with spasticity often lacks the ability to control or to respond appropriately to shifts in the center of gravity that should typically result in righting, equilibrium, or protective reactions. These children

Table 11-7 | INFLUENCE OF TONIC REFLEXES ON FUNCTIONAL MOVEMENT

TONIC REFLEX	IMPAIRMENT	FUNCTIONAL MOVEMENT LIMITATION
TLR in supine	Contractures	Rolling from supine to prone
	Abnormal vestibular input	Reaching in supine
	Limited visual field	Coming to sit
		Sitting
TLR in prone	Contractures	Rolling from prone to supine
	Abnormal vestibular input	Coming to sit
	Limited visual field	Sitting
ATNR	Contractures	Segmental rolling
	Hip dislocation	Reaching
	Trunk asymmetry	Bringing hand to mouth
	Scoliosis	Sitting
STNR	Contractures	Creeping
	Lack of upper and lower extremity dissociation	Kneeling
		Walking
	Lack of trunk rotation	

ATNR, asymmetric tonic neck reflex; STNR, symmetric tonic neck reflex; TLR, tonic labyrinthine reflex.

are fearful and often do not feel safe because they have such precarious static and dynamic balance. In addition, the child's awareness of poor postural stability may lead to an expectation of falling based on prior experience. The inability to generate sufficient muscle activity in postural muscles for static balance is further compounded by the difficulty in anticipating postural changes in response to body movement; these features make performance of movement transitions such as prone to sitting or the reverse, sitting to prone, more difficult.

Mobility and Ambulation

Impaired lower extremity separation hinders reciprocal leg movements for creeping and walking; therefore, some children learn to move forward across the floor on their hands and knees by using a "bunny hopping" pattern that pulls both legs together. Other ways that the child with spasticity may attempt to move is by "commando crawling," forcefully pulling the arms under the chest and simultaneously dragging stiff legs along the floor. The additional effort by the arms increases lower extremity muscle tone in extensor muscle groups and may also interfere when the child tries to pull to stand and to cruise around furniture. The child may attain a standing position only on tiptoes and with legs crossed (Fig. 11–8). Cruising may not be possible because of a lack of lower extremity separation in a lateral direction. Walking is also limited by an absence of separation in the sagittal plane. Adequate trunk control may be lacking to provide a stable base for the stance leg, and inadequate force produc-

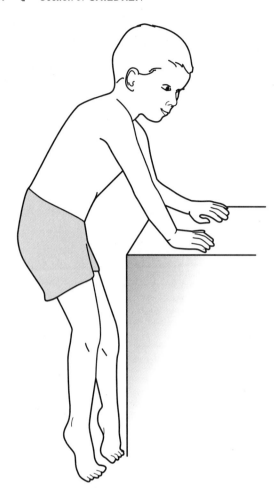

FIGURE 11-8 ■ Tiptoe standing.

Extremity Usage

Reaching in any position may be limited by an inability to bear weight on an extremity or to shift weight onto an extremity and produce the appropriate balance response. Weight bearing on the upper extremities is necessary for propped sitting and for protective extension when other balance responses fail. Lower extremity weight bearing is crucial to independent ambulation.

The child with spasticity is at risk of contractures and deformities secondary to muscle and joint stiffness and to muscle imbalances from increased tone. Spasticity may be present only in extremity muscles, whereas the trunk demonstrates low muscle tone. In an effort to overcome gravity, the child may try to use the abdominal muscles to attain sitting from a supine position. Excessive exertion can increase overall tone and can result in lower extremity extension and possible scissoring (hip adduction) of the legs through associated reactions.

Impairments and Functional Limitations in the Child with Athetosis or Ataxia

The most severe impairments and functional limitations in children with athetosis or ataxia are related to the lack of postural stability. These are listed in Table 11-8. The inability to maintain a posture is evident in the lack of consistent head and trunk control. The child exhibits large, uncompensated movements around the long axis of the body or extremities. In contrast to children with spasticity who lack movement, children with athetosis or ataxia lack postural stability. Because of this instability, the child with athetosis or ataxia may use abnormal movements such as an asymmetric tonic neck posture to provide additional stability for functional movements such as using a pointer or pushing a joystick. Overuse of this posture can predispose the child with CP to scoliosis or hip subluxation. Children with CP demonstrate impair-

tion may prevent controlled movement of the swing leg. Because of absent trunk rotation, arm movements are often used to initiate weight shifts in the lower extremities or to substitute for a lack of lower extremity movement. The arms may remain in a high-guard position to reinforce weak trunk muscles by sustaining an extended posture and thus delay the onset of arm swing.

Table 11-8 ▌ IMPAIRMENTS, FUNCTIONAL LIMITATIONS, AND FOCUS OF TREATMENT IN CHILDREN WITH ATHETOSIS

IMPAIRMENTS	FUNCTIONAL LIMITATIONS	TREATMENT FOCUS
Low or fluctuating muscle tone	Postural instability; poor balance and safety	Hold postures, cocontraction in midline
Wide, incoordinated movements	Poor movement transitions; unsafe movement	Control and direct movement with resistance; resist reciprocal movements
Lack of midrange control	Reaching, walking	Hold in midrange; work in small increments of range
Lack of use of hands for support	Poor movement transitions; unsafe movement	Weight bearing through arm; use upper extremity weight bearing for safe movement transitions
Lack of graded movement	Difficulty grasping; changing positions	Facilitate shoulder position; stabilize trunk or opposite extremity
Emotional lability	Poor judgment of balance risk	Modify behavior

ments, functional limitations, and movement dysfunction throughout their lifetime.

PHYSICAL THERAPY INTERVENTION

Four stages of care are used to describe the continuum of physical therapy management of the child with CP from infancy to adulthood. Physical therapy goals and treatment are presented within the framework of these four stages: early intervention, preschool, school age and adolescence, and adulthood.

Because the brain damage occurs in a developing motor system, the primary emphasis of physical therapy intervention is to foster motor development and to learn functional motor skills. When a child learns to move for the first time, the infant's own movements provide sensory feedback for the learning process to occur. If the feedback is incorrect or is incorrectly perceived, the movement may be learned incorrectly. Children with CP tend to develop stereotypical patterns of movement because they have difficulty in controlling movement against gravity. These stereotypical patterns interfere with developing functional motor skills. Inaccurate motor learning appears to occur in CP. The child (1) moves incorrectly, (2) learns to move incorrectly, and (3) continues to move incorrectly, thereby setting up a cycle for more and more abnormal movement. By assisting the child to experience more functional and normal movement, the clinician promotes functional movement and allows the child more independence within her environment.

The acquisition of motor milestones and of subsequent skills has to be viewed as the promotion of the child's highest possible independent level of function. Although the developmental sequence can act as a guide for formulating treatment goals and as a source of treatment activities, it should not be adhered to exclusively. Just because one skill comes before another in the typical developmental sequence does not mean that it is a prerequisite for the next skill. A good example of this concept is demonstrated by looking at the skill of creeping. Creeping is not a necessary prerequisite for walking. In fact, learning to creep may be more difficult for the child because creeping requires weight shifting and coordination of all four extremities. Little is to be gained by blindly following the developmental sequence. In fact, doing so may make it more difficult for the child to progress to upright standing.

The physical therapist is responsible for formulating and directing the plan of care. The physical therapist assistant implements interventions designed to assist the child to achieve the goals as outlined in the plan of care. Therapeutic interventions may include posi-

tioning, developmental activities, and practicing postural control within cognitively and socially appropriate functional tasks.

General Treatment Ideas

Child with Spasticity

Treatment for the child with spasticity focuses on mobility in all possible postures and transitions between these postures. The tendency to develop contractures needs to be counteracted by range of motion, positioning, and development of active movement. Areas that are prone to tightness may include shoulder adductors and elbow, wrist, and finger flexors in children with quadriplegic involvement, whereas hip flexors and adductors, knee flexors, and ankle plantar flexors are more likely to be involved in children with diplegic involvement. Children with quadriplegia can show lower extremity tightness as well. These same joints may be involved unilaterally in hemiplegia. Useful techniques to inhibit spasticity include weight bearing; weight shifting; slow, rhythmic rocking; and rhythmic rotation of the trunk and body segments. Active trunk rotation, dissociation of body segments, and isolated joint movements should be included in the treatment activities and home program. Appropriate handling can increase the likelihood that the child will receive more accurate sensory feedback for motor learning.

Advantages and Disadvantages of Different Positions

The influence of tonic reflexes on functional movement is presented in an earlier section of this chapter. The advantages of using different positions in treatment are now discussed. Both advantages and disadvantages can be found in Table 11–9. The reader is also referred to Chapter 8 for descriptions of facilitating movement transitions between positions.

Supine. Early weight bearing can be done when the child is supine, with the knees bent and the feet flat on the support surface. To counteract the total extension influence of the TLR, the child's body can be flexed by placing the upper trunk on a wedge and the legs over a bolster. Flexion of the head and upper trunk can decrease the effect of the supine TLR. Dangling or presenting objects at the child's eye level can facilitate the use of the arms for play or object exploration.

Side Lying. This position is best to dampen the effect of most of the tonic reflexes because of the neutral position of the head. Be careful not to allow lateral flexion with too thick a support under the head. It is also relatively easy to achieve protraction of the shoulders and pelvis, as well as trunk rotation, in preparation for rolling and coming to sit. The side the child is lying on is weight bearing and should be elon-

Table 11-9 ❚ ADVANTAGES AND DISADVANTAGES
OF DIFFERENT POSITIONS

POSITION	ADVANTAGES	DISADVANTAGES
Supine	Can begin early weight bearing through the lower extremities when the knees are bent and feet are flat on the support surface. Can work on elongating hamstrings in a bottoms-up position, which occurs normally in development, while counteracting STLR influence. Positioning of the head and upper trunk in forward flexion can decrease the effect of the STLR. Can facilitate use of the upper extremity in play or object exploration. Lower extremities can be positioned in flexion over a roll, ball, or bolster.	Effect of STLR can be strong and not easily overcome. Supine can be disorienting because it is associated with sleeping. The level of arousal is lowest in this position, so it may be more difficult to engage the child in meaningful activity.
Side lying	Excellent for dampening the effect of most tonic reflexes because of the neutral position of the head; achieving protraction of the shoulder and pelvis; separating the upper and lower trunk; achieving trunk elongation on the down side; separating the right and left sides of the body; and promoting trunk stability by dissociating the upper and lower trunk. Excellent position to promote functional movements such as rolling and coming to sit or as a transition from sitting to supine or prone.	It may be more difficult to maintain the position without external support or a special device such as a sidelyer. Shortening of the upper trunk muscles may occur if the child is always positioned on the same side.
Prone	Promotes weight bearing through the upper extremities (prone on elbows or extended arms); stretches the hip and knee flexors and facilitates the development of active extension of the neck and upper trunk. In young or very developmentally disabled children, it may facilitate development of head control and may promote eye-hand relationships. With the addition of a movable surface, upper extremity protective reactions may be elicited.	Flexor posturing may increase because of the influence of the PTLR; breathing may be more difficult for some children secondary to inhibition of the diaphragm, although ventilation may be better. Prone is not recommended for young children as a sleeping posture because of its relationship with an increased incidence of sudden infant death syndrome.
Sitting	Promotes active head and trunk control; can provide weight bearing through the upper and lower extremities; frees the arms for play; and may help normalize visual and vestibular input as well as aid in feeding. The extended trunk is dissociated from the flexed lower extremities. Excellent position to facilitate head and trunk righting reactions, trunk equilibrium reactions, and upper extremity protective extension. One or both upper extremities can be dissociated from the trunk. Side sitting promotes trunk elongation and rotation.	Sitting is a flexed posture. A child may be unable to maintain trunk extension because of a lack of strength or too much flexor tone. Optimal seating at 90-90-90 may be difficult to achieve and may require external support. Some floor-sitting postures such as cross-legged sitting and W sitting promote muscular tightness and may predispose to lower extremity contractures.
Quadruped	Weight bearing through all four extremities with the trunk working directly against gravity. Provides an excellent opportunity for dissociation and reciprocal movements of the extremities and a transition to side sitting if trunk rotation is possible.	The flexed posture is difficult to maintain because of the influence of the STNR, which can encourage bunny hopping as a form of locomotion. When trunk rotation is lacking, children often end up W sitting.
Kneeling	Kneeling is a dissociated posture; the trunk and hips are extended while the knees are flexed. Provides a stretch to the hip flexors. Hip and pelvic control can be developed in this position, which can be a transition to half-kneeling posture to and from side sitting or standing.	Kneeling can be difficult to control, and children often demonstrate an inability to extend at the hips completely because of the influence of the STNR.
Standing	Provides weight bearing through the lower extremities and a stretch to the hip and knee flexors and ankle plantar flexors; can promote active head and trunk control and may normalize visual input.	A significant amount of external support may be required; may not be a long-term option for the child.

PTLR, prone tonic labyrinthine reflex; STLR, supine tonic labyrinthine reflex; STNR, symmetric tonic neck reflex.
Adapted from Lemkuhl LD, Krawczyk L. Physical therapy management of the minimally-responsive patient following traumatic brain injury: coma stimulation. Neurol Rep 17:10–17, 1993.

gated. This maneuver can be done passively before the child is placed in the side lying position, or it may occur as a result of a lateral weight shift as the child's position is changed.

Prone. The prone position promotes weight bearing through the upper extremities, as well as providing some stretch to the hip and knee flexors. Head and trunk control can be facilitated by the development of

active extension as well as promoting eye-head relationships. Movement while the child is prone can promote upper extremity protective extension and weight shift.

Sitting. Almost no better functional position exists than sitting. Weight bearing can be accomplished through the extremities while active head and trunk control is promoted. An extended trunk is dissociated from flexed lower extremities. Righting and equilibrium reactions can be facilitated from this position. ADLs such as feeding, dressing, bathing, and movement transitions can all be encouraged while the child is sitting.

Quadruped. The main advantage of the four-point or quadruped position is that the extremities are all weight bearing and the trunk must work directly against gravity. The position provides a great opportunity for dissociated movements of limbs from the trunk and the upper trunk from the lower trunk.

Kneeling. As a dissociated posture, kneeling affords the child the opportunity to practice keeping the trunk and hips extended while flexed at the knees. The hip flexors can be stretched and balance responses can be practiced without having to control all the lower extremity joints. Playing in kneeling is developmentally appropriate, and with support, the child can also practice moving into half-kneeling.

Standing. The advantages of standing are obvious from a musculoskeletal standpoint. Weight bearing through the entire lower extremities is of great importance for long bone growth. Weight bearing can produce a prolonged stretch on heel cords and knee flexors while promoting active head and trunk control. Upright standing also provides appropriate visual input for social interaction with peers.

Child with Athetosis or Ataxia

Treatment for the child with athetosis focuses on stability in weight bearing and the use of developmental postures that provide trunk or extremity support. Useful techniques include approximation, weight bearing, and moving within small ranges of motion with resistance as tolerated. The assistant can use sensory cues that provide the child with information about joint and postural alignment, such as mirrors, weight vests, and heavier toys that provide some resistance but do not stop movement. Grading movement within the midrange, where instability is typically the greatest, is the most difficult for the child. Activities that may be beneficial include playing "statues," holding ballet positions, and holding any other fixed posture such as stork standing. Use of hand support in sitting, kneeling, and standing can improve the child's stability. Visually fixing on a target may also be helpful. As the child grows older, the assistant should help the child to develop safe movement strategies during customary ADLs. If possible, the child should be actively involved in discovering ways to overcome her own particular obstacles.

Valued Life Outcomes

Giangreco and colleagues (1993) identified five life outcomes that should be highly valued for all children, even those with severe disabilities:

1. Having a safe, stable home in which to live now and in the future
2. Having access to a variety of places within a community
3. Engaging in meaningful activities
4. Having a social network of personally meaningful relationships
5. Being safe and healthy

These outcomes can be used to guide goal setting for children with disabilities across the life span. Perhaps by having a vision of what life should be like for these children, we can be more future-oriented in planning and giving support to these children and their families. We must always remember that children with disabilities grow up to be adults with disabilities.

First Stage of Physical Therapy Intervention: Early Intervention (Birth to 3 Years)

Theoretically, early therapy can have a positive impact on nervous system development and recovery from injury. The ability of the nervous system to be flexible in its response to injury and development is termed *plasticity.* Infants at risk for neurologic problems may be candidates for physical therapy intervention to take advantage of the nervous system's plasticity.

The decision to initiate physical therapy intervention and at what level (frequency and duration) is based on the infant's neuromotor performance during the physical therapy evaluation and the family's concerns. Several assessment tools designed by physical therapists are used in the clinic to try to identify infants with CP as early as possible. Pediatric physical therapists need to update their knowledge of such tools continually. As previously stated, a discussion of these tools is beyond the scope of this text because physical therapist assistants do not evaluate children's motor status. However, a familiarity with tools used by physical therapists can be gained by reading the text by Campbell (1994) or Connolly and Montgomery (1993). Typical problems often identified during a physical therapy evaluation at this time include lack of head control, inability to track visually, dislike of the prone position, fussiness, asymmetric postures secondary to exaggerated tonic reflexes, tonal abnormalities, and feeding or breathing difficulties.

Early intervention usually spans the first 3 years of life. During this time, typically developing infants are establishing trust in their caregivers and are learning how to move about safely within their environment. Parents develop a sense of competence through taking care of their infant and guiding safe exploration of the world. Having a child with a disability is stressful for a family. By educating the family about the child's disability and by teaching the family ways to position, carry, feed, and dress the child, the therapist and the assistant practice family-centered intervention. The therapy team must recognize the needs of the family in relation to the child, rather than focusing on the child's needs alone. Intervention can be provided in many different ways during this time and in a variety of settings.

Periodic assessment by a pediatric physical therapist who comes into the home may be sufficient to monitor an infant's development and to provide parent education. Hospitals that provide intensive care for newborns often have follow-up clinics in which those children are evaluated at regular intervals. Instruction in home management, including specific handling and positioning techniques, is done by the therapist assigned to that clinic. Infants can be seen for ongoing therapy as outpatients in a center-based program (Easter Seals, United Cerebral Palsy) or a school, or they may be seen in the home as part of an early intervention program.

Role of the Family

The family is an important component in the early management of the infant with CP. Hanson and Lynch (1989) enumerated many factors that underscore the importance of family involvement in early intervention. These include the following:

1. Parents are the most important people in the child's life.
2. Parents have the right to make decisions regarding their child.
3. Parents have legal rights for input and decision making in the educational process.
4. Parent participation is essential for optimizing early intervention.
5. Positive parenting experiences support keeping children at home.
6. Parents can be empowered to use community resources effectively.
7. Parental involvement can ensure more fully coordinated services.
8. Parental involvement is economical.

Role of the Physical Therapist Assistant

The physical therapist assistant's role in providing ongoing therapy to infants is determined by the supervising physical therapist. The neonatal intensive care unit is not a place for a physical therapist assistant or an inexperienced physical therapist. Specific competencies must be met to practice safely within this specialized environment, and they usually require additional course work and supervised work experience.

These competencies have been identified and are available from the Section on Pediatrics of the American Physical Therapy Association.

The role of the physical therapist assistant in working with the child with CP is as a member of a team. The makeup of the team varies depending on the age of the child. During infancy, the team may be small and may consist only of the infant, parents, physician, and therapist. By the time a child is 3 years old, the rehabilitation team may have enlarged to include additional physicians involved in the child's medical management and other professionals such as an audiologist, an occupational therapist, a speech pathologist, a teacher, and a teacher's aide. The physical therapist assistant is expected to bring certain skills to the team and to the child, including knowledge of positioning and handling techniques, use of adaptive equipment, management of impaired tone, and developmental activities that foster motor abilities and movement transitions within a functional context. Because the physical therapist assistant may be providing services to the child in the home or at school, the assistant may be the first to observe additional problems or be told of a parental concern. These concerns should be communicated to the supervising therapist in a timely manner.

General goals of physical therapy in early intervention are to

1. Promote infant-parent interaction
2. Encourage development of functional skills and play
3. Promote sensorimotor development
4. Establish head and trunk control
5. Attain and maintain upright orientation

Handling and Positioning

Handling and positioning in the supine or "en face" (face-to-face) posture should promote orientation with the head in the midline and symmetry of the extremities. A flexed position is preferred so the shoulders are forward and the hands can easily come to the midline. Reaching is encouraged by making sure that objects are within the infant's grasp. Positioning with the infant prone is also important because this is the position from which the infant first moves into extension. Some infants do not like being prone, and the caregiver has to be encouraged to continue to put the infant in this position for longer periods. Carrying the infant in prone can increase the child's tolerance for the position. The infant should not sleep in prone, however, because of the increased incidence of sudden infant death syndrome in infants who sleep in this position (American Academy of Pediatrics, 1992). Carrying positions should accentuate the strengths of the infant and should avoid as much abnormal posturing as possible. The infant should be allowed to control as much of her body as possible for as long as possible before external support is given. The reader is referred to Chapter 8 for other carrying positions.

Most handling and positioning techniques are outlined in Chapter 8 and represent a neurodevelopmental treatment approach to the management of the child with CP popularized by the Bobaths. Although this approach appears to be prevalent in its use in this population, research evidence of its effectiveness over other, more eclectic approaches is minimal. As the reader is aware, neurologic development occurs at the same time at which the child's musculoskeletal and cognitive systems are maturing. Motor learning must take place if any permanent change in motor behavior is to occur. The infant should be encouraged to initiate reaching when in the supine position by being presented with visually interesting toys. Active head lifting when she is prone can be encouraged by using toys that are brightly colored or make noise.

Feeding and Respiration

A flexed posture facilitates feeding and social interaction between the child and the caregiver. The more upright the child is, the easier it is to promote a flexed posture of the head and neck. Although it is

---

Intervention 11–1 ▍ POSITIONING FOR FEEDING

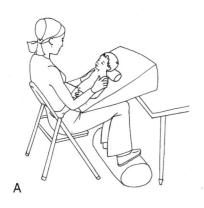

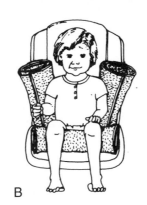

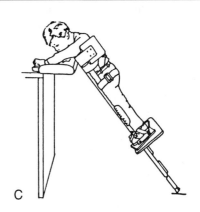

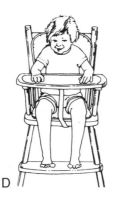

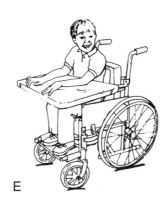

A. The face-to-face position can be used for a child who needs trunk support. Be careful that the roll does not slip behind the child's neck and encourage extension.

B. A young child is positioned for feeding in a car seat with adaptations using towel rolls.

C. A young child positioned on a prone stander is standing for mealtime.

D. A child is positioned in a highchair with adaptations for greater hip stability and symmetry during feeding.

E. A child is positioned in his wheelchair with an adapted seat insert, a tray, and hip stabilizing straps for mealtime.

A, Reprinted by permission of the publisher from Connor FP, Williamson GG, Siepp JM (eds). Program Guide for Infants and Toddlers with Neuromotor and Other Developmental Disabilities (New York: Teachers College Press, © 1978 by Teachers College, Columbia University. All rights reserved), p. 201. B through E, From Connolly BH, Montgomery PC. Therapeutic Exercise in Developmental Disabilities, 2nd ed. Chattanooga, TN, Chattanooga Group, 1993.

not appropriate for a physical therapist assistant to provide oromotor therapy for an infant with severe feeding difficulties, the physical therapist assistant could assist in positioning the infant during a therapist-directed feeding session. One example of a position for feeding is shown in Intervention 11–1A. The face-to-face position can be used for a child who needs trunk support. Be careful that the roll does not slip behind the child's neck and encourage extension. Other examples of proper body positioning for improved oromotor and respiratory functioning during mealtime are depicted in Intervention 11–1B. Deeper respirations can also be encouraged prior to feeding or at other times by applying slight pressure to the child's thorax and abdominal area prior to inspiration. This maneuver can be done when the child is in the side lying position, as shown in Intervention 11–2, or with bilateral hand placements when the child is supine. The tilt of the wedge makes it easier for the child to use the diaphragm for deeper inspiration, as well as expanding the chest wall.

Therapeutic Exercise

Gentle range-of-motion exercises may be indicated if the infant has difficulty in reaching to the midline, has difficulty in separating the lower extremities for

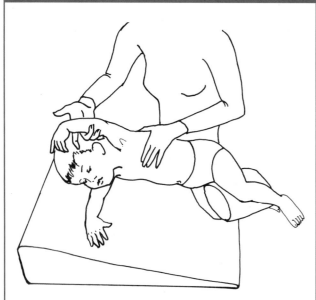

Intervention 11–2 ▌ FACILITATING DEEPER INSPIRATION

In side lying, slight pressure is applied to the lateral thorax to facilitate deeper inspiration.

diapering, or has tight heel cords. Infants do not have complete range of motion in the lower extremities normally, so the hips should never be forced into what would be considered full range of adduction or extension for an adult. Parents can be taught to incorporate range of motion into the daily routines of diapering, bathing, and dressing. The reader is referred to the instruction sheets by Jaeger (1987) as a good source of home program examples to use for maintenance of range of motion.

Motor Skill Acquisition

The skills needed for age-appropriate play vary. Babies look around and reach first from the supine position and then from the prone position, before they start moving through the environment. Adequate time playing on the floor is needed to encourage movement of the body against gravity. Gravity must be conquered to attain upright sitting and standing postures. Body movement during play is crucial to body awareness. Movement within the environment is necessary for spatial orientation to the external world. Although floor time is important and is critical for learning to move against gravity, time spent in supine and prone positions must be balanced with the benefits of being in an upright orientation. All children need to be held upright, on the parent's lap, and over the shoulder to experience as many different postures as are feasible. The reader is again referred to Chapter 8 for specific techniques that may be used to encourage head and trunk control, upper extremity usage, and transitional movements.

Functional Postures

The two most functional positions for a person are sitting and standing because upright orientation can be achieved with either position. Some children with CP cannot become functional in standing because of the severity of their motor involvement, but almost every child has the potential to be upright in sitting. Function in sitting can be augmented by appropriate seating devices, inserts, and supports.

When motor control is insufficient to allow independent standing, a standing program can be implemented. Upright standing can be achieved by using a supine or prone stander, along with orthoses for distal control. Standers provide lower extremity weight bearing while they support the child's trunk. The child is free to work on head control in a prone stander and to bear weight on the upper extremities or engage in play. In a supine stander, the child's head is supported while the hands are free for reaching and manipulation. The trunk and legs should be in correct anatomic alignment. Standing programs are typically begun when the child is around 12 to 16 months of age. The goals are to improve bone density and development and to manage contractures. Stuberg (1992) recommends standing for at least 60 minutes, four or five times per week, as a general guideline. Salter (1983) had previously reported that standing three times daily for 45 minutes controlled contractures and promoted bone development in children with CP.

Independent Mobility

Mobility can be achieved in many ways. Rolling is a form of independent mobility but one that may not be practical except in certain surroundings. Sitting and hitching (bottom scooting with or without extremity assistance) are other means of mobility and may be appropriate for a younger child. Creeping on hands and knees can be functional, but upright ambulation is still seen as the most acceptable way for a child to get around because it provides the customary and expected orientation to the world.

Ambulation Predictors

A prediction of ambulation potential can be made on the basis of the type and distribution of disordered movements, as well as by achievement of motor milestones (Table 11–10). The less of the body that is involved, the greater is the potential for ambulation. Children with spastic quadriplegia show the largest variability in their potential to walk. Children who display independent sitting by the age of 2 years or the ability to scoot along the floor on the buttocks have a good chance of ambulating (Goodman and Miedaner, 1998).

A child with CP may achieve independent ambulation with or without an assistive device. Children with

Table 11–10 ▌ PREDICTORS OF AMBULATION FOR CEREBRAL PALSY

PREDICTOR	AMBULATION POTENTIAL
By diagnosis:	
Monoplegia	100%
Hemiplegia	100%
Ataxia	100%
Diplegia	85–90%
Spastic quadriplegia	0–70%
By motor function:	
Sits independently by 2 years	100%
Sits independently by 3–4 years	50% community ambulation
Presence of primitive reactions beyond 2 years	Poor
Absence of postural reactions beyond 2 years	Poor
Independently crawled symmetrically or reciprocally by 2½–3 years	100%

From Goodman CC, Miedaner J. Genetic and developmental disorders. In Goodman C, Boissonnault WG (eds). Pathology: Implication for the Physical Therapist, Philadelphia, WB Saunders, 1998, p 580.

spastic hemiplegia are more likely to ambulate at the high end of the normal range, which is 18 months. Some researchers report a range of up to 21 months (Bleck, 1987). Typical ages for ambulation have been reported in children with spastic diplegia (Molnar and Gordon, 1976). We have observed a range of 2 to 6 years for achieving independent ambulation in this population. Other investigators have reported that if ambulation is possible, it usually takes place by the time the child is 8 years of age (Goodman and Miedaner, 1998).

Most children do not require extra encouragement to attempt ambulation, but they do need assistance and practice in bearing weight equally on their lower extremities, initiating reciprocal limb movement, and balancing. Postural reactions involving the trunk are usually delayed, as are extremity protective responses. Impairments in transitional movements from sitting to standing can impede independence. In children with hemiplegic CP, movements initiated with the involved side of the body may be avoided, with all the work of standing and walking actually accomplished by the uninvolved side.

Power Mobility

Mobility within the environment is too important for the development of spatial concepts to be delayed until the child can move on her own. Power mobility should be considered a viable option even for a young child. Some children as young as 17 to 20 months have learned to maneuver a motorized wheelchair (Butler, 1986, 1991). Just because a child is taught to use power mobility does not preclude working concurrently on independent ambulation. This point needs to be stressed to the family. Other mobility alternatives include such devices as prone scooters, adapted tricycles, riding battery-powered toys, and manual wheelchairs. The independence of moving on one's own teaches young children that they can control the environment around them, rather than being controlled.

Second Stage of Physical Therapy Intervention: Preschool Period

The major emphasis during the preschool period is to promote mobility and functional independence in the child with CP. Depending on the distribution and degree of involvement, the child with CP may or may not have achieved an upright orientation to gravity in sitting or standing during the first 3 years of life. By the preschool period, most children's social sphere has broadened to include day care attendants, babysitters, preschool personnel, and playmates, so mobility is not merely important for self-control and object interaction; it is a social necessity. All aspects of the child's being—mental, motor, and social-emotional—are developing concurrently during the preschool period in an effort to achieve functional independence.

Physical therapy goals during the preschool period are to

1. Establish a means of independent mobility
2. Promote functional movement
3. Improve performance of ADLs such as grooming and dressing
4. Promote social interaction with peers

The physical therapist assistant is more likely to work with a preschool-age child than with a child in an infant intervention program. Within a preschool setting, the physical therapist assistant implements certain aspects of the treatment plan formulated by the physical therapist. Activities may include promoting postural reactions to improve head and trunk control, teaching transitions such as moving from sitting to standing, stretching to maintain adequate muscle length for function, strengthening and endurance exercises for promoting function and health, and practice of self-care skills as part of the child's daily home or classroom schedule.

Independent Mobility

If the child with CP did not achieve upright orientation and mobility in some fashion during the early intervention period, now is the time to make a concerted effort to assist the child to do so. For children who are ambulatory with or without assistive devices and orthoses, it may be a period of monitoring and reevaluating the continued need for either the assistive or orthotic device. Some children who previously may not have required any type of assistance benefit from one now because of their changing musculoskeletal status, body weight, seizure status, or safety concerns. Their previous degree of motor control may have been sufficient for a small body, but with growth, control may be lost. Any time the physical therapist assistant observes that a child is having difficulty with a task previously performed without problems, the supervising therapist should be alerted. Although the physical therapist performs periodic reevaluations, the physical therapist assistant working with the child should request a reevaluation any time negative changes in the child's motor performance occur. Positive changes should, of course, be thoroughly documented and reported because these, too, may necessitate updating the plan of care.

Gait

Ambulation may be possible in children with spastic quadriplegia if disease involvement is not too severe. The attainment of the task takes longer, and gait may never be functional because the child requires assistance and supervision for part or all of the components of the activity. Therefore, ambulation may be considered only therapeutic, that is, another form of exercise done during therapy.

Specific gait difficulties seen in children with spastic diplegia include lack of lower extremity dissociation, decreased single-limb and increased double-limb support time, and limited postural reactions during weight shifting. Children with spastic diplegia have problems dissociating one leg from the other and dissociating leg movements from the trunk. They often fix (stabilize) with the hip adductors to substitute for the lack of trunk stability in upright necessary for initiation of lower limb motion. Practicing coming to stand over a bolster can provide a deterrent to lower extremity adduction while the child works on muscular strengthening and weight bearing (Intervention 11–3A). If the child cannot support all the body's weight in standing or during a sit-to-stand transition, have part of the child's body weight on extended arms while he practices coming to stand, standing, or shifting weight in standing (see Intervention 11–3B).

Practicing lateral trunk postural reactions may automatically result in lower extremity separation as the lower extremity opposite the weight shift is automatically abducted (Intervention 11–4). The addition of trunk rotation to the lateral righting may even produce external rotation of the opposite leg. Pushing a toy and shifting weight in step-stance are also useful activities to practice lower extremity separation. As the child decreases the time in double-limb support by taking a step of appropriate length, she can progress to stepping over an object, or to stepping up and down off a step. Single-limb balance can be challenged by using a floor ladder or taller steps. Having the child hold on to vertical poles decreases the amount of support and facilitates upper trunk extension (Fig. 11–9). Many children can benefit from using some type of assistive device such as a rolling reverse walker during gait training (Fig. 11–10). Orthoses may be needed to enhance ambulation.

Orthoses

The most frequently used orthosis in ambulatory children with CP is some type of ankle-foot orthosis (AFO). The standard AFO is a single piece of molded polypropylene. The orthosis extends 10 to 15 mm distal to the head of the fibula. The orthosis should not pinch the child behind the knee at any time. All AFOs and foot orthoses should support the foot and should maintain the subtalar joint in a neutral position. Hinged AFOs have been shown to allow a more normal and efficient gait pattern (Middleton et al, 1988). Ground reaction AFOs have been recommended by some clinicians to decrease the knee flexion seen in the crouch gait of children with spastic CP (Fig. 11–11). Other clinicians state that this type of orthotic device does not work well if the crouch results from high tone in a child with spastic diplegia (Ratliffe,

Intervention 11-3 ‖ COMING TO STAND OVER A BOLSTER

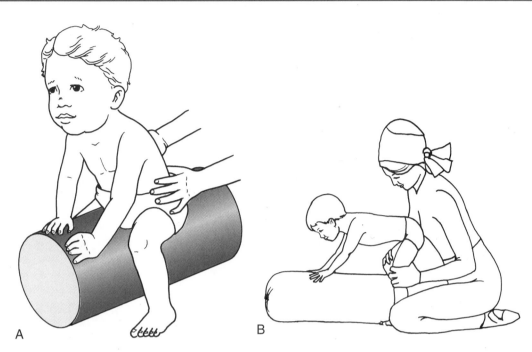

A. Practicing coming to stand over a bolster can provide a deterrent to lower extremity adduction and can work on lower extremity strengthening and weight bearing.

B. If the child cannot support all the body's weight in standing or during a sit-to-stand transition, part of the child's body weight can be borne on extended arms while the child practices coming to stand, standing, or weight shifting in standing.

A, From Campbell SK (ed). Physical Therapy for Children. Philadelphia, WB Saunders, 1994; B, Reprinted by permission of the publisher from Connor FP, Williamson GG, Siepp JM (eds). Program Guide for Infants and Toddlers with Neuromotor and Other Developmental Disabilities (New York: Teachers College Press, © 1978 by Teachers College, Columbia University. All rights reserved), p. 163.

1998). Knutson and Clark (1991) found that foot orthoses could be helpful in controlling pronation in children who do not need ankle stabilization. Dynamic AFOs have a custom-contoured soleplate that provides forefoot and hindfoot alignment.

An AFO may be indicated following surgery or casting to maintain musculotendinous length gains. The orthosis may be worn both during the day and at night. Proper precautions should always be taken to inspect the skin regularly for any signs of skin breakdown or excessive pressure. The physical therapist should establish a wearing schedule for the child. Areas of redness that last more than 20 minutes after brace removal should be reported to the supervising physical therapist.

A child with unstable ankles who needs medial lateral stability may benefit from a supramalleolar orthosis (SMO). This orthotic device allows the child to move freely into dorsiflexion and plantar flexion while restricting mediolateral movement. An SMO may be indicated for a child with mild hypertonia (Knutson

and Clark, 1991). In the child with hypotonia or athetoid CP, the SMO may provide sufficient stability within a tennis shoe to allow ambulation. General guidelines for orthotic use can be found in the article by Knutson and Clark (1991) and in the publication of Goodman and Miedaner (1998).

Assistive Devices

Some assistive devices should be avoided in this population. For example, walkers that do not require the child to control as much of the head and trunk as possible are passive and may be of little long-term benefit. When the use of a walker results in increased lower extremity extension and toe walking, a more appropriate means of encouraging ambulation should be sought. Exercise saucers can be as dangerous as walkers. Jumpers should be avoided in children with increased lower extremity muscle tone.

If a child has not achieved independent functional ambulation before the age of 3 years, some alternative type of mobility should be considered at this time. An

---

Intervention 11–4 ▍ **BALANCE REACTION ON A BOLSTER**

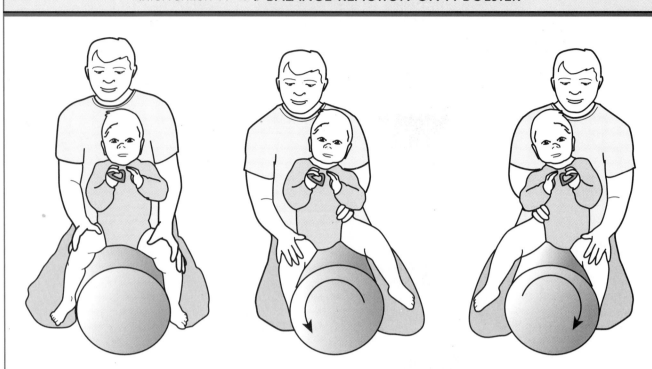

Practicing lateral trunk postural reactions may automatically result in lower extremity separation as the lower extremity opposite the weight shift is automatically abducted.

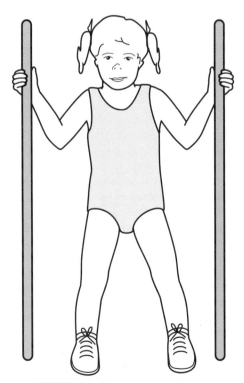

FIGURE 11-9 ■ Standing with poles.

adapted tricycle, a manual wheelchair, a mobile stander, a battery-powered scooter, and an electric wheelchair are all viable options.

Power Mobility

Children with more severe involvement, as in quadriplegia, do not have sufficient head or trunk control, let alone adequate upper extremity function, to ambulate independently even with an assistive device. For them, some form of power mobility, such as a wheelchair or other motorized device, may be a solution. For others, a more controlling apparatus such as a gait trainer may provide enough trunk support to allow training of the reciprocal lower extremity movements to propel the device (Fig. 11–12). M.O.V.E. (Mobility Opportunity Via Education, 1300 17th Street, City Centre, Bakersfield, CA 93301-4533) is a program developed by a special education teacher to foster independent mobility in children who experience difficulty with standing and walking, especially severely physically disabled children. Early work with equipment has been expanded to include a curriculum and an international organization that promotes mobility for all children. Much of the equipment is available through Rifton Equipment (P.O. Box 901, Rifton, NY 12471-1901).

For children already using power mobility, studies have shown that the most consistent use of the wheel-

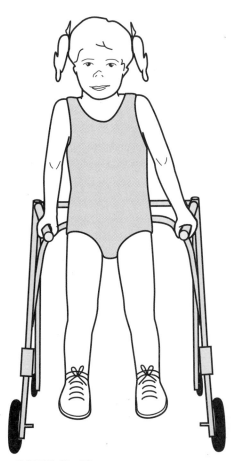

FIGURE 11-10 ∎ Walker (rolling reverse).

chair is at school. When parents and caregivers of children using power mobility were interviewed, two overriding issues were of greatest concern—accessibility and independence. Although the wheelchair was viewed as a way to foster independence in an otherwise dependent child, most caregivers stated that they had some difficulty with accessibility either in the home or in other local environments. To increase the benefit derived from a power wheelchair, the environment it is to be used in must be accessible, the needs of the caregiver must be considered, and the child must be adequately trained to develop skill in driving the wheelchair (Berry et al, 1996).

Medical Management

This section presents the medical and surgical management of children with CP because during this period of life they are most likely to require either form of intervention for spasticity or musculoskeletal deficits.

Medications

Medications used over the years to try to decrease spasticity in children with CP have met with little relative success (Pranzatelli, 1996). The most common drugs used include diazepam (Valium), baclofen (Lio-

resal), and dantrolene (Dantrium). The latter two drugs produce drowsiness as a side effect and increased drooling, which can interfere with feeding and speech (Pellegrino, 1997). The use of a pump to deliver baclofen directly to the spinal cord has been promoted. The youngest age at which a child would be considered for this approach is 3 years. It takes up to 6 months to see functional gains. The procedure is expensive, and the benefits are being studied. Because implantation of the pump is a neurosurgical procedure, further discussion is found under that heading.

Botulinum Toxin

Traditionally, spasticity has also been treated in the adult population with injections of chemical agents such as alcohol or phenol to block nerve transmission to a spastic muscle. Although this procedure is not routinely done in children with spasticity because of pain and discomfort, a new alternative has been gaining favor in the literature (Calderon-Gonzalez et al, 1994; Koman et al, 1993). Botulinum bacterium produces a powerful toxin that can inhibit a spastic muscle. If a small amount is injected into a spastic muscle group, weakness and decline of spasticity can be achieved for up to 3 to 6 months. These effects can make it easier to position a child, to fit an orthosis, to improve function, or to provide information about the appropriateness of muscle lengthening. More than one

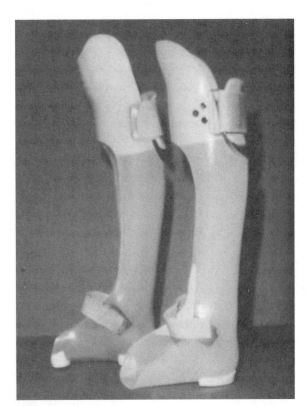

FIGURE 11-11 ∎ Ground reaction ankle-foot orthoses. (From Campbell SK [ed]. Physical Therapy for Children. Philadelphia, WB Saunders, 1994.)

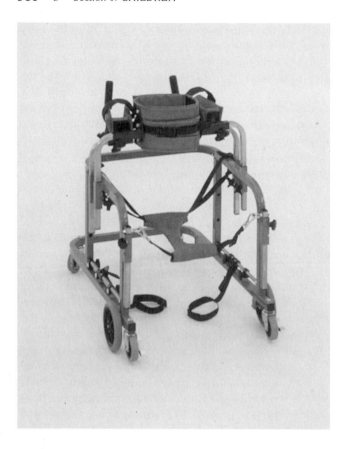

FIGURE 11–12 ■ Rifton gait trainer. (Courtesy of Rifton Equipment, Rifton, NY.)

muscle group can be injected. The lack of discomfort and ease of administration are definite advantages over motor point blocks using alcohol or phenol (Pellegrino, 1997).

Surgical Management

Orthopedic surgery is an often inevitable occurrence in the life of a child with CP. Indications for surgery may be to (1) decrease pain, (2) correct or prevent deformity, and (3) improve function. The decision to undergo an operation should be a mutual one among the physician, the family, the child, and the medical and educational team. Children with CP have dynamic problems, and surgical treatment may provide only static solutions, so all areas of the child's function should be considered. The therapist should modify the child's treatment plan according to the type of surgical procedure, postoperative casting, and the expected length of time of immobilization. A plan should be developed to address the child's seating and mobility needs and to instruct everyone how to move and position the child safely at home and school.

Surgical procedures to lengthen soft tissues are most commonly performed in children with CP and include tendon lengthening and release of spastic muscle groups. Surgical procedures to lengthen tight adductors or hamstrings may be recommended for the child to continue the best postural alignment or to maintain ambulatory status. In a *tenotomy,* the tendon is completely severed. A *partial tendon release* can include severing part of the tendon or muscle fibers or moving the attachment of the tendon. A *neurectomy* involves severing the nerve to a spastic muscle and thereby producing denervation. The child is usually placed in a spica cast or bilateral long leg casts for 6 to 8 weeks to immobilize the area.

A 3-week period of casting has been found to be useful in lengthening the triceps surae (Tardieu et al, 1982). A child with tight heel cords who has not responded to traditional stretching or to plaster casting may require surgical treatment to achieve a flat (plantigrade) foot. Surgical lengthening of the heel cord is done to improve walking (Fig. 11–13). The results of surgical treatment are more ankle dorsiflexion range and weaker plantar flexors. Overlengthening can occur, resulting in a calcaneal gait or too much dorsiflexion during stance. This condition may predispose the child to a crouched posture and the development of hamstring and hip flexion contractures (Styer-

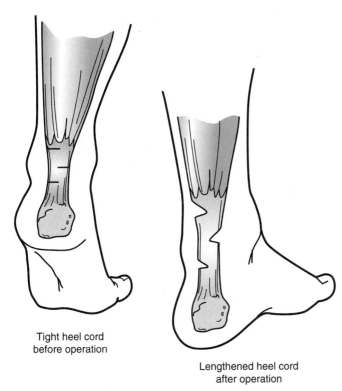

Tight heel cord
before operation

Lengthened heel cord
after operation

FIGURE 11-13 ■ Heel cord lengthening.

Acevedo, 1994). Rattey and colleagues (1993) reported that children who underwent heel cord lengthenings at 6 years of age or older did not have a recurrence of tightness.

More complex orthopedic surgical procedures may be indicated in the presence of hip subluxation or dislocation. The hip may subluxate secondary to muscle imbalances from an obligatory ATNR. The skull-side leg is pulled into flexion and adduction. Conservative treatment typically includes appropriate positioning to decrease the influence of the ATNR, passive stretching of tight muscle groups, and an abduction splint at night (Styer-Acevedo, 1994). If the hip becomes dislocated and produces pain and asymmetry, surgical treatment is indicated. The problem can be dealt with surgically in many ways, depending on its severity and acuity. The most minimal level of intervention involves soft tissue releases of the adductors, iliopsoas muscles, or proximal hamstrings. The next level requires an osteotomy of the femur in which the angle of the femur is changed by severing the bone, derotating the femur, and providing internal fixation. By changing the angle, the head of the femur is put back into the acetabulum. Sometimes, the acetabulum has to be reshaped in addition to the osteotomy. A hip replacement or arthrodesis could even be an option. Orthopedic surgical procedures are much more complex and require more lengthy immobiliza-

tion and rehabilitation. Loss of function must be considered a possible consequence of orthopedic surgical intervention.

Gait analysis in a gait laboratory can provide a clearer picture on which to base surgical decisions than visual assessment of gait. Quantifiable information about gait deviations in a child with CP is gained by observing the child walk from all angles and collecting data on muscle output and limb range of motion during the gait cycle. Video analysis and surface electromyography provide additional invaluable information for the orthopedic surgeon. This information can be augmented by temporary nerve blocks or botulinum toxin injections to ascertain the effects of possible surgical interventions.

Neurosurgery

Selective posterior or dorsal rhizotomy has become an accepted treatment for spasticity in certain children with CP (Pellegrino, 1997). Peacock and colleagues (1987) began advocating the use of this procedure, in which dorsal roots in the spinal cord are identified by electromyographic response (Fig. 11–14). Dorsal roots are selectively cut to decrease synaptic, afferent activity within the spinal cord, which decreases spasticity. Through careful selection, touch and proprioception remain intact. Candidates for this procedure have included children with spastic diplegia, hemiplegia, and quadriplegia with good cognitive abilities. Children with cerebellar or basal ganglia deficits are not good candidates. Gains in functional skills such as the ability to side sit, to stand, and to ambulate have been documented by multiple researchers (Abbott et al, 1989; Berman et al 1990; Peacock and Staudt, 1990). Other investigators, however, have been more cautious in interpreting the results and suggest the need for better controlled clinical trials because of the great variability in functional outcomes (McLaughlin et al, 1994). Following rhizotomy, a child requires intense physical therapy for 6 to 12 months postoperatively to maximize strength, range of motion, and functional skills (Ratliffe, 1998). Once the spasticity is gone, weakness and incoordination are prevalent. Any orthopedic surgical procedures that are still needed should not be performed until after this period of rehabilitation. If the child is to undergo neurosurgery, it should be completed 6 to 12 months before any orthopedic surgery (Styer-Acevedo, 1994).

Implantation of a baclofen pump is a neurosurgical procedure. "A disk-shaped pump is placed beneath the skin of the abdomen, and a catheter tunneled below the skin around to the back, where it is inserted through the lumbar spine into the intrathecal space" (Pellegrino, 1997). This placement allows the direct delivery of the medication into the spinal fluid (intrathecal space). The medication is stored inside the disk

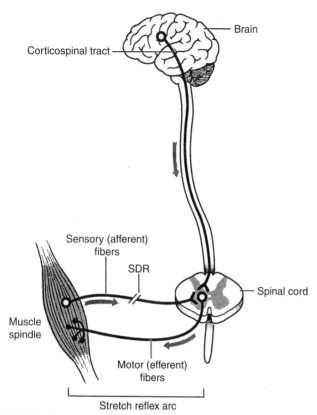

FIGURE 11–14 ▪ Selective dorsal rhizotomy (SDR). (From Batshaw ML [ed]. Children with Developmental Disabilities, 4th ed. Baltimore, Paul H. Brookes, 1997.)

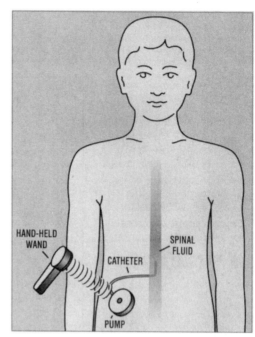

FIGURE 11–15 ▪ Baclofen pump. (Courtesy of Medtronic, Inc.)

and can be refilled by injection through the skin. It is continuously given, with the dosage adjustable and controlled by a computer (Fig. 11–15). According to Albright (1997), the greatest advantages are the adjustable dosages, with a resulting real decrease in spasticity. Lower amounts of medication can be given because the drug is delivered to the site of action, with fewer systemic complications.

Functional Movement

Strength and endurance are incorporated into functional movements against gravity and can be repeated continuously over the course of a typical day. Kicking balls, carrying objects of varying weights, reaching overhead for dressing or undressing, pulling pants down and up for toileting, and climbing or walking up and down stairs and ramps can be used to promote strength, endurance, and coordination. Endurance can be promoted by having a child who can ambulate use a treadmill (Fig. 11–16) or through dancing or playing tag during recess. Preschool is a great time to foster an appreciation of physical activity that will carry over to a lifetime habit.

Use of positioning can provide a prolonged static stretch. Manual stretching of those muscles most likely to develop contractures should be incorporated into

the child's functional tasks. Positions used while dressing, eating, and sleeping should periodically be reviewed with the parents by a member of the therapy team. Stretching may need to be part of a therapy program in addition to part of the home program conducted by the child's parents. The most important

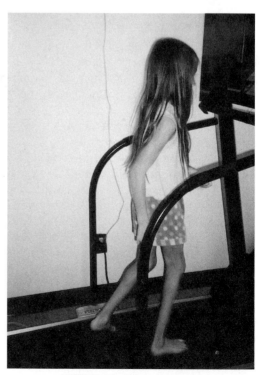

FIGURE 11–16 ▪ Treadmill.

positions for a preschooler are sitting in a chair, standing, lying, and sitting on the floor to play. Teachers should be made aware of the importance of varying the child's position during the day. If a preschooler cannot stand on her own, a standing program should be incorporated into the daily classroom and home routine. Such a standing program may well be carried over from a program started when the child was younger. Standing devices are pictured in Chapter 8.

Activities of Daily Living and Peer Interaction

While the child is in preschool, the ability to perform ADLs may not seem to be an important issue; however, if it takes a child with CP twice as long to toilet than her classmates, what she misses is the social interaction during snack time and on the playground. Social-emotional development depends on interactions among peers, sharing secrets, pretend play, and learning game playing. Making these opportunities available to the child with CP may be one of the most important things we can do in physical therapy because these interactions help to form the child's self-image and social competence. Immobility and slow motor performance can create social isolation. Always take the child's level of cognitive ability into consideration when you select a game or activity to incorporate into therapy. If therapy takes place in an outpatient setting, the clinician should plan an activity that will keep the child's interest and will also accomplish predetermined movement goals. When therapy is incorporated into the classroom, the activity to be carried out by the child may have already been selected by the teacher. The assistant may need to be creative by using an alternative position to assist the child to improve performance within the context of the classroom activity. Some classroom periods such as free play or story time may be more easily adapted for therapeutic intervention.

Function in sitting can be augmented by the use of assistive technology such as communication devices and environmental controls. The child can use eye, head, or hand pointing to communicate or to activate other electronic devices. Children with neuromotor dysfunction should also achieve upright orientation to facilitate social interaction. McEwen (1992) studied interactions between disabled students and teachers and found that when students with disabilities were in a more upright position, such as sitting rather than on the floor, the level of interaction increased.

Third Stage of Physical Therapy Intervention: School Age and Adolescence

During the next two major periods of development, the focus of physical therapy intervention is to safeguard all previous gains. This may be easier said than done because the school-age child may be understandably and appropriately more interested in the school environment and in friends than in physical therapy.

Self-Responsibility and Motivation

The school-age child should also be taking some degree of responsibility for her own therapy program. An exercise record in the form of a calendar may be a way to motivate the younger child to perform exercises on a routine basis. A walking program may be used to work on increasing endurance and cardiovascular fitness. Finding an activity that motivates the student to improve her performance may be as simple as timing an obstacle course, increasing the time spent on a treadmill, or improving the number of repetitions. Everyone loves a contest. Find out what important motor task the student wants to accomplish. Can she carry a tray in the cafeteria (Fig. 11–17)? Does she want to be able to dribble a basketball or pedal a bicycle?

Adolescents are notorious for ignoring adults' directions, so lack of interest in therapy can be especially trying during this period. However, adolescence can work in favor of compliance with physical therapy goals if the student becomes so concerned about appearances that she is willing to work harder to modify a gait deviation or to decrease a potential contracture. Some teenagers may find it more difficult to ambulate the longer distances required in middle school, or

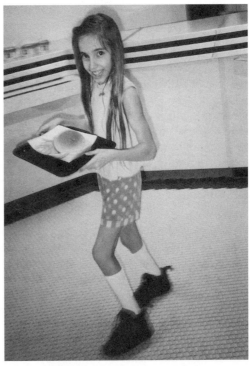

FIGURE 11–17 ■ Carrying a tray.

they may find that they do not have the physical stamina to carry books and make multiple trips to and from their lockers and still have energy to focus attention in the classroom. In addition to dealing with changing physical demands, the student at this age has to deal with the ever-present reality that she is different from the majority of her classmates. Poor endurance in performing routine self-care and personal hygiene functions can cause difficulty as the teen demands more privacy and seeks personal independence while still requiring physical assistance.

Physiologic Changes

Other great potential hazards to continued independent motor performance are the physical and physiologic changes brought on by adolescence. Greater growth of the lower extremities in relation to the trunk and upper body can produce a less stable gait. Growth spurts in which muscle length does not keep up with changes in bone length can cause problems with static and dynamic balance.

During periods of rapid growth, bone length may outstrip the attached muscles' ability to elongate, with resulting potential contracture formation. The development of such contractures may contribute to a loss of independent mobility or to a loss in movement efficiency. In other words, the student may have to work harder to move. Some teens may fall with increasing frequency. Others may limit distances walked in an effort to preserve function or to save energy for school-related tasks and learning. Any change in functional ambulation ability should be reported to the supervising physical therapist so the therapist can evaluate the need for a change in the student's treatment plan. The student may benefit from a change in either assistive device or orthosis. In some instances, the loss of functional upright ambulation is a real possibility, and a wheelchair evaluation may be warranted.

Another difficulty that can arise during this period is related to body mass changes secondary to the adolescent's growth. Increasing body weight compared with a disproportionately smaller muscle mass in the adolescent with CP can represent a serious threat to continued functional independence.

Physical therapy goals during the school years and through adolescence are to

1. Continue independent mobility
2. Develop independent ADL and instrumental ADL skills
3. Foster fitness and development of a positive self-image
4. Foster community integration
5. Develop a vocational plan
6. Foster social interaction with peers

Independence

Strength

Studies have shown that adolescents with CP can increase strength when they are engaged in a program of isokinetic resistance exercises (MacPhail, 1995). The use of traditional electrical stimulation or functional electric stimulation has also been reported in the literature (Carmick, 1993). More recently, therapeutic electric stimulation was promoted to improve muscle mass in children with CP, but few research data are available on this topic (Pape et al, 1993).

Fitness

Students with physical disabilities such as CP are often unable to participate fully in physical education. If the physical education teacher is knowledgeable about adapting routines for students with disabilities, the student may experience some cardiovascular benefits. The neuromuscular deficits affect the ability of a student with CP to perform exercises. Students with CP have higher energy costs for routine activities. Studies done in Canada and Scandinavia have shown improvements in walking speed and other motor skills when students were involved in exercise programs (Bar-Or, 1990; Berg, 1970; Sommer, 1971). Dresen and colleagues (1985) showed a reduction in the oxygen cost of submaximal activities after a 10-week training program. Fitness in all students with disabilities needs to be fostered as part of physical therapy, to improve overall health and quality of life.

Availability of recreation and leisure activities that are appropriate and accessible can be almost nonexistent for the student with a disability. It is no less important for the individual with a disability to remain physically active and to achieve some degree of health-related fitness than it is for a nondisabled person. Recreational and leisure activities, sports-related or not, should be part of every adolescent's free time. Swim programs at the YMCA, local athletic club, or elsewhere provide wonderful opportunities to socialize, develop and improve cardiovascular fitness, control weight, and maintain joint and muscle integrity. Wheelchair athletics may be an option for school-age children or adolescents in places with junior wheelchair sports programs.

Community Integration

Accessibility is an important issue in transportation and in providing disabled students easy entrance to and exit from community buildings. Accessibility is often a challenge to a teenager who may not be able to drive because of CP. Every effort should be made to support the teenager's ability to drive a motor vehicle, because the freedom this type of mobility provides is important for social interaction and vocational pursuits.

Fourth Stage of Physical Therapy Intervention: Adulthood

Physical therapy goals during adulthood are to foster

1. Independence in mobility and ADLs
2. Healthy lifestyle
3. Community participation
4. Independent living
5. A vocation

Even though five separate goals are identified for this stage of rehabilitation, they are all part of the life role of an adult. Society expects adults to live on their own and to participate within the community where they live and work. This can be the ultimate challenge to a person with CP or any lifelong disability. Living facilities that offer varied levels of assisted living are beginning to be available in some communities. Adults with CP may live on their own, in group homes, in institutions, or in nursing homes. Some continue to live at home with aging parents or with older siblings. Employment figures are almost nonexistent for this population (Olney and Wright, 1994). Factors that determine the ability of an adult with CP to live and work independently are cognitive status, degree of functional limitations, and adequacy of social and financial support.

The outcomes described by Giangreco and colleagues (1993) are repeated here to reinforce the need to use them as guides for goal-setting for persons with disabilities across the life span:

1. Having a safe, stable home in which to live now and in the future
2. Having access to a variety of places within a community
3. Engaging in meaningful activities
4. Having a social network of personally meaningful relationships
5. Being safe and healthy

When we have a vision of what life should be like for these children, we can be more future-oriented in planning and giving support to the children and their families. Children with disabilities grow up to be adults with disabilities, but when these five life outcomes are kept in mind, the person comes first, not the disability.

CHAPTER SUMMARY

The child with CP presents the physical therapist and the physical therapist assistant with a lifetime of goals to attain. These goals revolve around the child's achievement of some type of mobility and mastery of the environment, including the ability to manipulate objects, to communicate, and to demonstrate as much independence in physical, psychologic, and social function as possible. The needs of the child with CP and her family change in relation to the child's maturation and reflect the family's priorities at any given time. Physical therapy may be one of many therapies the child receives. Physical therapists and physical therapist assistants are part of the team working to provide the best possible care for the child within the context of the family, school, and community. Regardless of the stage of physical therapy management, the long-term goal must always be to maximize the individual child's capabilities to achieve a maximum level of function and an optimum quality of life.

REVIEW QUESTIONS

1. Why may the clinical manifestations of CP appear to worsen with age even though the pathologic features are static?
2. Name the two greatest risk factors for CP.
3. What is the most common type of abnormal tone seen in children with CP?
4. How may abnormal tonic reflexes interfere with acquisition of movement in a child with CP?
5. Compare and contrast the focus of physical therapy intervention in a child with spastic CP and in a child with athetoid CP.
6. What is the role of the physical therapist assistant when working with a preschool-age child with CP?
7. What type of orthosis is most commonly used by children with CP who ambulate?
8. At what age should a child with CP begin to take some responsibility for her therapy program?
9. What medications are used to manage spasticity in children with CP?
10. What are the expected life outcomes that should be used as a guide for goal setting with children with disabilities?

REHABILITATION UNIT INITIAL EVALUATION: JENNIFER

Chart Review: Jennifer is a 6-year-old girl with spastic diplegic CP. She was born at 28 weeks of gestation, required mechanical ventilation, and sustained a left intraventricular hemorrhage. She received physical therapy as part of an infant intervention program. She sat at 18 months of age. At 3 years of age, she made the transition into a school-based preschool program. She had two surgical procedures for heel cord tendon transfers and adductor releases of the hips. She is now making the transition into a regular first grade. Jennifer has a younger sister. Both parents work. Her father brings her to weekly outpatient therapy. Jennifer goes to day care or to her grandparents' home after school.

SUBJECTIVE

Jennifer's parents are concerned about her independence in the school setting.

OBJECTIVE

Physical Therapy Examination

Peabody Developmental Motor Scales (PDMS) Developmental Motor Quotient (DMQ) = 69.
Age equivalent of 12 months. Fine-motor development is average for her age (PDMS DMQ = 90).

Range of Motion

	Active		Passive	
	R	L	R	L
Hip				
Flexion	0–100°	0–90°	0–105°	0–120°
Adduction	0–15°	0–12°	0–5°	0–12°
Abduction	0–30°	0–40°	0–30°	0–40°
Internal rotation	0–25°	0–78°	0–83°	0–84°
External rotation	0–26°	0–30°	0–26°	0–40°
Knee				
Flexion	0–80°	0–80°	0–120°	0–120°
Extension	–15°	–15°	Neutral	Neutral
Ankle				
Dorsiflexion	Neutral	Neutral	0–20°	0–20°
Plantarflexion	0–8°	0–40°	0–30°	0–40°
Inversion	0–5°	0–12°	0–5°	0–20°
Eversion	0–30°	0–30°	0–50°	0–40°

Muscle Tone: Moderately increased tone is present in the hamstrings, adductors, and plantar flexors bilaterally.

Reflexes: Patellar 3+, Achilles 3+, Babinski present bilaterally.

Posture: Jennifer demonstrates a functional curvature of the spine with the convexity to the right. The right shoulder and pelvis are elevated. Jennifer lacks complete thoracic extension in standing. The pelvis is rotated to the left in standing.

Leg Length: Leg length is 23.5 inches bilaterally measured from ASIS to medial malleolus.

Postural Reactions: Incomplete trunk righting with any displacement in sitting. No trunk rotation present with lateral displacements in sitting. Upper extremity protective reactions present in all directions in sitting. Jennifer stands alone for 3 to 4 minutes every trial. She exhibits no protective stepping when she loses balance in standing.

Strength: Upper extremity strength appears to be WFL because Jennifer can move her arms against gravity and take moderate resistance. Lower extremity strength is difficult to determine in the presence of increased tone.

Mobility: Jennifer ambulates independently using solid polypropylene AFOs with a reverse-facing walker for short distances (15 feet). She can take five steps independently before requiring external support for balance. She goes up and down stairs alternating feet and using a hand rail. She can maneuver her walker up and down a ramp and a curb. Jennifer requires assistance to move about with her walker in the classroom.

Movement Transitions: Jennifer can roll to either direction and can achieve sitting by pushing up from side lying. She can get into a quadruped position from prone and can pull herself into kneeling. She attains standing by moving into half-kneeling with upper extremity support. She can come to stand from sitting in a chair without hand support but adducts her knees to stabilize her legs.

Self-care: Jennifer is independent in eating and in toileting with grab bars. She requires moderate assistance with dressing secondary to balance.

REHABILITATION UNIT INITIAL EVALUATION: JENNIFER *Continued*

ASSESSMENT

Jennifer is a 6-year-old girl with moderately severe spastic diplegic CP. She is independently ambulatory with a reverse-facing walker and AFOs for short distances on level ground. She attends a regular first grade class. Rehabilitation potential for the following goals is good.

Problem List

1. Dependent in ambulation without an assistive device
2. Impaired strength and endurance to perform age-appropriate motor activities
3. Impaired dynamic sitting and standing balance
4. Dependent in dressing

Short-Term Goals (actions to be achieved by midyear review)

1. Jennifer will ambulate independently within her classroom.
2. Jennifer will perform weight shifts in standing while throwing and catching a ball.
3. Jennifer will walk on a treadmill with arm support for 10 consecutive minutes.
4. Jennifer will ambulate 25 feet without an assistive device three times a day.
5. Jennifer will don and doff AFOs, shoes, and socks, independently.

Long-Term Goals (end of first grade)

1. Jennifer will ambulate independently without an assistive device on level surfaces.
2. Jennifer will be able to go up and down a set of three stairs, step over step, without holding onto a railing.
3. Jennifer will walk continuously for 20 minutes without resting.
4. Jennifer will dress herself for school in 15 minutes.

PLAN

1. Increase dynamic trunk postural reactions by using a movable surface to shift her weight and to facilitate responses in all directions.
2. Practice coming to stand while sitting astride a bolster. One end of the bolster can be placed on a stool of varying height to decrease the distance needed for her to move from sitting to standing. Begin with allowing her to use hand support and then gradually withdraw it.
3. Practice stepping over low objects, first with upper extremity support and again gradually withdraw the support. Then practice stepping up and down one step without the railing, by giving manual support at the hips.
4. Begin walking on a treadmill with hand support. Set at a slow speed for 5 minutes. Gradually increase the time. Once she can tolerate 15 minutes, begin to increase speed.
5. Time her ability to maneuver an obstacle course involving walking, stepping over objects, moving around objects, going up and down stairs, and throwing a ball and beanbags, and keep track of her personal best time. Vary the complexity of the tasks according to her latest motor accomplishments.
6. Participate in the family instruction and home exercise program.

FOLLOW-UP

Jennifer is now 12 years old. Secondary to rapid growth, especially in her lower extremities and extensive hip and knee flexion contractures, she is once again ambulating with a reverse-facing wheeled walker. She is able to stand independently for 5 seconds and to take 13 steps before falling or requiring external support. She has been evaluated for surgical releases, but the gait studies indicate significant lower extremity weakness and increased co-contraction of lower extremity muscles during gait. The orthopedist believes that she would not have sufficient strength to ambulate following surgery. Physical therapy goals are to increase hip and knee range of motion, gluteus maximus, quadriceps, and ankle musculature strength and to regain the ability to ambulate independently without an assistive device. What treatment interventions could be used to attain these functional goals?

Continued on following page

REHABILITATION UNIT INITIAL EVALUATION: JENNIFER *Continued*

QUESTIONS TO THINK ABOUT

- What interventions could be part of Jennifer's home exercise program?

- How is fitness being incorporated into her physical therapy program?

REFERENCES

Abbott R, Forem SL, Johann M. Selective posterior rhizotomy for the treatment of spasticity: a review. Childs Nerv Syst 5:337–346, 1989.

Aksu F. Nature and prognosis of seizures in patients with cerebral palsy. Dev Med Child Neurol 32:661–668, 1990.

Albright AL. Baclofen in the treatment of cerebral palsy. J Child Neurol 11:77–83, 1997.

American Academy of Pediatrics AAP Task Force on Infant Positioning and SIDS. Positioning and SIDS. Pediatrics 90:264, 1992.

Bar-Or O. Disease-specific benefits of training in the child with a chronic disease: what is the evidence? Pediatr Exerc Sci 2:384–394, 1990.

Bennett FC, Chandler SL, Robinson NM, et al. Spastic diplegia in premature infants: etiologic and diagnostic considerations. Am J Dis Child 135:732, 1981.

Berg K. Adaptation in cerebral palsy of body composition, nutrition and physical working capacity at school age. Acta Paediatr Scand Suppl 204, 1970.

Berman B, Vaughan CL, Peacock WJ. The effect of rhizotomy on movement inpatients with cerebral palsy. Am J Occup Ther 44:511–516, 1990.

Berry ET, McLaurin SE, Sparling JW. Parent/caregiver perspectives on the use of power wheelchairs. Pediatr Phys Ther 8:146–150, 1996.

Bleck EE. Orthopedic Management of Cerebral Palsy. Philadelphia, JB Lippincott, 1987.

Butler C. Effects of powered mobility on self-initiated behaviors of very young children with locomotor disability. Dev Med Child Neurol 28:325–332, 1986.

Butler C. Augmentative mobility: why do it? Phys Med Rehabil Clin North Am 2:801–815, 1991.

Calderon-Gonzalez R, Calderon-Sepulvedo R, Rincon-Reyes M, et al. Botulinum toxin A in management of cerebral palsy. Pediatr Neurol 10:284–288, 1994.

Campbell SK (ed). Physical Therapy for Children. Philadelphia, WB Saunders, 1994.

Capute AJ, Accardo PJ. Cerebral palsy: the spectrum of motor dysfunction. In Capute AJ, Accardo PJ (eds). Developmental Disabilities in Infancy and Childhood, vol 2: The Spectrum of Developmental Disabilities, 2nd ed. Baltimore, Paul H. Brookes, 1996, pp 81–94.

Carmick J. Clinical use of neuromuscular electrical stimulation for children with cerebral palsy. I. Lower extremity. Phys Ther 73:505–513, 1993.

Connolly BH, Montgomery PC. Therapeutic Exercise in Developmental Disabilities, 2nd ed. Chattanooga, TN, Chattanooga Group, 1993.

Dresen MH, de Groot G, Mesa Menor JR, et al. Aerobic energy expenditure of handicapped children after training. Arch Phys Med Rehabil 66:302–306, 1985.

Gersh ES. Medical concerns and treatments. In Geralis E (ed). Children with Cerebral Palsy: A Parent's Guide. Bethesda, MD, Woodbine, 1991.

Giangreco MF, Cloninger CH, Iverson VS. Choosing Options and Accommodations for Children: A Guide to Planning Inclusive Education. Baltimore, Paul H. Brookes, 1993.

Goodman C, Miedaner J. Genetic and developmental disorders. In Goodman C, Boissonnault WG (eds). Pathology: Implications for the Physical Therapist. Philadelphia, WB Saunders, 1998, pp 577–616.

Graham EM, Morgan MA. Growth before birth. In Batshaw M (ed.) Children With Disabilities, 4th ed. Baltimore, Paul H. Brookes, 1997, pp 53–69.

Hanson MJ, Lynch EW. Early Intervention: Implementing Child and Family Services for Infants and Toddlers Who Are At-Risk or Disabled. Austin, TX, Pro Ed, 1989.

Jaeger L. Home program instruction sheets for infants and young children, 1987. (Available from Therapy Skill Builders, 3830 East Bellevue, PO Box 42050, Tuscon, AZ 85733.)

Knutson LM, Clark DE. Orthotic devices for ambulation in children with cerebral palsy and myelomeningocele. Phys Ther 71:947–960, 1991.

Koman LA, Mooney JF III, Smith BP, et al. Management of spasticity in cerebral palsy with botulinum A toxin: report of a preliminary, randomized, double-blind trial. J Pediatr Orthop 14:299–303, 1993.

Kuban KCK, Leviton A. Cerebral palsy. N Engl J Med 330:188–195, 1994.

Long TM, Cintas HL. Handbook of Pediatric Physical Therapy. Baltimore, Williams & Wilkins, 1995.

MacPhail H. The effect of isokinetic strength training on functional mobility and walking efficiency in adolescents with cerebral palsy. Dev Med Child Neurol 37:763–776, 1995.

McEwen IR. Assistive positioning as a control parameter of social-communicative interactions between students with profound multiple disabilities and classroom staff. Phys Ther 72:534–647, 1992.

McLaughlin FJ, Bjornson KF, Astley SJ, et al. The role of selective dorsal rhizotomy in cerebral palsy: critical evaluation of a perspective clinical series. Dev Med Child Neurol 36:755–69, 1994.

Middleton EA, Hurley GR, McIlwain JS. The role of rigid and hinged polypropylene ankle-foot orthoses in the management of cerebral palsy: a case study. Prosthet Orthot Int 12:129–135, 1988.

Molnar GE (ed). Pediatric Rehabilitation. Baltimore, Williams & Wilkins, 1985.

Molnar GE, Gordon SU. Cerebral palsy: predictive value of selected signs for early prognostication of motor function. Arch Phys Med Rehabil 56:153–158, 1976.

Nelson KB. Epidemiology and etiology of cerebral palsy. In Capute AJ, Accardo PJ (eds). Developmental Disabilities in Infancy and Childhood, vol 2: The Spectrum of Developmental Disabilities, 2nd ed. Baltimore, Paul H. Brookes, 1996, pp 73–79.

Nelson KB, Ellenberg JH. Antecedents of cerebral palsy. I. Univariate analysis of risks. Am J Dis Child 139:1031–1038, 1985.

Olney SJ, Wright MJ. Cerebral palsy. In Campbell SK (ed). Physical Therapy in Children. Philadelphia, WB Saunders, 1994, pp 489–523.

Paneth N, Kiely JL. The frequency of cerebral palsy: a review of population studies in industrialized nations since 1950. Clin Dev Med 87:46–56, 1984.

Pape KE, Wigglesworth JS. Hemorrhage, ischemia and perinatal brain. Clin Dev Med 69/70, 1979.

Pape KE, Kirsch SE, Galil A, et al. Neuromuscular approach to the motor deficits of cerebral palsy: a pilot study. J Pediatr Orthop 13:628–633, 1993.

Pathways Awareness Foundation. Early Infant Assessment Redefined.

Chicago, Pathways Awareness Foundation, 1992. (Video available from Pathways Awareness Foundation, 123 North Wacker Drive, Chicago, IL 60606.)

Peacock WJ, Arens LF, Berman B. Cerebral palsy spasticity: selective dorsal rhizotomy. Pediatr Neurosci 13:61–66, 1987.

Peacock WJ, Staudt LA. Spasticity in cerebral palsy and the selective posterior rhizotomy procedure. J Child Neurol 5:179–185, 1990.

Pellegrino L. Cerebral palsy. In Batshaw ML (ed). Children with Developmental Disabilities, 4th ed. Baltimore, Paul H. Brookes, 1997, pp 499–528.

Pranzatelli MR. Oral pharmacotherapy for the movement disorders of cerebral palsy. J Child Neurol 11: S13–S22, 1996.

Ratliffe KT. Clinical Pediatric Physical Therapy. St. Louis, CV Mosby, 1998.

Rattey TE, Leahey L, Hyndman J, et al. Recurrence after Achilles tendon lengthening in cerebral palsy. J Pediatr Orthop 134:184–147, 1993.

Russman BS, Gage JR. Cerebral palsy. Curr Probl Pediatr 19:65–111, 1989.

Salter RB. Textbook of Disorders and Injuries of the Musculoskeletal System, 2nd ed. Baltimore, Williams & Wilkins, 1983, pp 5–14.

Schumway-Cook A, Woollacott MH. Development of postural control. In Schumway-Cook A, Woollacott MH (eds). Motor Control: Theory and Practical Applications. Baltimore, Williams & Wilkins, 1995, pp 143–168.

Sommer M. Improvement of motor skills and adaptation of the circulatory system in wheelchair-bound children in cerebral palsy. Lecture No. 11. In Simon U (ed). Sports as a Means of Rehabilitation. Netanya, Wingate Institute, 1971, pp 1–11.

Stanley FJ. Survival and cerebral palsy in low birth weight infants: implication for perinatal care. Paediatr Perinat Epidemiol 6:298–310, 1991.

Steer PJ. Premature labour. Arch Dis Child 66:1167–1170, 1991.

Steffenburg U, Hagberg G, Kyllerman M. Characteristics of seizures in a population-based series of mentally retarded children with active epilepsy. Epilepsia 37:850–856, 1996.

Stuberg WA. Considerations related to weight-bearing programs in children with developmental disabilities. Phys Ther 72:35–40, 1992.

Styer-Acevedo J. Physical therapy for the child with cerebral palsy. In Tecklin JS (ed). Pediatric Physical Therapy, 2nd ed. Philadelphia, JB Lippincott, 1994, pp 89–134.

Sweeney JK, Swanson MW. Neonatal care and follow-up for infants at neuromotor risk. In Umphred DA (ed). Neurologic Rehabilitation, 3rd ed. St. Louis, Mosby–Year Book, 1995, pp 203–262.

Tardieu G, Tardieu C, Colbeau-Justin P, et al. Muscle hypoextensibility in children with cerebral palsy. II. Therapeutic implications. Arch Phys Med Rehabil 63:103–107, 1982.

ANSWERS TO THE REVIEW QUESTIONS

Chapter 1

1. An impairment is an alteration in an anatomic, physiologic, or psychologic structure or function.
2. Factors that affect an individual's performance of functional activities include personal characteristics such as physical ability, emotional status, and cognitive ability; the environment in which the person functions; and expectations placed on the individual by family and the community.
3. Prior to delegating the care of any patient to the physical therapist assistant, the primary physical therapist must critically evaluate the patient's condition, consider the patient's medical stability, review the practice setting in which therapy will be provided, and assess the type of intervention the pa-

tient is to receive. In addition, the assistant's knowledge base and level of experience must also be considered to determine whether the patient's care should be delegated.
4. The physical therapist assistant is expected to provide therapeutic interventions to improve the patient's functional skills or, if working with a child, to assist the child in acquisition of functional motor skills and movement transitions. In addition, the physical therapist assistant participates in patient and family teaching and patient care conferences and provides input into the patient's discharge plan.

Chapter 2

1. The nervous system is divided into two parts, the central nervous system and the peripheral nervous system.
2. White matter is composed of myelinated axons that carry information away from cell bodies.
3. Primary functions of the parietal lobe include sensory processing, perception, and short-term memory.
4. Broca's aphasia is an inability to perform the motor components necessary for speech. The patient may experience weakness of the lips and tongue musculature.
5. The thalamus is a central relay station for sensory impulses traveling from other parts of the body and brain to the cerebrum. Motor information received from the basal ganglia and cerebellum is transmitted to the motor cortex through the thalamus.
6. The corticospinal tract is the primary motor pathway.

7. Anterior horn cells are neurons located within the gray matter of the spinal cord. They send axons out through the ventral root that eventually become peripheral nerves that innervate muscle fibers.
8. The peripheral nervous system is divided into the somatic and autonomic divisions. The somatic nervous system is under conscious control and is responsible for skeletal muscle contraction. The autonomic nervous system is an involuntary system that functions to maintain homeostasis, or an optimal internal environment.
9. The middle cerebral artery is the most common site of infarction.
10. Clinical signs of an upper motor neuron injury include spasticity, hyperreflexia, presence of a Babinski sign, and, possibly, clonus.

Chapter 3

1. Motor control is the ability to maintain and change posture and movement. It is the result of neurologic and mechanical processes. Motor learning is the process that brings about a permanent

change in motor behavior as a result of practice or experience.
2. Sensation is used in motor control as a means of feedback and as a way to prepare the body's pos-

ture in anticipation of movement. Sensation is needed to learn a new motor skill.

3. The stages of motor control can be used to guide intervention.

4. Balance is maintained by controlling posture. The postural control system is affected by the limits of stability (base of support), environmental demands, the flexibility and strength of the musculoskeletal system, the readiness of the posture for movement, motor coordination, and ability of the sensory systems to prepare and guide movement while maintaining balance.

5. The vestibular system provides the defining input to make a postural response when a conflict exists between the information from the visual system and that from the somatosensory system.

6. Children demonstrate consistent adult sway strategy responses between 7 and 10 years of age.

7. The highest amount of attention is needed in the initial stage of motor learning, with a decreasing amount of attention needed in subsequent stages.

8. Driving a car is an example of an open task, whereas riding on an escalator is an example of a closed task.

9. A closed loop is used to learn movement because feedback is required to perfect performance. An open loop is used to move quickly, with little or no feedback used.

10. Much practice is needed to learn a new motor skill. The best type of practice to use for learning is one that closely resembles the task to be learned, with feedback given intermittently.

Chapter 4

1. A theory has a life span perspective if it meets Baltes' five criteria that development is lifelong, multidimensional, plastic and flexible, contextual, and embedded in history.

2. Maslow describes a hierarchy of needs that an individual strives to achieve.

3. Major examples of the directional concept of development are that development proceeds from cephalic to caudal, from proximal to distal, from mass to specific, and from gross to fine.

4. Growth, maturation, and adaptation are the three processes that guide development.

5. The major milestones achieved during the first year of life are head control at 4 months, sitting alone at 8 months, walking alone by 12 months, hand regard at 2 months, voluntary grasp at 6 months, and superior pincer grasp at 12 months.

6. A typical 4-month-old's posture is symmetric regardless of position; head control, defined as an ability to keep the head in line with the body when the child is pulled to sit, is evident. The 6-month-old is mobile in a prone position and exhibits the ability to move from prone to supine with some trunk rotation. The infant at 6 months

can sit propping on arms if placed in that position; the upper trunk is extended, but the lower trunk is still rounded. The 6-month-old may make the transition to and from many different positions such as four point, propped sitting, prone, and supine.

7. Running, jumping, throwing, and catching are considered fundamental motor patterns.

8. Motor patterns continue to change across the life span because the patterns are the result of the interaction among the mover, the task, and the environment.

9. Decreased activity can accentuate the effect gravity has on an older individual's ability to remain erect. Extending against gravity, as in rising from a chair or walking with an erect posture, may become more difficult as a result of cumulative changes in body systems related to normal or pathologic aging.

10. Decreased speed of gait, shortened stride length, and increased double-limb support time may contribute to less function in stair climbing, stepping over objects, and crossing the street in a timely manner.

Chapter 5

1. Major impairments seen in patients who have had CVAs include motor impairments (flaccidity, spasticity, the presence of synergies, paresis, and apraxia), sensory impairments, communication impairments, orofacial deficits, respiratory dysfunction, bowel and bladder dysfunction, and functional limitations.

2. Risk factors for the development of CVA include hypertension, heart disease, hyperlipidemia, cigarette smoking, a prior history of CVA or TIA, gender (males), race (African Americans) alcohol consumption, physical inactivity, obesity, and age.

3. The flexion synergy pattern in the upper extremity is characterized by scapular retraction and eleva-

tion or hyperextension, shoulder abduction with external rotation, elbow flexion, forearm supination, and wrist and finger flexion. The extension pattern in the upper extremity consists of scapular protraction, shoulder adduction with internal rotation, elbow extension, forearm pronation, and wrist and finger flexion. The lower extremity flexion synergy pattern is characterized by hip flexion, hip abduction, and hip external rotation; knee flexion; ankle dorsiflexion and inversion; and dorsiflexion of the toes. The extension synergy pattern in the lower extremity consists of hip extension, hip adduction, and hip internal rotation; knee extension; ankle plantar flexion and inversion; and plantar flexion of the toes.

4. Proper positioning out of the synergy patterns assists in stimulating motor function, increases sensory awareness, improves respiratory and oromotor function, assists in maintaining normal range of motion, and decreases the risk of deformities and pressure ulcers.

5. Early physical therapy intervention for the patient with CVA includes cardiopulmonary retraining (diaphragm strengthening), positioning, motor relearning exercises for the upper and lower extremities, encouraging the use of the involved extremities, bed mobility activities (bridging, scapular mobilization), rolling activities, and transfers.

6. The basic principles behind the NDT approach to physical therapy care are to inhibit abnormal postural reflexes and movement patterns and to facilitate normal functional movement.

7. Activities that can be performed in a sitting position include posture correction, maintenance of a neutral pelvic tilt, weight bearing on the involved upper extremity and hand, weight-shifting activities, alternating isometrics and rhythmic stabilization, and performance of functional tasks such as ADLs and reaching activities.

8. To initiate gait activities with the patient who has had a CVA, the following sequence should be used: The patient must be able to stand and to bear weight equally on both lower extremities; this includes maintaining an upright erect posture. The patient must then be able to shift weight in standing in order to advance first the uninvolved lower extremity and then the involved lower extremity. Once the patient is able to step forward and back with either leg, several steps can be put together.

9. The following are considered advanced dynamic standing activities: walking outside on uneven surfaces, walking on a balance beam, side stepping, tandem walking, walking backward, braiding, throwing and catching, and marching in place.

10. Environmental factors that must be considered when preparing the patient for discharge include the type of dwelling the patient lives in, the type of entrance, interior accessibility, the type of carpeting present, and the patient's access to transportation.

Chapter 6

1. A subdural hematoma develops between the dura and the arachnoid. The patient's findings can fluctuate and are similar to those seen after a CVA. Patients can experience decreased consciousness, ipsilateral pupil dilation, and contralateral hemiparesis.

2. Signs and symptoms of increased intracranial pressure can include decreased responsiveness, impaired consciousness, severe headache, vomiting, irritability, papilledema, an increase in blood pressure, and a decrease in heart rate.

3. A patient who is in a coma is neither aroused nor responsive to what is occurring internally or within the external environment. The patient's eyes remain closed, and no distinction is made between sleep and wake cycles. A patient in a persistent vegetative state has a return of brain stem reflexes and sleep-wake cycles. If an individual remains unaware of his internal needs or external environ-

ment for a year or longer, he is said to be in a persistent vegetative state.

4. Acute care goals for a patient with a TBI include increasing the patient's level of arousal, preventing secondary complications, improving or preventing loss of function, and educating the patient and family.

5. Levels of cognitive function:
   I. No response
   II. Generalized response
   III. Localized response
   IV. Confused, agitated
   V. Confused-inappropriate
   VI. Confused-appropriate
   VII. Automatic-appropriate
   VIII. Purposeful and appropriate

6. Hand-over-hand modeling can assist patients to relearn automatic functional activities. During completion of a meaningful functional task, the pa-

tient receives proprioceptive and kinesthetic feedback from the clinician.

7. Too much sensory stimulation (lighting, sound, or the number of people present) may overstimulate the patient and cause the patient to become distracted or agitated.

8. For patients who are disoriented, the use of a script or memory book can help the patient fill in missing information about himself. Simple verbal instructions, redirection to the task, and preparing a number of different treatment activities can be used with patients who have attention deficits.

9. Patients who are disoriented can become agitated and may exhibit aggressive behaviors. Reorienting the patient may assist in calming him. If the patient becomes overstimulated, the clinician should try to remove the stimulus or remove the patient from the environment. If the patient's condition escalates to a crisis situation, the clinician's primary concern is to protect the patient from harming himself or others.

10. The following are examples of activities that incorporate both physical and cognitive components: counting the number of repetitions of an exercise completed, using a map or route-finding techniques, throwing and catching in a sitting or standing position, completing an obstacle course, and going on community outings.

Chapter 7

1. The four most common causes of spinal cord injuries are motor vehicle accidents, acts of violence, falls, and sports-related injuries.

2. In a complete injury, sensory and motor function will be absent below the level of the injury and in the S4 and S5 sacral segments. Incomplete injuries are characterized by the presence of some motor or sensory function below the level of the injury and in the lowest sacral segments. Perianal sensation must be present for an injury to be classified as incomplete.

3. Spinal shock is a condition of flaccidity, areflexia, loss of bowel and bladder function, and autonomic deficits including decreased blood pressure and poor temperature regulation.

4. Autonomic dysreflexia is a pathologic autonomic reflex that can occur in patients with injuries above the T6 level. A noxious stimulus causes autonomic stimulation, vasoconstriction, and a rapid increase in the patient's blood pressure. Signs and symptoms can include hypertension, severe and pounding headache, profuse sweating, flushing above the injury, constricted pupils, goose bumps, blurred vision, and a runny nose.

5. An individual with C7 tetraplegia has the potential to live independently.

6. The following activities improve pulmonary function: diaphragm strengthening, instruction in glossopharygeal breathing, incentive spirometry, postural drainage, and instruction in assistive cough techniques.

7. The three primary goals during the acute care phase of intervention are to prevent joint contractures and deformities, to maximize muscle and respiratory function, and to acclimate the patient to the upright position.

8. The mat program for a patient with C6 tetraplegia consists of the following exercises: passive range of motion to the lower extremities, diaphragm strengthening, assistive cough techniques, upper extremity strengthening to innervated musculature, rolling from supine to prone, making the transition from prone to prone on elbows, transferring from supine to long sitting, long-sitting activities with the elbows anatomically locked, instruction in pressure relief, increasing the patient's tolerance to upright, and instruction in wheelchair propulsion.

9. A patient with C7 tetraplegia should be able to perform a lateral transfer without a sliding board independently.

10. An aquatics program assists in decreasing abnormal muscle tone, increasing muscle strength, increasing range of motion, and improving pulmonary function. Therapeutic pools also provide the opportunity to practice standing and weight bearing and to exercise weak muscles more easily.

11. Initially, the patient will begin gait training in the parallel bars. The patient will work on finding his balance point (the point at which the orthoses will maintain the patient in an upright standing position). Once the patient finds his balance point, the patient works on weight shifting forward and back and to the right and left. Pushups on the bars and learning to jackknife are then practiced. Once the patient is able to complete these preparatory activities, the patient can begin to put steps together. Patients will be instructed in either a swing-to or a swing-through gait pattern. During gait training activities, the patient must also practice sit-to-stand and stand-to-sit transitions.

12. Important areas for patient and family teaching include instruction in patient transfers and range of motion exercises. In addition, families must be knowledgeable about the patient's injury, potential complications, any precautions, and the patient's likely functional outcome.

Chapter 8

1. Positioning and handling should always be included in therapeutic intervention.
2. Positioning is used to provide support and to encourage functional movement.
3. Touch and movement are important in developing body and movement awareness. All sensory input is used early on to learn to move.
4. The two most important handling tips are as follows: (1) the child should be allowed to do as much of any movement as possible; and (2) handling should be decreased as the child gains more control.
5. Key points of control are proximal joints from which to guide movement or reinforce a posture.
6. Adaptive equipment can be used to achieve postural alignment, to prevent contractures and deformities, and to provide mobility. (Other goals of adaptive equipment are found in Table 8–5.)
7. The two most functional postures are sitting and standing. Sitting is functional because so many activities of daily living can be performed in this position. Sitting provides a stable postural base for upper extremity movements. Standing is functional because it affords the ability to move through the environment in an erect posture, thus combining the mobility of the limbs with the stability of the head and trunk.
8. The major disadvantage of the quadruped position is that it is a flexed posture, and it is difficult for some children to learn to move in this position.
9. Side sitting is a difficult posture to master because it requires trunk rotation to have one's hands free. Because of the flexed lower extremities, the lower trunk is rotated in one direction. The upper trunk must be rotated in the opposite direction to free the hands.
10. Standing is an important activity because the loading forces placed on the long bones of the lower extremities produce positive physiologic changes. It is also important because it is socially acceptable to be at eye level with one's peers. Third, the sensory input from being upright is beneficial to perceptual development.

Chapter 9

1. The classic presentation is flaccid paralysis; however, if some innervation occurs below the level of the myelomeningocele, spastic paralysis can be present.
2. Complications related to skeletal growth can include tethered spinal cord, scoliosis, kyphosis, and lordosis.
3. Irritability, seizures, vomiting, and lethargy are common signs of shunt malfunction in a child.
4. Prone positioning is important to prevent development of hip and knee flexion contractures.
5. Areas of skin insensitivity should be protected by clothing and should be inspected on a routine basis.
6. Age, level of lesion, and strength of innervated musculature must be taken into account when choosing an orthosis for a child with myelomeningocele.
7. The lower the level of lesion, the more functional the level of ambulation will be and the more likely that level of ambulation will be continued through the life span.
8. The ultimate functional level of mobility can be determined during the school years when physical maturity peaks.
9. Changes in body weight, body proportions, immobilization from skin breakdown or orthopedic surgery, spinal deformity, joint pain, or ligamentous laxity can contribute to a loss of mobility in an adolescent with myelomeningocele.
10. Physical therapy intervention is crucial at an early age to teach functional movement and is important any time the child makes the transition from one mode of mobility to another or from one setting to another.

Chapter 10

1. DS is the leading chromosomal cause of mental retardation.
2. Each child has a 1 in 4 chance of having CF.
3. SMA is a progressive disease of the nervous system that produces muscle weakness but no mental retardation.
4. Chromosome abnormalities occur by one of three mechanisms: nondisjunction, deletion, and translocation.
5. Children with most genetic disorders commonly present with hypotonia and some degree of mental retardation.
6. The motor learning principles of practice and repetition are important to use in any intervention with a child with mental retardation.
7. Appropriate interventions for a child with low tone include approximation, weight bearing in proper postural alignment, and activities that increase muscular work against gravity.
8. Soft splints can be used to prevent elbow or knee hyperextension. Positioning can be used to encourage midline orientation. A strong balanced trunk can improve trunk control for controlled movement transitions that require trunk rotation and can support adequate respiratory function for breathing and phonation.
9. Interventions for children with OI should focus on developmental activities within safe limits. All rotations should be active. Orthoses are used to support and protect joints. Positioning should be used to minimize joint deformities. The pool is an excellent medium for exercise.
10. The ultimate physical therapy goal is to provide education and support for the family while managing the child's impairments. Management is a total approach with preventive and supportive aspects.

Chapter 11

1. The clinical manifestations of cerebral palsy may appear to worsen with age because the child's motor abilities cannot adapt to the increased environmental demands. The lack of function of the originally damaged areas of the brain can interfere with the function of other areas of the brain.
2. Prematurity and low birth weight are the two greatest risk factors for cerebral palsy.
3. Spasticity, or increased muscle tone, is the most common type of abnormal tone seen in children with cerebral palsy.
4. Tonic reflexes such as the ATNR, STNR, or TLR can interfere with the acquisition of coordinated movement because they can dominate a child's posture if they are obligatory. For example, an obligatory ATNR may prevent the child from rolling; an obligatory STNR may prevent the child from performing reciprocal extremity movements; and an obligatory TLR may prevent development of antigravity head and trunk control.
5. The focus of physical therapy intervention in children with spastic cerebral palsy is on mobility because their tone is increased and movements are limited to stereotypical patterns. The focus of physical therapy intervention in children with athetoid cerebral palsy is on stability because these children lack the ability to sustain static postures and maintain head and trunk stability while moving their extremities.
6. The physical therapist assistant implements certain aspects of the treatment plan formulated by the physical therapist. Activities can include those promoting postural reactions, transitional movements, strength, endurance, and self-care skills.
7. The most frequently used orthosis in ambulatory children with cerebral palsy is some type of AFO.
8. The school-age child should be taking some degree of responsibility for her own therapy program.
9. Many medications have been used to decrease spasticity in children with cerebral palsy. The medications of choice at this time appear to be botulinum toxin and baclofen.
10. Giangreco and colleagues (1993) identified five life outcomes that could be used as a guide for goal setting. These are

   ● Having a safe, stable home in which to live now and in the future.
   ● Having access to a variety of places within a community.
   ● Engaging in meaningful activities.
   ● Having a social network of personally meaningful relationships.
   ● Being safe and healthy.

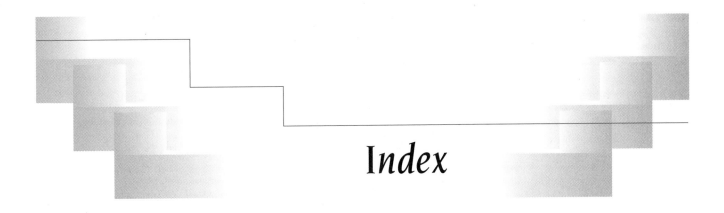

Index

Note: Page numbers in *italics* refer to illustrations; page numbers followed by t refer to tables.